Display 11-7 Nursing Interventions to Help Promote Normal Sexual Feelings in the Elderly
Display 11-8 Nursing Interventions to Help Relieve Spiritual Distress
Display 11-9 Nursing Interventions to Enhance Spiritual Well-Being

UNIT IV PHARMACOLOGY AND THE OLDER ADULT

CHAPTER 12 Effects of Medication on the Older Adult
Display 12-1 Selected Highly Protein-bound Drugs
Table 12-2 Examples of Selected Drugs, Therapeutic Levels and Symptoms of Toxicity

CHAPTER 13 Medication Administration Considerations
Figure 13-1 Picture of a Medication Administration Container
Table 13-1 Undesirable Drugs for Older Patients
Table 13-2 Considerations for the Elderly When Administering Commonly Prescribed Drugs
Display 13-1 Guide for Obtaining Important Drug Information
Display 13-2 Medication Usage in the Visually Impaired
Display 13-3 Patient Drug Monitoring System
Display 13-4 Self-Monitoring Check-Off Chart

UNIT V COMMON PROBLEMS AFFECTING THE OLDER ADULT

CHAPTER 14 Managing Physiologic Problems
Table 14-1 Drugs That Affect Incontinence
Table 14-2 Pain Management Flow Sheet
Table 14-3 Analgesics Commonly Used for Mild to Moderate Pain in the Elderly
Table 14-4 Comparisons of Depression, Dementia, and Delirium
Table 14-5 Nursing Strategies for Acute Confusion
Table 14-6 Clinical Signs of Vitamin and Mineral Deficiency
Display 14-1 Voiding and Incontinence Record
Display 14-2 Questions to Ask When Assessing Incontinence
Display 14-3 General Nursing Interventions for a Patient With Urinary Incontinence
Display 14-4 Nursing Interventions for a Bladder Training Program
Display 14-5 Questions to Ask When Assessing Sleep Patterns
Display 14-6 Nursing Interventions That Promote Sleep
Display 14-7 Nursing Interventions That Help Alleviate Pain
Display 14-8 Nursing Interventions to Use for Patients With Delirium
Display 14-9 Fall Prevention Precautions
Display 14-10 Nursing Interventions to Use if Physical Restraints are Used
Display 14-11 Determine Your Nutritional Health Checklist
Display 14-12 DETERMINE Guidelines
Display 14-13 10 Ways to Boost Caloric Intake
Display 14-14 Nursing Interventions to Help Restore Hydration

CHAPTER 15 Managing Psychosocial Problems
Table 15-1 Signs of Lithium Toxicity
Display 15-1 Drugs That May Precipitate Depression
Display 15-2 Geriatric Depression Scale
Display 15-3 General Nursing Interventions When Caring for a Depressed Individual
Display 15-4 Nursing Interventions when Caring for a Person in the Manic Phase of Bipolar Disorder
Display 15-5 Nursing Interventions That Foster Hope
Display 15-6 Nursing Interventions That Encourage Self-care
Display 15-7 Nursing Interventions to Promote Social Interaction
Display 15-8 Common Misunderstanding About Suicide
Display 15-9 Suicide Lethality
Display 15-10 Nursing Interventions for a Patient Considering Suicide
Display 15-11 What to Say When Someone is Grieving
Display 15-12 Interventions That Help Overcome Loneliness
Display 15-13 Nursing Interventions for Anticipatory Grief
Display 15-14 Nursing Interventions for a Patient With Dysfunctional Grief
Display 15-15 Nursing Interventions to Assist the Patient Abusing Alcohol to Cope More Effectively
Display 15-16 Nursing Interventions When Elder Abuse is Suspected
Display 15-17 Nursing Interventions to Assist the Patient in Developing Alternative Coping Mechanisms
Display 15-18 Nursing Interventions for Caregiver Role Strain

UNIT VI PHYSIOLOGIC CHANGES AFFECTING THE OLDER ADULT

CHAPTER 16 The Integumentary System
Table 16-1 Common Skin Lesions in the Elderly
Figure 16-1 Cross Sections of the Skin
Figure 16-2 Areas of Greatest Risk for Developing Pressure Ulcers
Figure 16-3 Examples of Shear and Friction
Figure 16-4 Sample Pressure Ulcer Assessment Guide
Figure 16-5 Sample Nutritional Assessment
Figure 16-6 Skin Self-Assessment Guide
Display 16-1 Interventions Suggested for Prevention of Pressure Ulcers
Display 16-2 Administering Collagenase Correctly
Display 16-3 Instructions for Prevention of Skin Cancer
Display 16-4 Descriptive Terms for Skin Lesions
Display 16-5 Using Lindane Correctly

CHAPTER 17 The Neurological System
Figure 17-1 Summary of Symptoms of Parkinson's Disease
Figure 17-2 Drawing of the Brain Denoting Areas Affected in Patients With Parkinsonism
Display 17-1 Hypothermia
Display 17-2 Criteria to Diagnose Alzheimer Patients
Display 17-3 Stages of Alzheimer's Disease
Display 17-4 Behavorial Symptoms Exhibited by Alzheimer Patients
Display 17-5 Nursing Interventions for Patients Who Wander
Display 17-6 Nursing Interventions to Manage Sundown Syndrome Patients
Display 17-7 Nursing Interventions to Manage Abusive Behavior by Residents
Display 17-8 Nursing Interventions to Manage Socially Inappropriate Disruptive Behavior
Display 17-9 Resources for Families and Patients With Alzheimer's Disease
Display 17-10 Questions to Ask When Choosing a Nursing Home
Display 17-11 Understanding Validation Therapy and Reality Therapy
Display 17-12 Resources for Patients With Parkinson's Disease
Display 17-13 Factors That Increase the Probability of Seizure Disorders

CHAPTER 18 The Cardiovascular System
Figure 18-1 Normal Heart
Figure 18-2 Systole and Diastole
Figure 18-3 Decision Tree for Cardiac Rehabilitation Services
Figure 18-4 Glasgow Coma Scale
Figure 18-5 Clinical Flow Design for Stroke Rehabilitation
Display 18-1 Symptoms of Heart Failure
Display 18-2 Nursing Interventions When the Patient Has Decreased Cardiac Output
Display 18-3 Suggested Topics for Patient, Family Education and Counseling and Caregiver
Display 18-4 Risk Factors for Coronary Heart Disease

Introductory Gerontological Nursing

Sally S. Roach RN, MSN
Associate Professor
University of Texas at Brownsville and
Texas Southmost College
Brownsville, Texas
Vocational Nursing Program Director and
Instructor
(1979–1998)

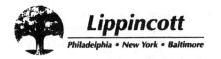
Lippincott
Philadelphia • New York • Baltimore

Acquisitions Editor: Lisa Stead
Editorial Assistant: Karin McAndrews
Managing Editor: Barbara Ryalls
Senior Production Manager: Helen Ewan
Production Coordinator: Mike Carcel
Art Director: Carolyn O'Brien
Cover Designer: Melissa Walters
Indexer: Ellen Brennan
Manufacturing Manager: William Alberti

9 8 7 6 5 4 3 2 1

Library of Congress Cataloging-in-Publication Data

Roach, Sally S.
     Introductory gerontological nursing / Sally S. Roach.
        p. cm.
     Includes bibliographical references and index.
     ISBN 0–397–55479–6
       1. Geriatric nursing. I. Title.

RC954.R62 2000
610.73'65--dc21   00–042804

Reviewers

Acknowledgments

My appreciation and sincere thanks to all of those individuals at Lippincott Williams & Wilkins who were in any way responsible for this book. A special thank-you goes to Susan Keneally, for her help and support in the early manuscript development. My sincere thanks to Lisa Stead, Acquisitions Editor, for her professional editorial assistance and for putting life back into this project. A special thank you to Karin McAndrews, Editorial Assistant, for answering my calls and taking care of all the obstacles that arose during the preparation of the manuscript. My deep appreciation to Doris Wray, Ancillaries Editor, for her valuable editorial assistance. Thank you, as well, to Helen Ewan, Senior Production Manager; Barbara Ryalls, Managing Editor; and Michael Carcel, Production Coordinator, who were responsible for the production of this text.

As always, my heartfelt thanks goes to all of my family and friends who are patient when I must work long hours and who are always supportive of my efforts. And last, but certainly not least, to Austin, who brings so much joy to my life.

Preface

The speciality of gerontological nursing provides an area of great opportunity and a host of challenges for the practical/vocational nurse. Practical nurses care for older adults in acute-care settings, such as the hospital; in long-term care settings, such as the nursing home; and in outpatient settings, such as adult day care centers, community centers, and outpatient clinics. These nurses have a profound influence on the type of care older adults in our society receive. *Introductory Gerontological Nursing* provides an easy-to-read, practical guide to providing basic nursing care to the most rapidly growing segment of our population . . . . . . those over the age of 65.

Purpose

The purpose of this text is to provide an understanding of the basic concepts of aging, the physiologic changes that occur with age, and how these changes impact nursing care. This text seeks to provide a sound knowledge base from which students can practice gerontological nursing and to cultivate within the student a respect and appreciation for the older adult.

Organization

This text is divided into **seven units,** with one or more chapters contained in each unit. While specific disease processes are presented in the unit pertaining to the body system affected, certain conditions may be presented in more than one chapter. For example, dementia is covered in the chapter concerned with common problems of the older adult as well as in the chapter on the neurological system. Medication administration is covered primarily within the unit on pharmacology and the older adult. However, pharmacologic considerations are discussed throughout the text when specific medications are addressed for a disease process.

Unit I: Foundations of Gerontological Care is composed of four chapters that provide basic information on the characteristics of the aging population, concepts of gerontological nursing care, and theories of aging. Ethical and legal aspects of gerontological care are also considered.

Unit II: The Role of the Gerontological Nurse contains five chapters that discuss ways to enhance communication with the older adult, how to apply the nursing process in gerontological care, and how to perform a functional assessment. One chapter within this unit is devoted to psychosocial aspects of gerontological care and another to the principles of restorative care in the older adult.

Unit III: Health and Wellness of the Older Adult contains two chapters that provide ways to promote physiologic and psychosocial health in older adults. Topics covered in these chapters include promoting cardiovascular health, principles of good nutrition, cancer prevention, stress management, increasing self-esteem, spirituality, and sexual health of the older adult.

Unit IV: Pharmacology and the Older Adult deals with the important responsibility of administering medications to the elderly and the effects of medications in the elderly. The nursing process and the "Six Rights" of medication administration provide the framework for the two chapters in this unit.

Unit V: Common Problems Affecting the Older Adult consists of two chapters that deal with common physiologic and psychosocial problems facing the elderly. Some of problems discussed include incontinence, sleep disturbances, pain, delirium, confusion, depression, falls, elder abuse, depression, grief, and substance abuse.

Unit VI: Physiologic Changes Affecting the Older Adult contains nine chapters dealing with each major body system. Each chapter includes normal anatomy of the system, age-related changes within that system, and the most commonly occurring diseases of that system in the older adult. A nursing process format is used to present nursing care.

Unit VII: Management Functions in a Gerontological Setting focuses on the increasingly important role the practical/vocational nurse plays in the management of unlicensed assistive personnel, particularly in a nursing home setting. Developing management and leadership skills in the practical nurse is critical if the practical nurse is to function competently in a leadership role. This chapter discusses the basic principles involved in leadership and gives practical guidelines for the nurse leader when managing others in a health care setting.

Pedagogic Aids

Several features are incorporated to help clarify the contents of each chapter. Every chapter has a *Chapter Outline,* a list of *Key Terms, Chapter Objectives,* and *Critical Thinking Exercises.* The key terms are identified in the text of the chapter and defined. Emphasis is placed throughout the text on the nursing process as a means of planning and implementing nursing care. *Assessment Alerts* are included in chapters dealing with physiologic or psychosocial care. Assessment Alerts include specific assessments that are of special concern in the older adult. When appropriate, the chapter contains a display with a list of *Resources* that provides specific resources for the student, family, or the older adult on the topic discussed in the chapter. The concept of caring, so important in all areas of nursing, is a thread throughout the text. **Critical Thinking Exercises** are presented at the end of the chapter and are based on the material presented in the chapter. A *Glossary* is included at the end of the book containing words that may be unfamiliar to the student.

Ancillary Material

The *Instructor's Manual for Introductory Gerontological Nursing* contains multiple-choice questions, critical thinking questions, and suggested learning activities. The multiple-choice questions are written in the format of the NCLEX-PN examination and pertain to material within the chapter. Answers to the multiple-choice questions are included in the Instructor's Manual.

The Instructors Manual correlates with the textbook chapter by chapter, with the exception of the last chapter in the Instructor's Manual. This contains a series of eight case studies to use either during or at the end of the course (whichever the instructor chooses). Specific recommendations for use of the case studies can be found in the Instructor's Manual.

Additional critical thinking exercises are provided in the Instructor's Manual. No answers are provided for the critical thinking exercises. To do so would stifle creativity and too narrowly define the answers. Vocational nurses must be prepared to think not only critically but creatively as well. Students are encouraged to develop their creative and critical thinking skills to formulate the best possible solutions to the exercises. By providing no set answer the instructor has the opportunity to explore different options with the student. The suggested activities provide an avenue for further growth and ways to enhance an appreciation of the uniqueness of the older adult.

Another activity to enhance learning are the Web activities included for each chapter. We are in the midst of the "information age," and students need to know how to use the technology necessary to obtain the latest information. The Web activities are designed to provide the student with credible sources for obtaining the most up-to-date health care information.

Contents

Introductory Gerontological Nursing

I Foundations of Gerontological Care

CHAPTER 1 Characteristics of the Aging Population 1
CHAPTER 2 Basic Concepts of Gerontological Nursing 12
CHAPTER 3 Theories of Aging 22
CHAPTER 4 Ethical and Legal Considerations 27

II The Role of the Gerontological Nurse

CHAPTER 5 Communicating with the Older Adult 39
CHAPTER 6 Applying the Nursing Process to Gerontological Care 52
CHAPTER 7 Performing a Functional Assessment 65
CHAPTER 8 Psychosocial Aspects of Gerontological Care 77
CHAPTER 9 Implementing Restorative Care 91

III Health and Wellness in the Older Adult

CHAPTER 10 Promoting Physiologic Health 102
CHAPTER 11 Promoting Psychosocial Health 116

IV Pharmacology and the Older Adult

CHAPTER 12 Effects of Medication in the Older Adult 130
CHAPTER 13 Medication Administration Considerations 137

V Common Problems Affecting the Older Adult

CHAPTER 14 Managing Common Physiologic Problems 150
CHAPTER 15 Managing Psychosocial Problems 172

VI Physiological Changes Affecting the Older Adult

CHAPTER 16 The Integumentary System 187
CHAPTER 17 The Neurologic System 200
CHAPTER 18 The Cardiovascular System 218
CHAPTER 19 The Musculoskeletal System 240
CHAPTER 20 The Respiratory System 259
CHAPTER 21 The Gastrointestinal System 276
CHAPTER 22 The Genitourinary System 293

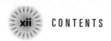

CHAPTER 23   The Endocrine System   313
CHAPTER 24   The Sensory Organs   330

VII Management Functions in a Gerontological Setting

CHAPTER 25   Developing Leadership and Management Skills   346

INTRODUCTORY GERONTOLOGICAL NURSING

CHAPTER **1**

Characteristics of the Aging Population

CHAPTER OUTLINE

KEY TERMS
CHAPTER OBJECTIVES
CHARACTERISTICS OF THE AGING POPULATION
    Life Expectancy
    Aging Women
    Aging Men
    Social Security
    Caregiving
    The Family
    Baby Boomer Cohort
    The 85-Year and Older Population
    Frail Elderly
ILLNESS IN THE OLDER POPULATION
HEALTH CARE FOR THE OLDER ADULT
    Financing Health Care
    Poverty
    Resources for the Aging Population
    National Council on the Aging
ATTITUDES TOWARD AGING
    Ageism
    Nurses Attitudes Toward Aging
REALITIES OF AGING
NURSES RESPONSIBILITY TO COMBAT AGEISM
CRITICAL THINKING EXERCISES
REFERENCES AND SUGGESTED READING

KEY TERMS

ageism
baby boomer
gerontological nursing
gerontocracy
health maintenance organizations (HMOs)
managed health care
Medicare
Medicaid
preferred provider organizations (PPOs)
provider sponsored organizations (PSOs)
sandwich generation

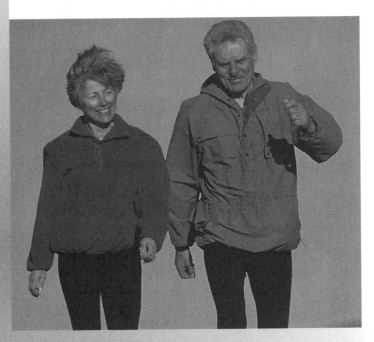

CHAPTER OBJECTIVES

At the completion of this chapter, the student will be able to

- Discuss characteristics and demographics of the aging population
- Describe the significance of the baby boomer cohort
- Identify characteristics of the 85-year and older population
- Describe the frail elderly
- Discuss important aspects of financing and managing health care for the older adult
- Discuss issues concerning the health care of the older adult
- Identify resources for the aging population
- Discuss various attitudes, myths, and realities regarding the aging population

In the early 1900s, less than 5% of the population lived to be 65 years of age. Today, individuals older than age 65 account for more than 12% of the U.S. population. By the year 2020, the U.S. Bureau of the Census estimates that the population older than 85 years of age will triple. Nurses must be prepared to meet the challenges of caring for this rapidly increasing segment of the population. The nurse must be aware of the characteristics of aging population, special concerns of these individuals, and issues of importance to those individuals who will most likely dominate nursing practice in the 21st century. **Gerontological nursing** (ie, care of the older adult) is the most rapidly growing nursing specialty area.

CHARACTERISTICS OF THE AGING POPULATION

There is no "typical" older person. Each older adult is as different as the experiences that person has encountered over a lifetime. Age 65 has long been considered the most suitable age for retirement and therefore as the beginning of "old age." In reality, age 65 is nothing more that an arbitrary age set by government for retirement with no real scientific data to support the decision. Some acknowledge Chancellor Otto von Bismarck of Germany as the initiator of this phenomenon, because he decided that age 65 was the best age to retire his military personnel. In our society, most older adults are active and healthy at age 65. Rather than conforming to the stereotypical image of sitting in a rocking chair and watching the world go by, older adults are energetic, vibrant, and influential members of society. They represent a very diverse group influenced by their past experiences. For example, those of the 85-year and older group are veterans World War II and lived through the Great Depression. These individuals have little in common with those of the younger members of the aging population who were influenced by the Vietnam War, the Civil Rights Movement, and economic growth.

Although older adults are diverse and dissimilar in many ways, certain common characteristics and problems are associated with aging. This and subsequent chapters seek to identify and discuss those common characteristics, problems, disease processes, and concerns of the aging population. However, when planning and implementing care for the older adult, the nurse must consider individual differences and characteristics.

Life Expectancy

In 1990, life expectancy at birth was 79 years for women and 72.1 years for men. With technologic advances in medicine, improved nutrition, and an emphasis on disease prevention and health promotion, an increasingly high quality of health and a longer lifespan can be attained. In the year 2040, the projected life expectancy will be 82.8 years for women and 75.9 years for men.

Aging Women

Women outlive men. There are approximately 18.3 million women and 12.6 million men who are 65 years or older. Older women outnumber older men by 3 to 2. As age increases, this number increases as well. The trend for a greater number of aging women continues and no doubt will increase in future years. These statistics bring with them potential problems:

- Widowhood
- Living alone
- Coping with the loss of a mate
- Difficulty finding another life companion
- Lack of a caregiver
- Financial problems

Older women who are widows are more likely than men to live below the poverty level. Minority women living alone have the most difficult time. Poverty rates are highest among elderly black women. Approximately 61% of elderly black women live in poverty. Hispanic women have the lowest median income.

Aging Men

Men in our society have a shorter life span and die at a younger age than women. Older men are more likely to remarry if widowed. Widows outnumber widowers by 5 to 1. Men who are widowers face problems similar to those of women who lose their husbands (ie, loneliness, lack of a caregiver, and living alone). However, men often remarry and have fewer financial problems than women. Men are more likely than women to have worked 30 years or longer and to qualify for full Social Security benefits.

Social Security

The Social Security Act of 1935, established during the administration of Franklin D. Roosevelt, provided for a federal government–sponsored retirement plan. This act established a program to provide retirement benefits for those who are 65 and older. When the law was first enacted, the life expectancy was 63 years, making the prospect of many years of benefit payments to any one individual unlikely. As life expectancy increased, however, a larger burden has been placed on this system.

In addition to retirement benefits, Social Security provides survivor benefits to widows, widowers, children, and dependent parents; death benefits to the surviving spouse; and disability benefits. A worker and employer make payments into a special fund during the participant's working years. After retirement (usually age 65 or in some cases age 62), monthly benefits are dispersed based on the length of time the individual made payments into the system and the amount of income before retirement.

Social Security benefits for women are generally less than the benefits received by men. Most women have a discontinuous work pattern, making Social Security benefits less than those for men. Women are more apt to quit their jobs for caretaking or family problems, to have low paying jobs, and to place other areas of life before that of maintaining a continuous work pattern.

For women depending on Social Security benefits in old age, a discontinuous work pattern presents problems. Men usually work for 30 plus years, but most women do not. Women often do work for long periods and are more likely to have large "gaps" in reported earnings during which no Social Security earnings are credited. A Social Security profile with a large number of years in which there are no reported earnings can result in lower benefits accrued. By the year 2030, it is estimated that less than 4 of 10 women between the ages of 62 and 69 will have worked for 35 years or more. Women who have a discontinuous work pattern or who work for less than 30 years will receive less from Social Security.

Women older than age 65 who qualify for Social Security benefits must select the benefits based on their own work record or the work record of their husband. Most elect to collect from the husband's Social Security because men usually have the largest continuous contribution.

The Social Security Act was amended in 1974 to mandate cost of living increases and has resulted in slight gains in economic status for some older adults. However, a significant number of older adults still live below the poverty level. More than 90% of the elderly receive some Social Security payment.

To ensure that Social Security will remain viable in the years to come, several changes have been made. For example, beginning with the year 2000, the retirement age increases gradually from age 65 until it reaches age 67 in the year 2022. To keep pace with increasing demands for payment of Social Security benefits, more changes may have to be made in the future.

Caregiving

Who is caring for older adults? Caregiving has traditionally been the woman's role. Many older men, however, are also taking care of wives or parents who develop chronic illnesses or disabilities. Many middle-aged adults are part of the so-called **sandwich generation.** These individuals are "sandwiched" between caring for two generations. They are responsible for raising and educating children and responsible for caring for aging parents.

Another caregiver role is that of the 65- to 70-year-old caring for an aging parent who may be 90 years old or older. Caregivers are responsible for a number of activities related to their own lives and have the responsibility of dependent, older family members. Family caregivers provide between 80% to 90% of the care needed by the elderly, such as shopping, transportation, and personal care. Although adult day care centers and other social services are available through community resources, these services are usually only adjuncts to the care of the elderly. The caregiver role takes an enormous toll emotionally, physically, and financially on the caregiver. Women have traditionally been the major caregiver, but as more and more women are entering the work force, the caregiver role may of necessity fall to other resources. More support systems for caregivers, more respite services (a place for the elderly to go for care to allow the caregiver to rest), and a more family responsive work place are needed.

The Family

In addition to family members in the caregiver role, the family is the cornerstone of social support. Most older people have frequent contact with their families. Women are more likely than men to live alone. Most older adults desire to remain independent with minimal support from other family members. Support within the family is provided by the expression of affection, emotional support, and material support (ie, money or gifts). Families with close supportive relationships continue to follow the same pattern. Families who have not remained close may provide only minimal support to older adults. When older adults do not receive close emotional and

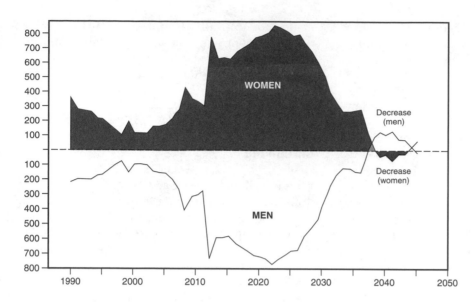

FIGURE 1-1. Annual increases in U.S. population, age 65 and over (projected for the years 1990 to 2045).

physical support from family members, other support systems must be developed to meet this need.

Older adults help the younger generation by serving as role models for coping with loss, for successful aging, and in the transmission of family values. Stress within the family may cause family dysfunction. Family dysfunction is manifested by elder neglect or abuse, burnout of caregivers, and depression. Nurses must continually assess and interact with the patient, caregiver, and other family members to detect any dysfunction or signs of elder abuse (see Chapter 15).

Baby Boomer Cohort

The most dynamic segment of our population is the baby boomer cohort (ie, population segment). **Baby boomers** are a population segment composed of individuals born during the period of prosperity after World War II between 1946 and 1964. During this timeframe, 76 million babies were born. Baby boomers currently compose one third of the U.S. population. They have and will continue to have a tremendous impact in all areas of our society. As a group, they are better educated, healthier, and more active than previous generations. Growth of the older population will peak between 2005 and 2030 as the baby boom generation reaches 65 years of age.

So many babies were born during the almost 20 years after World War II that the older population will swell within the 21st century. Some authorities describe the effect of the baby boomers on society as a "pig moving through a python" effect. The graph depicted in Figure 1-1 shows the fishlike pattern of population growth of those age

65 and older. The fish tail at the left depicts individuals born in the 1920s as the birth rates were increasing. The sharp dip represents the decline in birth rate during the Depression years. Notice that in the year 2022 the graph enlarges when the 1.2 million baby boomers born in 1955 reach age 65. However, in the next 10 years the "head" of the fish forms, representing the declining birth rates of the 1960s and the years following. This chart shows only the increase among people reaching age 65 in any given year and not the entire population of people age 65 or older.

This large increase in the older population leads some to believe that a gerontocracy could develop. A **gerontocracy** is a government ruled by older people. Certainly the older age group has become a strong political force. Groups such as the Gray Panthers, American Association of Retired Persons (AARP), and National Alliance of Senior Citizens exert tremendous political and social influence.

The 85-Year and Older Population

The magnitude of the number of individuals who will be in the 85 years or older within a relatively short time is mind boggling. For example, there were 3.2 million Americans older than age 85 in 1991. By 2020, this number is expected to double and, by 2040, to quadruple. Although many of these individuals older than 85 are not frail or dependent, a significant number will need the services of health care professionals. Currently, 22% of all nursing home residents are older than 85. Of the 85-year and older population who do not reside in nursing homes, nearly 50% need help with daily activities.

Frail Elderly

Individuals who, because of poor mental and physical health, are unable to care for themselves and need assistance are called the **frail elderly.** These individuals are generally from a low income and socioeconomic background and are predominantly female.

In general, the frail elderly spend more money on health care and medications and more time in the nursing home. The frail elderly are the most dependent and most vulnerable of our older population. They often need help in meeting basic needs such as food, shelter, and medical care. For those who do not live in nursing homes, these needs are met through family involvement and community resources such as day care centers, support groups, clinics, telephone support networks, and alternative residential care.

Health care services must match the needs of these older adults. Nurses must be prepared to give the type of care needed, including health promotion, disease prevention, and specialized nursing care.

ILLNESS IN THE OLDER POPULATION

Older adults have fewer acute illnesses than younger adults. When older adults do become ill with an acute illness, they usually require longer periods of recovery and experience more complications than younger people.

Mental illnesses common in the older adult include alcoholism, dementia, and depression. Suicide is the 10th leading cause of death in elderly men. Hypertension is a major health problem for all Americans but particularly for black Americans.

Chronic illness (ie, sickness of a long duration showing little change or slow progression) is a major concern for the older adult. Approximately 80% of older adults have at least one chronic illness, such as heart disease, diabetes, arthritis, or hypertension. Many elderly people have two or more chronic illnesses. Chronic illnesses are likely to cause disabilities. The incidence of chronic illness complicates care and makes nursing care an integral part of the health care of the older adult.

To combat the effects of chronic illness the elderly are challenged to reach their highest functional capacity. An emphasis on developing healthy lifestyles and the presence of health maintenance programs assist the elderly to deal with the impact of chronic illness.

HEALTH CARE FOR THE OLDER ADULT

People older than age 65 require more health care services than any other age group. Most patients in acute care hospitals are older than age 50, particularly in the states with large populations of older adults such as New Jersey, Michigan, Pennsylvania, Ohio, Texas, Illinois, Florida, and New York. Because of the escalating numbers of adults older than 65 years of age, most of the patients that nurses will care for in the future will be older. To properly care for this growing number of older adults, nurses must develop an awareness of the specific needs of the elderly. They must be knowledgeable about the diseases common to the elderly and about the physical and psychological changes that occur with aging.

Financing Health Care

Costs of health care are increasing substantially every year. The federal government sponsors two programs designed to help those in need of health care: Medicare and Medicaid.

Medicare

In 1965, the federal government enacted Medicare. **Medicare** is a national health insurance program for the elderly and for many who have disabilities. Medicare pays for approximately 45% of the health care costs of individuals age 65 or older. When Medicare was first established, there was no provision for reimbursement for nursing home care. This partly reflected a fear that long-term nursing home care would overburden and perhaps bankrupt the system. In-patient hospital care was covered under Medicare. As hospital stays increased in length and became more costly, Medicare was amended to include reimbursement for nursing home care after a lengthy hospital stay. Nursing home care was a more cost-effective alternative for those needing nursing care but not the full gamut of services offered in the hospital or acute care setting. Again fearful of the high costs of long-term care, the government set limits on the number of days Medicare would pay for long-term care. Currently, Medicare pays for skilled nursing home care for up to 100 days.

There are two parts to Medicare: Part A and Part B. Part A is hospital insurance that helps pay for inpatient hospital care, for certain follow-up services for persons age 65 or older, and for qualified individuals with disabilities. All 65-year-old adults who receive Social Security are automatically

DISPLAY 1-1. Expenses Not Covered by Medicare

Custodial care
Dental work
Eye examinations and glasses
Hearing test and hearing aids
Extended nursing home care
Prescription drugs
Routine physical examinations and related tests

enrolled in Part A. Those with disabilities and who have received disability benefits also are automatically enrolled in Medicare after 24 months of disability. Any 65-year-old person who plans to continue working should be instructed to contact the local Social Security office. There are many rules associated with Medicare and adults 65 years of age and older should be encouraged to keep up to date on the Medicare requirements to protect benefits already earned.

Most elderly people qualify for Part A or hospital insurance. Part A is paid for by the Social Security taxes that were collected during the working years. Part A helps pay up to 80% of the following services:

- Inpatient hospital care
- Skilled nursing home care
- Home health care
- Hospice

Part B of Medicare is medical insurance. This insurance plan helps to cover expenses for doctors' services, outpatient hospital services, home health visits, diagnostic tests such as x-ray procedures and laboratory tests, and other services and some supplies. Display 1-1 identifies services Medicare does not cover.

The federal government appears to be rethinking Medicare benefits. There is much interest in providing some type of payment for prescription drugs. Some elderly pay up to 60% of their income for prescription drugs.

When the elderly need extended nursing home care (more than 100 days) they must pay out of pocket, use private long-term care insurance (rare), or reduce their assets to a point of near poverty to qualify for Medicaid. Some older adults must use all of their savings, cash, retirement, and other resources until they "spend down" enough to qualify for Medicaid.

Medicaid

Medicaid is a government program designed to provide health insurance for the poor. Although Medicaid is federally funded, individual state govern-

ments manage it. Medicaid is an important funding source for older people who require long-term care or custodial care. Only approximately 10% of nursing home residents must spend down to be able to pay for long-term care, but for those 10%, the results can be financially devastating. With more and more elderly needing long-term care in the future, the need to spend down may become a more common problem, particularly because financial requirements must be met for the elderly to qualify for Medicaid. The need to spend down can force the elderly into poverty or near poverty to pay for nursing home care.

According to government statistics, approximately 48% of all nursing home revenues come from Medicaid, 4% from Veterans Administration, 4% from Medicare, 43% from patient and families, and only about 1% from long-term care insurance policies. Medicaid is an important source of financing for nursing homes.

Managed Health Care

Managed health care is an alternative method of delivering, coordinating, and financing health care. The emphasis of managed care is on providing comprehensive, high quality, cost-effective health care to a specific group of enrolled individuals. The holistic concept of health care is accentuated. The trend toward managed care as the means of obtaining health care is growing. According to the Health Care Financing Administration (HCFA), in 1997, more than 5.6 million Medicare beneficiaries (about 15% of the total Medicare population) have chosen managed health care plans to provide and manage their health care needs. Organizations delivering managed health care include health maintenance organizations (HMOs), preferred provider organizations (PPOs), and provider-sponsored organizations (PSOs).

HMOs are health care plans usually owned and administered by insurance companies that receive prepaid premiums for the delivery of health care. Services are provided from individuals employed by or under contract to the HMO. Recipients are generally required to select a primary care provider (PCP) who coordinates the patients care. A referral from the PCP is usually required before the patient can go to the hospital or see a specialist.

PPOs are composed of a group of independent physicians, hospitals, and other health care providers who contract with an insurance company to provide care at a reduced rate. Recipients are allowed to use services and physicians outside of the PPO but must pay a higher out-of-pocket cost. **PSOs** are similar to HMOs, except that instead of being owned by an insurance company they are owned and managed by a group of independent physicians and hospitals.

Medicare payments to managed health care plans are not uniform to all areas of the country. Payments are based on the average amount spent per person in that area. Medicare pays 95% of that amount for each older adult who joins the managed care organization. Payments are usually higher in urban areas and lower in rural areas. This disparity allows those who live in the city to receive extra benefits. The Budget Act of 1997 has certain provisions that help to alleviate some to this discrepancy. For example, payments to rural areas that have traditionally been the lowest will increase. The law also has certain provisions that allows Medicare recipients more options. Traditionally, only HMOs have been available to Medicare beneficiaries, but now options such as PPOs and PSOs are available. Since 1998, Medicaid provides more information on managed care and the options available to Medicare recipients by holding information seminars across the country. The trend toward managed health care continues to grow and will continue to evolve over the next decade.

Poverty

Of the 31.5 million Americans who are age 65 or older, approximately 20% are slightly above or below the poverty rate. Of those only slightly above the poverty rate, most are dangerously close to financial disaster should an emergency arise or catastrophic illness occur. Even with Medicare these individuals are paying as much for health care as they were before Medicare was established.

Minorities bear a disproportionate burden of poverty. Of older adults classified as poor, 10% were white, 31% were black, and 21% were Hispanic. With rapid increases in the 65-year and older population in the 21st century, these numbers will rise dramatically.

As the baby boomers age, single women will continue to be at the greatest risk for poverty. By the year 2030, it is projected that approximately 12% of older women will be poor or near the poverty level, but only 2.5% of the men are projected to live in poverty.

There is concern by many that, as increasing numbers of older Americans become dependent, a tremendous hardship will be placed on younger generations. The younger generation may be unable to provide the necessary funds to support and care for the growing number of elderly. Harold Sheppard, prominent gerontologist, points out that

---

> ### DISPLAY 1-2. How to Find an Area Agency on Aging
>
> Most Area Agencies on Aging (AAAs) are listed in the yellow pages of the local telephone directory, often under "senior services." It may be called the office, commission, department, or division on aging and can also be identified with the name of your city, town, county, or region. If there is difficulty in locating the AAA, call the state office on aging in the state capital for help. In 14 states or territories that are small or rural, there are no AAAs; in these, the state unit fulfills the area agency functions. If an older family member or friend lives in a distant community, it is possible to identify the AAA serving them by contacting the U.S. Administration on Aging, 330 Independence Avenue SW, Washington, DC (202-245-0641).
>
> These agencies were created and are funded through the Older Americans Act of 1965. Over the years, this act has been amended to better meet the changing needs of the elderly population. AAAs serve as visible focal points to administer services and to plan, develop, and coordinate a comprehensive range of services at the local level.

---

when children, who are dependent as well, are added to the equation the situation appears more balanced. Sheppard states that "by 2040, the total dependency ratio will be only 0.010 above the 0.831 ratio of 1920." Sheppard points out that the 1920 ratio included the large number of those younger than age 20 who were dependent on the working adult for care and education. Others are quick to reply that, in general, children and adolescents do not have the immense health care needs of the elderly.

Resources for the Aging Population

Community services are the heart of caring for the elderly. Each community offers programs through federal, state, and local governments; church groups; volunteer organizations; and social service agencies. Funding for these services comes from a variety of sources. About 675 communities have an Area Agency on Aging (AAA). Local AAAs have the responsibility to plan and coordinate services, provide information, and act as a referral source to other area agencies. When looking for available resources and services, families, caregivers, and nurses can turn to the local AAA for help. Help in locating a local AAA is given in Display 1-2.

DISPLAY 1-3. Goals and Purposes of the National Council of Aging

- Works to make our society more equitable, caring, and understanding about older persons so that their rights are protected, their opportunities advanced, and their needs met in a humane, effective, and efficient manner
- Conducts research, sets standards, disseminates information, and promotes the development of a continuum of opportunities and quality services with, by, for, and to older persons
- Develops and advocates improvement as well as new directions in public and private policies and practices that affect the aging
- Provides training, education, technical assistance, and consultation for those working with current and future generations of older persons
- Convenes and provides leadership and support services for a variety of professional constituent associations
- Develops relationships and coalitions with voluntary nonprofit, public, business, and labor organizations and with associations of older persons
- Can be contacted at NCOA, Inc., 409 Third Street SW, Washington, DC 20024 (202-479-1200)

National Council on the Aging

The National Council on the Aging (NCOA) was founded in 1950 as a national nonprofit organization. Membership in NCOA is open to individuals, voluntary agencies, business organizations, labor unions, and associations (ie, social, health, education, housing, religious, and civic). The guiding principle of NCOA is the belief that our nation's older people deserve lives of dignity and security and that they should have an opportunity for full participation in society. Display 1-3 identifies the goals and purposes of the NCOA.

In all its efforts, NCOA seeks to help meet the current and changing needs of all older persons, regardless or sex, race, color, creed, national origin or special handicap, and to tap the vast resource that older people offer the nation. NCOA can be reached.

ATTITUDES TOWARD AGING

Many in our society view aging as a topic to be avoided. Old age is associated with chronic illness, mental deterioration, and death. Aging is a topic that many are uncomfortable discussing. In reality, aging is like any other stage in life. It has certain problems and difficulties, but it also has joys and rewards.

Because of stereotyping by society and the desire to avoid discussing aging, there are many false ideas and misconceptions about older adults. Negative attitudes concerning aging are based partly on false ideas about what older people are like. Display 1-4 identifies some of the myths or incorrect beliefs concerning aging and the older adult that are common in our society.

Ageism

In the early days of our country, age was respected and revered (Display 1-5). Older men were sought after for advice gained through the experience of living a significant number of years. However, during era before and after world War II, age began to be viewed somewhat negatively. In the 1960s, when Medicare was instituted, and in 1973, when Social Security improvements were needed, many continued to view the elderly in a negative manner. The term ageism was coined to give meaning to the disapproving and prejudicial views of society toward the older population.

Ageism is a term used to describe discrimination against older people. Ageism is similar to racism and sexism. Racism is discrimination against someone because they belong to a certain race. Sexism is discrimination against someone because they are a male or a female. Ageism includes negative attitudes and stereotyping against people because of their age. Examples of stereotyping include viewing all elderly people as dependent, helpless, frail, demented, or needing assistance. Negative attitudes include not valuing the opinions, contributions, or ideas of the elderly; treating the elderly with disrespect; and ignoring or belittling them whenever possible.

With the rise of the tremendous number of aging baby boomers, attitudes toward aging seem to be changing once again. The pendulum that moved so far toward ageism appears to be moving toward a more humanistic view of the elderly. Studies indicating that age does not necessarily lead to physical and mental decline may help convince the skeptics that aging is not necessarily a negative experience. The activity of organizations like the Gray Panthers and AARP help mobilize this population group and focus attention on the positive aspects of aging (Display 1-6). This large and diverse group is now viewed by many as an untapped resource for society rather than a burden on society.

DISPLAY 1-4. Myths Concerning Older Adults

Myth: Most older people are confused and disinterested in the world around them.
Most older people have an interest in the world around them. They are knowledgeable, articulate, and eager to learn. Only a small portion of the aging population suffers from dementia and health problems that affect cognitive ability. Even with dementia and loss of cognitive functioning, many nursing interventions nurses can stimulate interest in the surrounding world and, in some cases, decrease confusion.

Myth: Most older people are unhealthy.
Most older persons view themselves as being in good health. They live full, active lives and practice health-promotion behaviors. Although most do have at least one chronic illness, they learn to manage their health care and live productively within the limitation caused by chronic illness.

Myth: Most older people are lonely and unhappy.
Some older people are lonely and unhappy, but chances are they were lonely and unhappy as young and middle-aged adults. Most older people are happy, active, and eagerly pursue pleasurable activities with friends and family. Many take advantage of the numerous opportunities to engage in volunteer activities through participation in various service organizations. The American Heart Association, the American Cancer Society, local hospitals, nursing homes, libraries, and many other organizations have active volunteer service programs. Older adults who express loneliness or unhappiness can be encouraged to participate in volunteer activities.

Myth: Most older people are disinterested in sex.
Interest in sex and sexual activity is an important aspect of life, regardless of the age. The need for closeness, intimacy, and love plays a vital role in an older person's life. Sexual feelings and activity do not automatically shut off at 65. Men are able to father children well into old age. Women are free to enjoy the sexual act without fear of becoming pregnant.

Myth: Most older people live in institutions.
Most older people live at home with help, support, and assistance coming from family members. Only 5% to 7% of older adults live in an institutional setting such as a nursing home.

Myth: The elderly are a useless segment of our society.
Countless contributions by older adults contribute to the betterment of our society. Many discover talents in old age that they were unaware of in their youth. See Display 1-6 for the contributions of older adults.

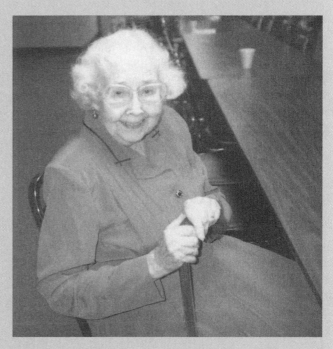

FIGURE 1-2. Most older adults are happy and well adjusted. They enjoy life and remain active and busy well into their 70s and 80s.

DISPLAY 1-5. An Earlier Attitude Toward Aging

Because the elderly could synthesize and share vital lessons garnered from the past and present, Americans between 1790 and 1860 considered it practical to heed an older person's counsel and to use his or her talents, even in periods of rapid change. The experience and wisdom of years seemed indispensable in nurturing the well-being of the republic. For this reason, most people before the Civil War believed that the aged, except those whose unseemly behavior provoked contempt, made essential contributions to their contemporaries. It should not be altogether surprising, therefore, that early Americans chose the image of a sinewy old man with long white hair and chin whiskers to symbolize their new land. Dressed in red- and white-striped pantaloons and a blue coat bespangled with stars and sporting an unabashedly old-fashioned plug hat, "Uncle Sam" seemed to personify the honesty, self-reliance, and devotion to country so deeply cherished in the early decades of our national experience.

—W. Andrew Achenbaum, *Old Age in the New Land: The American Experience Since 1790,* The University Press, 1978.

DISPLAY 1-6. Contributions of Older Adults

Gloria Stuart	At 87, she was nominated for an Oscar for her performance in the movie *Titanic.* This made her the oldest actress ever nominated for an Oscar.	**Claude Pepper**	A Democratic congressmen from Florida in his 80s, he was an advocate for the rights of senior citizens.
Voltaire	One of the greatest 18th-century European authors, he wrote his best works, including *Candide,* after the age of 64.	**James Michener**	Author of *Tales of the South Pacific* and other books, his writing continued into his 80s.
Benjamin Franklin	He was a framer of the constitution at the age of 81.	**Sohn Kee Chung**	Korea's greatest marathon runner, at age 76, he was still running and carried the Olympic torch in the 1988 Summer Games.
Verdi	An Italian composer, he wrote his opera, *Falstaff,* at age 80.	**Mary Martin**	She became the world's favorite Peter Pan on the stage at age 40 and returned to the stage at age 72.
William Harvey	An English physician, he described circulation of the blood and defined the heart as a pump when he was 73.	**Maggie Kuhn**	After her retirement, she founded the Gray Panthers, a political organization for older people. She described two advantages of being in her 80s: outliving her opposition and being able to speak her mind.
Disraeli	He was Prime Minister of Great Britain for the second time, at the age of 70.		
Golda Meir	At age 71, she became Prime Minister of Israel.	**Ronald Reagan**	At age 69, he was the oldest man ever sworn into office as President of the United States and served from 1981 to 1989.
Henry Ford	He introduced the V-8 engine at age 69.		

Nurses Attitudes Toward Aging

Ageism affects the attitudes of health care professionals and affects the care of the older adult. For example, if a nurse views aging as a negative experience with inescapable cognitive and physical decline, that nurse's care will reflect those views. The nurse may not see the need to work toward restoring or increasing functional ability because her view of aging is that of inevitable decline. This nurse may not treat the older adult with dignity and respect but instead treat them as individuals who are incapable of making self-care and health care decisions.

Ageism must be identified and eliminated for nursing care to be effective. Nurses can lead the way in defeating attitudes of ageism and set the example of caring in a respectful and considerate manner.

REALITIES OF AGING

Certain realities of aging must be accepted and understood to combat the attitudes that foster ageism. Display 1-7 identifies realities of aging that will assist the nurse in eliminating stereotypical thinking toward aging.

NURSES RESPONSIBILITY TO COMBAT AGEISM

Nurses have a responsibility to help dispel attitudes of ageism and misconceptions about aging. The first step is to identify and eliminate personal attitudes of ageism. Understanding the realities of aging and identifying common misconceptions about aging better equips the nurse to educate individuals and communities about characteristics of the aging population. Nurses can refer others to agencies that can provide accurate, current information on aging.

CRITICAL THINKING EXERCISES

1. Plan an in-service education program for the staff at an adult day care center about "The Aging Adult." What information would be most important to include for this audience?
2. How prevalent do you feel ageism is in our society? Give four examples of ageism. Do you see any indications that ageism is increasing or decreasing? Explain your answer.

DISPLAY 1-7. Realities of Aging

Reality: Aging is a life-long process.
Aging is a life-long process that begins at conception. Age-related changes are inevitable. These changes do affect lifestyle, but most changes can be managed in order for the older person to live a happy, productive life. A nurse who understands that aging is a normal, natural process that occurs in all individuals is more prepared to give nursing care than the nurse who views aging as a disease that must be tolerated.

Reality: Aging is highly individualized.
Aging is highly individualized and influenced by factors such as environment, genetics, health care, and health promotion activity. The aging population encompasses those between 65 and 100 plus years. There is great diversity in years and in mental, physical, and psychological ability. No two older adults are alike. Nursing care must be individualized to meet specific individual needs.

Reality: Health habits are reversible.
Disease is *not* inevitable. In some instances, disease is avoidable. Poor health habits are reversible. As the lifespan increases, more individuals older than 65 are interested in improving the quality of life and changing health habits to provide an even higher quality of life. More senior citizens are involved in exercise programs, eating the proper diet, stress reduction, and eliminating cigarette smoking.

3. Identify seven characteristics of an aging woman. Interview an elderly woman 70 years of age or older, and assess for the presence or absence of these characteristics.
4. A nursing assistant asks you what the term *frail elderly* means. How would you explain this term to the nursing assistant? What types of assistance does the frail elderly nursing home resident most often require?

REFERENCES AND SUGGESTED READING

American Nurses Association. (1995). *Scope and Standards of Gerontological Nursing Practice.* Publication no. GE-14. Washington, DC: American Nurses Publishing.

U.S. Department of Commerce. Bureau of the Census. (1998). *Population Profile of the United States: 1997*, no. 194. Washington, DC: Government Printing Office.

U.S. Department of Commerce. Bureau of the Census. (1997). *Sixty-Five Plus in the United States*, no. 190. Washington, DC: Government Printing Office.

RESOURCES ON THE WORLD WIDE WEB

http://www.census.gov

http://www.nih.gov/nia

(National Institutes of Health/National Institute on Aging)

Basic Concepts of Gerontological Nursing

KEY TERMS

CHAPTER OBJECTIVES

CHRONOLOGIC AND FUNCTIONAL AGE

IMPORTANT QUALITIES OF THE GERONTOLOGICAL NURSE

PRACTITIONERS OF CARE IN GERONTOLOGICAL NURSING

CARE SETTINGS FOR GERONTOLOGICAL NURSING

NURSING FACILITY STAFFING: A MULTIDISCIPLINARY TEAM

MASLOW'S HIERARCHY OF NEEDS

CRITICAL THINKING EXERCISES

REFERENCES AND SUGGESTED READINGS

RESOURCES ON THE WORLD WIDE WEB

KEY TERMS

chronologic age

frail elderly

functional age

geriatrics

gerontological nursing

gerontology

healthy elderly

nursing facility

Omnibus Budget Reconciliation Act

physiologic needs

residents

self-actualization

therapeutic relationship

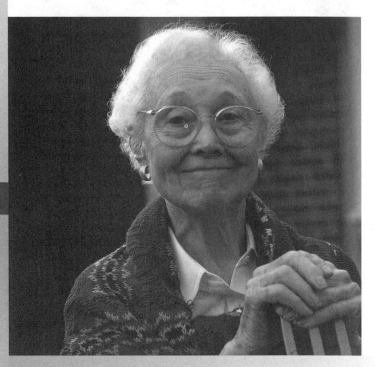

CHAPTER OBJECTIVES

At the completion of this chapter, the student will be able to

- Define gerontology, geriatrics, and gerontological nursing

- Distinguish between chronologic age and functional age

- Discuss important qualities for the geriatric nurse

- Describe the types of practitioners involved in the care of geriatric patients

- Discuss the various health care settings used for geriatric care

- Identify the important aspects of the Omnibus Budget Reconciliation Act (OBRA)

- Discuss the use of Maslow's Hierarchy of Needs in gerontological nursing

Gerontology is the study of all aspects of aging, including the physical, psychological, social, and economic problems of older adults. **Geriatrics** focuses on diagnosis and treatment of diseases common in aging. **Gerontological nursing** is a specialized area of nursing that focuses on providing care to elderly patients through the use of the nursing process (ie, assessment, planning, implementation, and evaluation). When using the nursing process in planning care, the gerontological nurse considers the needs and characteristics unique to the older adult.

CHRONOLOGIC AND FUNCTIONAL AGE

Chronologic age, the number of years since birth, is a simple method of evaluating age. Although the easiest method, it is not the most effective method. For example, two people the same chronologic age can function quite differently. One can be alert and independent, whereas the other is dependent and confused. This discrepancy of functioning among people of the same age leads to the second method of evaluating age, the functional method. **Functional age** evaluates age in terms of functional performance. The functional ability of the elderly person is compared with the standard adult performance. Adults who fail to meet the criteria for standard adult performance are considered "old."

Display 2-1 provides age classification for the older population. Those falling within the young-old age group are generally healthy and function independently. Young-old persons may require assistance when ill for short periods, but overall, they function independently.

The term **frail elderly** refers to those older than 75 years or those older than 65 years who have some type of functional impairment. Elderly persons with functional impairment need help with activities of daily living, caring for themselves, or making decisions. The term **healthy elderly** usually means individuals without functional impairment who maneuver well within the environment and need minimal assistance.

IMPORTANT QUALITIES OF THE GERONTOLOGICAL NURSE

Caring for the older adult is a specialized area of nursing, and certain qualities in the nurse are important. Display 2-2 identifies attributes that are of special importance when caring for the elderly.

> **DISPLAY 2-1. Classification of the Older Population by Chronologic Age**
>
> Young-old: 65 to 74 years
> Middle-old: 75 to 84 years
> Old-old: 85+ years

> **DISPLAY 2-2. Attributes of Importance for the Gerontological Nurse**
>
> - Ability to form a therapeutic relationship with elderly adults
> - Appreciation of the uniqueness of elderly adults
> - Clinical competence in basic nursing skills
> - Good communication skills
> - Knowledge of physical and psychosocial changes that occur with age
> - Ability to work with and supervise others

Ability to Form a Therapeutic Relationship

One of the most important qualities of the gerontological nurse is the ability to form a therapeutic relationship with an older adult. The **therapeutic relationship,** also referred to as the nurse-patient relationship or a trusting relationship, is defined as an association between the patient and the nurse designed to produce a healing and caring atmosphere that fosters health or health-seeking behaviors. Chapter 5 provides more information on developing a therapeutic relationship with older adults.

Nurses sometimes do not feel comfortable with older adults. Many of these nurses have not cultivated an appreciation for the wisdom and uniqueness of the older adult. Nurses must be willing to take the time to develop a therapeutic or trusting relationship. Developing this type of relationship requires more time and effort than developing a trusting relationship with a younger adult. Older adults may not be accustomed to someone listening to them and may be distrustful, particularly during the initial stages of the therapeutic relationship. Older adults have a longer health history than younger adults. Sixty five or more years of living, often with a number of significant health-altering events, requires that the nurse be willing to spend sufficient time to obtain a thorough health history.

Nurses are sometimes reluctant to spend the time necessary to develop a trusting relationship. Nurses may be too busy with the daily hospital routine or nursing home responsibilities to take the time to listen to the older adult. Some nurses may be afraid of growing older themselves and mistakenly assume that avoidance of the older adult can perpetuate their own youth.

Personal feelings about the aged and aging must be explored, because negative or stereotypical feelings can hinder the care the nurse provides. Stereotypical attitudes such as feeling that all older people are confused, sick, or have nothing to contribute to society sabotage the development of a therapeutic nurse-patient relationship. Failure to invest the time to develop a good nurse-patient relationship is a mistake that can foster noncompliance or an uncooperative attitude in the older adult. To develop the type of relationship that allows the nurse to provide the care the elderly person needs and deserves, the nurse must be in touch with personal feelings and eliminate stereotypical attitudes.

Appreciation of the Uniqueness of Elderly Adults

Recognition of individual attributes and characteristics of each older adult enables the nurse to plan care to meet specific needs rather that follow a "canned" plan of care. An accurate assessment allows the nurse to develop an individualized plan of care that meets the patient's specific needs. Identified problems and weaknesses become the foundation for care. Individual strengths are emphasized and past coping skills reinforced. An appreciation of qualities and characteristics present in the older adult assists the nurse in developing a therapeutic rapport with the older adult. A therapeutic relationship increases patient compliance and enhances all aspects of care from the assessment process to the evaluation of care.

Clinical Competence

Nurses caring for the elderly must be skilled in assessment and practice. Catheterizing patients, administering medications, monitoring patients for adverse reactions to medications, and managing feeding tubes are important skills for the nurse caring for elderly patients. Competence in the performance of basic nursing skills gives the patient confidence in the nurse and enhances the nurse-patient relationship.

Knowledge of Physical and Psychosocial Changes

Understanding the physical and psychosocial aspects of aging is important for the nurse in giving holistic care. Knowledge of changes that occur within the body as a result of age enhances assess-

ment. Psychosocial problems contribute to feelings of depression and anger, which leads to physical problems. Chapters 8 and 11 provide more information on the psychosocial needs of the older adult.

Ability to Communicate

The ability to communicate with patients, family members, and other health care providers is essential (see Chapters 5 and 25). Practicing good communication techniques is vital when determining health care needs or when teaching the older adult about health care regimens. Nurses must be capable of discussing delicate issues with the patient and family members. For example, issues related to death and dying require caring and empathetic communication.

Ability to Work With and Supervise Others

Practical nurses may be in a supervisory role in a nursing home or geriatric day care center. The supervisory role requires good communication skills and the ability to work closely with other members of the health care team such as the registered nurse, the geriatric nurse practitioners, the clinical nurse specialist, and the physician. The practical nurse working in a nursing home must be able to supervise others (eg, nurse assistants, other unlicensed assistive personnel) in the care of the elderly. Chapter 25 provides more information on leadership and the management skills needed by the practical nurse.

The Art of Caring

Caring is the core of all nursing care, particularly gerontological nursing care. The art of caring is the ability of the nurse to apply the principles of nursing care in a meaningful and tender manner. A caring nurse views the older adult from a holistic perspective: physically, mentally, emotionally, and socially (Fig. 2-1). In our fast-paced, highly technologic world, the simple art of caring is often neglected. Older adults are sometimes ignored, hurried, belittled, or treated with disrespect. Display 2-3 identifies ways in which holistic care can be implemented.

Nurses working with older adults have a unique opportunity to practice the art of caring. Although many older adults are hesitant to respond at first, they usually eagerly reciprocate when the nurse is perceived as caring. Sincerity is a vital component of caring because the elderly are quick to detect a false attitude of caring. A nurse who cares is able to make

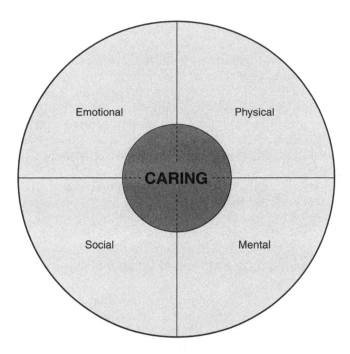

FIGURE 2-1. Holistic care of the older adult. Caring is the center for holistic care. Care is given in four areas: physical, mental, social, and emotional.

DISPLAY 2-3. **Providing Holistic Care**	
Holistic Component	**Interventions**
Mentally	Provide stimulating activities
	Encourage participation in community continuing education classes
	Provide opportunities to learn new skills
	Allow and encourage decision making regarding life situations
Physically	Meet basic physiologic needs
	Keep clean and comfortable
	Encourage exercise suitable for health status and physical abilities
Socially	Assist in building healthy relationships
	Assist in resolving relationship conflicts
	Encourage formation of new relationships
	Encourage participation in social activities
Emotionally	Encourage participation in reminiscence therapy and life review
	Encourage expression of feelings (positive and negative)

DISPLAY 2-4. Ways for the Nurse to Exhibit Caring

- Treating the older adult with dignity and respect
- Valuing the life and contributions of older adults
- Actively listening and responding to older adults in a positive manner
- Talking and spending time with older adults
- Practicing patience and kindness
- Meeting basic physiologic needs promptly and competently
- Assisting older adults to be self-directed to help reach their highest functional capacity

a "connection" or form a bond with the patient. Display 2-4 identifies ways that caring is exhibited.

Cultural Considerations

The United States is a melting pot for many cultures. Members of a certain culture or ethic group have similar attributes such as language, customs, and beliefs about health and aging. An appreciation for the differences of various cultures is needed for the nurse to be sensitive to the needs of others. The wise nurse discusses with the patient, family members, or significant others the ethnic and cultural practices that have meaning to the patient. Chapter 8 provides information on how to perform a cultural assessment.

PRACTITIONERS OF CARE IN GERONTOLOGICAL NURSING

Several types of practitioners provide care in gerontological settings:
- Licensed practical or vocational nurse (LPN, LVN)
- Registered nurse (RN)
- Geriatric nurse practitioner (GNP)
- Clinical nurse specialist (CNS)

The GNP and CNS work independently in areas such as hospitals, nursing homes, senior citizen centers, rehabilitation centers, and other areas where elderly patients need specialized nursing care. In some states, the GNP and CNS have some form of prescriptive authority. RNs usually work as directors of nursing in nursing homes, and a licensed nurse (LPN, LVN, or RN) is on duty at all times. Each state has specific standards regarding staffing of nursing homes, adult day care centers, and other areas requiring nursing services.

CARE SETTINGS
FOR GERONTOLOGICAL NURSING

Most older adults live at home. They are able to care for themselves, or they are cared for by their families. Only 5% to 7% of the people older than age 65 live in nursing homes or long-term care facilities. However, as the population of older adults, especially those older than 85 years, increases in number, more facilities will be needed to provide long-term care. Nearly one fourth of older adults older than age 65 need some help with self-care.

Several types of facilities are available as options for the elderly and their families to choose from. Various names used for the different facilities denote the type of care provided. Examples include independent living, assisted living, continuing care communities, nursing homes, adult day care centers, and senior citizen centers. The choice of facility depends on the type of care needed by the elderly person. Home health care services are a rapidly growing segment of the health care system. Home health care enables the person to receive health care at home while allowing the individual to retain some measure of independence.

Independent Living Retirement Communities

Independent living communities are residential communities for active older adults who want an enjoyable lifestyle free of the worries and trouble of home maintenance. Dwellings are similar to an apartment or single-family unit. Most independent living communities have security (ie, individuals to greet and screen all visitors around the clock). Shopping trips, outings to cultural events, and organized gatherings are typical activities. Some independent living communities have tennis courts, swimming pools, recreational rooms, and various other amenities. Some independent living communities are rental communities, but a few require residents to purchase their own units or homes.

Assisted Living Community

A variety of names are used to identify assisted living communities, such as adult homes, personal care homes, retirement residences, or sheltered housing. For individuals who want to remain independent but who are ready to relinquish the major chores of maintaining a home, an assisted living community may be the best choice. Assisted living communities usually offer help with bathing, dressing, meals, and housekeeping. The amount of help provided depends on individual need. A variety of other services such as meals, housekeeping, laundry, transportation, health care, and long-term care are options for the elderly when living in a sheltered housing facility. In some assisted living centers, these services can be purchased for a fee. Nurses are available to monitor health problems, provide health screening, and identify psychosocial problems. Residents usually have private apartments and live alone or with their spouse. The elderly often feel safer and more secure in an assisted living setting.

Continuing Care Retirement Community

Another type of assisted living is called continuing care retirement communities (CCRCs). CCRCs are residential facilities where older adults can live independently. They offer seniors long-term contracts that guarantee lifelong shelter and access to specified health care services. The older adult pays an initial fee and a monthly maintenance fee. Residents usually are expected to move into the community while they are still independent. If, in the future, assistance is needed with meals or long-term nursing care is required, these services can be obtained on site. CCRC residents enjoy an independent lifestyle with the knowledge that their needs will continue to be met if they become sick or frail. The cost of CCRC is generally less than the cost of traditional nursing home care.

Home Health Care

Home health care services are available for elderly people who need assistance in the home. Home care services can be categorized as skilled care or home support services. Services include skilled nursing, social services, nutritional counseling, home health aides, and occupational and physical therapy. A registered dietitian helps plan special diets. Therapists perform physical, speech, respiratory, and occupational therapies in the home.

Home health agencies may also provide home health aides to assist the older adult with activities such as shopping, meal preparation, and light housekeeping. Home support services include personal care (eg, bathing, dressing, eating, exercising), homemaker services (eg, meal preparation, light housekeeping, shopping), and companion services (ie, sitter). These services can be paid for by the individual or through Medicare or Medicaid if the elderly person meets the eligibility requirements. The RN usually performs the initial assessment and develops a plan of care. The care plan outlines services needed, staff required to carry out the services, and a timeframe to meet the identified goals. In some states, practical nurses can then perform the nursing care, with the RN periodically monitoring the care and updating the plan of care. Home health care agencies may be hospital based or privately owned.

Adult Day Care Centers

Adult day care centers are community-based centers where the elderly and physically or mentally challenged people older than age 60 go during the day to engage in social activities. These individuals need supervision and care during the day but not the 24-hour care provided in a nursing facility. The center provides the participant transportation from home to the center and back home at the end of the day. Activities include card games, dominos, trips to the supermarket, shopping, and social activities such as weekly dances (Fig. 2-2). An activity director plans the activities. The licensed nurse monitors health status and vital signs such as blood pressure and blood glucose levels, makes referrals for social services, and sometimes arranges transportation for medical care. These centers assist the elderly in maintaining functional ability and provide relief for care givers.

Adult day care is funded through Medicaid in some states or paid for by the family. These programs are cost-effective. Studies show that as many as 25% of people in nursing homes could be cared for at home with the supportive assistance of an adult day care center.

Community Senior Citizen Centers

Community senior citizen centers are community-sponsored centers that provide a place where elders congregate to socialize and have fun. The services of the center are usually provided for a minimal fee or may be free of charge. For example, one center provides a daily meal free of charge for everyone, but it asks for a small donation if the older adult feels he can afford it. Elderly people meet for meals, social activity, and support. These adults provide their own transportation and function independently.

Transitional Care Setting

Another care setting is the transitional care setting. Transitional care units are often extensions of the

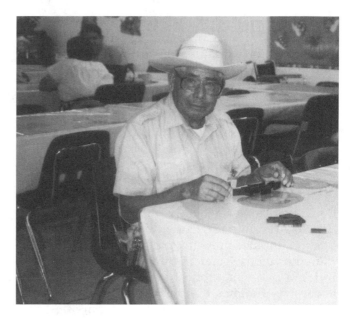

FIGURE 2-2. This elderly man attends an adult daycare center where he socializes and participates in activities offered at the center, such as playing dominos or cards.

hospital where individuals receive nursing care similar to the care received in a nursing facility. Individuals in a transitional unit do not require the more highly skilled care and monitoring given in the acute care setting. Patients in the transitional unit are preparing to return home or to a nursing home.

Hospital Care

Acute care is given in hospital settings. In acute care settings, health problems are treated that require immediate attention and pose a threat to life. Hospital stays usually are relatively short (eg, 8 or 9 days for the elderly) compared with stays in a nursing facility. Acute diseases such as pneumonia or diabetic ketoacidosis are too complex to handle in outpatient settings such as physicians' offices, home health care settings, or the nursing home and require hospitalization. Elderly people are hospitalized more often than younger adults and stay for longer periods. Many older adults are dismissed from the hospital to a nursing facility for a short stay of restorative care or extended care.

Nursing Homes

Nursing homes are facilities that care for patients with chronic illnesses and physical impairments who do not need hospitalization but require at least one form of skilled care, such as feeding tubes, injections, physical therapy, or Foley catheters. For example, an older adult after fracturing a hip may be hospitalized for immediate care and stabilization. She may be dismissed to a nursing home for convalescence, physical therapy, or occupational therapy. Within several months, the person may progress to the point that she can be dismissed to go home or live with a family member. Other people, such as those with Alzheimer's disease may be totally unable to regain the ability for self-care. These individuals make their homes permanently in the nursing home. Because the nursing home does become the older persons' home, they are called **residents** (ie, people who live in a nursing home or a nursing facility), not patients, in most facilities. Resident more accurately denotes the position of the older adult in the nursing home. The typical nursing home resident is 85 years or older, female, white, and widowed.

Omnibus Budget Reconciliation Act

The federal government passed the **Omnibus Budget Reconciliation Act** (OBRA) in 1987. A portion of that legislation is called the Nursing Home Reform Act, but the legislation is most commonly referred to as OBRA. OBRA is viewed as an important milestone in improving the quality of care in nursing homes. OBRA has as its goal that every resident in a nursing home be functioning at the highest possible level of physical, mental, and psychosocial well-being. OBRA requires that resident's rights be respected and that the resident be treated with dignity. A resident assessment form must be completed within 14 days of admission and care plan developed from that assessment that is continually evaluated and revised. A comprehensive assessment must be done at least annually thereafter or whenever there is a significant change in the resident (ie, improvement or deterioration of the patient's condition).

Nursing Facility

Nursing facility is the term given to facilities caring for Medicare or Medicaid residents and providing nursing care, medical services, and rehabilitative care to these residents. In this book, nursing facility and nursing home are used interchangeably. A nursing facility or nursing home provides 24-hour nursing care by RNs, licensed practical nurses, and

nurse assistants. Federal law requires that an RN be on duty 8 hours each day for 7 days per week in nursing facilities (see Registered Nurses section). LPNs manage unlicensed assistive personnel and delegate the work load.

Nurses provide various types of nursing care at a nursing facility:

- Observing patients with an acute or unstable condition
- Administering nasogastric or enteral feedings
- Monitoring intravenous fluids
- Administering oral, intramuscular, subcutaneous, or intravenous medications
- Changing sterile dressings

Occupational therapy, physical therapy, and services of social workers may also be a part of the care. Nursing facilities provide restorative care for patients who have the potential to regain functional ability (eg, walking, toileting, dressing, other self-care activities). Chapter 9 provides more information on restorative care.

NURSING FACILITY STAFFING: A MULTIDISCIPLINARY TEAM

Nursing facilities use a multidisciplinary approach to planning and providing care. Health care providers forming the multidisciplinary team include RNs, LPNs or LVNs, nursing assistants, the medical director, pharmacist, dietitian, occupational therapist, physical therapist, social worker, restorative aid, and an activity director. Each member of the team provides input when planning the care of the resident.

Registered Nurses

OBRA requires that an RN be on duty in a nursing facility for a minimum of 8 hours per day for 7 days each week and that an LPN be on duty 24 hours per day. Some nursing facilities are unable to meet this requirement and request a waiver for this standard. The waiver applies to the RN requirement on weekends. A "good faith" effort must be made to hire the required staff.

The director of nursing (DON) is an RN who works full time and is responsible for all nursing staff and nursing care. The director of nursing implements OBRA requirements, provides and monitors nursing care, participates in the development of the care plan, and helps to recruit and manage the staff.

Additional RNs are sometimes part of the staff. Their responsibilities vary with each facility but usually include developing policies and procedures within OBRA guidelines, working with quality assurance, performing resident assessments, and supervising and directing care.

GNPs and the geriatric CNS are advanced-practice RNs with a master's degree in nursing. These individuals practice nursing in a nursing facility or other agency that specializes in care of the older adult. In many states, advanced-practice nurses receive independent reimbursement for the services they perform. GNPs provide primary care. Their presence helps to provide early identification and intervention for acute and chronic illnesses. Early intervention by the GNP or CNS is cost-effective and greatly improves the quality of care that an elderly person receives.

Licensed Practical or Vocational Nurses

The practical nurse provides most of the day to day management of nursing assistants and monitoring of resident care in a nursing facility. The term LVN is used in some states. This places the practical or vocational nurse in a supervisory role for which he or she is often unprepared. Practical or vocational nursing schools increasingly are including concepts of management and leadership to the curricula to better prepare the nurse for this important role (see Chapter 25).

The role of the assistant director of nursing is filled by an RN or a practical nurse. The assistant director of nurses is responsible for staffing, quality improvement, and other duties assigned by the organization.

Nursing Assistants

More than 90% of direct care in a nursing facility is given by nursing assistants. OBRA has mandated certain minimal standards for training nursing assistants. Students complete a specified number of training hours and demonstrate proficiency through an evaluation determined by each state. After meeting educational standards and demonstrating competency through an evaluation process, these nursing assistants are certified. After becoming certified, their names are placed on the state's registry. Titles vary, but often they are called certified nurse assistants.

Other Members of the Multidisciplinary Team

Nursing facilities must have a medical director or physician who establishes administrative and clinical practice standards. Ideally, the physician is board certified in geriatrics. In addition to administrative responsibilities, the physician may also have a case load of patients within the facility and a private practice outside of the facility.

Another member of the multidisciplinary staff is the pharmacist. The pharmacist monitors medication regimens to reduce polypharmacy (ie, taking more drugs than are needed), monitors adverse reactions, and recommends dosage adjustments. Medication orders and records are periodically reviewed to evaluate effectiveness of the drug therapy.

Other members of the multidisciplinary team include the registered dietitian (RD), the occupational therapist (OT), the physical therapist (PT), the restorative aid, the social worker, and the activity director. An RD is needed to plan meals and evaluate nutritional status of the residents. The OT, PT, and restorative aide work together as a part of the multidisciplinary team to improve the functional ability of the older adult.

A social worker is required in all Medicare and Medicaid approved nursing facility with more than 120 beds. The social worker helps explain the rules and regulations of Medicare and Medicaid, participates in the development of a plan of care, and plans group activities. The activities director plans a schedule of daily activities that are stimulating, interesting, and motivating for elderly adults. Activities include games such as dominos or cards, parties, special outings, exercise programs, special guests, and religious services.

MASLOW'S HIERARCHY OF NEEDS

A orderly, systematic method of identifying the needs of the older adult is necessary if care is to be individualized and problems addressed in an effective manner. Psychologist Abraham Maslow developed a psychosocial development theory based on the potential of the individual to become fully mature and self-actualized (ie, totally fulfilled). Maslow's theory provides a systematic framework for recognizing individual needs and planning nursing care.

Maslow's theory is based on a hierarchy of needs (Fig. 2-3), which can be used to prioritize and plan nursing care. Maslow's needs are ranked in ascending order, with the most basic needs first.

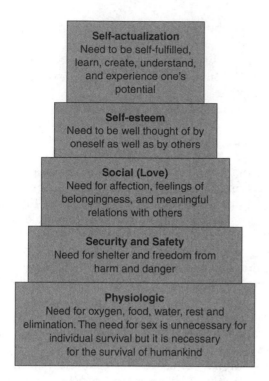

FIGURE 2-3. According to Maslow, basic physiologic needs, such as food and water must be met before a person can move on to meeting higher-level needs. Nursing is based on helping people to meet needs they cannot meet by themselves because of age, illness, or injury.

Physiologic Needs

The lower or most basic needs are the **physiologic needs.** Maslow believed that the most basic physiologic needs such as the need for oxygen, food, water, rest, and elimination must be satisfied before proceeding to higher needs such as love and belonging or esteem needs. Physiologic needs are sometimes called survival needs, because they must be met for the survival of the person. After survival needs are met or at least partially met, higher needs can be pursued.

Safety Needs

Safety needs are the second level in this hierarchy. These needs are particularly important for the elderly. In working with elderly patients, safety needs are closely related to physiologic needs. A patient must feel safe and secure to heal. Elderly adults who do not feel safe may become confused, agitated, or angry. Frequent contact with people the elderly person loves and trusts can increase feelings of safety and security. An important aspect of fulfilling safety needs of the older adult is to develop a trusting nurse-patient relationship.

Love and Belonging

When physiologic and safety needs are met, the individual is ready to address other needs such as love and belonging. All individuals have the need to feel special, to be loved, and to belong to a group. A significant and meaningful relationship with others increases the feeling of belonging. When the older adult loses loved ones and friends who are members of their peer group, they can lose the sense of being loved and belonging to a special group. For example, an elderly person may have several siblings, but with age and time, she may find herself the sole surviving member of the family. Loss of individuals in the older adult's peer group can cause loneliness and depression. New relationships must be cultivated that are satisfying and fulfilling. The need for love and belonging sometimes can be transferred from people to an animal, a special project, or working for charitable organizations. For example, an older adult who volunteers with the American Cancer Society or for a hospital auxiliary group can develop a renewed sense of belonging.

Esteem Needs

Esteem reflects the feelings a person has for himself. When these feelings are positive, good self-esteem follows. Negative thoughts and feelings concerning self lead to a low self-esteem. Although self-esteem comes from within, the acceptance of others contributes. Approval from those we love and trust enhances self-esteem. Family members, friends, and loved ones are encouraged to express their approval and admiration of the older adult. To assist elderly individuals in meeting their esteem needs, nurses must convey acceptance and approval. Nurses should listen attentively to what the older adult is saying, and encouraging her to reminisce about past experiences and successes can enhance self-esteem.

Self-Actualization

Self-actualization is a growth process in which the individual strives to "be all that he can be," to reach the highest potential possible, and to be totally fulfilled. Although self-actualization is a worthy goal, only a few people are able to become fully self-actualized. Exploring avenues such as religion or philosophy can help the individual in the search for self-actualization. Life is fulfilled to the greatest extent with the elderly person being able to do with his life what he desires to do and what he is best suited to do. Pursuing self-actualization is often as fulfilling as achieving it.

The need to acquire knowledge and understanding is a part of self-actualization. Older adults who remain intellectually active have a greater opportunity to become self-actualized. Opportunities to learn are available through continuing education classes, lectures, self-study groups, and study clubs. Some older adults attend colleges or universities. Baring a physical condition that affects mental functioning (eg, Alzheimer's disease), stimulating the mind is something that all older adults can do. Evidence indicates that using the mind is a form of mental exercise that helps to perpetuate efficient mental functioning.

Aesthetic needs (ie, need for beauty and creativity) are among the highest needs postulated by Maslow. Aesthetic needs can be met through perfecting a talent such as playing the piano or by an artist expressing himself creatively through painting. Some may achieve aesthetic satisfaction through an appreciation for music, art, or beauty.

Meeting Maslow's Hierarchy of Needs

Rarely does any individual have all of his needs met. Maslow estimated that fewer than 1% of the population reach full self-actualization. People move up and down this hierarchy throughout life, responding positively or negatively to external and internal stimuli.

Death usually occurs because of an inability to meet a physiologic need, such as the occurrence of an illness or a decline in functional ability. Death can result from an unmet safety need, such as a fall or an automobile accident. Rarely, death occurs because of an unmet need to feel loved or self-esteem. When esteem needs remain unmet and the individual is unable to compensate, depression can develop, making suicide a real possibility.

☀ CRITICAL THINKING EXERCISES

1. Have a brainstorming session to identify at least 10 caring behaviors of the nurse in a nursing facility. After the list is complete, select three behaviors you feel are the most important and give a rationale for your choice.

2. Mr. Jefferies recently was admitted to the nursing facility. The nurse notices that he has some difficulty breathing, bruises easily, and has an unsteady gait when ambulating. His wife has recently died, and his children felt he could be better cared for in a nursing facility because he was unable to care for himself at home. Using Maslow's hierarchy, identify Mr. Jefferies needs in each area. Give a rationale for each need selected.

3. Obtain job descriptions for a nurse working in a nursing facility, hospital, adult day care center, or another geriatric facility. Compare the job descriptions. What responsibilities are unique to each job represented?

4. What ways are Maslow's needs met in your life? Begin with the physiologic needs and proceed to the higher needs. Are you a self-actualized individual? Give a rationale for your answer.

REFERENCES AND SUGGESTED READING

Allen, J. (2000). *Nursing home federal requirements and guidelines to surveyors* (4th ed.). New York: Springer Publications.

Burger, S., Fraser, V., Hunt, S., & Frank, B. (1996). *Nursing homes: Getting good care there.* San Luis Obispo, CA: American Source Books.

Grossman, D. (1996). Cultural dimensions in home health nursing. *American Journal of Nursing, 96 (7),* 33–36.

Timby, B., Scherer, J., & Smith, N. (1999). *Introductory medical-surgical nursing* (7th ed.). Philadelphia: Lippincott Williams & Wilkins.

RESOURCES ON THE WORLD WIDE WEB

http://seniors-site.com/nursing/index.html (nursing home information)

http://www.hcfa.gov (OBRA regulations)

CHAPTER 3

Theories of Aging

CHAPTER OUTLINE

KEY TERMS
CHAPTER OBJECTIVES
LIFESPAN VERSUS LIFE EXPECTANCY
SENESCENCE AND THE AGING PROCESS
BIOLOGIC THEORIES OF AGING
    Genetic Theory of Aging
    Free Radical Theory of Aging
    Cross-Linking Theory of Aging
    Immunologic Theory of Aging
    Wear and Tear Theory of Aging
PSYCHOSOCIAL THEORIES OF AGING
    Disengagement Theory of Aging
    Activity Theory of Aging
    Continuity Theory of Aging
FINDING A COMMON THEORY OF AGING
CRITICAL THINKING EXERCISES
REFERENCES AND SUGGESTED READING

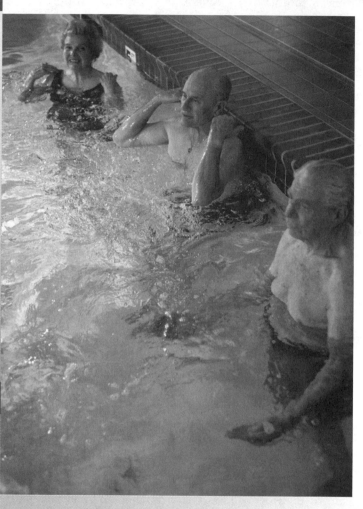

KEY TERMS

cell-mediated immunity
centenarian
collagen
free radical
humoral immunity
life expectancy
lifespan
lipofuscin
senescence
T cells

CHAPTER OBJECTIVES

At the completion of this chapter, the student will be able to

- Identify four basic characteristics of the aging process

- Distinguish between lifespan and life expectancy

- Identify basic components of the biologic and psychosocial theories of aging

What causes aging? Can the aging process be altered? These still unanswered questions have plagued scientists for many years. This chapter examines some of the more common theories of aging.

There are four basic characteristics of the aging process:

The aging process is universal. All people age except when death occurs at a young age.

The aging process is progressive, but all individuals do not necessarily show the signs of aging at the same chronologic age.

The aging process is intrinsic in nature; it appears to originate from within the body.

Aging is affected by extrinsic factors, which originate outside the body and affect the aging process. Extrinsic factors include the environment, standard of living, and coping mechanisms.

These four characteristics interact to determine the aging process for each individual. Although the basic pattern of aging is universal, the rate that one ages is influenced by extrinsic factors such as the environment or standard of living. Intrinsic factors, such as genetic makeup, also affect the rate of aging. Some individuals remain young looking with few signs of aging until an older chronologic age than other individuals. The reasons for the wide variations in the aging process are not fully understood.

LIFESPAN VERSUS LIFE EXPECTANCY

Lifespan can be defined as the potential maximum number of years a person can live. Maximum human lifespan is 110 to 125 years. Diseases such as cancer or cardiovascular disease can shorten the lifespan. These diseases become more prevalent as the aging process continues. **Life expectancy** is the average number of years one can expect to live. Currently, the life expectancy is 72 years for men and 79 years for women.

Centenarian is a word used to denote a person who has reached 100 years of age. There are approximately 56,000 Americans older than 100 years of age. With more individuals living longer, some authorities estimate that those older than 100 will become the most rapidly increasing age group in the 21st century.

SENESCENCE AND THE AGING PROCESS

Senescence can be defined as the end stage of life or the process of growing old. Theoretically, aging begins at birth and progresses at varying rates throughout senescence. Senescence brings these

---

> **DISPLAY 3-1. Biologic Theories of Aging**
>
> - Genetic theory: individuals inherit a genetic program that determines life expectancy.
> - Free radical theory: aging is caused by the buildup of products called free radicals as a result of oxygen use within the cell.
> - Cross-linking theory: aging is a result of decreased cellular division because a cross-linking agent attaches to a deoxyribonucleic acid (DNA) strand.
> - Immunologic theory: aging occurs as a result of a decrease in the activity of the immune system.
> - Wear and tear theory: aging occurs as the result of normal "wear and tear" or use of the body and body systems.

age-related changes to the forefront, because this is the time that the most noticeable changes associated with aging occur. Noticeable changes include changes such as the loss of subcutaneous tissue leading to wrinkling of the skin or loss of melanin (a black or brown pigment) in the hair follicles leading to graying of the hair. Various theories have been suggested to explain these changes, but no one theory is thought to account totally for the aging process. For the purposes of this text, the theories of aging are divided into two broad categories: biologic theories of aging and psychosocial theories of aging.

BIOLOGIC THEORIES OF AGING

Biologic theories define aging as an involuntary process that over time causes changes in cells and tissues of the body. Other biologic theories explain the aging process as a result of interactions with the environment. Biologic theories of aging include the genetic theory, free radical theory, cross-linking theory, immunologic theory, and wear and tear theory (Display 3-1).

Genetic Theory of Aging

Genetic theorists believe that individuals inherit a genetic program that determines life expectancy. The premise of this theory is that an internal mechanism or "genetic clock" determines senescence. Cells are programmed to divide a certain number of times. The longer the lifespan, the greater is the number of cell divisions. Supporting the genetic theory is the fact that some families have a strong predisposition for longevity. Identical twins have very similar life expectancies, even more similar than the life expectancy among siblings. Related theories propose that aging occurs because of a finite number of fixed incidents within the body, such as a finite number of heart beats.

Free Radical Theory of Aging

The basis of the free radical theory of aging is the accumulation of products called free radicals as a result of oxygen use within the cells. Oxidation of fats, protein, and carbohydrates results in the formation of oxygen compounds with highly reactive electrons. **Free radicals** are formed from covalently bonded atoms when unpaired valence electrons are released as the bond is broken by some form of energy such as heat, light, or ionizing radiation. Although most free radicals have only microseconds of independent existence before they recombine with other atoms, the transitory forms can initiate many kinds of biochemical reactions, including oxidation, combustion, photolysis, and polymerization. Free radicals can generate other free radicals, and aging results from the progressive disruption of cellular function. The cumulative effects in cells can interfere with normal body function. Environmental contaminants also increase the production of free radicals and interfere with the function of cells.

Lipofuscin is a yellowish brown pigment partially composed of lipids and proteins and found in the cells of the muscle, heart, liver, and nerves. This pigmented material appears to have some relation to the free radicals and develops as a result of the oxidation of certain lipids. Some theorists think that lipofuscin is the byproduct of cellular wear and tear. Regardless of the cause, the amount of lipofuscin increases in affected organs with age and is thought to be responsible for aging.

Cross-Linking Theory of Aging

This theory holds that aging is a result of a decrease in cellular division caused by a cross-linking agent attaching itself to a deoxyribonucleic acid (DNA) strand. DNA is the genetic material of the cell. Crosslinking prevents the DNA strand from functioning normally. When crosslinking occurs, changes take place in the collagen tissue within the body. **Collagen** is a protein bundle that forms the framework for the body and supports the tissue. Collagen gives strength and resilience to connective tissue such as bone and cartilage. Collagen is also found in the heart, lungs, vessels, and muscles.

Crosslinking decreases mobility and causes a loss of elasticity in these organs resulting in degenerative changes. The organs affected are the skin, blood vessel walls, musculoskeletal system, and the lens of the eye. Certain proteins in the eye are particularly sensitive to cross-linking changes contributing to the development of opacity (loss of transparency) of the lens of the eye and the development of cataracts.

Immunologic Theory of Aging

The immunologic theory states that aging occurs as a result of a decrease in the activity of the immune system. The immune system, particularly the T cells, protects the body against disease. **T cells** originate in the thymus and make up about 80% of the lymphocytes (ie, white blood cells that function in immunity) in the circulating blood. The T cells produce a type of immunity called **cell-mediated immunity.** Cell-mediated immunity defends the body against cancers and some viruses. T cells work by destroying foreign cells directly, stimulating other cells to assist in immunity, and by initiating a rapid immune response if repeated invasion occurs by certain antigens (ie, foreign substances).

After young adulthood, the immune system declines. With age, tissue of the thymus gland is replaced with fatty tissue, and the gland changes color from a pinkish gray to yellow. The production of T cells decreases, and the body has greater difficulty fighting disease.

Humoral immunity is another type of immunity used by the body to fight disease. In humoral immunity, the body produces a specific antibody to destroy a specific antigen such as a type of bacteria or virus. This reaction is called that antigen–antibody response. Humoral immunity also declines with age causing an increased susceptibility to disease. Some theorists believe that with aging the body does not recognize its own aging cells and attacks them as if they were antigens.

Wear and Tear Theory of Aging

The wear and tear theory states that aging occurs as the result of normal use of the body and body systems. With age, these systems wear out and no longer function to capacity. If this theory is accepted, chronologic age does not determine whether a person is old. The cumulative damage from continuous use and abuse leads to the death of tissues, cells, organs, and the organism.

In the wear and tear theory of aging, some authorities theorize that each individual is supplied with various amounts of adaptive energy. This adaptive energy is used to adjust to personal and environmental stressors. As the adaptive energy declines aging occurs and when this energy is no longer available, the organism dies.

PSYCHOSOCIAL THEORIES

Psychosocial theories attempt to explain aging in terms of a person's cognitive function such as intelligence, memory, and emotions; coping ability; and social changes. Aging is viewed as an interaction between the person and his mental function and physical environment. Examples of psychosocial theories include the disengagement theory, activity theory, and continuity theory (Display 3-2).

Disengagement Theory of Aging

The disengagement theory views aging as a process of withdrawal from life. Society withdraws from the elderly, and the elderly person withdraws from society. This withdrawal is acceptable to the individual and to society because it prohibits frustration in the elderly when faced with role changes that occur with aging. It also facilitates an easier transition of power from the older generation to the younger generation. As the elderly person withdraws, younger people take on greater responsibility and assume leadership roles. This theory is controversial, and critics point out that many older adults do not disengage themselves from life. These adults remain active, productive members of society. Individuals who withdraw appear to do so out of choice, not as a part of the natural aging process.

Activity Theory of Aging

The activity theory states that society should have the same expectations of older adults as it does for middle-aged adults. Aging should be denied as long as possible. As losses occur that are associated with aging, they should be replaced with new and different roles, interests, or people. For example, loss of the ability to engage in strenuous activity can be replaced with intellectual activities. After retirement, new and different roles can be cultivated. Many older adults are unknowingly believers of this philosophy. More and more older adults are refusing to be stereotyped into acting old. They have an active, productive, and fun-filled life.

DISPLAY 3-2. Psychosocial Theories of Aging

- Disengagement theory: Views aging as a process of withdrawal or disengagement from life
- Activity theory: States that society should have the same expectations for older adults as it does for middle-aged adults
- Continuity theory: Also referred to as the developmental theory of aging because it deals with the individual's developmental patterns throughout life, says that successful aging depends on the individual's ability to maintain and continue previous behavior patterns

Continuity Theory

The continuity theory of aging is also referred to as the developmental theory of aging because it deals with the individual's developmental patterns throughout life. According to this theory, successful aging depends on the individual's ability to maintain and continue previous behavior patterns. The perseverance of lifestyle and behavior patterns, whatever they may be on an individual basis, predicts the response to aging.

The basic personality and patterns of behavior remain unchanged as aging progresses. A person who was withdrawn and socially isolated at a young age will most likely be the same in old age. Similarly, an individual who is people oriented and fun loving in youth will mostly likely bring these characteristics into old age. Coping mechanisms and behavior patterns that remain intact allow the person to adjust and adapt to aging successfully. Nursing interventions that encourage greater social interaction are not therapeutic for an individual who spends the greater part of life somewhat socially isolated. Likewise, spending more time alone for reflection and introspection may not be appropriate for fun-loving, socially active individuals.

Continuity theorists relate behavior and coping patterns of aging with similar patterns during other phases of the life cycle. This theory allows for a wide range of individual adaptation in aging, but some authorities think its simplistic nature does not allow for the more complex aspects of aging.

FINDING A COMMON THEORY

For many years, scientists have studied aging, but the exact causes of the aging process remain a mystery. No one theory explains all aspects of aging. The various theories appear to be interrelated and may support or refute one another. More research is needed to gain increased information on this complex topic.

CRITICAL THINKING EXERCISES

1. Select two of the theories of aging discussed in this chapter and discuss the aging process, taking into consideration the interrelatedness of the two theories.
2. Explain each of the two theories from a holistic viewpoint (ie, the physical, mental, and emotional components).

REFERENCES AND SUGGESTED READING

Hoyer, W., Rybash, J., & Roodin, P. (1998). *Adult Development and Aging* (4th ed.). Dubuque, IA: Brown & Benchmark.

Matteson, M., McConnell, E., & Linton, A. (1997). *Gerontological Nursing: Concepts and Practice* (2nd ed.). Philadelphia: W.B. Saunders.

CHAPTER 4

Ethical and Legal Considerations

CHAPTER OUTLINE

KEY TERMS

CHAPTER OBJECTIVES

ETHICAL AND LEGAL CONSIDERATIONS

    Ethical Aspects of Care

    Patient Advocacy

LEGAL ASPECTS OF CARE

    Negligence and Malpractice

    Informed Consent

    Determining Competence

    Patient Self-Determination Act

    Medical Directive to Physician

    Medical Power of Attorney for Health Care

    Nursing Responsibility Concerning Advanced
       Directives

ARTIFICIAL NUTRITION AND HYDRATION

USE OF RESTRAINING DEVICES

    Physical Restraints

    Chemical Restraints

    Behavior Symptoms

    Managing Behavior Symptoms

    When and How to Use Restraints

CRITICAL THINKING EXERCISES

REFERENCES AND SUGGESTED READING

RESOURCES ON THE WORLD WIDE WEB

KEY TERMS

advanced directives

behavioral symptoms

chemical restraints

ethical nursing care

ethics

malpractice

Medical Directive to Physician

Medical Power of Attorney for Health Care

negligence

patient advocate

physical restraints

proxy

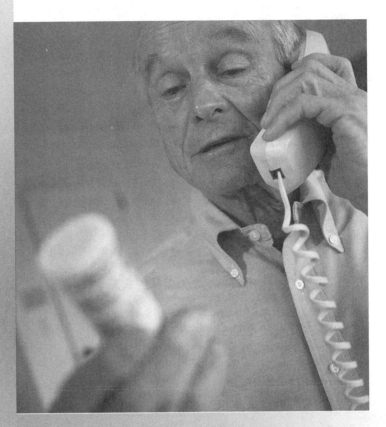

CHAPTER OBJECTIVES

At the completion of this chapter, the student will be able to

- Describe ethical and legal aspects involved in providing care to the older adult

- Discuss the role of the nurse as a patient advocate

- Identify malpractice and negligence in nursing

- Discuss the importance of informed consent

- Discuss the issue of determining competence

- Describe important considerations complying with the Patient Self-Determination Act of 1990

- Discuss the issue of providing artificial nutrition and hydration

- Discuss the use of restraints in the care of the older adult

More and more practical nurses are moving from the acute care setting to practice in outpatient settings, such as adult day care centers, home health, and outpatient clinics. This shift in employment settings places the nurse in roles requiring independent decision making without the support of other health care providers. Gerontological nurses practicing in the nursing home are accountable for the actions of nursing assistants and ancillary staff under their supervision. This increased responsibility requires a thorough understanding of ethical and legal issues to protect the nurse and provide high-quality care. Nursing practice is guided by ethical standards and legal parameters.

ETHICAL AND LEGAL CONSIDERATIONS

Ethical and legal considerations must be adhered to when caring for the elderly. **Ethics** refers to the practices, principles, and guidelines that guide moral decision making and behaviors in a society. In an effort to protect society, especially those who cannot protect themselves, ethical standards may be translated into law. Ideally, the care provided to elderly patients is ethically sound as well as legal. Ethical care of the elderly person is an area of growing concern throughout our nation. The elderly, particularly the frail elderly, are one of the most vulnerable segments of our population. These older adults are at increased risk for neglect, social isolation, oversedation, and excessive use of restraining devices. This increase in vulnerability of the older adult makes ethical and legal issues an important aspect in the care of the elderly.

Ethical Aspects of Care

Ethical standards are set forth as codes for nurses that provide guidelines for determining ethical nursing practice. Ethical standards also include personal ethics that develop within each individual over a lifetime. Each nurse brings a set of personal ethics that plays a role in ethical decision making. Sometimes, nurses have a difference of opinion on issues pertaining to health care. For example, on the issue of withholding food and fluids from a terminally ill person, one nurse may feel that to withhold food and fluids is unacceptable and constitutes unethical care, while another nurse feels that the withholding of food and fluids is a humane and compassionate option that allows for a more peaceful death.

DISPLAY 4-1. Code for Nurses

- The nurse provides services with respect for human dignity and the uniqueness of the client, unrestricted by considerations of social or economic status, personal attributes, or the nature of health problems.
- The nurse safeguards the client's right to privacy by judiciously protecting information of a confidential nature.
- The nurse acts to safeguard the client and the public when health care and safety are affected by the incompetent, unethical, or illegal practice of any person.
- The nurse assumes responsibility and accountability for individual nursing judgments and actions.
- The nurse maintains competence in nursing.
- The nurse exercises informed judgment and uses individual competence and qualifications as criteria in seeking consultation, accepting responsibilities, and delegating nursing activities to others.
- The nurse participates in activities that contribute to the ongoing development of the profession's body of knowledge.
- The nurse participates in the profession's efforts to implement and improve standards of nursing.
- The nurse participates in the profession's efforts to implement and maintain conditions of employment conducive to high quality nursing care.
- The nurse participates in the profession's effort to protect the public from misinformation and misrepresentation and to maintain the integrity of nursing.
- The nurse collaborates with members of the health professions and other citizens in promoting community and national efforts to meet the needs of the public.

From American Nurses Association. (1985). *Code for Nurses with Interpretive Statements.* Kansas City: American Nurses Association.

Ethical nursing care is the type of care provided when adhering to the principles established by nurses in the code of ethics. In 1976 the American Nurses Association (ANA) first published its Code for Nurses. This code provides a framework for delivering care for all nurses (see Display 4-1).

The International Council of Nurses developed a code for nurses that encompasses nurses and their relationship to other people, practice, society as a whole, coworkers, and to the profession (Display 4-2). Every nurse, regardless of the practice setting, should examine these codes for nurses because they

DISPLAY 4-2. International Council of Nurses Code for Nurses

- The fundamental responsibility of the nurse is fourfold: to promote health, to prevent illness, to restore health, and to alleviate suffering.
- The need for nursing is universal. Inherent in nursing is respect for life, dignity, and rights of man. It is unrestricted by considerations of nationality, race, creed, color, age, sex, politics, or social status.
- Nurses render health services to the individual, the family, and the community and coordinate their services with those of related groups.

Nurses and People
- The nurse's primary responsibility is to those people who require nursing care.
- The nurse, in providing care, promotes an environment in which the values, customs, and beliefs of individuals are respected.
- The nurse holds in confidence personal information and uses judgment in sharing this information.

Nurses and Practice
- The nurse carries personal responsibility for nursing practice and for maintaining competence by continual learning.
- The nurse maintains the highest standards of nursing care possible within the reality of a specific situation.

- The nurse uses judgment in relation to individual competence when accepting and delegating responsibilities.
- The nurse when acting in a professional capacity should at all times maintain standards of personal conduct that reflect credit on the profession.

Nurses and Society
- The nurse shares with other citizens the responsibility for initiating and supporting action to meet the health and social needs of the public.

Nurses and Coworkers
- The nurse sustains a cooperative relationship with coworkers in nursing and other fields.
- The nurse takes appropriate action to safeguard the individual when his care is endangered by a coworker or any other person.

Nurses and the Profession
- The nurse plays the major role in determining and implementing desirable standards of nursing practice and nursing education.
- The nurse is active in developing a core of professional knowledge.
- The nurse, acting through the professional organization, participates in establishing and maintaining equitable social and economic working conditions in nursing.

Adapted from The International Council of Nurses. (1973). *ICN Code for Nurses: Ethical Concepts Applied to Nursing.* Geneva: Imprimeries Populaires.

are representative of the standards of behavior expected of all nurses.

Patient Advocacy

Perhaps one of the most important ethical roles for the nurse is that of **patient advocate.** A patient advocate is an individual who speaks or acts on behalf of the patient. Gerontological nurses are the elderly person's strongest advocate. An informed nurse is aware of the hospitalized patient's rights and the rights of the resident of the nursing home.

Being an advocate involves informing the older person of his rights in the health care setting. Being an advocate may require intervening when inappropriate care is delivered. For example, suppose a practical nurse working in a nursing home observes a nursing assistant mistreat a resident by using abusive language. The practical nurse must intervene to correct this situation. To allow the nurse assistant to behave in this unethical manner is to fail as

the resident's advocate. It is important for the elderly to have an advocate to speak or act for them when there is illegal or unethical behavior or when inappropriate conduct occurs from another health care worker, friend, or family member.

Patients in hospitals and residents of nursing homes are viewed as consumers with certain rights. The rights of the health care consumer are outlined in numerous documents prepared by organizations such as the National League for Nursing, the American Hospital Association, and the American Nursing Home Association. See Appendix A for the Bill of Rights prepared by the American Hospital Association.

The Nursing Home Reform Law and many state laws contain specific provisions to protect the rights of nursing home residents. Display 4-3 lists the general rights of nursing home residents. When caring for patients in the hospital or in nursing homes, great consideration must be taken so that individual rights are not lost among the busy routines and tasks involved in the care.

> **DISPLAY 4-3. General Rights of Patients in Nursing Homes**
>
> - Be fully informed of all rules and regulations of the facility and of services and charges
> - See the state survey reports on the nursing home
> - Participate in planning their own care
> - Review medical records
> - Participate in activities of the community inside and outside the facility, have visitors, make and receive telephone calls, and share a room with a spouse
> - Vote
> - Participate in a resident council
> - Have privacy in caring for personal needs
> - Be treated with respect, consideration, and dignity
> - Present grievances without fear of reprisal
> - Manage their own financial affairs
> - Know their personal possessions are safe and secure
> - Remain in the facility as long as their needs can be met

LEGAL ASPECTS OF CARE

Nursing is also guided by legal parameters. The practice of nursing is regulated in each state through the individual state governments. States have nurse practice acts that establish boards of nursing with the authority to make and enforce administrative law. The laws are the rules and regulations for the practice of nursing in that particular state. Every nurse has a legal responsibility to be knowledgeable about the rules and regulations of the state in which he or she is practicing and to practice within the limitations of those rules. States have the power to grant a license to practice nursing to individuals meeting the minimum standards. Likewise, states have the power to remove a license if the nurse does not practice within the guidelines established by the nurse practice act of that state.

Negligence and Malpractice

Negligence is a legal term for performing an action that causes harm to another person or neglecting to perform an act that would have prevented harm. **Malpractice** is a form of negligence that implies failure to act as a "reasonably prudent nurse." The standard of care of any nurse must be comparable to that of a nurse who is reasonable and prudent. Care of a reasonable nurse implies that the care must be

rational, logical, and sensible. Prudent care suggests care that is wise, careful, and knowledgeable. The student nurse is held to the level of accountability of a "wise and prudent nurse."

A guiding principle in determining malpractice issues is a comparison of the type of care a nurse with a similar educational background would provide in a similar situation. If the standard of care is vastly different than the nurse's action, the behavior may be deemed inappropriate. When the standard of care is not met the nurse can be held liable for negligence. Examples of negligence include injury resulting from falls, burns to a patient, medication errors resulting in harm to a patient, and inappropriate management of feeding tubes.

Informed Consent

Before any care is given, the person must agree to the treatment or procedure. The person receives a full explanation of all the facts needed to make an intelligent and informed decision. Included in this explanation are the risks and benefits involved, any alternatives to the treatment, and what can be expected if the treatment is refused. All questions concerning risks, benefits, and alternatives must be answered to the person's satisfaction. Informed consent must be voluntarily obtained without any coercion.

Although it is the physician's responsibility to obtain informed consent, the task of having the consent form signed is often delegated to the nurse. If any questions of competency arise or if the person expresses any misgivings or concerns about the procedure, signing is delayed until these issues are resolved. Families and patients need to receive timely information concerning any treatment, even if consent has been obtained. Questions concerning treatment, the medication regimen, and care are answered to the satisfaction of the family and the patient.

The one signing the consent form must be mentally and physically competent. Determining mental and physical competence sometimes becomes a problem in obtaining consent from the elderly. Comatose persons and those with obvious cognitive loss, such as those in the later stages of Alzheimer's disease, are considered incapable of giving informed consent. However, there often are borderline cases for which establishing competence is difficult. Individuals who are unable to make competent decisions are represented by another individual who makes decisions in the incompetent person's best interest. This individual may be court appointed or designated by the individual before he or she became incompetent (see section on Medical Power of Attorney for Health Care).

Determining Competence

Making competent decisions requires the ability to express desires and understand information. Age alone cannot be the determining factor of establishing competency. Many 90-year-old or older individuals are capable of making intelligent decisions.

Competency issues are of particular interest to those working in nursing homes. These residents have the right to be involved in decisions about their care. Often, nurses and other staff are unsure about the competence of some residents to participate in decision making. There exists no consensus on the best method to determine a person's ability to make competent decisions. The capability to understand relevant information and the ability to communicate reasonable choices are two criteria often cited to determine competence. The person also must be able to evaluate various treatment options and understand the potential consequences of each of those options.

An important aspect of care that assists the nurse in determining competence is the development of a positive nurse-patient relationship. The patient must feel comfortable talking with the nurse and trust the nurse. Nurses working with the elderly document in the medical record any condition or occurrence that affects competence such as incidents of poor judgment, inability to participate in decision making, or disorientation.

Patient Self-Determination Act

In 1990, federal law established the Patient Self-Determination Act (PSD) under the Omnibus Budget Reconciliation Act (OBRA) of 1987. This federal law mandates the right of all individuals to be involved in making decisions concerning their medical care. The PSD act is intended to assist people in making decisions about their health care before they are faced with the trauma of life threatening situations. Under this law, the patient has the right to make medical decisions, including the right to refuse or accept treatment and to formulate advanced directives. This allows individuals to make treatment desires known and to prepare written advanced directives to protect the right to have their desires carried out. **Advanced directive** is a term that encompasses all documents that allow individuals to make decisions about their health care if they should become incapacitated (ie, mentally and physically unable to function). This includes medical directives (ie, living wills) and Medical Power of Attorney for Health Care. Standard forms for advanced directives are usually available at each institution.

This PSD Act affects any institution receiving Medicare or Medicaid funds. This act requires institutions to comply with the following stipulations:

Provide on admission written information that outlines the state laws concerning advanced directives including the right to accept or refuse treatment.

Document in the patient's record whether the patient received information about advanced directives and whether they have executed advanced directives. (Those who say yes are requested to provide a copy for their medical record.)

Educate the staff and community about state laws concerning advanced directives.

Keep up to date written policies about state laws concerning advanced directives.

This law affects all federally funded institutions such as hospitals, nursing homes, health maintenance organizations, and hospices in the United States. Laws about living wills and medical power of attorney vary from state to state. Each institution is required to become knowledgeable about their specific state law and to educate staff members of the important aspects of that law. Generally, an attorney is not needed to execute an advanced directive.

Choice in Dying is a national, not-for-profit organization dedicated to serving the needs of dying patients and their families. The organization pioneered the living will more than 30 years ago and has distributed more than 10 million living wills since that time. Information concerning each state law concerning advanced directives can be obtained from Choice in Dying, 1035 30th Street, Washington, D.C. 20007 (1-800-989-9455).

Medical Directive to Physician

In some states, the Natural Death Act allows a person to request the withholding or withdrawal of artificial measures to prolong life in the event of a terminal illness. This document is called a **Medical Directive to Physician** or living will. Although specific requirements vary from state to state, in general the Medical Directive to Physician addresses only the withholding or withdrawal of medical treatment that would artificially prolong life. This medical directive or living will becomes effective when the primary physician and one other doctor attest in writing that an individual is in a terminal or irreversible condition and that death will occur without the use of life-sustaining medical care. The physician has a responsibility to make a reasonable effort to transfer the responsibility for care to another physician if he or she chooses not to follow the directive. See Appendix B for an example of a Medical Directive to Physician.

Some states may require that the Medical Directive to Physician be notarized; others do not. In addition to the individual making the living will, two witnesses must sign the document. In general these witnesses cannot be

Related to the individual by blood or marriage

A beneficiary to any part of the individual's estate

The attending physician or an employee of the physician

An employee of the health care facility where the individual is a patient (in some states, members of the health care team can witness advanced directives)

A fellow patient in the health care facility (in some states, this is not the case)

Someone who has a claim against the person's estate

In some states, personal instructions can be added as part of the document under "Other Instructions." In this section, the individual may add specific instructions such as refusal of cardiopulmonary resuscitation, a respirator, artificial feeding, or antibiotics. Statements requesting that pain medication be used as necessary to provide comfort may also be added.

The directive can be revoked at any time by an oral statement indicating the desire to revoke the directive, signing a written revocation, or destroying the directive. The physician must be notified of the person's decision to revoke the directive.

Medical Power of Attorney for Health Care

A **Medical Power of Attorney for Health Care,** formerly called Durable Power of Attorney, is a type of advanced directive that allows an individual to appoint representatives and alternates to make health care decisions if he or she becomes incapacitated. The document affects only health care and should not be confused with granting power of attorney for other matters.

Although the Medical Directive to Physician becomes effective only when the person becomes terminally ill, the Medical Power of Attorney for Health Care becomes effective at any time the person becomes incapacitated. This means that conditions such as Alzheimer's disease, anesthesia, and unconsciousness all constitute situations in which the Medical Power of Attorney for Health Care becomes effective. This expansion of conditions allows control over more health care situations.

Selection of a **proxy** (ie, agent to make health care decisions) is an important decision. The proxy or agent may be a family member, close friend, an attorney, or anyone the individual trusts to make health care decisions. A second or third person may be named as alternates in case the first person selected is unavailable. The Medical Power of Attorney for Health Care, like the Medical Directive to Physician, must be signed in front of witnesses, usually two, who attest to the fact that the person is of sound mind and that the document was signed voluntarily. The proxy must have a clear understanding of the person's wishes concerning health care. Appendix C offers an example of a Medical Power of Attorney for Health Care.

Choice in Dying, a national organization that protects the rights of dying patients, recommends that no instructions be added to this document, because any instruction could limit the flexibility of the proxy to make decisions. This document, like the living will, can be revoked at any time and in the same manner.

Nursing Responsibility Concerning Advanced Directives

Nurses must be knowledgeable about state laws concerning Advanced Directives. Patients in hospitals and residents of nursing homes must be made aware of their right to direct their health care. Although written information is provided, patients or residents look to the nurse to answer questions, and the nurse must be prepared to answer. The topic of advanced directives is addressed when an individual enters a health care facility. Some people may misinterpret this topic and not wish to discuss the issue. They may feel that this topic is indicative of a poor prognosis. The nurse must be careful to ensure that all persons are asked the same questions and given similar information, regardless of their prognosis or medical condition.

For those wanting to prepare an advanced directive before entering a health care institution, the nurse or another individual can provide the necessary forms. For those already hospitalized or living in the nursing home, the nurse can refer them to the staff member designated to assist with advanced directives. The nurse encourages the person to decide what care is wanted in case of a permanent unconscious condition, terminal illness, or other serious condition. They should discuss with their proxy and alternates any and all information about health care desires such as the use of life-sustaining medical treatments (eg, cardiopulmonary resuscitation, intubation, intravenous lines). The proxy must agree to serve as the agent.

After the directive is completed, instruct the individual to place the original in a safe place, provide a copy for the medical record and give copies to family members, the agents, and the physician. The nurse is responsible to answer questions and provide information, not to give personal or legal advice about advanced directives.

Perhaps the most difficult decision with the elderly lies in deciding when the Medical Power of Attorney becomes effective. Nurses working with the elderly will assist in determining competence of the older adult. Careful assessment and documentation of the resident's orientation, judgment, behavior, decision-making ability, and functional ability can assist in determining competence.

When the elderly person is no longer capable of decision making, the proxy is called. The physician, family members, and the agent may be involved in the decision. Advanced directives must be honored. For any questions concerning the validity of the advanced directives, an attorney is consulted.

The nurse working in a nursing home may be responsible to educate the staff concerning advanced directives. This can be accomplished through in-service education sessions, employee orientation, or staff meetings. If the need arises and there is no advanced directive, the spouse or other family members may be asked to make decisions about the use of life-sustaining measures.

ARTIFICIAL NUTRITION AND HYDRATION

An important ethical and legal issue facing many families and health care providers is that of withholding or withdrawal of nutrition (food) and hydration (fluid) to terminally ill or irreversibly comatose individuals. Artificial nutrition is the administration of a chemically balanced mix of nutrients and fluid through a feeding tube such as a nasogastric tube (NGT), gastrostomy tube, percutaneous endoscopic gastrostomy (PEG), or jejunostomy tube. Many families and health care professionals feel compelled to continue the administration of artificial nutrition and hydration, even when the loved one has a terminal condition. Feelings about withholding food and fluids are emotionally charged and often have religious connotations. In our world of high technology and aggressive medicine, it is difficult for many to "do nothing."

Others feel that research has demonstrated that death occurs naturally and free of pain when patients receive no artificial hydration and nutrients. These individuals point out that feeding tubes can cause abdominal bloating, cramping, or diarrhea. Confused or agitated patients can pull on the tubing, causing it to dislodge. There is a danger of aspiration in patients receiving NGT feedings. If restraints are used to control the movements of the hands, agitation is increased. These individuals feel that feeding tubes can prolong the agony of dying and increase discomfort (see Appendix D).

The U.S. Supreme Court has upheld the right of patients to accept or reject the administration of artificial nutrition and hydration. Decisions to withhold food and fluids must be made by families and physicians unless the individual has made his or her wishes known through a Medical Directive to Physician or Medical Power of Attorney for Health Care. Regardless of personal feelings, nurses are responsible to provide the family with accurate, current information on this issue. When a decision is made, the nurse supports the patient and the family in their decision.

USE OF RESTRAINING DEVICES

According to OBRA, a resident in a nursing home has the right to be free from restraints not needed to treat a medical condition. To use restraints for any medical condition, the resident or the family must give consent before restraints are used. There are two types of restraints. **Physical restraints** restrict a person's movement in some way. **Chemical restraints** are drugs used to control behaviors that should be managed in other ways. The use of restraints requires adherence to certain criteria, and there are several acceptable uses of restraints:

- To ensure the physical safety of the resident or other residents
- Only on the specific written order of a physician, which must include the duration and circumstances in which restraints can be used
- In emergency situations until a physician's order can reasonably be obtained

Research indicates that restraining agitated, confused, or combative residents tends to increase behavior problems rather than calm and soothe the residents. Restraints can result in fractures, concussions, contusions, and bruises. Display 4-4 offers a more complete listing of potential harm caused by the use of physical restraints. Studies demonstrate that falls occurring in unrestrained residents result in less serious injuries than in those who are

DISPLAY 4-4. Potential Harm Caused by Physical Restraints

Decreased appetite
Malnutrition
Dehydration
Pneumonia
Urinary tract infection
Constipation
Incontinence
Decreased bone strength
Decreased muscle strength
Contracted muscles
Bruising, cuts, or redness of skin
Pressure sores
Fall-related injuries
Death by asphyxiation

From National Citizens' Coalition for Nursing Home Reform. (1993). *Avoiding Physical Restraint Use: New Standards in Care.* Washington, DC: 15.

restrained. Display 4-5 identifies some suggestions useful in minimizing the need for chemical or physical restraints.

Physical Restraints

The OBRA interpretive guidelines for nursing homes define physical restraints as "any manual method of physical or mechanical device, material or equipment attached or adjacent to the resident's body that the resident cannot remove easily which restricts free movement or normal access to one's body." Examples of physical restraints include arm and leg restraints, soft ties or vests, hand mitts, and lap trays or cushions that the resident cannot move.

Other devices that may qualify as restraints include wheelchairs, bed rails, or sheets. An example of using a wheelchair as a restraint is when the safety bars are used to prevent a resident from getting out of a chair. Tying sheets to the back of a wheelchair to prevent the resident from rising out of the chair is also considered a restraint. The use of physical restraints often leads to the use of chemical restraints, because physical restraints are likely to increase agitation, combativeness, and confusion.

Chemical Restraints

Chemical restraints are drugs, particularly psychotherapeutic drugs, that are used to control behavior or for discipline or convenience and that are not required to treat a medical problem. Any of the psychotherapeutic drugs, such as the antipsychotic drugs, sedatives, hypnotics, antianxiety drugs, or antidepressants, can be used inappropriately to treat behavior symptoms. Side effects of these drugs increase the older person's risk of falling, developing pressure sores, and becoming confused. Psychotherapeutic drugs should only be used when ordered by the physician as a part of the individualized written care plan to treat a medical problem (see Chapter 13).

Behavior Symptoms

Older adults with dementia cannot adequately express themselves verbally and nonverbally. **Behavioral symptoms** are behaviors used by those with certain medical conditions, such as dementia (ie, loss of cognitive function) or psychiatric diseases (eg, schizophrenia, bipolar disorder, depression) to express feelings of discomfort or distress that they cannot otherwise communicate. Display 4-6 identifies behavior symptoms that may indicate an older person is in distress. Behavioral symptoms should alert the nurse that something is wrong. Any of these behaviors require investigation by the nurse to determine what type of distress the patient is communicating with the behavior. Display 4-5 offers interventions that help manage behavioral problems without the use of restraints.

Certain conditions increase the chance that behavioral symptoms will develop. Risk factors for the development of behavioral symptoms include infection, acute or chronic illness, stress, adverse reactions to medications, and unmet physiologic needs (eg, food, fluid, comfort, sleep, elimination).

The nurse determines whether the resident has experienced one or more of the risk factors. If risk factors are identified, the nurse plans interventions that address the risk factor. For example, if the resident has an unmet physiologic need such as constipation (ie, need for elimination of body wastes), the discomfort from the constipation may be causing the behavioral symptom. Interventions to relieve the constipation, such as increasing fluids, increasing exercise, or administering a stool softener are planned. These interventions can alleviate the constipation, meeting the patient's physical need and decreasing the behavioral symptom.

Managing Behavior Symptoms

Managing behavioral problems can be a challenge for the nursing personnel. Assessment of the resident and the environment for clues to the cause of the behavior is important before successful interventions

DISPLAY 4-5. Restraint Alternatives for Common Challenges

Reasons people are typically restrained can be identified in terms of four problematic behaviors: unsafe mobility/postural instability; wandering; agitated, confused, and/or disruptive behavior; and interference with life support measures.

A successful restraint reduction program requires total staff support and an interdisciplinary team approach. The resident's capabilities, rather than deficits, are the focus of the care plan and treatment interventions.

Promote Resident's Function

• Identify reasons for the resident's unsteadiness, need to get up, poor trunk control, or other problems (eg, what medication is this person on; how much exercise has the individual been getting; is the individual hungry or thirsty; has the person been sitting too long; is the individual experiencing pain; does the resident need to go to the bathroom?).
• Eliminate medications or combinations of medications whose side effects distort resident's balance, perceptions, and/or cognitive function.
• Increase ambulation skills by giving resident opportunities to exercise (eg, walking to and from meals or activities, developing formal exercise groups).
• Be sure resident wears comfortable, well-fitting shoes or sneakers and has appropriate foot and nail care.
• Provide supportive devices to maximize function (eg, transfer disk, modified walkers, grab-safety bars in bathroom, elevated toilet seat, nonslip floors).
• Address resident's vision and hearing impairments.

Minimize Likelihood of Resident's Need to Get Up Unaided

• Be familiar with the resident's lifelong roles and habits to anticipate personal needs and interests, such as when he or she usually goes to the bathroom, preferred snack times, or leisure activities.
• Provide the resident with meaningful activity such as listening to music, assisting staff with simple tasks, or executing a repetitive task that satisfies a personal need.
• Offer resident adequate stimulation such as reading materials, talking books, or an activities cart placed strategically on each unit.
• Vary the locations where an individual sits. Sometimes, quiet areas are appreciated, but residents often want to be "where the action is."
• Explore possible alerting strategies or devices (eg, attach call bell to resident's garment or use of portable battery-operated alarms that monitor the individual's movements).

Customize Seating for Individual Postural Needs

• Provide flexion at hips and knees and lateral support with wedge cushions, positioning pillows, and/or deep inclined seats to minimize slumping, falling to the side, or sliding out of chair.

• Ensure that the most comfortable seating is available and that the resident is not expected to sit for prolonged periods. Offer a variety of sitting arrangements, such as Lay-Z-Boys, Barc-a-loungers, rockers, deep-seated and high-backed chairs, or soft comfortable wing chairs.
• Prevent tipping of wheelchairs with anti-tipping devices that are commercially available.
• Wheelchairs are for transportation only. If a resident is unable to propel the wheelchair independently, he or she should be seated in it solely for transportation purposes.

Ensure a Safe Environment for the Resident

• Monitor environment for safety hazards.
• Modify environment with optimal lighting in resident's room and bathroom, appropriately placed safety bars, removal of wheels from overbed table and other furniture (the resident may lean on for support).
• Keep beds as low to the floor as possible. Low beds are commercially available.
• Use one-half or three-quarter siderails on bed to prevent the resident from climbing over rails or footboards to get out of bed. It may be necessary to pad floor area for resident at risk of falling.
• Put the mattress directly on the floor and make the bed for a temporary period during crisis situation.

Make the Environment as Homelike as Possible

• Allow resident to surround self with personal furniture and possessions. This helps in recognition of one's room and provides a comfortable, secure haven in an often strange environment.
• Allow nursing staff to wear ordinary clothing rather than uniforms.
• Eliminate or reduce the use of a public address system. Voices coming over these systems are stressful and confusing for frail residents.

Decrease the Risks Associated with Residents Wandering

• Provide opportunities for the resident to have a sense of purpose.
• Schedule activities that are consistent with the resident's interest and cognitive ability.
• Offer opportunities for the resident to phone, listen to tapes or view videos of persons he or she wants to find.
• Provide companionship and one-on-one attention. Identify the emotional needs the resident is trying to meet by wandering. Listen to and validate the resident's feelings.
• Enlist *all* staff to do their part in keeping track of a wandering resident. **It is not just a nursing responsibility.** Make it a shared responsibility of all departments by assigning one staff member to supervise a wanderer for short periods.
• Provide comfortable rocking chairs to offer relaxation and satisfy the need for constant motion.

Continued

DISPLAY 4-5. CONTINUED

- Give the resident opportunities to exercise.
- Modify the environment to discourage people from wandering into inappropriate areas and/or exiting the facility:

    Create a grid with masking tape on the floor in front of a doorway.

    Put a mirror on the door.

    Camouflage the door with wallpaper or a window treatment.

    Install an alarm system.

    Attach an 18-inch wide barrier strip across the doorway with Velcro.

    Put a dark mat or felt circle on the floor in front of doors.

    Place a stop sign on the door.

Accept the Fact that Restless, Anxious Residents Must be Allowed to Walk When Able

- Make the environment as safe as possible, and allow them freedom to wander.
- Place a resident's name and picture on door of his or her room (preferably a photo taken 20 to 30 years earlier).
- Learn the resident's daily routines and patterns of movement. Provide an activity that makes use of the wandering "agenda behavior." For example, allow the resident to assist the staff in simple tasks such as folding napkins, setting the table, decorating a bulletin board, sorting papers, dusting, or pushing a laundry cart.
- Install a curtained, swinging cafe door with a buzzer on the entrance of the resident's room. (serves to alert staff of resident's movement, especially at night).
- Provide a safe, enclosed area outside with a walking path and shaded benches for rest stops.

Educate Staff in Techniques for Managing Agitated or Disruptive Behavior

- Use a calm approach when addressing the resident. Be gentle and consistent.
- Increase communication with the resident.
- Seek underlying causes for behavior (ask the person what is the matter; check medications; is individual experiencing discomfort?).
- Be familiar with the clinical stages of dementia to ensure that activity programs are appropriate for each resident's cognitive ability.

- Engage the resident in structured activity—provide meaningful activity throughout the day such as occupational therapy, physical therapy, recreation, or special sessions for special needs.
- Have the resident listen to relaxation tapes.
- Respect the resident's need for personal space. "Back off" from the resident who is acting in an aggressive manner until he or she feels calmer.
- Provide for a consistent caregiver to ensure continuity of care. This can decrease the likelihood of agitated behavior and increase sensitivity to the individual's needs.

Reevaluate Life Support Measures

- Consider wisdom and ethics of an approach.
- Encourage residents to make a Living Will or Durable Power of Attorney for Health Care while they are competent.
- Explore with physicians about the resident's right to dignity, comfort, and autonomy.
- Discuss resident's rights with family members. Talk about what the resident wants.
- Evaluate the need for a feeding tube; consider alternatives such as oral hydration.
- Evaluate the need for urinary catheters; allow incontinence or attempt a rigorous bladder training program.
- Remove tubes that appear to be causing the resident major distress.
- Consider insertion of tube directly into stomach instead of nasogastric tubes.
- Cover intravenous tubing with long sleeves.
- Disguise a gastrostomy tube with flextone binders over the abdomen.
- Fit a stockinette over a small Nerf ball held in the hand or to prevent resident from pulling a nasogastric tube as a ***temporary*** measure.

Nurture a Positive Staff-Resident-Family Relationship

- Provide primary nursing care and avoid rotation of caregivers.
- Maintain communications with family members. Family input is invaluable in understanding resident behavior and developing appropriate care plans.
- Understand each resident as an individual with personal needs and desires. Care plans must be individualized and flexible to meet the ever-changing status of the resident.

Used and adapted with permission from *Untie the Elderly*, The Kendal Corporation, Kennet Square, PA, 1991.

can be planned. Clues can be subtle and difficult to identify. The clues may be related to habits, practices, or lifestyles of the past. For example, Mr. Jones was wandering in and out of the other residents' rooms for several hours each morning. After talking with his family, the nurse discovered that he was a mailman for 30 years. The staff provided a path for the resident to walk, keeping him out of other residents' rooms. This solution was helpful in promoting Mr. Jones' strength through walking. A picture of Mr. Jones was placed on the door of his room to provide a cue to help him identify his room. A safe and more controlled walking regimen resulted, and other residents were not disturbed.

DISPLAY 4-6. Behavior Symptoms of Older Adults

Agitation
Anger
Continuous wandering
Crying
Decreased appetite
Delusions
Fears (eg, bathing)
Hitting
Pacing
Repetitive actions
Sadness
Screaming
Spitting
Swearing
Undressing

Consider the cause of the behavioral symptom by observing for a pattern. For example, ask what is happening before, during, and after the symptom. Who is present, and what time of the day does the behavior occur? Treat the suspected cause with nursing interventions before requesting psychotropic drugs. Use medication only when all other methods fail.

An evaluation of the resident's medication regimen may provide clues to the occurrence of behavioral symptoms. Psychotropic drugs such as tranquilizers, antidepressants, and antipsychotics may increase behavior symptoms. Dosages of these medications should be the lowest dose that produces the desired effect.

When and How to Use Restraints

Short-term use of restraints in emergency situations may be beneficial. Before restraining, the hospital or nursing home must identify a specific medical condition that necessitates the use of restraints. Restraints should assist the resident to reach maximal physical and emotional potential. For maintaining proper body alignment, devices such as pillows, pads, or lap trays may be used in lieu of restraints. Display 4-7 identifies interventions used when restraining devices are necessary.

Situations that may warrant the use of restraints include situations such as a resident with a hip fracture who will not stay in bed, a severely dehydrated resident who is pulling out the intravenous line, or a delirious resident so that a physician can perform an examination to determine the cause of the delirium.

Hospitalized patients are restrained for the same reasons as older adults are restrained in the nursing

DISPLAY 4-7. Interventions to Use When Restraining Devices are Necessary

- Use the least restrictive device possible (eg, use a vest restraint or mitten restraints rather than wrist restraints).
- Check restrained limbs or body parts every 30 minutes to 1 hour. Remove them from the restraint and provide range of motion for the extremity.
- Assess for the presence of pain from the restraint, any interference with circulation, or abrasions on the skin. Use padding if necessary.
- Provide an opportunity to participate in activities and socialization.
- Assess for basic needs (eg, toileting, thirst, hunger) at least every 2 hours.
- Document the assessment and any actions or interventions used.
- Remove restraints as soon as the emergency is over.
- Make sure that there is a written order from the physician that specifies the duration and the circumstances under which the restraints are to be used. The only exceptions are restraints used in emergency situations until a physician's order can be obtained.

home. Comparable guidelines concerning when to restrain and how to manage patients or residents when they are restrained apply regardless of the health care setting.

CRITICAL THINKING EXERCISES

1. Carefully examine the code for nurses. Give examples of how each ethical standard of behavior would apply to you. Are there any of the standards that you would not be able to follow?
2. Ms. Jefferys, 69 years old, is interested in making an advanced directive for health care. She tells you that several of her friends have advanced directives and that she feels that she should make plans for her health care. However, Ms. Jefferys states that she does not understand what an advanced directive is and what options she has when making one. Develop a teaching plan to help Ms. Jefferys understand this very important topic.
3. Plan an in-service education session that addresses the topic of the appropriate and inappropriate use of chemical restraints.

4. Develop two specific scenarios that would necessitate the use of restraints. Explain the rationale for the restraint. Describe exactly what type of restraint would be necessary.

5. Mr. Stovall has been in the nursing home for 2 months. His daughter tells you that he is missing two pairs of pants, three shirts, and some personal belongings. The nursing assistant had previously told the daughter that she would "just have to get used to it because that's how things are in the nursing home." How would you deal with this situation?

REFERENCES AND SUGGESTED READING

Blatt, L. (1999). Working with families in reaching end-of-life decisions. *Clinical Nurse Specialist, 13 (5)*, 36.

Burger, S., Fraser, V., Hunt, S., & Frank, B. (1996). *Nursing Homes: Getting Good Care There.* San Luis Obispo, CA: American Source Books.

Chichin, E., Burack, O., Olsen, E., & Likourezos, A. (2000). *End-of-Life Ethics and the Nursing Assistant.* New York: Springer Publishing.

DePalma, J. (1998). Communication between facilities affects continuity of advanced directives. *American Journal of Nursing, 98 (8)*, 46.

Department of Health and Human Services. Health Care Financing Administration. (1995). Medicare and Medicaid programs: Advanced directives. Final rule. *Federal Register*, 33262–33298.

Duffield, P. (1998). Advanced directives in primary care. *American Journal of Nursing, 98 (4)*, 16.

Haynor, P. (1998). Meeting the challenge of advanced directives. *American Journal of Nursing, 98 (3)*, 26.

Jansson, L., Norberg, A., Sandman. P., & Astrom, G. (1995). When the severely ill elderly patient refuses food: Ethical reasoning among nurses. *International Journal of Nursing Studies, 32 (1)*, 68–78.

Jenson, B., Hess-Zak, A., Johnston, S., Otto, D., Tebbe, L., Russel, C., & Sheffeld-Waller, A. (1998). Restraint reduction. *Journal of Nursing Administration, 28 (7)*, 32.

RESOURCES ON THE WORLD WIDE WEB

http://www.rights.org/deathnet/lwc.html
(living will center)

http://www.choices
(information on living wills and advanced directives)

CHAPTER **5**

Communicating With the Older Adult

CHAPTER OUTLINE

KEY TERMS
CHAPTER OBJECTIVES
THE COMMUNICATION PROCESS
TYPES OF COMMUNICATION
LIMITATIONS TO COMMUNICATION
THERAPEUTIC COMMUNICATION TECHNIQUES
ANGER
DEVELOPING AND MAINTAINING A THERAPEUTIC
    RELATIONSHIP
PHASES OF THE NURSE-PATIENT RELATIONSHIP
COMMUNICATING EFFECTIVELY WITH THE OLDER
    ADULT
CRITICAL THINKING QUESTIONS
REFERENCES AND SUGGESTED READING

KEY TERMS

active listening
communication
empathy
feedback
genuineness
message
nonverbal communication
receiver
sender
therapeutic nurse-patient relationship
verbal communication

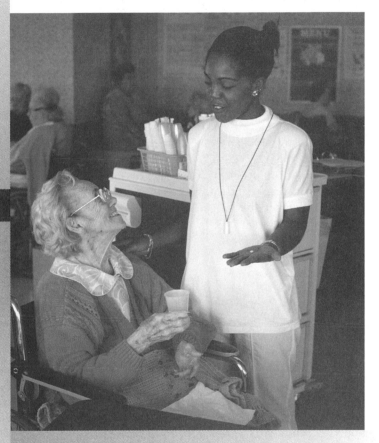

CHAPTER OBJECTIVES

At the completion of this chapter, the student will
be able to

- Discuss the communication process

- Describe various types of nonverbal
  communication

- Identify limitations to communication

- Use therapeutic communication techniques
  when working with older adults

- Discuss important aspects in developing and
  maintaining the therapeutic nurse-patient
  relationship

Communication is in many ways the very core of nursing. It is the foundation on which a helping or therapeutic relationship is established and the medium by which the nursing process is achieved. All phases of the nursing process, including assessment, planning, implementation, and evaluation, require good communication skills. Communication in nursing is not simply talking to a patient, but rather using words, behaviors, gestures, and body language to convey to the patient that the nurse truly cares. All nurses must strive to learn the basic communication skills necessary to develop a therapeutic relationship and to communicate a caring attitude.

THE COMMUNICATION PROCESS

Communication is a two-way process involving sending and receiving messages. Actions, feelings, behavior, and words are all involved in the communication process. Figure 5-1 shows a model of the communication process. The basic components of communication include the sender, message, receiver, and feedback.

Sender

The **sender** is the communicator (ie, one conveying the message). The sender has the responsibility to convey actions, words, and feelings that are congruent (ie, give the same message). Without congruent messages, the receiver is unsure of the message. For example, if you are using words to indicate you are pleased with a situation, be certain that your facial expression and body language convey the same message. The sender uses mental images and nonverbal feelings to influence the way the message is communicated.

Message

The **message** is the information conveyed by the sender. The receiver changes the message back into feelings and mental images. A clear message expressed in terms familiar to the receiver has the best chance of being understood correctly.

Receiver

The **receiver** is the individual who listens and interprets the message. The clearer the message, the easier the message is to understand. The receiver's interpretation is influenced by the mental images, thoughts, and feelings contributed by the environment. For example, telling an older widow with a fractured hip that nursing home care is essential may cause mental images of loneliness, fear, and abandonment for the widow with many friends in the apartment complex where she lives. To the nurse, the same message may bring mental images of an efficient, well-organized health care facility that can facilitate the patient's recovery. Verbal and nonverbal clues are given by the elderly widow that an astute nurse can identify to clarify the message and alleviate the older woman's anxiety.

Feedback

Feedback is the mechanism by which the receiver in some way communicates the message back to the sender. Feedback enables the sender to determine whether the message was correctly interpreted. Simply having the receiver restate the message is a type of feedback. The sender may also ask questions that allows the sender to clarify any misunderstandings concerning the intended message. When the mental image and the feelings of the sender and the receiver match, true communication has occurred. When this does not occur, the meaning of the message is muted or inaccurate.

Two-Way Communication

Most communication is a two-way process. Two-way communication is a dynamic process in which the exchange or ideas and thoughts occurs as a continuous, ongoing process. This type of communication demands that the receiver give feedback and become actively involved in communication. By having the receiver actively involved in the process, the sender can determine the receiver's understanding of the message. If the message was not understood, the sender has the opportunity to clarify the message.

One-Way Communication

One-way communication allows the sender to remain in control of the situation. In one-way communication, the receiver remains passive. This type of communication is not the most effective type of communication and is usually not the preferred method of communication. One-way communication can be effective when used to announce that visiting hours are over or to give a patient report to a group of nurses.

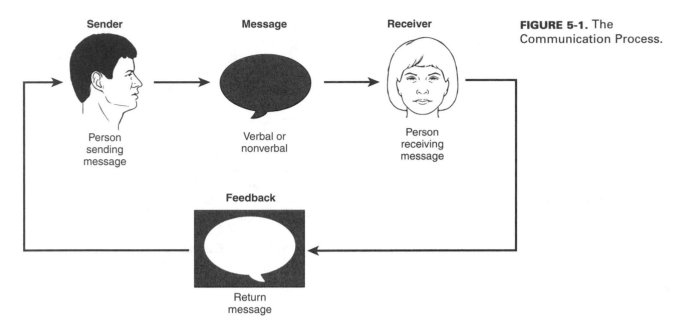

FIGURE 5-1. The Communication Process.

Sender — Person sending message

Message — Verbal or nonverbal

Receiver — Person receiving message

Feedback — Return message

Sometimes, one-way communication is used when the nurse is too busy to interact with the patient. Giving commands to the patient without allowing feedback is one-way communication. For example, suppose an elderly nursing home resident is sitting in the recreation room in a wheelchair. As a busy nursing assistant walks by, he anxiously calls out for the nursing assistant to take him back to his room. Without asking why he wants to go back to his room, the nursing assistant says "Oh Mr. Tankersley, you know the doctor wants you to stay up for most the morning." Mr. Tankersley slumps back in his chair, waiting for someone else to come by. Within 10 minutes, Mr. Tankersley, who wanted to go to his room to use the bathroom, has a large puddle of urine under his wheelchair. This situation would never have happened had the nursing assistant taken the time to have more than a one-way conversation with Mr. Tankersley.

Unclear Messages

Ideally, the message sent by the sender is the one received by the receiver. When this occurs, communication is said to be effective. Unfortunately, messages can become clouded by factors such as emotions (ie, fear or anxiety), pain, various knowledge levels, and differences in culture or language. Environmental factors such as excessive warmth or coldness can also influence sending or receiving a message. Nurses must assess the patient to identify any areas that may disrupt communication. For example, an elderly person in pain may not be able to communicate an accurate history of the illness until the pain is relieved. An elderly person who reluc-

tantly allows himself to be admitted to a nursing home may not, at least initially, fully communicate with the nursing home staff. Memory impairment can complicate communication as well. Depression, unhappiness, or anger are emotions that disrupt communication. The sender, the receiver, or both can be the cause of an unclear message.

TYPES OF COMMUNICATION

The two types of communication are verbal and nonverbal. Approximately 10% of all communication is verbal, and 90% is nonverbal. The tremendous influence of nonverbal communication is astonishing and places a tremendous responsibility on the nurse to pay close attention to the patient's nonverbal behavior as well as the nonverbal communication by the nurse. Remember, communication is a two-way process!

Verbal Communication

Verbal communication is the use of words to convey messages. Words are used to express thoughts, feelings, attitudes, and beliefs. Words bring mental images to mind. The nurse must not assume that these mental images are the same for every patient or even every nurse. Different backgrounds, experiences, and cultures influence the images that each person envisions when hearing words. This is particularly true with the elderly because they are of a different generation than a young nurse or nursing assistant. Words may bring about unlike images in the elderly and younger adults.

To ascertain the meaning of verbal communication as intended by the sender, feedback is essential. The nurse can have the older person repeat in his own words what was said or ask questions that would indicate understanding. Another way to obtain feedback is to explore thoughts of the older adult and ask for a more detailed explanation.

Nonverbal Communication

Some authorities believe that nonverbal communication is the most accurate form of communication. **Nonverbal communication** is communication without the use of words. People communicate nonverbally by their facial expressions, eye contact, gestures, and body language. Nonverbal behavior reveals feelings and attitudes without using words that may contradict or confirm verbal communication. The person's innermost feelings cannot be separated from the communication process.

Facial Expression
Facial expression is one of the most important aspects of nonverbal communication. The mouth, eyebrows, eyes, and mouth are all capable of providing nonverbal cues. Older adults often look for signs of approval and understanding in a nurse's face. Many older adults have a hearing impairment and the facial expression of the nurse may be the most significant form of communication. A sign of interest in what is being said comes when the nurse sits leaning forward with the eyes wide open and head tilted forward. Smiling and nodding the head conveys a positive message to the older adult and helps to boost self-esteem. Raising one eyebrow often indicates skepticism or a question. It is important to validate facial expressions because they can sometimes be misinterpreted. For example, a grimace may be interrupted as a way to brush off the nurse trying to feed a patient, although the grimace occurred because the patient was experiencing pain. Exploring the meaning of the grimace by asking "Is something troubling you, Ms. Walker?" allows the patient to provide the nurse with more information on current thoughts and feelings of the patient.

Eye Contact
Maintaining eye contact is necessary when communicating with older adults. It conveys the nonverbal message of being interested in what the older adult is saying. Many older adults complain that no one listens to them. Having eye contact

helps convey to the older adult that you are interested in what is being said.

The eyes also convey fear, anger, or embarrassment. Regardless of the culture, eye contact conveys a message. It is important for the nurse to know what culture the older adult is a part of so the appropriate nonverbal message from the eyes can be identified. In some cultures, such as the Native American and Asian cultures, eye contact is considered inappropriate and rude. In other cultures, a lack of eye contact is considered a sign of dishonesty or disrespect. Maintaining eye contact for several seconds at a time conveys interest, respect, and attentiveness in Western cultures.

Gestures and Body Language
Hand gestures convey meaning. Pointing a finger, the thumbs-up sign, and a handshake are used as nonverbal communication. Body language is movement by a body that convey messages. Folding the arms together across the chest convey a message of sternness or a closed mind. Quick jerky movements often indicate nervousness. Directly facing the individual when one is talking to indicates interest. Sitting when interviewing the older adult puts the person at ease and indicates that time is to be spent with the older adult. Standing in a position where the nurse is looking down on the older adult gives the nurse an air of authority and places the patient in a dependent and powerless position.

The physical position of two individuals is important. In general, the space between two individuals communicates the degree of emotional intimacy between them. Most individuals have a "personal space" of 12 to 18 inches. When this area is encroached on, the person feels uncomfortable or threatened. If this occurs, the individual immediately moves back several feet or moves a safe distance to the side, establishing a personal space in which he feels comfortable. Maintaining a personal distance of approximately 2 to 3 feet allows comfortable speech and is less threatening to the older adult. Display 5-1 gives some guidelines for use of body language, eye contact, and gestures when communicating with the older adult.

Silence
Silence can be used as a powerful nonverbal communicating method. Silence at appropriate times allows the other person time to think about a reply or collect their thoughts. When silence continues too long, the individual may become distracted or anxious. If distraction or anxiety occurs, help the individual overcome this anxiety by speaking.

Sometimes the nurse may come into the patient's room and offer support through physical presence and silence. If silence is used as a therapeutic tech-

DISPLAY 5-1. Guidelines to Enhance Nonverbal Communication

- Avoid crossing the arms and legs when communicating because these postures are associated with a closed mind.
- Sit with knees and feet slightly apart with the hands not touching the body.
- Lean slightly forward, and maintain frequent eye contact.
- Assume a position similar to that of the other person.
- Smile frequently.
- Do not invade the person's personal space. Maintain a distance of 2 to 3 feet.
- Nod frequently to encourage continued communication.
- Use facial expressions, gestures, and body postures that are congruent with the desired message.

nique, limit the periods of silence to no more than 5 minutes. Tell the older adult, "I will just sit here with you quietly for a few minutes." This type of silence conveys caring and unconditional acceptance.

Nurses who are afraid of silence often talk excessively or engage in work to appear too busy to be quiet and still. Nurses can learn to be comfortable with periods of silence to allow silence to have a positive effect on the patient.

Deciphering the Meaning of Nonverbal Behavior

Deciphering the meaning of nonverbal behavior is not always easy. Care must be take not to jump to conclusions with nonverbal behavior. Nonverbal behaviors are clues that need validation and investigation to determine the exact message that the individual's behavior is communicating. Giving the older adult the opportunity to express feelings, anxiety, and concerns provides the nurse with the opportunity to explore the meaning of nonverbal behaviors. Active listening (discussed in the next section) is an important skill for the nurse who is seeking to interpret the meaning of nonverbal and verbal communication. All behavior has meaning, particularly nonverbal behavior. When nurses learn to really listen to the older adult and delve below the surface, meaningful communication can occur.

Active Listening

Listening is perhaps the most important element of communication for the nurse. Many older adults believe that "no one listens" to them. Unfortunately, that belief has some merit. How many times has an older adult been seen trying to communicate, only to have a younger person brush them off or ignore them? The feeling that no one listens is one reason that the older adult is reluctant to talk or responds inappropriately to the nurse. Past experiences have taught them not to trust.

Active listening is a form of therapeutic listening in which the nurse pays close attention to verbal and nonverbal communication with the goal of truly understanding the message the patient is trying to convey. The nurse uses clarifying techniques to determine if the message was fully understood. Sentences with phrases such as "I think I understand you to say . . ." or with "is that what you are saying" help to clarify the message.

The art of active listening must be developed. It is easy when someone is talking to allow the mind to wander, to think of a clever response, or to jump to erroneous conclusions. The mind works faster than an individual speaks, making it possible to think a variety of thoughts during one short conversation with an older adult. Avoid the temptation to let the mind wander; give your full attention to the message that the older adult is attempting to communicate. Use your knowledge of nonverbal communication, such as eye contact and facial expressions, to help get the full meaning of the message. The process of listening to the message includes the interpreting of feelings of the patient and the body language used. The goal of active listening is to understand the message from the patient's frame of reference and to be able to understand the thoughts, feelings, and ideas of the patient.

For example, Ms. Chambers, an elderly woman who is recovering from a stroke that has left her with left sided hemiparesis has been cared for by the same nurse for the past 3 days. John is the nurse caring for Ms. Chambers. One afternoon, while John helped Ms. Chambers up to a chair, she began to open up to him by saying, "You know I used to paint beautiful pictures with this old limp hand of mine." John quickly responded with "Oh, yes, you'll soon be back to normal again, painting up a storm. Don't fret over that right now." Ms. Chambers looked down at her limp hand resting in her lap and did not respond to John's comments. She never discussed her feelings with John again. John did not really listen to Ms. Chambers. He heard her words but did not respond to her gestures and nonverbal clues. His response blocked any further discussion of feelings and fears. Ms. Chambers needed a nurse who would actively listen to her thoughts, feelings, and fears of never being able to use her left hand again.

The nurse must work to improve active listening skills. Display 5-2 offers suggestions to improve active listening skills.

- Forget self and really concentrate on what the patient is saying
- Give your full attention to what the patient is saying
- Be interested and concerned
- Allow the conversation to flow naturally (do not rush the conversation)
- Maintain eye contact
- Use appropriate facial expressions and gestures (eg, nod to indicate you are paying attention)
- Observe for nonverbal behaviors
- Avoid the pretence of listening
- Think before responding

LIMITATIONS TO COMMUNICATION

Certain types of communication do not encourage openness or expression of feelings but rather limits good communication among the nurse, the patient, and family members. By learning these limitations, nurses can avoid their use and substitute techniques that encourage openness and the development of trust between the nurse and the patient.

Limitations to Good Communication

Inappropriate reassurances
Making judgments
Giving advice
Challenging
Belittling or scolding
Patronizing
Changing the subject
Improper questioning
Defending

Inappropriate Reassurance

Words that are spoken to reassure the patient do very little to make the patient feel better. They are usually more reassuring to the nurse than the patient. For example, a daughter says of her elderly mother, "I am afraid for my mother. She is so confused. I think that she may have Alzheimer's disease." The nurse replies, "Oh, don't worry; your mother is probably going through a difficult period. She will snap out of it soon." This type of false reassurance disassociates the nurse from having to deal with the daughter's fears and trivializes the specific feelings of the other individual. Any further discussion is stifled.

On the surface, statements such as "things could be worse" or "at least it's not . . ." seem reassuring, but they are not. They belittle the individual's feelings and can cause resentment, frustration, and guilt. The nurse must remember that all people have unique feelings and fears. The nurse must never be guilty of trivializing or belittling an older person's feelings.

Making Judgments

Nurses have the responsibility of accepting each individual patient and appreciating his uniqueness. When judgments are made, the nurse labels the patient or the patient's actions as good or bad. Making judgments includes giving approval ("That's good"), disapproval ("That's bad" or "I don't think you should"), or agreeing or disagreeing. Making judgments can make the patient defensive and implies rejection if the person does not agree with the nurse. When the person is accepted unconditionally, the patient is free to grow emotionally.

Giving Advice

Giving advice or telling the person what to do should be avoided. Statements that begin "I don't think you should . . ." or "If you want my opinion . . ." discourage independent thinking. Older adults should be encouraged to think for themselves and make decisions involving their own care.

Challenging

Challenging or demanding proof from an elderly patient is never appropriate. Elderly patients are sometimes easily confused or may have illogical thoughts. They may require validation of feelings rather than validation of the facts (see Chapters 8 and 17). For example, saying to an elderly person who is crying to go see her mother, "Mrs. James, don't you remember? Your mother has been dead 20 years. How can you see her?" is challenging her words. Although it may be true, trying to convince Mrs. James with challenging words can hinder further communication. It is better for the nurse to validate her feelings by saying, "Mrs. James, do you miss your mother?"

Belittling or Scolding

Nurses have been overheard belittling or scolding older adults. The elderly are often vulnerable, particularly the frail elderly, and nurses sometimes inappropriately use scolding or belittling to manipulate older adults. For example, saying "Oh, come on, Mr. Taylor; lots of older people break their hip, and they aren't afraid to walk" to an older adult who is reluctant to walk after a hip fracture is a form of belittling. Belittling humiliates and embarrasses the older adult. A more appropriate response to this situation would be to say, "You're finding it difficult to try to walk. Would you like to talk about it?"

Changing the Subject

Changing the subject under discussion by a nurse or a patient indicates that the topic is in some way anxiety provoking. The person who changes the subject is seeking a safer, more comfortable topic. Nurses must be aware of these situations. Dealing first with

> **TIPS FOR COMMUNICATING WITH THE OLDER ADULT**
>
> Example of the nurse changing the subject:
> Older adult: "I would rather die than spend the rest of my life in a nursing home."
> Nurse: "Where is your grocery list for shopping?"

the anxiety allows discussion of the topic to proceed with less anxiety.

If the nurse would take the same time to explore the older adult's feelings, the topic could be explored. The nurse could appropriately ask, "Tell me what you fear most about living in a nursing home."

Improper Questioning

When questioning older adults, avoid questions that require a "yes" or "no" answer. These types of questions prohibit open expression of feelings. For communication to be effective, questioning should be phrased to encourage verbalization of thoughts and feelings.

> **TIPS FOR COMMUNICATING WITH THE OLDER ADULT**
>
> Example of improper questioning:
> Nurse: "Did you eat your lunch today?"
> Nursing home patient: "Yes, I did."

Rather than provide sufficient information, this question leaves several unanswered questions: "How much of the meat did you eat?" or "What foods did you eat?" and "Was the amount of food enough to satisfy your hunger?"

The question is sufficient for the nurse to place a check mark in the blank of a flow sheet, indicating that the patient did eat. However, good nutrition depends on the types of food eaten, the amount, and whether the food was satisfying. A better question may be "Tell me about your lunch."

Questions beginning with "Why" are also best avoided because they place the person on the defensive. Questions such as "Why didn't you ask for help to the bathroom?" are uncomfortable for the older adult. This type of question places the person in a position of feeling the need to make up an excuse rather than risk disapproval for an honest answer.

Defending

Defending is commonly used by nursing staff to explain or make excuses for behaviors rather than investigating the situation. For example, an elderly nursing home patient complains to the practical nurse that the nursing assistant was unnecessarily rough when helping her out of the bed to a chair. The practical nurse states, "That's impossible; Ms. Martin is my best nursing assistant. She is always careful with patients." More than likely, this conversation will end with this defensive statement. The elderly patient is left to deal with anxiety and fear without support from the nurse. The practical nurse indicates to the patient that any disagreement with this assessment of the situation will not be considered. A better response by the nurse is "That's unacceptable. I'll look into the situation. What can I do for you now?"

THERAPEUTIC COMMUNICATION TECHNIQUES

Miscommunication is responsible for much of the frustration and stress of working with elderly patients. Almost every nursing function requires the use of a good communication technique. With the use of these techniques, communication is enhanced, and the nurses' frustration is decreased.

> **TIPS FOR COMMUNICATING WITH THE OLDER ADULT**
>
> Techniques that enhance communication:
> Offering general leads
> Making observations
> Using broad opening statements
> Being available
> Using silence
> Restating
> Presenting reality
> Clarifying
> Reflecting

Offering General Leads

The older adult sometimes needs encouragement to continue talking. Phrases such as "Go on" or "Tell me more about . . ." allow the patient to direct the conversation in a way that is meaningful to him. Statements that offer general leads also indicate that the nurse is interested in the conversation. For example, an elderly patient is describing symptoms he is experiencing during the night. Suddenly, he stops talking. The nurse needing to obtain the rest of the information says, "Yes, go on."

Making Observations

Nurses are continually making observations about the patient. This is part of collecting data. Sometimes, it is important to call attention to observations made of the patient's behavior. This focuses the patient's attention on the behavior and helps the patient identify feelings associated with the behavior, such as "Mr. Jones, you appear tense when your family leaves. . . ." Other phrases to use when making observations often involve reflecting to the patient the nonverbal behavior observed.

> **TIPS FOR COMMUNICATING WITH THE OLDER ADULT**
>
> Phrases to use when making observations:
> "I notice you appear tense."
> "I notice you are clenching your fist."
> "You seem angry."
> "You seem frustrated."

Using Broad Opening Statements

Broad opening statements, sometimes called open-ended questions, are excellent statements to use to encourage verbalization. These statements allow the patient to elaborate or describe the situation in question. The patient can then take the initiative in the discussion and explain the situation using their own words.

> **TIPS FOR COMMUNICATING WITH THE OLDER ADULT**
>
> Examples of broad opening statements:
> "You seem to be thinking about something."
> "Where would you like to begin?"
> "Tell me about . . ."

For example, asking "Mr. Cauley, tell me about you daughter's visit" allows more freedom for verbalization of thoughts than asking a question that can be answered with a one-word answer such as yes or no. Asking "Did you enjoy you daughter's visit?" does not provide as great an opportunity for the expression of feelings.

Questions beginning with what, which, where, when, and who are avoided. Questions beginning with these interrogatives put the patient on the defensive and are not considered therapeutic. For the same reason, questions beginning with why are avoided because these questions belittle the older adult.

> **TIPS FOR COMMUNICATING WITH THE OLDER ADULT**
>
> Examples of "why" questions that belittle or humiliate:
> "Why are you wearing two sweaters?"
> "Why don't you use that call light when you need help?"
> "Why are you acting like this?"

Although the intention may simply be to obtain information, "why" questions usually imply that the nurse thinks the behavior is childish or foolish.

Being Available

Loneliness is a constant companion for many elderly people, especially the elderly living in a nursing home. The nurse who takes the time to be available is communicating to the older adult that this nurse cares. Offering self communicates interest in the individual and a desire to understand. This technique involves offering the nurse's presence; it is not a method to get the older adult to talk or communicate verbally.

> **TIPS FOR COMMUNICATING WITH THE OLDER ADULT**
>
> Examples of statements that convey the nurse is available:
> "I'll sit with you for awhile."
> "I would like to spend some time with you."

Using Silence

A powerful but often uncomfortable therapeutic technique is remaining silent. Silence is the absence of verbal communication. Silence offers support and encouragement. It gives the person time to collect thoughts or think through a problem or a situation. When using silence, remember that even a minute can seem like an eternity to a nurse who is constantly involved in the daily routines of a busy hospital or nursing home. Be willing to commit 10 to 15 minutes to this form of communication.

Restating

Restating is a technique used to force the patient to clarify a statement. In restating, the nurse repeats the main idea expressed by the patient. The patient hears the main idea and can clarify or expand if he has been misunderstood.

> **TIPS FOR COMMUNICATING WITH THE OLDER ADULT**
>
> Example of restating:
> Patient: "I can't eat this food. It makes me sick."
> Nurse: "The food makes you ill?"

The nurse's statement forces the patient to agree with the statement or to restate the message.

Clarifying

Clarification is a communication technique that seeks to make clear communication that is vague. Clarification should be used regularly when communicating to maximize understanding. In clarification, the message is acknowledged and even elaborated on. After an attempt to clarify, the patient is asked to verify the statement.

> **TIPS FOR COMMUNICATING WITH THE OLDER ADULT**
>
> Example of clarifying:
> Patient: "I can't sleep at night. That doctor doesn't care whether I sleep or not."
> Nurse: "I think you're saying you want your physician to prescribe something to help you sleep."

> **TIPS FOR COMMUNICATING WITH THE OLDER ADULT**
>
> Example of statements that encourage clarification:
> "I am not sure I follow you."
> "Can you elaborate on . . ."
> "I understood you to say . . ."

Reflecting

A reflective response accurately repeats, paraphrases, or rephrases the message. Messages have three components; words, thoughts, and feelings. When reflecting, the nurse responds to all three components. This technique directs feelings, thoughts, and ideas of the message back to the patient and encourages exploration of ideas and feelings.

> **TIPS FOR COMMUNICATING WITH THE OLDER ADULT**
>
> An example of reflecting:
> Caregiver: "Do you think I should place Mom in a nursing home?"
> Nurse: "Do you think your mother should be placed in a nursing home?"

The nurse should care not to overuse this technique, or she may simply appear as an echo and cause irritation rather than enhance communication.

ANGER

Anger is an emotion that limits communication. Stress from being in a new environment, unfamiliarity with hospital policies, prolonged waiting time for procedures, decline in physical ability, increased dependency on others, and separation from loved

DISPLAY 5-3. Tips For Calming an Angry Patient or Family Member

- Keep calm and speak softly.
- Show respect and treat the patient with dignity.
- Remain quiet and allow verbalization of anger.
- Accept the feelings and emotions expressed.
- Acknowledge feelings and express regret or understanding of the situation.
- Do not defend personal actions or the actions of others.
- Do not argue, intimidate, or belittle the patient or family members.
- Offer suggestions and alternatives to the problem.

ones are factors that contribute to an older person's anger and frustration. Careful assessment and observation can alert the nurse that a patient's anger is on the rise. Signs of anger include an increasingly loud voice, making demands of the nursing staff or other health care providers, clenched jaws, or a change in previous behavior. When signs of anger occur, the nurse must use good communication skills to defuse the situation. When the patient or family becomes angry, the nurse must not to respond with anger. By remaining calm, the nurse is better able to handle the situation in a constructive manner. Display 5-3 offers suggestions to help calm an angry patient. The following phrases may be helpful when communicating with an angry patient or family member:

"You seem upset. Can you tell me what's wrong?"

"Please help me understand why you are troubled."

"I understand your anger."

"I see your point."

DEVELOPING AND MAINTAINING A THERAPEUTIC RELATIONSHIP

The act of nursing demands that the nurse communicate with the patient. The nurse uses verbal and nonverbal communication to develop a therapeutic or helping relationship. A therapeutic nurse-patient relationship is important when working with the gerontological patient. Too often, older adults are faced with attitudes of ageism such as prejudice and rudeness. These attitudes may cause older adults to build a wall of stoicism and withdraw to protect themselves from hurtful remarks and negative attitudes. The nurse must communicate in a caring and genuine manner to break through the barriers established over a long period and establish a therapeutic relationship with the geriatric patient.

A **therapeutic nurse-patient relationship,** sometimes simply referred to as the therapeutic relationship, may be defined as an interpersonal process between the nurse and the patient in which the nurse uses specific communication skills to help the patient solve mental, physical, emotional, or spiritual problems, or eliminate potential problems. In the therapeutic relationship, the nurse and the patient are partners and establish goals based on the patient's perceived and real needs. By working together, the patient is more likely to comply with the therapeutic regimen because there is the feeling of "ownership" in helping to develop the plan of care. Although this feeling of ownership is important is any setting, it is particularly important in a nursing home.

Some older adults welcome the nurse with open arms and are eager to have someone who will listen and show an interest in them. Others are wary and slow to warm to the nurse's overtures. The therapeutic relationship differs from a social relationship in that a social relationship is focused on friendship, enjoyment, or meeting a specific goal; the therapeutic relationship is concerned with meeting the patient's needs. In the social relationship, there is a mutual benefit for both parties. In a therapeutic relationship, the focus is on the patient and the patient's needs. The nurse's needs are not directly addressed in a therapeutic relationship.

The nurse must remember that every act, gesture, and facial expression is communicating a message to the older adult. Most older adults eagerly embrace the opportunity to develop a relationship with the nurse. The nurse has the responsibility to continually evaluate and reflect on the communicating skills used. Modification of communication techniques may be needed to enhance the therapeutic relationship. Factors that enhance the nurse-patient relationship include genuineness, caring, and empathy.

Genuineness

Genuineness can be described as being sincere and honest. The nurse must have these qualities and convey this genuineness to the older adult. One way to do this is to be sure that nonverbal messages agree with the verbal messages. Patients, especially older adults, are quick to detect a lack of sincerity and inconsistency on the part of the nurse. It is important to be honest with the older adult. If the nurse cannot answer a question, that must be acknowledged and an answer sought. For example, the nurse may say, "I don't know the answer to that question, but I'll contact the social worker. She will be able to help you."

Explaining the care to be given or the procedure to be done in words that can be understood shows the patient you are genuinely concerned. Having an adequate explanation of what is being done promotes feelings that the nurse is genuinely concerned and reduces stress and anxiety. Active listening is also an important tool to convey genuineness. When the person feels the words he says are important to the nurse and feels that the nurse is sincerely trying to understand, genuine concern is conveyed.

Caring

When the older adult feels that the nurse truly cares, the door is opened for a meaningful therapeutic relationship. Caring is difficult to define, but when experienced by the patient, it can be the impetus to develop a therapeutic relationship. The patient feels cared for when the nurse goes beyond "just doing my job" and seeks every opportunity to assist the patient in meeting his needs. Often, it is the little things that may go unnoticed by others that are the very acts that convey that the nurse truly cares. The caring nurse approaches the patient in an accepting and nonjudgmental manner. Older patients are treated with the respect and dignity. Calling the patient by name, such as "Mr. Harrison" or "Miss Cobb," is one way the nurse shows respect and promotes dignity. Regardless of the patient's state of mind (eg, alert, oriented, confused, delirious), the patient is addressed with respect. Terms such as "Gramps," "Honey," or "Sweetie" are unprofessional and demeaning to older adults. Using the name the patient prefers and pronouncing the name correctly are also important. Taking the time out of a busy schedule to sit and talk, providing an extra portion of that favorite food, or giving a back rub to help a patient relax are simple but effective ways to exhibit caring.

Good nursing care depends on clinical expertise, a sound knowledge base, and the ability to convey an attitude of caring. Although each of these qualities is important, caring can be the one most appreciated by the family. For example, a new graduate nurse was assigned to care for a seriously ill patient in the acute care setting. The new nurse was uncertain of many of the technical aspects of this patient's care and was carefully supervised by an experienced nurse. The new graduate nurse was attentive to the physical needs of the patient and took time to talk with the family members. The patient recovered and

was discharged. Several weeks later, the nursing supervisor received a letter from this patient's family. The letter praised the new graduate for her caring attitude, her genuineness, and her ability as a nurse.

This letter from the patient and family emphasizes how important it is for the nurse to convey the message "I care about you." Although the newly graduated nurse did not have the clinical expertise of the other, more experienced nurses, the family's perception of the new nurse was positive because time was taken to convey the message, "I truly care about you."

Empathy

Empathy is the ability to understand the patient's pain or anguish and to convey that understanding to the patient. A young nurse with limited life experiences may have difficulty empathizing with an elderly patient. It is important to distinguish between empathy and sympathy. Sympathy is used in social settings to share emotional experiences. Sympathy involves feeling "sorry for" or having compassion for an elderly patient. For example, suppose an elderly women is upset because she recently had to leave her home of 60 years to enter a nursing home. A nurse shows sympathy by saying "I am so sorry that you had to leave your home. I know it must be awful." The nurse may then begin to cry with the patient. Many young adults can have sympathy (ie, feel sorry for another person or have compassion for another person's problem or situation), but few can empathize (ie, understand or feel another's sorrow and pain). A nurse showing empathy in the same situation may say "You must feel very sad about having to leave your home of many years. Would you like to talk about it?"

Being sensitive to the older person's words, maintaining eye contact, leaning forward toward the patient during the conversation, and maintaining a calm unhurried environment helps convince the older person that the nurse is truly trying to understand. It is important that the nurse not be overwhelmed by sadness, anger, or other emotions. When the nurse is too emotionally involved, there is an inability to respond appropriately and listen objectively.

Empathy is expressed by allowing the expression of feelings, being nonjudgmental, and respecting the patients need for privacy. Touch can be used to express empathy. Holding a patient's hand during a difficult procedure, giving a hug, or just a slight touch to the shoulder can tell the patient "I understand, and I'm here to help you through this."

PHASES OF THE NURSE-PATIENT RELATIONSHIP

The nurse-patient relationship is one that is therapeutic (ie, for the benefit or the good of the patient). The effectiveness of the nursing process (see Chapter 6) is enhanced when the nurse is successful in developing and maintaining a therapeutic relationship with the patient. The therapeutic nurse-patient relationship has three phases: developing phase, working phase, and terminating phase.

Each phase is essential for the nurse-patient relationship to have a full therapeutic effect. The relationship begins when the patient has needs that the nurse can meet or help the patient to meet. The therapeutic relationship ends when the goals established have been met and the patient can function independently.

Developing Phase

The key to developing a therapeutic relationship is to establish trust. During the period when the nurse and the patient are getting acquainted, if the nurse is able to convey a genuineness and a caring attitude, the patient will respond by identifying health needs. The nurse uses therapeutic communication techniques such as active listening and proper questioning to keep a positive tone within the relationship. The atmosphere within the relationship must be one in which trust can grow. The patient must be certain of the nurse's commitment to confidentiality (within the ethical framework discussed in Chapter 4). If the patient discloses information that, if kept within the confines of the nurse-patient relationship, would be harmful to the patient or someone else, the nurse must inform the appropriate individuals who can deal with the situation.

It is particularly important for patients who live in the nursing home to have a positive nurse-patient relationship. These relationships are long term, and a positive nurse-patient relationship can greatly enhance the patient's well-being and quality of life.

Working Phase

During the working phase, the patient is assisted to identify goals. In planning goals for the gerontologic patient, it is important to include the nurse, the patient, and family members. Family members often have special insight to the needs of the older adult. This also gives the nurse the opportunity to observe the family members and the patient interact. Strengths and weaknesses of the relationship may be identified.

In a nursing home, the resident and family may be asked to come to a care planning conference. When the family members are participating in developing the plan of care, it is important for the nurse to talk to the patient and include the patient. At times, the nurse directs conversation to the family member, and the patient becomes the topic of conversation and is "talked about" rather than "talked to." In other words, don't talk to the family member as if the patient was not there. The patient is the focus of the care conference.

During the working phase, goals of the patient are identified (see Chapter 6), and ways to meet these goals are explored. The nurse and the family must be careful not to stifle the patient's independence and self-care ability but to plan interventions that promote independence and self-care. Doing too much for the patient can be as harmful as doing too little. In the working phase, the nurse, the patient, and the family are viewed as partners working together for the good of the patient.

Terminating Phase

The therapeutic relationship is self-limiting and usually ends when the immediate goals have been met and the patient regains independence. In a nursing home environment, the therapeutic relationship terminates only when the nurse leaves the facility (or is transferred to another area), the patient is discharged, or the patient dies. Nurses who work in extended care areas develop long-term nurse-patient relationships that must be continually maintained and nourished. The working phase becomes an ongoing phase with problems identified and resolved or new interventions tried to solve needs that remain unmet.

When the nurse realizes that the nurse-patient relationship will end, it should be discussed with the patient. It is best if termination can be mentioned and discussed in the first stage, the developing stage. For example, if a patient is admitted to the nursing home for rehabilitation after a hip fracture, it is best to say, "Mrs. Talley, I am Miss Hartford, and will be your nurse for the next 4 to 6 weeks while you are recuperating from your hip injury." This lets Mrs. Talley know that her stay is limited and that goals must be accomplished within a certain time frame. It also lets Mrs. Talley know when this nurse-patient relationship will end.

Preparing the patient for termination of the nurse-patient relationship is important. Knowing when the relationship will end gives the patient and the nurse time to prepare and find closure. If the time of the termination phase is unknown in the beginning, the nurse must wait until the time is known.

During the termination phase, the patient, the nurse, and the family must agree that the goals have been met. In some instances, the nurse must facilitate the patient's transition of care to other health care services, such as home health. Most patients and families are pleased to see improvement and regain independence. These patients move easily move through the termination phase. However, some patients may be reluctant to let go of the nurse-patient relationship. These patients may withdraw or regress. Some patients withdraw and refuse to say goodbye. Others may become sarcastic, irritable, or depressed.

If a patient or family member appears uncomfortable with terminating the relationship, the nurse encourages the patient to verbalize feelings about the termination. For example, the nurse may say, "Goodbyes are difficult. Tell me how you feel about my leaving." This use of a broad opening statement allows the patient (or family) to express feelings about the end of the nurse-patient relationship.

COMMUNICATING EFFECTIVELY WITH THE OLDER ADULT

Communicating effectively with the older adult is not different from communicating with a younger adult. Each older adult is a unique individual with unique needs. By using the therapeutic communication techniques discussed in this chapter, better communication will occur.

Nonverbal communication is just as important as the spoken word. To understand what message the individual is trying to communicate through nonverbal behavior, remember that all behavior has meaning. To understand the message that the patient is trying to communicate, ask yourself the following questions:

Why is the patient behaving in this way?

What is the patient feeling?

What is the patient thinking?

Family members may be helpful in deciphering behavior cues (see Chapters 15 and 17). Communication is the key to developing a therapeutic nurse-patient relationship. Nurses who think before com-

municating, reflect on the methods used to communicate, and make modifications when necessary will have a major impact on their patient's recovery.

CRITICAL THINKING EXERCISES

1. Mr. Walker, age 85, is a resident in a nursing home. He is upset about losing his clothes after sending them to the laundry last week. He is accusing the nursing staff of the theft and angrily states that he wants something done about this situation. What communication techniques would you use? What would you say to Mr. Walker to calm him down in this situation? Give a rationale for your answer.
2. A nursing assistant complains to you that one of the nurses is "just sitting in Ms. Cantu's room, not saying anything." The nurse assistant states "that nurse is just wasting time and needs to quit loafing and do something to help out around here." How would you handle this situation? What would you say to the nursing assistant and to the nurse?
3. You notice that Mr. Scoggins, an elderly nursing home resident, likes to collect the unused sugar packets after each meal. He takes them to his room and stores them in his bedside table. Today, when he is collecting the sugar packets, one of the other residents becomes upset and follows Mr. Scoggins to his room. How would you handle this situation? What would you say to each of the residents? What communication techniques would be most effective?

REFERENCES AND SUGGESTED READING

Boyd, S. (1997). Listen up! *Nursing, 97 (5)*, 60.

Droppleman, P.G., & Thomas, S.P. (1996). Anger in nurses: Don't lose it, use it. *American Journal of Nursing, 96 (4)*, 26–32.

Fiesta, J. (1998). Failure to communicate. *Nursing Management, 29 (2)*, 22–25.

Grensing-Pophal, L. (1997). Eight signs of poor communication. *Nursing, 97 (10)*.

Sherman, K. (1996). *Communication and Image in Nursing*. Albany, NY: Delmar Publishing.

Zook, R. (1996). Take action before anger builds. *RN, 4*, 46–50.

CHAPTER 6

CHAPTER OUTLINE

KEY TERMS

CHAPTER OBJECTIVES

THE NURSING PROCESS

    Assessment

    Nursing Diagnosis

    Short-Term and Long-Term Goals

    Developing the Care Plan

    Implementation

    Evaluation

USING THE NURSING PROCESS IN A NURSING
FACILITY

    Resident Assessment Instrument

    Quarterly Review

    Minimum Data Set

    Resident Assessment Protocols

    Assessment

    Care Planning Conference

    Implementation and Evaluation

USING THE NURSING PROCESS TO DEVELOP A
TEACHING PLAN

    Assessment

    Nursing Diagnosis

    Planning and Implementation

    Evaluation

CRITICAL THINKING EXERCISES

REFERENCES AND SUGGESTED READING

KEY TERMS

assessment

collaborative problem

evaluation

goals

implementation

Minimum Data Set

nursing process

nursing diagnosis

objective data

Resident Assessment Instrument

Resident Assessment Protocol

subjective data

Applying the Nursing Process to Gerontological Care

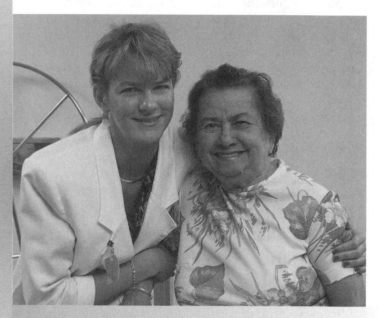

CHAPTER OBJECTIVES

**At the completion of this chapter, the student will
be able to**

- **Use the nursing process to assess and develop
a plan of care for older adults**

- **Distinguish between subjective and objective
data**

- **Discuss the use of the Resident Assessment
Instrument, the Minimum Data Set, and
Resident Assessment Protocols in developing a
plan of care for the nursing home resident**

The nursing process was introduced in the 1950s as
a three-step process of interrelated steps of assessment, planning, and evaluation. During the past
several decades, this process has evolved into the
five-step process used today.

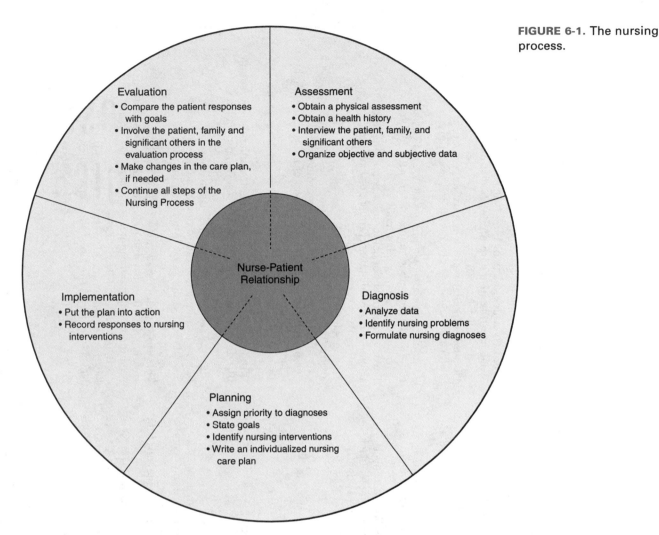

FIGURE 6-1. The nursing process.

THE NURSING PROCESS

The **nursing process** is a systematic, ongoing method of planning and managing patient care. This process has five essential components: assessment, diagnosis (sometimes called analysis), planning, implementation, and evaluation. The nursing process results in a care plan that individualizes patient care. The most significant patient problems are identified, and interventions are planned to solve or diminish these problems. The nurse-patient relationship is at the center of the nursing process (Fig. 6-1). A therapeutic relationship based on mutual trust provides the nurse with an avenue to use the nursing process to the fullest.

Assessment

The nursing process begins with assessment. **Assessment** is the collection of information or data concerning the patient. Data are subjective or objective. **Objective data** are collected through observation, diagnostic tests, laboratory or x-ray examination, and physical examination. Examples of objective data include vital signs (eg, temperature, pulse, respiration), the patient's hemoglobin or hematocrit, and the presence of a rash.

Subjective data refer to feelings and emotions such as fear or anxiety or to patient complaints of pain or nausea. Subjective data are obtained from the patient, family, or significant others. These individuals are asked to describe symptoms, feelings, and emotions expressed by the individual being assessed. It is important to involve the family in the assessment phase. Family members can provide information and insight that assists in the next phase, that of analysis. Subjective and objective data form the database to plan patient care and are obtained by interviewing the patient, family, and significant others and through observation.

A head to toe or systems physical assessment by the nurse is necessary to establish a baseline assessment and identify symptoms of diseases or illness. Table 6-1 provides a guide for a systems assessment for the elderly person based on information in the chapters on the various body systems.

TABLE 6-1. Physical Assessment Findings in Older Adults

Assessment Actions	Normal Findings	Abnormal Findings
HEAD AND NECK		
Inspect hair and scalp. Note lesions, redness, sensitivity of scalp; describe exact location and measurement.	Gray, dry, thinning hair Men: baldness	Coarse, dry, brittle hair (hypothyroidism) Excessively oily hair (poor grooming practices, parkinsonism) Irregular patches of hair loss (fungal infection) Smooth, round nodules (sebaceous cysts) Nodular, ulcerative, raised, glossy, painless growth (melanoma, basal cell carcinoma) Red patches of dry skin with silver-white, light gray, or brown scale, less than 1 cm (solar [actinic] kerotoses)
Inspect and palpate carotid pulse.	Regular, strong carotid pulse	Weak carotid pulse with diminished stroke volume (left ventricular failure)
Inspect jugular veins.	No distention of jugular vein when patient erect or with head elevated 45 degrees	Distended jugular veins when patient erect or with head elevated 45 degrees (congestive heart failure, pericarditis)
Inspect face. Note symmetry, scars, rashes, and lesions.	Symmetrical features; freckles, lines, wrinkles, decreased skin elasticity	Asymmetry, paralysis, numbness (CVA. Bell's palsy) Raised, circumscribed pigmentation with papules within lesion (malignant melanoma)
Inspect eyes. Note drooping eyelids, moisture of eyes, discharge, unusual movements, discoloration of sclera.	Loss of tissue elasticity around eyes, "baggy" eyelids; white sclera; black-skinned persons can have slightly yellow discoloration	Ptosis (impairment of oculomotor nerve, edema) Edematous eyelids (allergy, infection, nephrosis, heart failure) Yellow sclera (liver disease) Protruding eyes (hyperthyroidism) Excessively dry eyes (Sjögren syndrome) Eye pain, dilated pupils, perception of halos around lights (acute glaucoma) Tearing, headaches, complaint of "smeared" or unclear vision (chronic glaucoma) Blind spot in visual field: scotoma (macular degeneration) Blindness in same half of both eyes: homonymous hemianopsia (CVA)
Ask about visual capacity and changes, symptoms.		Inability to see small print (far-sightedness)
Inspect ears. Ask about pain, itching, discharge, care of ears. Note hearing capacity and patient's ability to hear a watch tick.	Increased cerumen accumulation Larger lobes, greater protrusion of ears Increased hair growth in ear. Atrophy of tympanic membrane (appears white or gray) Increased difficulty hearing high-pitched sounds	Itching (cerumen, chronic external otitis) Small, crusted ulcerated lesion on pinna (basal or squamous cell carcinoma) Tinnitus (hypertension, adverse drug reaction) Hearing deficit (sensorineural or conductive hearing loss, cerumen impaction, upper respiratory or ear infection, ototoxic drugs, diabetes)
Inspect nares. Note lesions and masses. Ask about nosebleeds, feeling of obstruction, pain, and other symptoms.	Drier nasal cavity	Obstructed nasal breathing (mass, polyp, dried crusts) Nosebleeds, hypertension, vitamin C deficiency, irritation from picking)

Assessment	Normal Findings	Abnormal Findings/Significance
Inspect face and mouth area.	Vertical wrinkling of skin surrounding mouth Drier, thinner, less vascular buccal mucosa Decreased secretion of salivary ptyalin Dark-skinned persons may have bluish hue to lips and brownish markings on gum as normal findings.	Dryness of lips and oral cavity (dehydration) Fissure at corner of mouth (vitamin B complex deficiency, infection, overclosure of mouth due to missing teeth or poorly fitting dentures) Bluish, black line along gumline (lead, arsenic, or mercury poisoning) Smooth, red tongue (iron, vitamin B_{12}, or niacin deficiency) White patches on tongue (moniliasis, leukoplakia)
Note voice tone and quality, articulation, and speech pattern.	Interpret and use language appropriately	Aphasia (neurologic disease, altered cognition) Monotonous, slurred speech (parkinsonism) Slurred speech (hypoglycemia, intoxication, neurologic disease)
Note breath odor.		Sweet, fruity smelling breath (ketoacidosis) Breath odor of urine (uremic acidosis) Breath odor of clover (liver failure) Foul breath odor (halitosis, decaying teeth, lung abscess)

RESPIRATORY SYSTEM

Assessment	Normal Findings	Abnormal Findings/Significance
Ask patient about ease of breathing, symptoms, coughing, sputum production. Inspect bare chest. Note coloring, symmetrical expansion during respiration. Evaluate scars, structural abnormalities. Evaluate respiratory rate, rhythm, depth, and length. Note anteroposterior and lateral chest diameter.	Reduced efficiency of cough response Slight increase in anteroposterior chest diameter	Orthopnea, dyspnea, shortness of breath (respiratory infection or disease) Ruddy, pink coloring of face, trunk, limbs (COPD) Bluish gray hue to face and neck (chronic bronchitis) Asymmetric lung expansion (acute pleurisy, pleural fibrosis, pleural effusion, pain, fractured rib) Significant increase anteroposterior diameter that is greater than lateral diameter (COPD) Crepitus (crunchy feeling to skin resulting from air getting trapped under epidermis)
Auscultate to assess pitch, intensity, quality, and duration of breath sounds.	Bronchial breath sounds over trachea (short inspirations; long expirations); vesicular breath sounds over entire lung field (long inspirations; short expirations; bronchovesicular breath sounds over sternum and scapula (equal inspiratory and expiratory phase)	Crackles, rales (extrainterstitial fluid due to CHF, pulmonary edema, bronchitis, pneumonia) Rhonchi, rattling (increased mucus production and partial airway obstruction due to bronchitis, bronchiectasis) Wheezes (presence of large amounts of thick mucus or narrowing of airway due to asthma, pulmonary stenosis)

CARDIOVASCULAR SYSTEM

Assessment	Normal Findings	Abnormal Findings/Significance
Note generalized coloring, energy level, breathing pattern, mental status. Inspect veins; note varicosities. Note condition of nails, presence of hair on extremities, color and temperature of extremities.	No distress, symptoms, or discoloration Extremities warm, hair present	Pallor, confusion, fatigue, dyspnea (cardiac disease) Confusion, blackouts, fatigue, dizziness (decreased carotid blood flow, aortic stenosis, reduced cardiac output, digitalis toxicity) Coughs, wheezes (left-sided heart failure) Hemoptysis (pulmonary embolus, heart failure)
Assess blood pressure. Palpate the radial pulse.	BP levels must be elevated individually and in relationship to physical and mental status at various BP levels.	Repeated BP >160/95 (hypertension)
Assess the blood pressure in lying, sitting, and standing positions.	Positional drops <20 mm Hg	
Assess rate, rhythm, and volume of pulse.	Pulse rate can range 60–100 beats. Some tachycardia may be present, related to stress of being examined; reevaluate in several hours.	Arrhythmias (digitalis toxicity, hypokalemia, infection, hemorrhage, cardiac disease)

Continued

TABLE 6-1. Physical Assessment Findings in Older Adults *continued*

Assessment Actions	Normal Findings	Abnormal Findings
GASTROINTESTINAL SYSTEM Ask about appetite, diet, swallowing problems, indigestion, regurgitation, pain, nausea, vomiting, flatus, and constipation.		Bleeding, irritation of esophagus (esophageal varicosities) Excessive salivation, hiccups, dysphagia, anemia, thirst Heartburn, dysphagia, belching, vomiting, regurgitation, pain Weight loss >5% in last 30 days; >10% in last 6 months
Inspect abdomen. Note discoloration, asymmetry, dilated vessels, bulges, distention, rashes, scars, and strong contractions. Ask the patient to raise head, and note herniations that may become evident.	Symmetrical sides, rounded, adipose tissue Silver-white striae from pregnancy, weight changes	Pink or blue striae (recent stretching due to tumors, ascites, obesity) Jaundice (cirrhosis, gallstones, pancreatitis) Rashes (irritation, drug reaction) Small painless nodules (skin cancer)
Auscultate abdomen before touching it for percussion or palpation to avoid stimulating bowel activity. Listen for bowel sounds over intestines using diaphragm portion of stethoscope. If sounds are not heard, listen for 5 minutes and then flick finger against abdominal wall to stimulate intestinal motility.	Peristaltic sounds every 5–15 seconds Continuous bowel sounds if food has been ingested within past several hours	Absent or reduced bowel sounds (late bowel obstruction, peritonitis, electrolyte imbalances, handling of bowel during surgery) Increased bowel sounds (early bowel obstruction, gastroenteritis, diarrhea)
Auscultate vascular sounds by placing bell portion of stethoscope over major arteries.	Heartbeat can be heard	Murmurs over abdominal aorta (aneurysm)
Ask about the pattern of bowel elimination.	Regular passage of moist, formed stool without straining	Infrequent passage of stool, abdominal fullness and discomfort, lethargy, poor appetite (constipation) Diarrhea or seepage of stool, palpable mass in rectum (fecal impaction) Dark, tarry stools, (hemorrhoids, lower GI cancer, diverticulitis) Gray, tan, unpigmented stool (obstructive jaundice) Pale, fatty stool (malabsorption) Mucus in stool (inflammation) Small worms in stool or rectal area (pinworms)
GENITOURNARY SYSTEM Inspect genitalia. Note inflammation, irritation, discharge, lesions, prolapse. Palpate genitalia for masses and tenderness.	Loss of pubic hair; flattening of labia; dry vaginal canal; smaller-sized uterus (may not be palpable)	Vaginal discharge, odor, irritation, soreness, itching (vaginitis, moniliasis, trichomoniasis) Protrusion of vaginal wall outside vulva, pelvic pressure or heaviness, urinary tract symptoms (prolapsed uterus, cystocele, rectocele) Palpable mass (cancer)
Inspect and palpate breasts for discharge, masses, abnormalities.	Atrophy of breast tissue	Dimpling and retraction of nipple; nontender, nonmovable hard mass in breast (carcinoma)

GENITOURINARY SYSTEM continued

For men, ask about sexual function, symptoms, date of last prostate examination. Inspect genitalia for lesions, edema, discharge, masses, or deformity. Palpate scrotum for symmetry of testicles, tenderness, and masses.

- Decreased frequency of sexual activity
- Potency
- Reduced size and firmness of testes
- Some degree of prostatic enlargement present in most older men

Impotency (stress, depression, drug side-effects, fatigue, overeating, neuropathy, long period of sexual inactivity)
Penile discharge (urethritis, prostatitis, venereal disease)
Crooked, painful erection (Peyronie's disease)
Mass (carcinoma)
Scrotal pain, swelling (epididymitis, orchitis, carcinoma)
Prostatic enlargement (benign prostatic hypertrophy, cancer)
Painful, edematous, reddened breasts (irritation from suspenders, restraints)

Ask about pattern, frequency, and characteristics of bladder elimination; history of incontinence.
Obtain urine specimen for evaluation.

- Urinary frequency, nocturia
- Continence

Incontinence (urinary tract infection, prostatic enlargement, neurogenic bladder, tumor, cerebral cortex lesion, calculi, medications, altered cognition)
Increased urinary frequency (urinary tract infection, diuretic therapy, increased fluid intake, diabetes, hypocalcemia, anxiety)
Cloudy, alkaline, odorous urine; temperature elevation; frequency (urinary tract infection)
Hematuria, pain, signs of urinary tract infection (renal calculi)
Painless hematuria, signs of urinary tract infection [bladder cancer)
Yellow-brown or green-brown urine (jaundice, obstructive bile duct)
Pink, red, or rust-colored urine (presence of bile, ingestion of phenazopyridine [Pyridium])

MUSCULOSKELETAL SYSTEM

Ask about joint pain, restricted movement, tremors, spasms; inquire as to how the patient manages these problems. Place all joints through active and passive range of motion.

- Reduction in muscle mass and strength
- Range of motion adequate to perform activities of daily living

Back pain (degenerative arthritis, muscle strain, osteoporosis)
Joint pain, stiffness, crepitus, bony nodules/Heberden nodes (osteoarthritis)
Joint pain, stiffness, redness, warmth, subcutaneous nodules over bony prominences, atrophy of surrounding muscle, flexion contractures (rheumatoid arthritis)
Calf cramps during exercise, relieved by rest (intermittent claudication)
Red, dry, thickened piece of skin over bony prominence (corn)
Medial allocation of first metatarsophalangeal joint (digiti flexus [hammer toe])

Adapted from Eliopoulos, C. (1996). *Gerontological Nursing* (4th ed.) Philadelphia: Lippincott-Raven.

Most nursing homes use the **Minimum Data Set** (MDS) (see Appendix E) as an assessment tool to obtain necessary information for patients entering a nursing home. The MDS is an assessment form provided by the federal government for use in nursing homes receiving federal funds. The MDS provides an easy to use format for obtaining minimum data. A more in-depth discussion of the MDS occurs later in this chapter.

Nursing Diagnosis

Analysis results in identifying unmet needs. An analysis of the data is obtained from the assessment and enables the nurse to formulate a nursing diagnosis. A **nursing diagnosis** identifies a health problem or a potential problem that can be solved or prevented by nursing interventions or nursing actions. Nursing diagnoses are *not* medical diagnoses, medical treatments, or diagnostic tests. They are problems that can be alleviated, prevented, or lessened in severity as a result of planned nursing actions.

A nursing care plan may have one or more nursing diagnoses. A potential problem may be stated as "risk for" diagnosis. For example a patient may have the diagnosis "Risk for Impaired Skin Integrity." This means that the patient's skin is a especially high risk for trauma and damage.

The North American Nursing Diagnosis Association (NANDA) developed a list of diagnoses that is periodically updated. The diagnoses identified by NANDA have been generally accepted by nurses as a method to identify nursing problems and needs. These diagnoses continue to evolve as they are used in the clinical area and are validated through nursing research. Some examples of common nursing diagnoses related to nursing care of the older adult are given in Display 6-1.

Nursing diagnoses are specific to the problems identified in analysis of the data and identify the problems that are to be addressed in the care plan. **Collaborative problem** is a term used to identify potential problems or complications that are medical in nature. Collaborative problems require medical and nursing interventions and collaboration between nursing and medical staff. Interventions focus on monitoring for the onset of complications or a change in status related to treatments, disease, diagnostic tests, or medications.

Nursing diagnoses are prioritized according to the most important or immediate need of the patient. Maslow's hierarchy of needs provides a framework to prioritize needs (see Chapter 2). The

---

> **DISPLAY 6-1. Common Nursing Diagnoses Related to Caring for the Older Adult**
>
> - Altered Thought Processes, related to (specify)
> - Ineffective Individual Coping, related to life crisis, inadequate support system, personal vulnerability, other (specify)
> - Risk for Injury, related to altered mobility, cognitive impairment, other (specify)
> - Impaired Skin Integrity, related to physical immobilization, altered nutritional state, other (specify)
> - Self-Care Deficit, related to activity, bathing, hygiene, toileting, feeding, cognitive impairment, other (specify)

---

physiologic or basic needs such as the needs for oxygen, food, water, and sleep are considered the most important and must be met or at least partially met before other needs can be addressed. For example, the need for adequate oxygen must be met before the need for esteem or love and belonging can be addressed. An elderly resident who is unable to breathe is not concerned with learning how to self-administer insulin until breathing is adequate.

When planning care, incorporate the patient's values, customs, or habits. As much as possible, involve the patient and the family in developing a plan of care. This makes the care plan individualized and pertinent to the patient or resident (if in a nursing facility). Residents of nursing facilities and their families are invited to care planning sessions in a nursing facility.

Short-Term and Long-Term Goals

Goals are short statements of expected outcomes. There are two types of goals: short-term goals and long-term goals to address the identified problems. After nursing diagnoses are prioritized, the next step is to identify short-term goals. In the hospital, setting short-term goals requires that goals can be met within a few days to a week. This timeframe may be increased in a nursing facility. In nursing facilities, short-term goals may be considered goals that can be met within 2 to 3 weeks or longer. Goals from the hospital setting may be carried over to the nursing facility to provide continuity of care. Display 6-2 gives examples of short-term goals.

When planning patient goals in an acute care facility or hospital, the goals can extend beyond

---

DISPLAY 6-2. Examples of Short-Term Goals

- Resident will walk to the dining room without assistance within 2 weeks.
- Pressure ulcer will measure less than 2 cm within 4 weeks.

DISPLAY 6-3. Examples of Goals Set in Increments

- Week 1 goal: Resident will walk to the bathroom with assistance at least twice each day.
- Week 2 goal: Resident will walk with assistance to the nurses station at least twice each day.
- Week 3 goal: Resident will walk with assistance to the cafeteria for lunch and dinner each day for the next 10 days.

---

hospitalization. Goals that are met over a longer period are long-term goals. In a nursing home, goals are reassessed every 3 months or when any significant change occurs in the resident's condition. Goals must have these three characteristics:

Goals must be measurable.

Goals must be specific.

Goals must be attainable.

For example, "The resident will eat 75% of each meal for the next 10 days" is a measurable, specific, and attainable goal. However, the goal "The resident will eat adequate food" is neither measurable nor specific.

To be successful in meeting goals, the resident's input is important. A goal that the resident does not see as attainable or beneficial will likely not be met. Some goals are set in increments (Display 6-3).

Developing the Care Plan

The care plan identifies nursing interventions to accomplish the goals. Nursing interventions are nursing actions that assist the patient to meet the identified goals and are written for each nursing diagnosis. Interventions are specific enough so that all members of the health care team understand exactly what action to take. For example, when the nursing diagnosis is "Impaired Skin Integrity, related to a 3-cm stage II decubitus ulcer on left buttock," a vague or inappropriate nursing intervention is "decubitus care tid." This provides no guidelines for intervention and no consistency of care.

With this type of intervention, one nurse may choose to apply a skin spray such as Granulex and no dressing, and another nurse may provide decubitus care by cleaning with normal saline and applying a dressing. There would be no consistency in treatment, and if healing occurred, it would not be as a result of the nursing care but reflect chance and the body's ability to heal itself. A more specific nursing intervention is "cleanse skin to affected area with normal saline, apply Granulex spray, and leave open to air at 8:00 AM, 1:00 PM, and 8:00 PM." This type of intervention leaves a little doubt about what should be done for the decubitus ulcer. Sometimes, the physician orders a specific treatment regimen for care of a decubitus ulcer. In other instances, the nursing facility or hospital may have protocols for the care of pressure ulcers.

Care plans change as the patient's condition or status changes or a problem is solved and new problems are identified. A well-developed care plan is one that is individualized, specific for each patient, and is written so that everyone involved in the care can understand. Display 6-4 provides an example of a care plan. The care plan is continually updated to meet the patient's changing condition.

Implementation

Implementation is carrying out the written plan of care. During implementation, nursing interventions are performed and documented. The patient's responses are documented as well.

Patient and family teaching is also included in implementation. Teaching is an important component of all areas of gerontological nursing (see Chapter 5). Teaching is done in adult day care centers, nursing facilities, or any setting where older adults congregate. For example, foot care for a diabetic patient is an important topic for teaching the elderly in any outpatient setting, nursing facility, acute care facility, or rehabilitation center.

Evaluation

The effectiveness of the plan is continually evaluated. Data are gathered, and the effectiveness of each intervention is analyzed. The nurse determines if the goals were met and if there is a need for a change in approach to care. Display 6-5 shows the results of the ongoing evaluation. Because the nursing process is ongoing, adjustments are made at any point new data indicate the need for revision.

DISPLAY 6-4. **Developing A Care Plan**

Situation: Mr. Taylor was admitted to the nursing facility a week ago. He has fallen two times in the last week when walking to the bathroom at night. His daughter is concerned that he is not adjusting well. The nurse informs Mr. Taylor and his daughter that a care conference will be held and invites Mr. Taylor and his daughter to attend. At the conference, Mr. Taylor reveals that he is unhappy with his roommate, Mr. Garcia. Mr. Garcia stays up late listening to a radio, and he seldom goes to sleep before midnight. Mr. Taylor likes to go to bed at 9 PM and awaken for his coffee at 6 AM. He feels lonely and isolated, and he misses playing cards with his friends at the adult day care that he previously attended.

Solution: One problem can easily be solved. Mr. Taylor was moved to another room with a roommate who also likes to go to bed early and awaken early in the morning. After this problem was addressed, the staff at the care conference developed the following plan to help Mr. Taylor adjust to living at the nursing facility.

Problem/Need	Goal	Interventions
Falling when attempting to walk to the bathroom at night	*Goal:* Mr. Taylor will call for assistance in ambulation to the bathroom every night for the next 2 weeks. *Reevaluation date:* April 10 (in 2 weeks) *Disciplines responsible:* Nursing	1. Keep a nightlight in bathroom at night. 2. Place the call light within easy reach. 3. Instruct on the use of call light *every* night. 4. Check the room every 2 hours. 5. Answer the call light within 2 minutes and assist with ambulation to the bathroom.
Feels lonely and isolated	*Goal:* Mr. Taylor will express greater satisfaction within 1 week and will participate at least three times in a social activity of his choice. *Reevaluation date:* April 3 (in 1 week) *Disciplines responsible:* Nursing, social services, activity coordinator, daughter	1. Encourage Mr. Taylor to participate in weekly socials. 2. Nurse assistant will walk with Mr. Taylor to the game room every day at 10 AM and 3 PM. 3. Have Mr. Taylor's daughter contact friends and invite them to the facility to play cards.
Likes to have coffee at 6 AM	*Goal:* Mr. Taylor will have coffee every morning at 6 AM if he desires. *Reevaluation date:* April 3 (in 1 week) *Disciplines responsible:* Nursing, dietary	1. Inform Mr. Taylor that coffee is available in the cafeteria beginning at 5:30 AM. 2. Have nurse assistant walk with Mr. Taylor every morning for 1 week to obtain coffee. 3. Encourage Mr. Taylor to walk to the cafeteria for coffee every morning.

DISPLAY 6-5. **Ongoing Evaluation Findings**

- The goals were met, and the problem is resolved.
- The plan needs revision based on new data.
- The plan needs to be continued with minor revisions.

USING THE NURSING PROCESS IN A NURSING FACILITY

Planning care in a nursing facility may be somewhat different that in an acute care setting. Nursing facil-ities that accept Medicare and Medicaid funds must use a set of standardized forms to assess residents and to plan care. The guidelines are established by the federal government in the Omnibus Budget Rec-onciliation Act. Federal law requires that nursing facilities conduct a comprehensive assessment of each resident using standardized forms called the **Resident Assessment Instrument** (RAI). The state can require the use of the RAI specified by the Health Care Financing Administration (HCFA), or it can develop one of its own provided it receives approval from HCFA. The state must obtain approval from HCFA before using any instrument. All state-designed instruments must include the minimum data set of core elements, common defini-tions, and use guidelines specified by the HCFA.

DISPLAY 6-6. Examples of Significant Decline and Improvement in Function

Decline in functioning is evidenced by:
- Increased occurrence of behavior symptoms (eg, wandering, agitation)
- Decreased functional ability (eg, ability to perform activities of daily living)
- Unexplained weight loss of 5% in 30 days or 10% in 180 days
- Change in continence of bladder or bowel
- Decreased cognitive function
- Development or worsening of depression or anxiety
- Occurrence or worsening of pressure ulcers

Improvement in functioning is evidenced by:
- Increased ability to perform activities of daily living and to function within the environment
- Decreased severity or number of behavioral symptoms
- Increased cognitive function
- General improvement in physical or mental condition

DISPLAY 6-7. Areas of Assessment in the Minimum Data Set

- Identification information
- Customary routine
- Communication on hearing patterns
- Physical functioning
- Psychosocial well-being
- Activity patterns
- Health conditions
- Oral or dental status
- Medication use
- Background information
- Cognitive patterns
- Vision patterns
- Continence
- Mood and behavior problems
- Disease diagnoses
- Oral or nutritional status
- Skin condition
- Special treatments or procedures

Resident Assessment Instrument

The RAI is a comprehensive and standardized assessment tool composed of two distinct but related parts: the Minimum Data Set (MDS) and the Resident Assessment Protocols (RAP). The MDS is the information (ie, facts) about each resident that the nursing home personnel must gather. The RAP is the information provided to guide the personnel in assessing the resident. The same or similar format is used throughout the nation, providing a method of standardized written communication about the resident, problems, medications, history, and demographic data that can be used within facilities, between facilities, and other agencies.

According to HCFA, a RAI must be completed at the following times:

Within 14 days of the resident's admission

After a significant change in the resident's
    condition

At least once each year

A significant change in the resident's condition is defined as a change that does not resolve itself within a short time (usually 10 to 14 days) without intervention by the nursing staff. A significant change can be a decline in physical or mental function or an improvement in physical or mental function. Examples of a decline in function or an improvement in function are found in Display 6-6.

Any time a significant change occurs, a comprehensive assessment is performed, and adjustments are made in the care plan that reflect the change in status. Significant changes usually affect more than one area of the resident's health status and require review by the entire multidisciplinary team.

Quarterly Review

Every 3 months, a quarterly assessment is performed on each resident to ensure that the care being given reflects the current problems. The quarterly assessment is called the quarterly review and is a subset of items on the MDS.

Minimum Data Set

Included in the RAI is the MDS (Appendix E). Federal regulations defines MDS as "a core set of screening & assessment elements, including common definitions and coding categories that form the foundations of the comprehensive assessment for all residents of long-term care facilities certified to participate in Medicaid and Medicare." Areas to be examined or screened in the MDS are identified in Display 6-7.

Resident Assessment Protocols

Resident Assessment Protocols are the second part of the Resident Assessment Instrument. This portion of the forms helps to analyze the information obtained in the MDS to identify problems, potential problems, and the potential for improvement. Certain MDS items provide triggers to alert the nurse that additional evaluation is necessary. Examples of trigger areas include a change in cognitive status, visual function, behavioral symptoms, falls, and feeding tubes. Trigger worksheets provide links to the possible cause of a problem. For example, the RAP may link a change in the resident's mood to the use of a psychotropic drug. The RAPs help the nurse to obtain the entire picture of the resident and avoid missing factors important for care that could otherwise be easily overlooked.

Assessment

The MDS and the RAPs assist the nurse in determining the resident's needs. During the assessment, information about the resident's life, likes and dislikes, preferences, and functional abilities are obtained. The registered nurse coordinates the assessment process, obtaining information from the appropriate health care professional, nursing assistants, family members, and close friends. Most important is the information obtained from the resident through interviews, observation, and demonstration of abilities. The resident, the multidisciplinary team (including the nursing assistants), and the resident's family or close friends participate in the assessment process and in implementation.

The assessment provides the foundation for planning care. Nurses must remember that the MDS is a *minimum* data sheet, and a head to toe or systems physical assessment is also important to establish a baseline assessment, identify symptoms of disease or illness, and monitor for the development of adverse reactions to medications.

Care Planning Conference

A multidisciplinary care planning conference is used to develop the plan of care and to address individual resident needs. Ideally, the resident is the focus of the care planning conference. When residents and family members participate in developing a care plan, the results are a more comprehensive individualized care plan that focuses on what the resident feels is important. The resident and the family are informed ahead of time to make plans to attend and write down questions or concerns that need to be addressed. Residents and family members should be encouraged to take an active role in developing the plan of care. By becoming directly involved in the decisions concerning care, the plan can be more specific and individualized. Even residents with cognitive impairment or dementia should be encouraged to attend the care planning conference. Although their input may be limited, they may be able to indicate certain preferences.

The entire multidisciplinary team is involved in care planning. The physician, nurse, social worker, nursing assistant, dietitian, occupational therapist, physical therapist, and pharmacists are all part of the care planning team. Members of the team who are unable to attend are encouraged to submit their ideas or observations in writing. The care plan identifies needs or problems of the residents, sets a goal for each problem or need, and lists interventions to attain the goal. All information on the care plan is very specific, written in language that all members of the health care team can understand, and contains a timeframe for meeting the goal. Wording of identified problems in a nursing facility is often stated in terms of the problem or the need rather than as a nursing diagnosis.

Implementation and Evaluation

The evaluation process is ongoing on a daily basis. As changes occur or goals are met, the care plan is updated or changed to meet new needs or problems. A care planning conference is held any time an assessment is completed or any time a change occurs in the resident's condition that requires a multidisciplinary approach to developing a plan of care. In general, a care conference occurs at least every 3 months for each resident.

Regardless of whether care is given in a nursing facility (nursing home) or an acute care facility (hospital), the nursing process is the most efficient and effective method of planning and implementing care. The nursing process can be used in a formal way with all steps written and identified. At other times, a more informal approach is used, such as stating a problem or need rather than writing a specific NANDA-approved nursing diagnosis.

USING THE NURSING PROCESS TO DEVELOP A TEACHING PLAN

Patient and family teaching is an important component of gerontological nursing care. When health care needs are identified, nurses must be prepared to intervene. Sometimes, intervention is in the form of nursing care; at other times, intervention focuses on providing information that will enable others to care for themselves. Patient and family teaching may occur informally at the bedside or in an outpatient setting, such as a community center or an adult day care center. Formal teaching is done when learning needs are identified and teaching strategies are planned appropriate to the individual's learning needs. When planning a formal teaching session the nursing process provides an appropriate format.

Assessment

In assessing learning needs, the nurse must first identify what information needs to be taught. Does the patient have a newly diagnosed condition? Has a new medication been prescribed? Is the patient noncompliant with the present health care regimen?

After determining learning needs, the nurse assesses the individual's physical ability to learn. Age does not necessarily decrease the ability to learn new information unless a pathologic condition such as Alzheimer's disease or stroke is present. Changes in the elderly that may affect learning include decreased short-term memory, slowed mental functioning, and decreased reaction time. These changes may be accompanied by the presence of a chronic disease that contributes to a decreased ability to learn.

Assess the elderly for sensory changes. Sensory changes such as a loss of visual acuity or hearing loss affect the teaching method selected. If possible, include a family member or friend in the teaching session for all elderly people.

The patient's or family members' readiness to learn is assessed. Individuals must feel the need to learn or be motivated to learn before any teaching is effective. A person who denies the presence of a disease process or one who is in pain is not ready to learn. Determine the person's health beliefs and behaviors. An individual who does not believe the therapeutic regimen prescribed by the health care provider is appropriate will not comply with the regimen no matter how well the information is taught.

Nursing Diagnosis

The nursing diagnosis is formulated after analyzing the information obtained during the assessment phase. Nursing diagnoses associated with learning needs are identified in Display 6-8. Other nursing diagnoses may be appropriate for individual patients experiencing various learning needs.

DISPLAY 6-8. Nursing Diagnoses Associated With Learning Needs

- Ineffective Management of Therapeutic Regimen, related to complexity of therapeutic regimen, lack of knowledge, health belief conflicts, financial cost of regimen, side effects of therapy, other (specify)
- Knowledge Deficit (learning need), regarding condition, prognosis, treatment needs, other (specify)
- Noncompliance with Therapeutic Regimen, related to lack of knowledge of condition, medication regimen, other (specify)

Planning and Implementation

Because each patient is unique and has needs specific to her own situation, teaching plans are individualized. Examples of teaching strategies include lectures, group teaching, and demonstration and practice. Select the teaching strategy that is most appropriate based on the analysis of the assessment findings. Keep the sessions short, and provide frequent repetition of the information when teaching the elderly. When small amounts of information are presented at a time, learning is enhanced. Older adults require a slower pace to learn. The information presented must be relevant, with frequent feedback from the teacher (nurse) to reinforce learning. Allow sufficient time for demonstration and practice if a skill is taught. Be certain that the patient has the manual dexterity to perform a skill. For example, the elderly with arthritis may not be able to draw up insulin. Another individual may not have the visual acuity to see the markings on a syringe. In incidences such as these, specialized equipment may be obtained for the patient's use. For example, specialized insulin syringes are available for those with loss of visual acuity. If specialized equipment is not available, adjustments may be made that allow the patient to be involved in self-care.

Provide written information in an easy to read format for all individuals, if possible. Written information reinforces teaching and gives the patient and family a resource to refer when at home or when a health care provider is not present.

Make adjustments for sensory deprivation. For example, provide information sheets with large print for those with a loss of visual acuity. For the hearing impaired, use techniques to improve communication (eg, speak distinctly, face the person, use a low-pitched voice). Make sure the hearing aid, if used, is in good working order. Include family members in the teaching session when sensory deprivation is present.

The nurse may obtain teaching aides from various sources in the form of pamphlets, picture, films, or models. These can be used for teaching sessions or as reinforcement.

Evaluation

If teaching is successful, learning occurs, and a change is behavior is seen. This change is evidenced by improved health, compliance with the health care regimen, or an increase in knowledge. Evaluation is done by talking with the patient, observing changes in health care behavior, or observing a return demonstration. If no changes occur, the process begins again with an assessment of the situation.

CRITICAL THINKING EXERCISES

1. Mr. Thompson, age 78, is a non–insulin-dependent diabetic. He states that he becomes short of breath when walking and has fallen twice in the past week. He appears very anxious and states he is a "nervous wreck." His vital signs include a temperature of 99°F, respiration rate of 28, pulse of 100, and blood pressure of 170/84. His skin feels warm and dry to the touch, except for the lower extremities, which are cool to the touch. Divide the data into subjective and objective data. After analyzing the data, name at least two diagnoses that can be used in planning Mr. Thompson's care. What additional assessments need to be made? How would these assessments help you in planning care?

2. Ms. Galvan, age 87, is a resident in a nursing home. The results of a recent assessment indicate that Ms. Galvan has begun to wander in the evenings. She is confused and has difficulty understanding simple commands. She persistently seeks attention and reassurance from the nursing staff. In developing Ms. Galvan's care plan, what problems can you immediately identify? What additional assessments may give more information concerning Ms. Galvan's behavior? Name some possible nursing interventions for the problems identified.

3. Select a patient that you have cared for who has a learning need. Used the nursing process format to develop a teaching plan for this patient.

REFERENCES AND SUGGESTED READING

Allen, J. (1997). *Long Term Care Facility Resident Assessment Instrument User's Manual* New York: Springer Publishers.

Alfaro, R. (1997). *Applying Nursing Process: A Step-by-Step Guide* (4th ed.). Philadelphia: Lippincott Williams & Wilkins.

Bickley, L., & Hoekelman, R. (1999). *Bates' Guide to Physical Examination and History Taking* (7th ed.). Philadelphia: Lippincott Williams & Wilkins.

Carpenito, L.J. (1999). *Nursing Diagnosis: Application to Clinical Practice* (8th ed.). Philadelphia: Lippincott Williams & Wilkins.

CHAPTER 7

CHAPTER OUTLINE

KEY TERMS
CHAPTER OBJECTIVES
WHY A FUNCTIONAL ASSESSMENT IS NECESSARY
DEFINITION OF FUNCTIONAL ASSESSMENT
COMPONENTS OF A FUNCTIONAL ASSESSMENT
    Physical Health Assessment
    Health History
    Self-Care Assessment
    Katz Index
    PULSES Profile and the Barthel Index
PSYCHOLOGICAL ASSESSMENT
    Cognitive Functioning
    Folstein Mini-Mental State Examination
    Affective Function
    Beck Depression Inventory
    Social Assessment
CONCLUDING THE FUNCTIONAL ASSESSMENT
CRITICAL THINKING EXERCISES
REFERENCES AND SUGGESTED READING

KEY TERMS

affective function
cognitive function
functional assessment

Performing a Functional Assessment

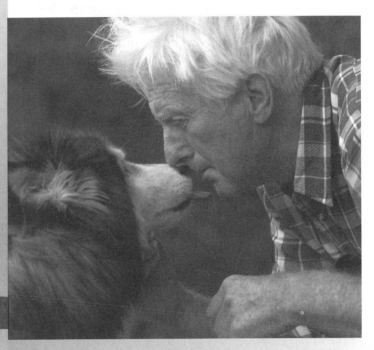

CHAPTER OBJECTIVES

At the completion of this chapter, the student will be able to

- **Define functional assessment**

- **Describe the importance of a functional assessment**

- **Discuss the components of a physical health assessment, a self-care assessment, a psychological assessment, and a social assessment**

A functional assessment is used to evaluate the overall health and well-being of the older adult. The major emphasis is on how well the older adult functions within the environment. The functional assessment is important for the nurse in planning the care of the elderly patient. Without a good functional assessment, the older adult may not obtain the health care needed or may receive more help than is necessary. Unnecessary or unneeded health care can foster dependency or be financially devastating to individuals on a fixed income.

WHY A FUNCTIONAL ASSESSMENT IS NECESSARY

The functional assessment identifies the self-care abilities and deficits of the older adult in order for needs to be matched with services. For example, if the elderly client is functionally unable to cook meals, a method of providing meals, such as Meals on Wheels, must be made available. If the elderly client is unable to perform any self-care, provisions must be made to see that care is obtained, such as providing a care giver or admittance to a nursing home. Display 7-1 identifies important uses of the information obtained from the functional assessment.

DEFINITION OF FUNCTIONAL ASSESSMENT

A **functional assessment** is a systematic method of evaluating the older adult's ability to function within the environment. There are many standardized functional assessment tools to assist the nurse with this assessment. This chapter discusses several tools used to assess the individual's functional ability such as the Katz Index of Activities of Daily Living, the Folstein Mini-Mental State Examination, the PLUSES Profile, the Barthel Index, Beck Depression Inventory, and the Social Dysfunction Scale.

The most widely used functional assessment tool is a tool developed by the federal government called the Minimum Data Set for Nursing Home Resident Assessment and Care Screening (MDS) (see Chapter 6). This tool is a comprehensive assessment that assesses the patient's physical, mental, social, and psychosocial function. The MDS must be used in all nursing homes that receive federal funding. This includes all facilities who care for patients on Medicare and Medicaid. Most facilities use this standardized form for all patients. Some states have developed their own forms to supplement the MDS. These forms must be approved by the federal government before use.

DISPLAY 7-1. Important Uses of Functional Assessment Findings

- Acquisition of a database to use as a basis for comparison
- Identification of individual patient needs
- Identification of specific self-care deficits
- Providing a foundation to develop an individualized care plan
- Providing data for referral to special services to promote independent health care, day care, or housekeeping services to promote independent living
- Providing a means to evaluate treatment and rehabilitation

According to the Omnibus Budget Reconciliation Acts (OBRA), a federal law that establishes guidelines for nursing homes, the MDS must be completed within 14 days of admission to a nursing facility. OBRA also requires that the entire assessment be revised when a significant change in a resident's mental or physical condition occurs. The practical nurse is the licensed health care provider who has the most contact with the resident and must continually assess and evaluate the resident for any change in condition.

COMPONENTS OF A FUNCTIONAL ASSESSMENT

Assessment of the older adult is challenging. The older adult is unique because she has had many years and experiences in which to develop her own distinctiveness. A functional assessment allows identification of particular qualities in each individual that affect the ability to function in the environment and perform activities of daily living (ADLs). The importance of an accurate functional assessment cannot be overemphasized. The functional assessment has four basic components: physical health assessment, self-care assessment, psychological assessment, and social assessment.

Physical Health Assessment

The goal of the physical health assessment is to determine the overall health and fitness of the gerontological client. The health history obtained provides much of the information needed for this portion of the functional assessment.

When an older person is admitted to the nursing home or extended care facility, the nurse performs the admission interview to obtain the overall health history. When interviewing the older person, the nurse must allow more time for the interview because the health history spans more than 50 years. More time is required because the older adult's responses are slower as a result of age-related changes. The nurse should remember that the events of the health history may not be regarded as important, and the older adult therefore may not mention certain health problems. Perhaps the client has adapted to the problem or the event was so long ago that it has been forgotten. The nurse may need to validate information from the interview with a family member or significant other.

The health assessment is obtained as soon after admittance to the facility as possible, usually within the first few hours. Topics addressed include disease conditions, medical diagnoses, handicaps, medications prescribed, and type and amount of medical services used in the past several years. Any history of heart disease, vascular disease, respiratory disease, neurologic disease (eg, dementia), or cancer is noted. A functional assessment tool selected by the facility such as the MDS may be used as a guide to obtain the needed information.

Health History

The health history is obtained as part of a planned interview to determine the person's overall health. There are numerous health history formats to guide the nurse in the interview. Questions in Display 7-2 may be used as a guide when interviewing the patient to obtain information for the health history. These types of questions can provide a framework for gaining information about the overall health of the elderly person.

Self-Care Assessment

The self-care (ie, functional status) assessment tells the nurse how well the older person is able to care for himself (ie, perform ADLs) in his environment. It identifies what self-care activities could be performed before entering the facility and how much help, if any, was needed in performing self-care activities.

Nursing facilities sometimes foster dependence. In an effort to complete tasks such as eating, bathing, or toileting, nursing assistants and sometimes nurses provide residents with more assistance in ADLs than is needed. Using a wheelchair for ambulatory residents, feeding residents who can feed themselves, and bathing residents who can bathe themselves can create dependence. The nurse must encourage the nurse assistant to provide an unhurried atmosphere that allows the elderly resident time to perform these tasks. "Doing for" the resident rather than allowing the resident to "do for himself" results in decreasing the levels of functional ability. A self-care assessment allows those involved in the care of the older adult to have a baseline assessment of functional ability for comparison. Any deterioration of function can then be identified in a timely manner.

Katz Index

One method of assessing function is to use the Katz Index of Activities of Daily Living (Display 7-3). This assessment provides a baseline from which goals can be set and improvement measured. There are six basic areas included in the self-care assessment:

Bathing
Dressing
Toileting
Transfer
Continence
Feeding

When using the Katz Index to assess self-care or functional ability, *independence* means without supervision or personal assistance. The person is scored according to the performance of the activity. Any patient who refuses to perform a self-care activity is considered dependent, even if he appears to have the ability. As with any assessment, the ability to perform self-care activities and any limitations must be carefully documented.

These activities are listed in a hierarchy. The higher-level functional skills include bathing, dressing, and toileting. Feeding is the most basic of the functional abilities. This is the ability that is learned first as a child and the functional ability that is generally lost last. Bathing, dressing, and toileting are the higher skills lost first as the individual declines in functional ability.

Bathing

In evaluating the ability of the older person to bathe, shower, or take a sponge bath, the amount of assistance needed is considered. If the person requires no assistance (ie, gets in and out of the bath tub or shower without help or is able to give herself a sponge bath), the person is considered independent in bathing. If assistance is needed for only one body part, such as the back, or if assistance is needed

---

DISPLAY 7-2. **Guidelines for Obtaining a Health History**

General Instructions
- General requests for information may prompt a discussion of health information, making some or all of the following questions unnecessary.
- Social, cultural, developmental, and educational levels are assessed throughout the interview.
- During the interview note the individual's openness and readiness to learn.

I. Current Health
Suggested opening statement: "Please tell me about your current health."
- How would you describe your general health?
- Do you have any chronic problems, such as diabetes, high blood pressure, arthritis, or heart disease?
- Have you had any weight loss or gain within last year? Within the last several weeks?
- Do you have any pain, unusual sensations, or lack of sensation?
- Do you have any cough, shortness of breath, other trouble breathing? Do you cough up any sputum? If yes, describe the sputum.
- Do you have any headaches, dizziness, weakness, fainting spells, or excessive sweating?
- Do you have any swelling?
- Are there any discharges or drainage from anywhere?
- Does your heart ever race, pound, skip a beat, or have any other unusual sensations?
- Tell me all the medications you take, including prescription, over-the-counter, or home remedies.

II. Past Health
Suggested opening statement: "It would help in planning your care if you tell me about your past health."
- Were you immunized, (given shots or vaccinated) for any disease?
- Have you had a tetanus vaccination?
- What childhood diseases did you have? Examples are measles and chickenpox.
- As an adult, what illnesses have you had that came and went, such as pneumonia or blood clots?
- Were you ever treated for any mental problems, such as depression?
- What surgeries have you had?

- Did you ever injure yourself and then receive treatment? Do you ever fall?
- Were you ever in the hospital for any reason?
- Have you ever had an allergic reaction to medicine, such as penicillin? Do you have any other allergies?

III. General Health Habits
Suggested opening statement: "Please tell me about your general health habits."
- Are you on a special diet? What food do you normally eat?
- Do you have any problem eating, such as trouble swallowing or have nausea or vomiting after eating?
- Do you drink caffeinated beverages such as coffee, tea, or carbonated drinks?
- How many glasses of water do you drink in 1 day?
- How many hours do you usually sleep at night?
- Do you take naps? Do you have any problems sleeping? What type of sleeping problems?
- What are your bowel habits? Do you use laxatives, suppositories, or enemas? Do you ever have diarrhea?
- Tell me about your bladder habits. Do you urinate often during the day? How much do you urinate? Small amounts or fairly large amounts? Do you have any problems urinating? Do you get up at night to go to the bathroom?
- What type of exercise do you engage in? How often do you exercise?
- Do you drink any alcoholic beverages? If so, what kind and how often?
- Do you smoke? If so, what and how often?
- Do you wear glasses, a hearing aid, or dentures? Describe hearing loss and any vision loss.
- Do you use a cane, crutches, or walker?
- Tell me about your memory.

IV. Nursing Focus
Suggested opening statement: "Please tell me about your needs."
- What are your strengths? Your weaknesses?
- What concerns do you have?
- What questions can I answer for you?
- What kinds of help do you need?
- What could the nursing staff do to be the most helpful to you?

Adapted from Smeltzer, S., & Bare, B. (1996). *Brunner and Suddarth's Textbook of Medical and Surgical Nursing* (8th ed.). Philadelphia: Lippincott-Raven, 30.

---

with the entire bath or shower, the person is considered dependent.

Dressing
An elderly person who is able to obtain clothing and personal items from closets and drawers and can completely dress herself is considered independent.

Dressing independently includes the ability to manage buttons, zippers, fasteners, braces, prosthesis, shoes, and other items required in getting dressed.

Toileting
Independent toileting involves the ability to get to the toilet, get on and off the toilet, and to clean one-

DISPLAY 7-3. Katz Index of Activities of Daily Living (ADL)

Independence means without supervision, direction, or active personal assistance, except as specifically noted below. This is based on actual status and not ability. A patient who refuses to perform a function is considered as not performing the function, even though he or she is deemed able.

Bathing (Sponge, shower, or tub)
Independent: assistance only in bathing a single part (back or disabled extremity) or bathes self completely
Dependent: assistance in bathing more than one part of body; assistance in getting in or out of tub; does not bathe self

Dressing
Independent: gets clothes from closets and drawers; puts on clothes, outer garments, braces; manages fasteners; act of tying shoes is excluded
Dependent: does not dress self or remains partly undressed

Going to Toilet
Independent: gets to toilet; gets on and off toilet; arranges clothes, cleans organs of excretion (may manage own bedpan used at night only and may or may not be using mechanical supports)

Dependent: uses bedpan or commode or receives assistance in getting to and using toilet

Transfer
Independent: moves in and out of bed and in and out of chair independently (may or may not be using mechanical supports)
Dependent: assistance in moving in or out of bed and/or chair; does not perform one or more transfers

Continence
Independent: urination and defecation entirely self-controlled
Dependent: partial or total incontinence in urination or defecation; partial or total control by enemas, catheters, or regulated use of urinals and/or bedpans

Feeding
Independent: gets food from plate or its equivalent into mouth (precutting of meat and preparation of food, as buttering bread, are excluded from evaluation)
Dependent: assistance in act of feeding (see above); does not eat at all or parenteral feeding

Evaluation Form

Name _____ Date of Evaluation _____

For each area of functioning listed below, circle description that applies (the word "assistance" means supervision, direction, or personal assistance).

Bathing—sponge bath, tub bath, or shower
Receives no assistance (gets in and out of tub by self if tub is usual means of bathing)
Receives assistance in bathing only one part of body (eg, back or a leg)
Receives assistance in bathing more than one part of body (or does not bathe self)

Dressing—gets clothes from closets and drawers; puts on clothes, including underclothes and outer garments; manages fasteners (including braces, if worn)
Gets clothes and gets completely dressed without assistance
Gets clothes and gets dressed without assistance except for tying shoes
Receives assistance in getting clothes or in getting dressed or stays partly or completely undressed

Toileting—going to the "toilet room" for bowel and urine elimination; cleaning self after elimination and arranging clothes
Goes to "toilet room," cleans self, and arranges clothes without assistance (may use object for support such as cane, walker, or wheelchair and may manage night bedpan or commode, emptying same in morning)

Receives assistance in going to "toilet room" or in cleansing self or in arranging clothes after elimination or in use of night bedpan or commode
Does not go to room termed "toilet" for the elimination process

Transfer
Moves in and out of bed and in and out of chair without assistance (may use object for support such as cane or walker)
Moves in or out of bed or chair with assistance
Does not get out of bed

Continence
Controls urination and bowel movement completely by self
Has occasional "accidents"
Supervision helps keep urine or bowel control; catheter is used or is incontinent

Feeding
Feeds self without assistance
Feeds self except for getting assistance in cutting meat or buttering bread
Receives assistance in feeding or is fed partly or completely by tubes or intravenous fluids

From Katz S., Ford, A.B., Moskowitz, R.S., et al. (1963). Studies of illness in the aged. The index of ADL: A standardized measure of biological and psychosocial function. *Journal of the American Medical Association* 185, 914–918.

self afterward. Canes, wheelchairs, or walkers are sometimes used to assist the elderly person in independent toileting. The elderly person is considered dependent if assistance is required with any activity involved in toileting, including re-dressing.

Transfer

Independent transfer includes moving in and out of the bed and chair without assistance from another individual or nurse. Mechanical supports such as canes or walkers may be used to enhance independence. The person is considered dependent if any assistance is needed in transferring.

Continence

Continence means that urination and bowel function are completely self-controlled. The elderly person is considered dependent if partially incontinent or control is maintained with the use of a catheter or other device. Observe the extent of the incontinent episodes, such as only occasional accidents or total incontinence. The person may be incontinent of bowel or bladder or both.

Feeding

The ability of the person to feed herself is considered independent when she can get the food from the plate to the mouth without assistance. The ability to cut food in preparation for eating, buttering bread, opening milk cartons, or other activities involved in setting up the food is not considered in determining functional ability. The person is considered dependent when she is unable to feed herself or when feeding is accomplished partially or completely through tubes.

Using the Katz Index

The Katz Index of ADL uses the six functions listed to determine functional ability. The functions are scored according to the person's actual perform of the functions rather than the person's ability to perform the functions. One point is given for each dependent function. For each function, an intermediary description is given. This intermediary abilities are designated as independent for some functions and independent for other functions. The index can be used to evaluate change and as indicators for the need for nursing home care. The higher the total score the greater the loss of function.

PULSES Profile and the Barthel Index

The PULSES Profile (Display 7-4) and Barthel Index (Table 7-1) assessment tools are also available to assess functional ability. These tools measure physical capabilities that the person can and cannot do and how much assistance the elderly person needs. Display 7-5 explains the meaning of the PULSES acronym.

The best possible score is 6, and the worst score is 24. A score of 16 or more indicates severe disability. The PULSES Profile gives an overview of mobility, self-care, and psychosocial functioning. The PULSES Profile can be used to monitor changes in function.

The Barthel Index focuses on self-care abilities in areas that range from drinking from a cup to controlling bowel movements and a person's mobility. A score of 100 is the maximum possible score and indicates independence in all items listed. Areas of judgment and cognitive function are not assessed, and problems in these areas may prohibit the elderly person from living alone. Scores less than 60 indicate the need for assistance in a significant number of activities. Individuals with scores below 60 may need to be in a nursing facility. The Barthel Index and the PULSES Profile are used in conjunction with other assessments to help determine functional ability and the amount of assistance needed.

PSYCHOLOGICAL ASSESSMENT

Psychological assessment determines the function of the mind. The two areas assessed are cognitive (mental) functioning and affective (emotional) functioning. **Cognitive functioning** estimates how well the mind works in areas such as orientation, memory, concentration, and judgment. **Affective function** describes the emotional feelings or mood of the person.

Cognitive Functioning

The most basic cognitive function assessed is orientation. Often, nurses document that the patient is "oriented" or "oriented × 3," which means oriented to person, place, and time. However, nurses must be aware that statements such as these concerning orientation do not necessarily mean that cognitive function is intact. Patients may have a vague awareness of who and where they are and the date, but they have a cognitive deficit in concentration or judgment.

Accurate cognitive assessment is particularly important when done as part of a functional

DISPLAY 7-4. PULSES Profile*

P—Physical condition: includes diseases of the viscera (cardiovascular, gastrointestinal, urologic, and endocrine) and neurologic disorders:
1. Medical problems sufficiently stable that medical or nursing monitoring is not required more often than 3-month intervals
2. Medical or nurse monitoring is needed more often than 3-month intervals but not each week
3. Medical problems are sufficiently unstable as to require regular medical and/or nursing attention at least weekly
4. Medical problems require intensive medical and/or nursing attention at least daily (excluding personal care assistance only)

U—Upper limb functions: self-care activities (drink/feed, dress upper/lower, brace/prosthesis, groom, wash, perineal care) dependent mainly on upper limb function:
1. Independent in self-care without impairment of upper limbs
2. Independent in self-care with some impairment of upper limbs
3. Dependent on assistance or supervision in self-care with or without impairment of upper limbs
4. Dependent totally in self-care with marked impairment of upper limbs

L—Lower limb functions: mobility (transfer chair/toilet/tub or shower, walk, stairs, wheelchair) dependent mainly on lower limb function:
1. Independent in mobility without impairment of lower limbs
2. Independent in mobility with some impairment in lower limbs, such as needing ambulatory aids, a brace, or prosthesis, or else fully independent in a wheelchair without significant architectural or environmental barriers
3. Dependent on assistance or supervision in mobility with or without impairment of lower limbs, or partly independent in a wheelchair or when there are significant architectural or environmental barriers
4. Dependent totally in mobility with marked impairment of lower limbs

S—Sensory components: relating to communication (speech and hearing) and vision:
1. Independent in communication and vision without impairment
2. Independent in communication and vision with some impairment such as mild dysarthria, mild aphasia, or need for eyeglasses or hearing aid, or regular eye medication
3. Dependent on assistance, an interpreter, or supervision in communication or vision
4. Dependent totally in communication or vision

E—Excretory functions (bladder and bowel):
1. Complete voluntary control of bladder and bowel sphincters
2. Control of sphincters allows normal social activities despite urgency or need for catheter, appliance, or suppositories; able to care for needs without assistance
3. Dependent on assistance in sphincter management or else has accidents occasionally
4. Frequent wetting or soiling from incontinence of bladder or bowel sphincters

S—Support factors: consider intellectual and emotional adaptability, support from family unit, and financial ability
1. Able to fulfill usual roles and perform customary tasks
2. Must make some modification in usual roles and performance of customary tasks
3. Dependent on assistance, supervision, encouragement, or assistance from a public or private agency because of any of the above considerations
4. Dependent on long-term institutional care (eg, chronic hospitalization, nursing home) excluding time-limited hospital for specific evaluation, treatment, or active rehabilitation

*PULSES total: best score is 6, worst score is 24.
From Granger, C.V., Albrecht, G.L., & Hamilton, B.B. (1979). Outcome of comprehensive medical rehabilitation: Measures of PULSES profile and the Barthel index. *Archives of Physical Medicine and Rehabilitation* 60, 145–154.

assessment. Cognitive dysfunction may be manifested by confusion, disorientation, generalized slowing of intellectual activity, or difficulty with abstract thinking. If a cognitive deficit is determined, some home support and supervision may be needed at least part of each day from family, friends, or through visits from a nurse with a home health care agency.

Reasoning, memory, and judgment can be assessed through direct questioning requiring specific answers.

Reasoning is assessed by asking for the interpretation of a proverb (ie, common saying expressing a truth) such as "the early bird catches the worm" or "a stitch in time saves nine." Evaluate distant memory by asking questions about well-known past events or about well-known people, such as "What is the name of the president who was assassinated in Dallas, Texas?" Assess recent memory with questions such as "What did you have for lunch today or supper last night?"

TABLE 7-1. Barthel Index With Corresponding Values for Independent Performance of Tasks*

Index	"Can Do By Myself"	"Can Do With Help of Someone Else"	"Cannot Do at All"
SELF-CARE INDEX			
1. Drinking from a cup	4	0	0
2. Eating	6	0	0
3. Dressing upper body	5	3	0
4. Dressing lower body	7	4	0
5. Putting on brace or artificial limb	0	−2	0 (not applicable)
6. Grooming	5	0	0
7. Washing or bathing	6	0	0
8. Controlling urination	10	5 (accidents)	0 (incontinent)
9. Controlling bowel movements	10	5 (accidents)	0 (incontinent)
MOBILITY INDEX			
10. Getting in and out of chair	15	7	0
11. Getting on and off toilet	6	3	0
12. Getting in and out of tub or shower	1	0	0
13. Walking 50 yards on the level	15	10	0
14. Walking up/down one flight of stairs	10	5	0
15. If not walking: propelling or pushing wheelchair	5	0	0 (not applicable)

*Barthel total: best score is 100; worst score is 0.
From Granger, C.V., Albrecht, G.L., & Hamilton, B.B. (1979). Outcome of comprehensive medical rehabilitation: Measures of PULSES profile and the Barthel index. *Archives of Physical Medicine and Rehabilitation* 60:145–154.

DISPLAY 7-5. PULSES Acronym

Physical condition
Upper limbs
Lower limbs
Sensory components
Excretory function
Support factors

Assessment of the ability of the elderly person to make sensible or sound judgments is done by asking one or more questions that require a decision. Questions such as "If a pan of grease catches fire in the kitchen, what would you do?" or "If you have no car for transportation, what would you do to obtain groceries?" are examples of questions that test judgment. Other methods to test cognitive function involves asking the older person to solve simple mathematical calculations, requiring the writing of a sentence or having the person recall a set of words given by the tester.

Folstein Mini-Mental State Examination

The Folstein Mini-Mental State Examination (Display 7-6) evaluates orientation, registration, attention and calculation, recall, and language. The maximum score is 30. Scores are evaluated in the following manner:

24–30: no cognitive impairment
18–23: mild cognitive impairment
0–17: severe cognitive impairment

Additional methods of evaluating cognitive ability may be needed for certain individuals. For example, educational levels below the eighth grade may produce an inaccurate result because accurate evaluation requires at least an eighth grade level of education. Cultural background, visual impairment, and age may also result in some individuals being misidentified as cognitively impaired. However, overall, the Folstein Mini-Mental State Examination is considered a very reliable method to determine cognitive functioning.

Affective Functioning

Affective functioning is the second part of psychological function. In assessing affective or emotional functioning, the nurse determines whether the elderly person's emotional state seems appropriate with the life situation. The nurse should be especially alert for depression or self-destructive thoughts or behavior.

DISPLAY 7-6. The Mini-Mental State Examination

Patient _____   Examiner _____   Date _____

Maximum Score	Score	
		ORIENTATION
5	( )	What is the (year) (season) (date) (day) (month)?
5	( )	Where are we (state) (county or neighborhood) (town) (hospital) (floor)?
		REGISTRATION
3	( )	Name 3 objects: 1 second to say each. Then ask the patient all 3 after you have said them.
		Give 1 point for each correct answer. Then repeat them until he/she learns all 3.
		Count trials and record.
		Trials _____
		ATTENTION AND CALCULATION
5	( )	Serial 7s. 1 point for each correct answer. Stop after 5 answers. If the patient refuses to *attempt* serial 7s, spell "world" backward.
		RECALL
3	( )	Ask for the 3 objects repeated above. Give 1 point for each correct answer.
		LANGUAGE
2	( )	Name a pencil and watch. (2 points)
1	( )	Repeat the following "No ifs, ands, or buts." (1 point)
3	( )	Follow a 3-stage command:
		"Take a paper in your hand, fold it in half, and put it on the floor." (3 points)
1	( )	Read and obey the following:
		CLOSE YOUR EYES. (1 point)
1	( )	Write a sentence. (1 point)
1	( )	Copy design. (1 point)
____		Total Score
		ASSESS level of consciousness along a continuum _____
		Alert Drowsy Stupor Coma

From Folstein, M.E., Folstein, S.E., & McHugh, P.R. (1975). Mini-mental state: A practical method for grading the cognitive state of patients for the clinician. *Journal of Psychiatric Research* 12, 189–198.

Depression is thought to be significantly underreported in the elderly population. Considering the losses and changes that come about with advancing age, it is easy to see how depression develops. Because some of the symptoms of depression are similar to dementia, a careful assessment is essential. Symptoms of depression include a loss of interest in life, a negative self-image, guilt, remorse, and a pessimistic attitude. A depressed person can be confused, have decreased cognitive function, or use poor judgment. Problems with sleep patterns (ie, sleeping too much or the inability to sleep) and eating problems (ie, not eating or overeating) are common in persons with depression. Depression can cause fatigue, headaches, or constipation. Certain types of statements indicate depression:

"I feel the future is hopeless."

"I feel like a complete failure."

"I hate myself."

"I am just too tired to do anything."

Somatic complaints such as anorexia or constipation are more common in the elderly and may not be the result of depression. Careful documentation of the psychological assessment (see Chapter 8) is important. If symptoms of depression are apparent, the elderly person may need counseling, antidepressant drugs, or psychotherapy. A more complete discussion of depression is found in Chapter 15.

DISPLAY 7-7. Beck Depression Inventory, Short Form

Instructions: This is a questionnaire. On the questionnaire are groups of statements. Please read the entire group of statements in each category. Then pick out the one statement in that group that best describes the way you feel today, that is, *right now!* Circle the number beside the statement you have chosen. If several statements in the group seem to apply equally well, circle each one.

Be sure to read all the statements in each group before making your choice.

A. (Sadness)
3 I am so sad or unhappy that I can't stand it.
2 I am blue or sad all the time and I can't snap out of it.
1 I feel sad or blue.
0 I do not feel sad.

B. (Pessimism)
3 I feel that the future is hopeless and that things cannot improve.
2 I feel I have nothing to look forward to.
1 I feel discouraged about the future.
0 I am not particularly pessimistic or discouraged about the future.

C. (Sense of failure)
3 I feel I am a complete failure as a person (parent, husband, wife).
2 As I look back on my life, all I can see is a lot of failures.
1 I feel I have failed more than the average person.
0 I do not feel like a failure.

D. (Dissatisfaction)
3 I am dissatisfied with everything.
2 I don't get satisfaction out of anything anymore.
1 I don't enjoy things the way I used to.
0 I am not particularly dissatisfied.

E. (Guilt)
3 I feel as though I am very bad or worthless.
2 I feel quite guilty.
1 I feel bad or unworthy a good part of the time.
0 I don't feel particularly guilty.

F. (Self-dislike)
3 I hate myself.
2 I am disgusted with myself.
1 I am disappointed in myself.
0 I don't feel disappointed in myself.

G. (Self-harm)
3 I would kill myself if I had the chance.
2 I have definite plans about committing suicide.
1 I feel I would be better off dead.
0 I don't have any thought of harming myself.

H. (Social withdrawal)
3 I have lost all of my interest in other people and don't care about them at all.
2 I have lost most of my interest in other people and have little feeling for them.
1 I am less interested in other people than I used to be.
0 I have not lost interest in other people.

I. (Indecisiveness)
3 I can't make any decisions at all anymore.
2 I have great difficulty in making decisions.
1 I try to put off making decisions.
0 I make decisions about as well as ever.

J. (Self-image change)
3 I Feel that I am ugly or repulsive-looking.
2 I feel that there are permanent changes in my appearance and they make me look unattractive.
1 I am worried that I am looking old or unattractive.
0 I don't feel that I look any worse than I used to.

K. (Work difficulty)
3 I can't do any work at all.
2 I have to push myself very hard to do anything.
1 It takes extra effort to get started at doing something.
0 I can work about as well as before.

L. [Fatigability]
3 I get too tired to do anything.
2 I get tired from doing anything.
1 I get tired more easily than I used to.
0 I don't get any more tired than usual.

M. (Anorexia)
3 I have no appetite at all anymore.
2 My appetite is much worse now.
1 My appetite is not as good as it used to be.
0 My appetite is no worse than usual.

Scoring: 0–4 = None or minimal depression
5–7 = Mild depression
8–15 = Moderate depression
16 + = Severe depression

From Beck, A.T., Ward, C.H., Mendelson, M., et al. (1961). An inventory for measuring depression. *Archives of General Psychiatry* 4, 561–571.

Beck Depression Inventory

The Beck Depression Inventory (Display 7-7) is a 13-item assessment to determine mood, self-esteem, and any physical symptoms the individual is experiencing. A score of 16 or higher indicates severe depression. The inventory can be administered by the nurse or self-administered and requires less than 10 minutes to complete.

Social Assessment

Assessment of social functioning reveals how well the individual is functioning within the environment. Social aspects assessed include the various social groups (eg, church groups, clubs, neighbors, volunteer agencies) that the individual belongs to and the support that is received from these groups. Areas of importance include frequency and number

DISPLAY 7-8. Social Dysfunction Rating Scale

Directions: Score each of the items as follows:
1. Not present
2. Very mild
3. Mild
4. Moderate
5. Severe
6. Very severe

SELF-ESTEEM

1. _____ Low self-concept (feelings of inadequacy, not measuring up to self-ideal)
2. _____ Goallessness (lack of inner motivation and sense of future orientation)
3. _____ Lack of a satisfying philosophy or meaning of life (a conceptual framework for integrating past and present experiences)
4. _____ Self-health concern (preoccupation with physical health, somatic concerns)

INTERPERSONAL SYSTEM

5. _____ Emotional withdrawal (degree of deficiency in relating to others)
6. _____ Hostility (degree of aggression toward others)
7. _____ Manipulation (exploiting of environment, controlling at other's expense)
8. _____ Overdependency (degree of parasitic attachment to others)

9. _____ Anxiety (degree of feeling of uneasiness, impending doom)
10. _____ Suspiciousness (degree of distrust or paranoid ideation)

PERFORMANCE SYSTEM

11. _____ Lack of satisfying relationships with significant persons (spouse, children, kin, significant persons serving in a family role)
12. _____ Lack of friends, social contacts
13. _____ Expressed need for more friends, social contacts
14. _____ Lack of work (remunerative or nonremunerative, productive work activities) that normally give a sense of usefulness, status, confidence
15. _____ Lack of satisfaction from work
16. _____ Lack of leisure time activities
17. _____ Expressed need for more leisure, self-enhancing and satisfying activities
18. _____ Lack of participation in community activities
19. _____ Lack of interest in community affairs and activities that influence others
20. _____ Financial insecurity
21. _____ Adaptive rigidity (lack of complex coping patterns to stress)

Patient: _____ Rater: _____ Date: _____

From Linn, M.W., Sculthorpe, W.B., Evje, M., et al. (1969). A social dysfunction rating scale. *Journal of Psychiatric Research* 6, 299–306.

of social contacts, amount of support offered, and types of support offered (ie, emotional or financial). All social groups do not provide the same amount of kind of support. Adequate social support helps the elderly person face stressors, provides emotional support, and offers an avenue for enjoyment and activity.

When doing a social functioning assessment, question the elderly person about the number of social contacts within the past week, the type of support from those contacts, who they could call on for help if needed, and how often they visit their family. Social relationships should be fairly satisfying, and the elderly should be able to identify at least one person who would care for them indefinitely.

Display 7-8 gives an example of the Social Dysfunctioning Rating Scale, which is a 21-item scale with each item receiving a score from 1 to 6 points, depending on the amount of dysfunction observed. This scale requires subjective interpretation and is best done by one who is familiar with the scale. The Social Dysfunctioning Rating Scale is helpful in identifying individuals dealing with personal, interpersonal, and geographic environments in a mal-

adaptive manner. The scale is useful in assessing the need for treatment change or as a measure of social dysfunction. Because social networks change often assessment of social functioning is repeated often, particularly if the older adult is faced with a particularly stressful situation.

CONCLUDING THE FUNCTIONAL ASSESSMENT

After the four areas of physical health, self-care, psychological functioning, and social functioning have been assessed, careful documentation is made of all areas. Specific deficiencies in any area are noted. Any information that appears to be inconsistent must be clarified and validated with a spouse, family member, or friend. This information provides a foundation for planning care of patients admitted to nursing homes, extended care facilities, or acute care settings. The information obtained also provides baseline data to use for comparison in the days, weeks, and months ahead. When there is a change in the functional status document, report the change, and follow the institutional protocol for reassessment. Functional assessment tools are useful in assisting with the assessment, but their value must be carefully determined within the patient's total environment or situation.

In addition to a functional assessment, a nursing physical assessment is done. Chapter 6 provides an overview of the nursing physical assessment. Specific aspects of the physical assessment related to the older adult are included in the chapters pertaining to body systems.

CRITICAL THINKING EXERCISES

1. Perform a functional assessment on an elderly person. After completing the assessment document your findings. Identify three nursing diagnoses based on the data from your assessment.
2. Explain why simply asking someone to name the date, time, and place is not necessarily a good method of determining an elderly person's orientation. Give an example of how determining orientation by only asking the individual to name the date, time, and place could cause a problem.

REFERENCES AND SUGGESTED READING

Dubin, S. (1998). The Mini-Mental state exam. *American Journal of Nursing, 98 (11)*, 16D.

Leslie, J. (1998). Current functional assessment tools. *Home Healthcare Nurse, 16 (11)*, 766.

O'Hanlon-Nichols, T. (1998). Basic assessment series. *American Journal of Nursing, 98 (6)*, 48.

Restrepo, A. (1999). The Katz activities of daily living scale. *American Journal of Nursing, 99 (1)*, 24BB.

CHAPTER **8**

CHAPTER OUTLINE

KEY TERMS
CHAPTER OBJECTIVES
PSYCHOSOCIAL DEVELOPMENT
PSYCHOSOCIAL ASSESSMENT
IMPACT OF CULTURE ON PSYCHOSOCIAL CARE
PSYCHOSOCIAL ADJUSTMENTS
SOCIAL SUPPORT ADJUSTMENTS
PSYCHOLOGICAL ADJUSTMENTS
COGNITIVE FUNCTIONING
CRITICAL THINKING EXERCISES
REFERENCES AND SUGGESTED READING

KEY TERMS

affective functioning
cognitive functioning
crystallized intelligence
culture
developmental task
ethnocentrism
fluid intelligence
life review
primary memory
psychosocial
reminiscence
respite care
secondary memory
self-esteem
transcultural health care
transcultural nursing

Psychosocial Aspects of Gerontological Care

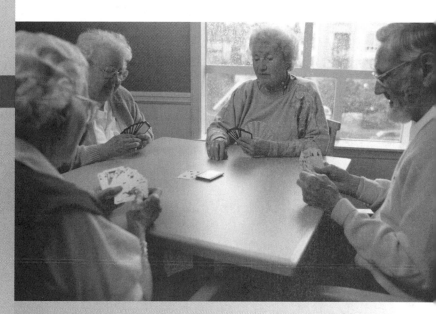

CHAPTER OBJECTIVES

At the completion of this chapter, the student will
be able to

- Identify major components of psychosocial
  development of the older adult

- Describe the importance of performing a
  psychosocial assessment

- Perform a psychosocial assessment on an
  older adult

- Discuss the impact of culture on psychosocial
  care

- Apply principles of transcultural nursing when
  providing nursing care to older adults

- Discuss psychosocial adjustments including role-
  related adjustments, social support adjustments,
  and psychological adjustments of the older adult

Psychosocial issues involve psychological and social aspects of aging. Older adults face many psychosocial concerns because of the emotional responses that occur as a result of the normal aging process, acute and chronic disease, changes in role or status, problems with housing, or problems obtaining medical services. Any of these psychosocial concerns produce stress and can lead to psychosocial problems. For example, a patient may become depressed when forced to leave home to enter a nursing facility. This becomes a psychosocial issue as the nurse seeks to help the patient adjust to a new social environment and to cope with the feelings of helplessness associated with the depression. Examples of psychosocial problems are listed in Display 8-1.

Psychosocial assessment involves assessing the functioning of the psychological aspects and social aspects of the older person's life. A psychological assessment involves evaluation of the psyche or mind and includes cognitive functioning and affective functioning. **Affective functioning** refers to the emotional responses such as happiness, sadness, fear, pain, anger, and confusion. **Cognitive functioning** refers to memory, learning, and intelligence. The social aspect of psychosocial care involves how the elderly person copes within the environment.

PSYCHOSOCIAL DEVELOPMENT

Psychosocial development continues throughout the life span. Physical and behavioral changes continually occur and contribute to the psychosocial development of the individual. Several theories about psychosocial development have been described using specific life stages and developmental tasks associated with each stage.

TABLE 8-1. Erikson's Developmental Stages

Developmental Stage	Positive Outcome	Negative Outcome
Stage I: Infancy	Trust	Mistrust
Stage II: Toddler	Autonomy	Shame and doubt
Stage III: Preschool	Initiative	Guilt
Stage IV: School age	Industry	Inferiority
Stage V: Adolescence	Identity	Identity confusion
Stage VI: Adulthood	Intimacy	Isolation
Stage VII: Middle adulthood	Generativity	Stagnation
Stage VIII: Old age	Integrity	Despair

Eric Erikson identified eight stages within the life cycle that represent major turning points in the life of the individual. The term psychosocial is used because Erikson believed that each stage is influenced by social relationships. Each stage has a specific **developmental task** or major achievement that must be accomplished to prepare the individual to meet the challenges of the future. A positive or a negative outcome can occur depending on how successful the individual is in accomplishing the major task. Positive resolution of the developmental task results in increased in life satisfaction (Table 8-1).

According to Erikson, the major developmental task for an adult 65 years or older is "ego integrity versus despair." An older adult who feels satisfied with life and feels that life was worthwhile has successfully met the criteria for ego integrity. This individual feels that, although all decisions may not have been ideal, the decisions made were the best possible at the time. With ego integrity, the individual feels a sense of peace with life and maintains a sense of dignity. There is the feeling of still being in control of one's life. The individual who feels that his life is a failure and is unhappy with the outcome of his life is in despair.

DISPLAY 8-1. Examples of Psychosocial Problems

Poor adjustment to role changes*
Poor adjustment to lifestyle changes
Family relationship problems
Coping with grief
Low self-esteem
Anxiety and depression
Aggressive behavior
Problems with sexuality
Elder abuse

*Some of these problems are discussed in this chapter. Others are discussed in subsequent chapters.

PSYCHOSOCIAL ASPECTS OF NURSING: EFFECTS OF DESPAIR IN THE ELDERLY

- Fear of the future and of dying
- Feeling discouraged and disappointed about life's failures
- Feeling that life has no meaning
- Withdrawing and having a negative attitude toward life in general

According to Erikson's theory, successful attainment of the previous developmental tasks facilitates the successful resolution of the last task. The older adult often engages in a life review, by which the person verbally and intellectually relives the significant and sometimes seemingly insignificant events of his life. Ultimately, the outcome of this life review results in feelings of ego integrity or in despair.

Developmental psychologist Robert Havighurst identified six developmental tasks as necessary for successful aging:

1. Adjusting to declining health and physical strength
2. Adjusting to retirement and reduced income
3. Adjusting to the death of a spouse
4. Establishing associations with others in the same age group
5. Maintaining a satisfactory living arrangement
6. Adapting to changes in social roles

When these developmental tasks are not met, frustration or emotional crisis may occur, leading to psychosocial problems. The older adult is helped to accept aging as a part of life and adjust to the realities of death. The goal of the nurse in dealing with psychosocial problems is to assist the patient to meet the highest potential possible within the realm of normal psychosocial functioning.

PSYCHOSOCIAL ASSESSMENT

The psychosocial assessment is an essential component of the overall health assessment. However, it is not routinely incorporated into the health assessment for two reasons. First, an accurate psychosocial assessment depends on the development of a trusting relationship between the patient and the nurse. Second, a psychosocial assessment requires more time to perform than a physical assessment. For these reasons, it is not always appropriate to perform a psychosocial assessment on admission. A good psychosocial assessment takes some time.

However, a psychosocial assessment is done as soon as possible to plan care to meet psychosocial needs. Nurses in long-term care settings have more time to collect psychosocial data and make accurate assessments. Nurse assistants can contribute important and relevant information about the psychosocial needs of residents. The nurse should consult with nurse assistants as a source of psychosocial information.

The purpose of a psychosocial assessment is to obtain information about the persons usual personality, mood, emotions, feelings, coping patterns, and cognitive abilities. The psychosocial assessment also determines how the elderly person is functioning within her social atmosphere or environment. There is no "normal" older adult. Each individual is unique, and findings are specific for that individual. Care is taken not to generalize or stereotype. To stereotype is to make a generalization about an individual or a group of individuals, such as believing that "all old people become senile with age."

PSYCHOSOCIAL ASPECTS OF NURSING: INFORMATION TO INCLUDE IN A PSYCHOSOCIAL ASSESSMENT

- Mental or cognitive abilities
- Social support
- Affective functioning and emotional status
- Current roles and role changes
- Financial resources
- Family patterns and structure
- Community resources used

Display 8-2 identifies specific components to be evaluated in the psychosocial assessment. The nurse must be careful not to label changes or alterations in status discovered in the psychosocial assessment as "normal for age." Until proven otherwise, view any changes in functioning as having an underlying disease or condition related to the environment or as an adverse reaction to a medication. In this way, any underlying disease condition is not overlooked, and interventions can be initiated that result in improvement.

The functional assessment discussed in Chapter 7 contributes data about psychosocial functioning. For example, the Folstein Mini-Mental Examination is an excellent resource to use to determine cognitive ability, the Social Dysfunction Rating Scale helps assess the need for social support, and the Beck Depression Inventory is an adjunct to assess affective functioning. The Social Dysfunction Rating Scale and other screening instruments that assess social support and activity are particularly helpful in assessing the psychosocial needs of the frail elderly. The Minimum Data Set (MDS) also addresses psychosocial well-being. Areas of psychosocial assessment in the MDS include how well the resident interacts with others, performs structured activities, or deals with uncomfortable or conflictual relationships and the person's past roles and life status.

DISPLAY 8-2. Components of a Psychosocial Assessment

Mental or Cognitive Ability
Determine orientation, alertness, and memory for remote events, recent past events, and immediate memory. Assess ability to read and follow directions and to make decisions (see Chapter 6).

Social Support
Have the person describe a typical day. Ask if she lives alone. What does she do for fun? Does she have frequent contact with others, belong to any club, or organizations? Is she involved with a church? Does she attend church regularly? Is she employed? Does she have someone she can talk with about personal matters? Does she have someone to depend on if she is ill, needs transportation, or needs assistance in the home?

Affective Functioning and Emotional Status
How does the person feel about life in general? Is he happy? How would he want his life to change? Does he enjoy living?

Current Roles and Role Changes
What roles does the person currently play? Has she suffered any losses recently, such as the death of close friends, family, or a spouse? Is she recently retired? Has

she moved recently? Has she had any major life changes within the past year?

Usual Coping Mechanisms
How does the person cope with life's problems? What does he do when he feels "uptight," irritable, or angry? How does he react to a new situation? Does religion help him to cope with life's problems?

Financial Resources
Is income sufficient to meet needs for food, housing, medical attention? Does the person have insurance? Is she on Medicaid or Medicare?

Family Patterns and Structure
Does the person live close to his family? How frequently does he see family members? What family member sees him the most often? What types of care do family members provide?

Resources Used in the Environment or Community
What community resources does the person use— Meals on Wheels, adult day care centers, senior citizen discounts, home health care, medical financial assistance, or others?

IMPACT OF CULTURE ON PSYCHOSOCIAL CARE

There are hundreds of cultures in our society, including those of the Native American, Alaskan Eskimo, and Vietnamese immigrant. With each culture comes a diversity of beliefs and perceptions that affect a person's view of health and illness. Each culture has its own set of beliefs, morals, and customs that can influence health care.

Transcultural Nursing

Culture encompasses all of the components that make up a society, such as knowledge, beliefs, customs, laws, art, diet, language, and religion. Culturally influenced lifestyle and health practices are learned behaviors that are taught by parents, grandparents, and other members of the culture.

The part of health care that seeks to identify cultural influences on health is called **transcultural health care.** Nurses who strive to become culturally sensitive in their care and interaction with patients and families are practicing **transcultural nursing.** Other terms used for transcultural nursing are crosscultural nursing and multicultural nursing. To become culturally sensitive, nurses must recognize that diver-

sity exists among various groups and must respect these differences. Regardless of the view of the nurse, it is important to know how the individual views health and illness and to incorporate those views into the care plan whenever possible.

When reviewing psychosocial issues related to health and illness of the elderly, the impact of culture is carefully examined. Even when individuals have been away from their homeland and cultural influences for many years, illness often brings to consciousness cultural practices that were learned years ago. This resurfacing of cultural beliefs can occur even if these individuals have been exposed to the mainstream culture for many years. Other individuals continue to retain and practice the health care practices that they learned within their ethnic background. These cultural practices must be respected and retained while giving nursing care if at all possible. Cultural practices provide comfort and add a stabilizing influence to the older adult's life. Nurses who are sensitive to the cultural and ethnic differences that exist among older adults are better able to provide a caring atmosphere, foster self-esteem, and gain cooperation from the patient and the family. A more meaningful and individualized care plan is created if cultural beliefs and practices are taken into consideration.

Ethnocentrism is viewing other ethnic or cultural groups from the perspective of one's own cultural background. This type of thinking prevents the development of cultural sensitivity and results in

TABLE 8-2. **Performing a Cultural Assessment: Nursing Care for the Ethnic Elder**

	Assessment	Interventions
Ethnicity	Number of years living in United States Age at immigration (immigrant vs refugee) Degree of affiliation with ethnic group or assimilation to U.S. culture	Be sensitive to historical events that influence elders' perception of self and authority of health care providers. Demonstrate respect for elder by using surname and providing care in a manner sensitive to cultural norms.
Communication	English as primary or secondary language Level of fluency Barriers to communication such as sensory deficits, lack of privacy, distractions Meaning of nonverbal gestures	Use of translator for exchange of health information. Document system for communicating basic needs between patient and staff. Provide patient access to sensory aids (glasses, hearing aids, pocket talkers). Eliminate background noise and provide optimum lighting. Smile and offer assistance with basic needs (warm blanket, glass of water).
Health perception	Perception of health problem, causes, and prognosis Response to pain, illness, and death	Educate patient/family about disease process and medical treatments. Identify and document reasons for behavior. Develop system for identifying and rating pain.
Folk practices	Use of cultural healers, herbal medicines, alternative health practices, and beliefs	Obtain order for use of folk remedies as indicated. Educate patient regarding contraindications for folk remedy and discourage use if dangerous.
Health care system	Previous hospitalization experiences Current hospitalization planned or emergency?	Encourage patient to express fears regarding hospitalization and treatments. Keep patient/family informed of patient's progress.
Religion	Spiritual practices and beliefs Level of incorporation of spiritual practices into healing or dying process	Allow privacy and space for religious articles and practices. Arrange for visit from spiritual leader. Refer patients to hospital chaplain. Document beliefs about death and burial.
Food	Beliefs regarding food and healing Use of hot/cold system Specific food preferences	Obtain consultation with dietician. Incorporate food preferences into menu selection. Ask family to supply familiar foods. Document use of hot/cold practices as they relate to nursing care.
Social support	Current living situation Support of family and/or community	Encourage family participation in care. Encourage visits or phone calls with peers.
Decision making	Primary decision maker for health care How does the patient make decisions? Who is needed for decisions?	Involve family when providing patient with health care information. Arrange for family conference if disparity exists between goals of patient, family, and/or health care team.
Discharge planning	Expectations for care after hospitalization and during future years of aging Financial status that affects discharge planning and long-term health status Ability of patient/family to support discharge needs	Involve family in discharge planning. Obtain consult for social services. Refer patient to community resources for legal advice, transportation, meals, shopping, and emotional support.

Adapted from Evans, C.A., & Cunningham, B.A. (1996). Nursing care for the ethnic elder. *Geriatric Nursing, 17 (3),* 107.

inadequate care for those with cultural differences. An open-minded and interested attitude on the part of the nurse when performing a cultural assessment helps prevent ethnocentrism. The assessment allows the nurse to explore the person's feelings and beliefs.

The areas to be evaluated when performing a cultural assessment include ethnicity, communication, health perception, folk practices, health care system, religion, food preferences, social support, and decision making. Table 8-2 provides an assessment framework

---

DISPLAY 8-3. Suggestions to Overcome Language Barriers

- Greet the patient using the last or complete name. Avoid being too casual or familiar. Gesture to yourself and say your name. Smile.
- Proceed in an unhurried manner. Pay attention to any effort by the patient or family to communicate.
- Speak in a low, moderate voice. Avoid talking loudly. Remember that there is a tendency to raise the volume and pitch of your voice when the listener appears not to understand. The listener may perceive that you are shouting or angry.
- Organize your thoughts. Repeat and summarize frequently. Use audiovisual aids when feasible.
- Use short, simple sentence structure and speak in the active voice.
- Use simple words, such as "pain" instead of "discomfort." Avoid medical jargon, idioms, and slang. Avoid using contractions such as don't, can't, or won't.
- Use nouns repeatedly instead of pronouns. For example, do not say: "He has been taking his medicine, hasn't he?" Do say: "Does Juan take medicine?"
- Pantomime words and simple actions while verbalizing them.
- Give instructions in the proper sequence. For example, do not say, "Before you rinse the bottle, sterilize it." Do say: "First, wash the bottle. Second, rinse the bottle."

- Discuss one topic at a time and avoid giving too much information in a single conversation. Avoid using conjunctions. For example, do not say: "Are you cold and in pain?" Do say: "Are you cold?" (while pantomiming) "Are you in pain?"
- Validate if the person understands by having him or her repeat instructions, demonstrate the procedure, or act out the meaning.
- Use any words you know in the person's language. This indicates that you are aware of and respect the patient's primary means of communicating.
- Try a third language. Many Indo-Chinese speak French. Europeans often know three or four languages. Try Latin words or phrases, if you are familiar with the language.
- Ask who among the patient's family and friends could serve as an interpreter. Be aware of culturally based gender and age differences and diverse socioeconomic, educational, and tribal or regional differences when choosing an interpreter.
- Obtain phrase books from a library or bookstore, make or purchase flash cards, contact hospitals for a list of interpreters, and use formal and informal networking to locate a suitable interpreter. Although costly, some telecommunication companies provide translation services.

From Smeltzer, S., & Barre, B. (1996). *Brunner and Suddarth's Medical-surgical nursing* (8th ed.). Philadelphia: Lippincott-Raven Publishers, 136.

---

and nursing interventions to assist the nurse when caring for an elder from a different culture.

Overcoming Language Barriers

Speaking the same language facilitates the assessment. Even minimal competence in speaking a language the patient understands can be beneficial, particularly in developing a therapeutic relationship. However, if the nurse cannot speak the language well enough to be understood, an interpreter can be a valuable resource. Certain dangers exist when using an interpreter. For example, the interpreter may not understand what is being said and may incorrectly translate the information. If family members or friends are acting as interpreters, any fear or concerns that they may have can influence the interpretation. Fears, such as the manner in which a patient will receive certain news, can influence the way in which an interpreter interprets the information to the patient. Sometimes, words pertaining to health care are difficult to translate, and no comparable word exists. Interpreters are invaluable if the nurse does not speak the language, but care must be

taken that the correct message is received when using an interpreter. Display 8-3 gives some suggestions to overcome language barriers.

PSYCHOSOCIAL ADJUSTMENTS

With age comes many psychosocial adjustments. These adjustments occur in three major areas: role-related adjustments, social support adjustments, and psychological adjustments.

Role-Related Adjustments

Many roles are enacted within the life span, such as those of child, parent, spouse, homemaker, breadwinner, and caretaker. With age, each of these roles change to some extent. Alternations in roles occur as a result of changes:

Change in the role of an individual (eg, retirement)
Change in the role of a close relationship (eg, death of a spouse)

Loss of social group members (eg, moving to a new location)

Decline physical or mental health.

Spousal Role

Perhaps the major life role is that of spouse. The spousal role encompasses many subroles, such as companion, sexual partner, confidante, cook, housekeeper, provider, or handyman. Spousal roles are interdependent; the relationship is reciprocal, with each partner giving as well as receiving. When the role of one partner changes, the role of the other partner of necessity also changes. For example, if the wife becomes ill, the role of the husband changes. In this case, the husband may take on more of a caregiver role or play a larger role in maintaining the home (ie, housekeeper role).

Loss of a spouse is a highly stressful experience that often causes significant psychosocial problems such as loneliness, change of status or income, or depression. There is an increase in the mortality rate of widows within the first 2 years after the loss of a spouse. Widowed men are especially lonely and often remarry after the wife's death.

Sexual Role

The role of the sexual partner is an important role regardless of chronologic age. Sexual intimacy continues to be a significant aspect of an elderly person's life, and sexual activity continues well into old age. There is, however, a gradual decline in sexual activity. Sexual intimacy does not have to culminate in sexual intercourse but can be expressed through touch (Fig. 8-1), massage, stroking, kissing, talking, or caressing each other.

Loss of the sexual role can result in psychosocial problems such as depression or anger. The nurse carefully assesses the sexual role of each elderly person. Medication sometimes may be the cause of impotence or loss of libido (ie, sexual desire). If this is the case, the physician may need to substitute a different medication or use a reduced dose. Nurses who stereotype the elderly as nonsexual beings with little or no sexual needs may overlook this very important role. A more detailed discussion of sexuality of the older adult is provided in Chapter 11.

Work Role

A change in the work role comes with retirement. Retirement causes a major role change. It changes the way time is managed and daily activities are carried out. Retirement alters identity, status and sometimes friendships. New relationships must be developed. If the person is ready to retire, has

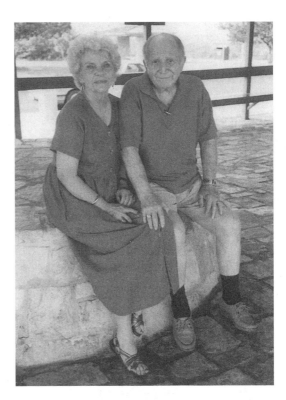

FIGURE 8-1. Older adults have the same psychosocial needs as those of younger adults. The need for friendship, intimacy, closeness, and expression of sexuality remain an important part of living regardless of the age.

developed hobbies, enjoys certain leisure activities, or has a variety of interests, retirement can be rewarding. However, if financial problems exist or the person received much emotional satisfaction and esteem from work, psychosocial problems may occur. Some older adults discover they miss working and find part-time jobs. Others work to supplement their income. Older workers are competent, efficient, and capable. In jobs that require minimal physical demands, older workers are more accurate and more consistent in their work performance than younger adults. They also tend to have fewer accidents and are absent less than their younger counterparts.

Adjusting to retirement is easier if activities that will become prominent after retirement are begun during the working years. Counseling and planning before retirement are offered by some companies. Sometimes, companies allow the worker to gradually decrease the work load over a period of several months or years. Decreasing the workload from 5 days to 3 days each week and then to 2 days per week can help even the most resistant person anticipate retirement.

Retirement brings an array of opportunities for older adults with adequate income. There is freedom to pursue long-anticipated leisure activities such as traveling, hobbies, or learning new skills. However, for others with limited income or for those in poor health, retirement can be a time of hardship and concern.

Family Roles

Family roles include the role of parent, sibling, and grandparent. With advancing age, these roles become more prominent. Although the parent role plays a significant role throughout, an interesting phenomenon occurs as the adult ages. A form of role reversal occurs in the parent–child relationship in which the parent becomes increasingly dependent on the adult child to help with decision making, for support, and for physical care. The adult child then plays the role of parent.

The sibling role, which was very strong in the early developmental years, again becomes more important. During the young adult and middle adult years, raising a family, career development, and planning for the future often placed sibling relationships in the background. The sibling relationship is the longest of all relationships. It surpasses the time spent in the marriage relationship, the time spent with children, and usually the time spent with parents. As the person ages, relationships with siblings who share the same family history become significant again and (barring any conflicts within the relationship) a source of support.

The grandparent role is generally one that brings great satisfaction and contentment. In general, the grandparent role can be enjoyed to the fullest without the responsibility of raising the child. Several types of grandparents have been identified: traditional, substitute parent, distant, and recreational. The traditional grandparent is bound by rigid and stereotyped role expectations for themselves and the grandchildren. More and more grandparents are abandoning this type of grandparenting role and developing their own grandparenting style. The grandparent who is a substitute parent assumes the major caregiver role and the responsibility for raising the child. Distant grandparents may talk on the phone or write letters, but visits are infrequent. They may maintain a certain special quality, but distance prevents frequent, face-to-face interaction. Recreational grandparents are in frequent contact with their grandchildren and engage in many pleasurable and recreational activities with their grandchildren. As more baby boomers become grandparents, the grandparenting role will become increasingly diverse and nontraditional.

SOCIAL SUPPORT ADJUSTMENTS

With increasing age, adjustments are made in social support. Social support comes from a variety of sources, such as family, friends, churches, clubs, volunteer groups, and governmental organizations. Family and friends form the framework for social support. The spectrum of social support ranges from an occasional telephone call to daily contact for social interaction to providing financial and physical care. Support systems provide the elderly with a wide range of services such as advice and guidance in dealing with problems, an avenue for companionship, and nursing care needs.

Adjustments are made in social support systems as roles change with age. For example, the retired executive may find that he has less and less in common with his old friends in the company and more and more interest in being with friends he plays with in his weekly golf game. After breaking a hip, an older woman who had always been very independent may find she must depend on her daughter for help.

Family

The family is the basic social unit and provides the primary support system for most elderly people. Most elderly people are close to their family and have frequent contact. Support is give and take and generally flows in all directions. It may take the form of affection, emotional support, and material support such as money and gifts. The older adult helps the younger generation by serving as a role model for successful aging, coping with stress, and imparting values and standards.

The family consists of the immediate family members (ie, parents, children, and grandchildren) and the extended family (ie, siblings, aunts, uncles, nieces, and cousins). Most elderly couples live at home and require minimal assistance from family. Children generally assist with the care, if necessary. Other relatives may provide support, care, and assistance if children are not available.

Most often, one family member is unofficially declared as the major caregiver. This person makes most of the decisions, keeps in frequent contact with the health care providers, and assumes most of the responsibility for seeing that an elderly family member receives the proper care. Many families do not have anyone who can be the primary caregiver if the elderly family member requires total care. Family members have jobs of their own or other responsibilities that make the caregiver role an impossible task. This poses a significant problem because most children do not want to place their parent in a nursing home. Caregiving can place a tremendous burden on the family emotionally, physically, and financially.

A form of care called respite care is available in some areas to give caregivers a much needed respite (ie, temporary relief) from the daily stresses of caregiving. **Respite care** is short-term care for the elderly or chronically ill to give caregivers some relief from the physical and emotional strain of 24-hour care. The caregivers can leave their loved ones for a few hours to a few days to receive some much needed rest.

Friends

Friends may be lifelong friends, new friends, neighbors, or acquaintances. They may engage in similar leisure activities or be members of the same club, church, or volunteer organization. They may see each other daily or only occasionally. These informal support systems can be very beneficial in meeting social support needs.

Some dependency needs, such as shopping or transportation, can be met by friends. If some dependency needs are met by friends or neighbors within the same age group, the loss of self-esteem from increased dependency is not as severe. Elderly people often form a mutually dependent bond. They look out for each other, help each other, encourage each other, and provide support.

Loneliness and depression arise when the elderly lose family or friends through death or a change of home location. Children may not be able to provide the needed support because they are involved in raising their own families. Family relationships may be strained. Other friends or siblings may have died or moved away and no support network is established to meet social needs. Hearing and speech deficits may add to the problem. Feelings of insecurity, loneliness, and isolation create psychosocial problems.

Interventions that Promote Social Support

Assessment of social contacts and social needs is the first step in intervention. Information to include when interviewing an older adult includes:

    Memberships in church or social clubs and the amount of contact with each group

    Amount and type of contact with children or other relatives

    Amount and type of contact with friends or neighbors

    Feelings of loneliness

    Activities engaged in

    Types of support needed

Encouraging older people to participate in social support groups is an important nursing intervention. After assessment, the amount and type of social support groups needed can be explored. Some elderly have strong social networks, and minimal intervention is necessary. Others need encouragement to examine different social groups to enhance social support. For many, increased social contact provides the necessary support. For others, social support may take the form of help with transportation, housekeeping services, or nursing care.

There are many different types of social support groups and services. Careful appraisal of each group or service allows the elderly to choose the services that best meet individual needs. Services vary from community to community. Knowing the local community and the services offered is important for the nurse.

Adult day care facilities and some senior citizen centers provide transportation, recreational activities, meals, mutual support, and minor medical assistance such as monitoring of blood pressure and blood glucose levels. Home health care agencies provide skilled nursing care and other services such as housekeeping, elder-sitters, and home health aides. Case management, counseling, and self-help groups are available in some areas for support. Nursing facilities are options when families can no longer continue caring for an elderly relative at home.

Senior citizens are often afforded senior citizen discounts on public transportation or on meals at restaurants. The American Association for Retired Persons (AARP) offers a variety of services from information to support networks. Health care insurance, life insurance, and a prescription drug service are also made available through the AARP.

Conflictual Relationships

When support from family and friends is strong, social support needs can more easily be met. However, family or friends sometimes are not able to provide the needed support. Family members may have long-standing relationship problems that prevent supportive care. Unexpressed feelings of hostility, anger, anxiety, or guilt create situations in which family members cannot effectively support each other. Display 8-4 identifies what the nurse should do when family coping is compromised.

DISPLAY 8-4. Actions of the Nurse When Family Coping is Compromised

- Establish a trusting relationship with the family and patient.
- Encourage verbalization of the problems.
- Encourage expression of feelings, (eg, anger, frustration, hostility, hopelessness).
- Identify underlying situations that contribute to the inability to provide support.
- Listen attentively to all parties involved in the conflict.
- Notice nonverbal behaviors.
- Avoid placing blame on any of the parties involved.
- Use problem solving techniques to deal with the problem (see Chapter 25).

PSYCHOLOGICAL ADJUSTMENTS

The psyche or the mind plays a role in how the older adult adjusts to age. Mental adjustments involve affective function and cognitive function. Affective function refers to the mood, emotions, and the expression of emotions. Cognitive function refers to intelligence, memory, and learning. Cognitive and affective functioning affect the person's self-esteem.

Affective Functioning

Affective functioning is influenced by the way an individual views the world and self. A positive view of self and the surrounding environment promotes a positive expression of mood and emotions. Self-esteem is the cornerstone for healthy affective functioning.

Self-Esteem

Self-esteem is the way a person views herself. A positive view of self promotes health and enables the elderly person to cope better with the changes and challenges of growing older. Age-related changes and losses that occur with aging contribute to a decrease in self-esteem. Chronic illness leads to increased dependency and decreased role competence, resulting in a loss of self-esteem. Stereotypes and a negative view by society toward the older person represents a threat to self-esteem. The elderly person with a high self-esteem feels good about himself, is satisfied with life, and has accepted himself as an aging person. Dependence, depersonaliza-tion, functional impairment, and lack of control over the person's environment can result in a loss of self-esteem. Many of these situations occur for the elderly, especially if they are placed in nursing homes.

Self-Esteem and Independent Functioning

Self-esteem is closely tied to independence and the ability to care for oneself. Chronic illness, disability, increased dependency, and role changes all contribute to a risk for decreased self-esteem. When the elderly are placed in nursing homes, they may not be encouraged to continue self-care activities such as bathing, dressing, or feeding themselves. Nursing homes are highly structured environments, and efficiency in accomplishing tasks sometimes takes precedence over individual need. It is often easier and quicker to have the nurse assistant give a bath or dress the resident than to allow the resident to bathe himself with some assistance. Older people need more time to perform daily activities and tend to become confused when rushed or hurried. Helping residents to provide self-care activities can give them more control over their environment and a sense of self-control.

Reminiscence and Life Review

Reminiscence and life review are two separate nursing interventions used primarily with older adults. **Reminiscence** is a nursing intervention that encourages the elderly person to recall or remember past events with the purpose of attaining a specific goal. For example, the nurse may use reminiscence to increase self-esteem or life satisfaction. In this intervention, the elderly person is encouraged to reminisce or discuss memories and past experiences. In general, reminiscence is a pleasurable experience that allows the older adult to relive past successes and pleasurable experiences, increases social interaction, and improves communication skills.

Reminiscence can be done formally, perhaps once or twice each week, in a group setting with the nurse acting as facilitator. Participants discuss different topics from their past, such as significant events, birth of their children, travel, places they have lived, and holidays. The goal of reminiscence is not to gain insight or to psychoanalyze behavior. Although most often focusing on pleasurable experiences, sad or uncomfortable experiences may surface during reminiscence. The individual is allowed to express these memories and feel the pain but not to stagnate in these areas. Reminiscence therapy is also done between the nurse and the older adult, with no others present. Actively listening, encouraging verbalization, asking open-ended questions, and giving positive feedback is the role of the nurse during reminiscence.

Life review is a nursing intervention that assists the older adult to positively resolve Erikson's major developmental task for the older adult and gain integrity. In life review, the older adult examines his life somewhat critically and reviews all aspects. The nurse is the audience in this process and has the role of active listener, questioner, and sometimes prober. As with reminiscence, active listening and asking open-ended questions are important roles for the nurse.

Life review is not a group process; it is done on an individual basis between the nurse and the participant. A structured approach is taken, with a specific time allowed to focus on a review of the different life periods, such as 1 to 2 weeks on childhood, 1 to 2 weeks on the teenage years, and so forth. Life review is mostly a pleasurable experience, resulting in the participant feeling a sense of integrity about his life.

Reminiscence and life review are similar in some respects; both use memory as a tool for therapeutic intervention, both are used predominately with older adults, and both are basically pleasurable experiences. However, the goals of each intervention are different. Life review helps the older adult to fulfill the major developmental task of aging. A by-product of life review may be increased self-esteem, but that is not the primary goal. Reminiscence is used with a specific goal in mind: increase self-esteem, increase socialization, or decrease depression.

Use of Positive "I" Statements

The use of positive statements about oneself helps to reframe thinking patterns and increases self-esteem. Positive "I" statements help the resident to see her specialness and uniqueness. Too often, the elderly focus on the negative: "I can't get around like I used to" or "I am no good to anyone anymore." Encourage positive self-talk, and assist the resident in eliminating statements that are self-derogatory, such as "I'm just too old to be good for anything" or "I can't do anything right anymore." Redirect these statements to a positive view by saying, "Let's identify some of your talents. Many people view your ability to crochet that beautiful afghan as a special talent." Explore the statement by saying, "Tell me more about how you feel. Let's think of some things you do right."

Self-Esteem and Decision Making

Older people are often left out of decision-making processes, particularly decisions that can profoundly affect on their lives (eg, going to live in a

---

> **DISPLAY 8-5. Nursing Interventions to Increase Self-Esteem**
>
> - Develop a trusting relationship.
> - Treat the person with dignity and respect.
> - Allow sufficient time for the performance of daily activities of self-care.
> - Encourage verbalization.
> - Practice active listening.
> - Encourage the use of positive self-statements rather than praise.
> - Give positive reinforcement for progress.
> - Use reminiscence therapy.
> - Be alert for opportunities to include the patient in decision making.
> - Use verbal and nonverbal communication techniques that convey positive feelings toward the patient.
> - Encourage socialization.

nursing home). The more older individuals participate in decisions that directly affect them, the more in control they feel, adding to feelings of a positive self-esteem. Nurses must be alert for opportunities to involve the elderly in the decision-making process. It is often easier to make simple decisions without consulting the patient. However, taking a little extra time to consult with the patient can foster self-esteem and enhance the nurse-patient relationship. Nursing interventions that enhance self-esteem are included in Display 8-5.

Figure 8-2 illustrates a method to enhance self-esteem. The foundation for enhancing self-esteem is helping patients to have as much control as possible within the limitations of disease and age. The use of positive self-talk, recognizing positive traits, and improving self-care ability results in increased self-esteem.

Personality

The individual's basic personality does not change as a result of the aging process but remains consistent throughout life. Nevertheless, sometimes certain traits seem to be accentuated with age. A woman who is kind and sweet throughout life may seem to be even sweeter and kinder with age. Likewise, a cranky, negative young person will likely become a cranky, negative older person. Negative traits seem to be the traits most pronounced with age. Unless a person suffers from a disease process the personality remains intact. Display 8-6 identifies nursing interventions that enhance personality.

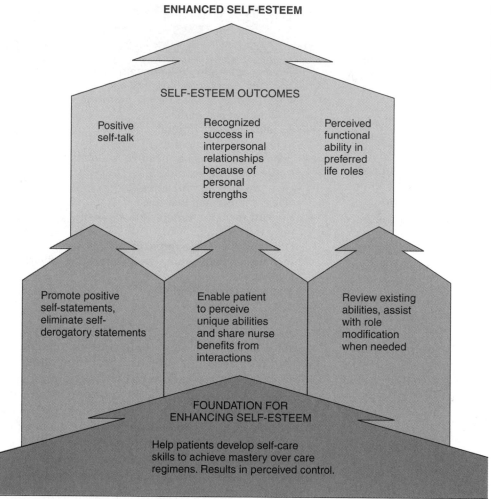

ENHANCED SELF-ESTEEM

SELF-ESTEEM OUTCOMES

Positive self-talk

Recognized success in interpersonal relationships because of personal strengths

Perceived functional ability in preferred life roles

Promote positive self-statements, eliminate self-derogatory statements

Enable patient to perceive unique abilities and share nurse benefits from interactions

Review existing abilities, assist with role modification when needed

FOUNDATION FOR ENHANCING SELF-ESTEEM

Help patients develop self-care skills to achieve mastery over care regimens. Results in perceived control.

FIGURE 8-2. Interventions for enhancing self-esteem. (From Miller, J.F. (1983). *Coping with chronic illness: Overcoming powerlessness.* Philadelphia: F.A. Davis)

DISPLAY 8-6. Nursing Interventions That Foster Positive Personality Traits in the Elderly

- Accept the patient.
- Identify the positive attributes of each patient.
- Encourage verbalization.
- Reward positive behavior.
- Avoid a judgmental attitude.

COGNITIVE FUNCTIONING

Intelligence, learning, and memory are all related to cognitive functioning and how well the mind is able to reason and make sound judgments.

Intelligence

Intelligence is mental alertness and includes the ability to learn new material, make wise decisions, and deal with stressful situations. Barring a disease process, fundamental intelligence is preserved. An elderly person does not become less intelligent with age. Verbal comprehension and arithmetic computation abilities remain intact. The presence of many intelligent and knowledgeable older people attest to the fact that intelligence and cognition do not automatically decrease with age. For example, Jerome Lemelson at the age of 72 is one of the most creative inventors in our time. He has more than 500 patented inventions and is ranked as the fourth largest patent holder in U.S. history.

Two types of intelligence are significant: fluid intelligence and crystallized intelligence. **Fluid intelligence** controls emotions, aesthetic appreciation, retention of nonintellectual information, creative functioning, and special perceptions. Fluid intelligence depends primarily on inherited abilities. **Crystallized intelligence** allows the person to use past experiences and knowledge for problem solving. This type of intelligence is acquired through culture, education, and life experience. Crystallized intelligence does not decline until very old age. Nursing interventions to enhance mental alertness are found in Display 8-7.

DISPLAY 8-7. Nursing Interventions to Enhance Mental Alertness

- Allow the patient to do as many tasks for himself as possible.
- Encourage use of the mind in problem solving.
- Encourage use of numbers and calculations (eg, balancing checkbook).
- Encourage creative activities (eg, painting, story telling).
- Encourage the discovery of new talents and abilities.

DISPLAY 8-8. Nursing Interventions When Caring for a Patient with a Short-Term Memory Loss

- Identify yourself each time there is an interaction with the patient.
- Give instructions in simple, direct terms.
- Repeat instructions several times.
- Explain everything that is happening, even if the patient does not seem to understand.
- Perform only one activity at a time.
- Report any sudden confusion. Confusion that appears suddenly is not normal and must be reported to the physician immediately.

Memory

Memory is composed of primary and secondary memory. **Primary memory** is for storage of information that can be easily accessed and actively processed for immediate use. The storage capacity for primary memory is limited. This type of memory is not affected by the aging process. **Secondary memory** is a type of memory that holds information in storage. The ability to retrieve secondary memory declines with age.

The most noticeable memory loss is that of short-term memory. For example, the older patient cannot remember whether her daughter visited her this morning or not, or an elderly man cannot remember what he had for supper last night. Short-term memory requires the use of primary and secondary memory. The decline in short-term memory is attributed to difficulty retrieving secondary memory. Long-term memory is also called remote memory and does not experience significant change with age.

Memory loss is significant in older adults who have dementia as a result of diseases such as Alzheimer's disease. Memory loss in Alzheimer's disease is thought to result from a lack of acetylcholine. Acetylcholine is a neurotransmitter released at autonomic nerve endings that facilitates the transmission of the nerve impulse. Acetylcholine is necessary for short-term memory. As the level of acetylcholine is reduced, less information is stored until all short-term memory is lost. Nursing interventions to enhance short-term memory are identified in Display 8-8.

Learning

Learning is the acquisition of new knowledge or skills. The ability of the mind to learn and retain new information remains unaltered, particularly when the mind is stimulated through regular use. However, the ability to solve complex problems declines with age.

Older people must be motivated to learn and are generally most interested in learning information

---

DISPLAY 8-9. Teaching an Older Person New Information

- Assess current knowledge. For example, if the teaching is to focus on taking an antihypertensive medication, determine whether the patient has been on antihypertensive medications before. If so, what was the medication? Did he experience any adverse reactions? Does he understand what hypertension is?
- Evaluate for any visual or hearing deficit. Make sure the hearing aid is working or glasses are available, if indicated.
- Determine the person's ability to learn.
- Identify any language barrier.
- Determine if the information to be taught is thought to be important or relevant to the elderly person.
- Begin by reviewing familiar information and then move to new information.
- Teach the spouse or family member as well as the elderly person if possible.
- Plan teaching over several days, with small increments of information presented at one time.
- Actively involve the patient in the learning process.
- Allow time for feedback to evaluate knowledge.

---

that is related to real life and that they feel is useful. They prefer to learn one task at a time and master each task before progressing on to another task.

Hearing and visual deficits related to the aging process can affect learning. Visual deficits that affect learning new material or a new task include presbyopia (ie, inability of the eye to accommodate for close work), difficulty distinguishing blues and greens, decreased color vision, and decreased depth perception. The elderly have difficulty hearing, especially hearing high-pitched sounds (see Chapter 24). Background noises may increase hearing disability and interfere with hearing in a classroom setting. Nursing interventions to enhance learning are found in Display 8-9.

CRITICAL THINKING EXERCISES

1. Jose Reyna, age 78, is from Mexico. He has been living in this country with his son for the past 5 years. Mr. Reyna speaks Spanish as his primary language but seems to understand most of what you are saying to him in English. How would you go about establishing a therapeutic nurse-patient relationship with Mr. Reyna. What are the most important aspects of Mr. Reyna's care? Explain your answer.

2. Using the guidelines in Display 8-2 assess an elderly person's psychosocial needs. From your assessment, identify this person's most important or significant psychosocial needs. What interventions would you use to alleviate these needs?

3. Plan an inservice education program on reminiscence and life review. Include the differences between the two and the most effective ways to incorporate both interventions into practice in the nursing home and in the outpatient setting.

4. James Gleason, age 65, is withdrawn and appears depressed. He has recently retired and is coming to the community center with his wife, June, several times each week. June comes to you for advice because she is worried about her husband. She tells you that, since retiring, James feels worthless and is having difficulty sleeping at night. What suggestions would you make to June? How could Mr. Gleason's self-esteem be enhanced?

5. Perform a cultural assessment on at least two individuals using the guidelines in Display 8-3. Discuss any cultural differences you notice between the two individuals.

REFERENCES AND SUGGESTED READING

Eliopoulos, C. (1996). *Gerontological nursing* (4th ed.). Philadelphia: Lippincott-Raven.

Feil, N. (1996). *The validation breakthrough.* Baltimore: Health Professions Press.

Gorman, L., Sultan, D., & Raines, M. (1996). *Davis's manual of psychosocial nursing for general patient care.* Philadelphia: F.A. Davis.

Haight, B., & Burnside, I. (1993). Reminiscence and life review: Explaining the differences. *Archives of Psychiatric Nursing, VII (2),* 91–98.

Hall, P. (1996). Providing psychosocial support. *American Journal of Nursing, 96 (10),* 16N.

Hartz, G., & Splain, D. (1997). *Psychosocial interventions in long term care: An advanced guide for social workers and nurses.* Binghamton, NY: Haworth Press.

McDougall, G., Blixen, C., & Suen, L. (1997). The process of life review psychotherapy with depressed homebound older adults. *Nursing Research, 46 (5),* 277.

Swanson, E., & Trip-Reimer, T. (1999). *Life transitions in the older adult: Issues for nurses and other health professionals.* New York: Springer Publishing.

CHAPTER 9

Implementing Restorative Care

CHAPTER OUTLINE

KEY TERMS
CHAPTER OBJECTIVES
REHABILITATION
    Care Settings for Rehabilitation
    Restorative Care
PROVIDING RESTORATIVE CARE
    Promoting Mobility
    Assistive Devices
    Promoting Personal Care
HOME MANAGEMENT
    Roles of the Physical and Occupational
        Therapists
CRITICAL THINKING EXERCISES
REFERENCES AND SUGGESTED READING

KEY TERMS

active assistive range of motion
custodial care
learned helplessness
rehabilitation
restorative care
self-care activities

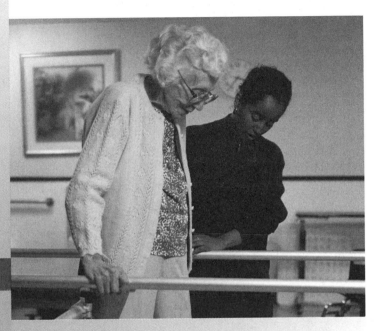

CHAPTER OBJECTIVES

At the completion of this chapter, the student will be able to

- Differentiate between rehabilitation and restorative care

- Identify care settings for rehabilitation and restorative care

- Identify members of the rehabilitation team

- Describe how to evaluate potential for rehabilitation

- Discuss the role of the nurse in rehabilitation

- Discuss the concept of restorative care versus custodial care

- Define learned helplessness

- Discuss methods to promote mobility

- Discuss ways to promote self-care in feeding, dressing, grooming, bathing, and toileting and in the home environment

- Identify situations where a referral to the physical therapist or occupational therapist would be beneficial to the patient

Restorative care is the focus of all gerontological nursing. The gerontological nurse is continually looking for ways to preserve the older person's ability to function in the environment and improve his quality of life. Restorative care is a specialized type of care that assists the older adult to reach maximum functional capacity, physically, mentally, emotionally, and socially. Restorative care ultimately enables the older adult to be as independent as possible. Even small gains toward independence can be viewed as successful restorative care. For example, suppose an elderly person does not have the functional ability to walk and is confined to a wheelchair. Through arm strengthening exercises, this person develops the necessary arm strength to successfully transfer from the bed to the wheelchair and back. Although viewed by some as a small achievement, this increased mobility allows greater independence in living skills and is an important part of restorative care.

REHABILITATION

Rehabilitation is the process of assisting disabled individuals to return to optimum health and a satisfactory level of independence. When entering the rehabilitation process, the participant has some form of disability (ie, a physical or mental inability to function normally). Examples of situations requiring rehabilitation include after a myocardial infarction, replacement surgery, cerebrovascular accident (ie, stroke), or in elderly patients recovering from a hip fracture.

Care Settings for Rehabilitation

Rehabilitation is done in a number of health care settings by a variety of health care professionals. Rehabilitative care can occur in an acute care setting, a rehabilitation center, or a nursing facility. Some hospitals have an inpatient rehabilitation unit. Other hospitals exist for the sole purpose of rehabilitation. These settings provide the advantage over a general hospital of an expert multidisciplinary staff and specialized equipment.

Sometimes an elderly person's limited rehabilitation potential may not warrant a special rehabilitation center. In these cases, the elderly person is dismissed from the hospital to a nursing home or transitional care unit for rehabilitation. A nursing facility that provides rehabilitation sometimes is called a subacute rehabilitation facility. The quality of rehabilitative care provided by a nursing facility varies according to the facility. Some nursing facilities provide mainly custodial care. Others provide high-quality restorative care that enables the older person to increase functional ability to a point where the individual is able to return home. If an older adult goes to the nursing facility for rehabilitation purposes, the nurse and the family should stress that he may be able to return home or to the prehospital setting. This helps to decrease the anxiety sometimes associated with going to a nursing facility.

Restorative Care

Restorative care is the specialized care given during rehabilitation. When caring for older patients, restorative care is an ongoing type of care in which nurses strive to maintain the older person's function in all areas of life, particularly activities pertaining to daily living and self-care. When a person is able to function independently, there is a greater sense of well-being and life satisfaction. Nurses in nursing facilities or in nursing homes work to maintain the patients' bladder and bowel function and ability to feed, bathe, and toilet themselves. Restorative care has a broad range of activities that covers all aspects of self-care.

Theoretically, rehabilitation ends when the patient has reached her maximum functional ability. However, the gerontological nurse is continually looking for ways to maintain and increase the functioning ability of older adults. During rehabilitation, restorative nursing measures are incorporated into the care, but the restorative care given by a gerontological nurse is done for all patients, regardless of whether the patient is participating in a formal rehabilitation program.

Settings for Restorative Care
Restorative care can occur in any health care setting, such as nursing facilities, adult day care centers, or anywhere elderly people are cared for. When caring for residents in nursing facilities restorative care is almost always a part of patient care. Bladder training programs, ambulation, proper positioning, helping the patient to feed, dress and care for himself are important aspects of restorative care. Adult day care centers provide activities that enhance restorative care such as maintaining orientation, providing social support systems and exercise programs and stimulating creativity through arts and crafts.

The Restorative Care Team
Providing restorative care requires a multidisciplinary team. The team consists of various types of

nurses, physical therapists, occupational therapists, recreational therapists, speech therapists, social workers, and physicians. Not every member of the team is needed with each patient. For example, if restorative care involves only the institution of a bladder training program (see Chapter 14), the physical therapist, occupational therapist, and speech therapist are not needed. The most important members of the team are the patient and the family. Without their cooperation, rehabilitation is virtually impossible.

The patient must have the desire and the motivation to participate in the rehabilitative process. The nurse coordinates the care, promotes functional independence, prevents complications, and provides patient and family teaching. The patient participates in the formulation of goals, in learning how to maximize the disability, and in adjusting to any limitations. The family, especially if the patient will be leaving the facility or the rehabilitation center, must be knowledgeable about caring for the patient and about the program established for rehabilitation so that progress will continue after dismissal. The therapist generally evaluates the patient and develops a restorative care plan. A restorative aid or a physical therapy assistant often carries out the plan on a daily basis. The patient may receive therapy once or twice each day while in the facility. When seen on an outpatient basis, treatment varies from one time each week to every other day to 5 days per week, depending on the patient's needs.

Assessing Potential for Restorative Care

When planning restorative care, it is important to assess the patient's potential to successfully participate in restorative care. The patient is evaluated mentally, physically, and emotionally.

Evaluation of mental status is more comprehensive than assessing for orientation to person, place, and time. For certain aspects of restorative care to be effective, the person must be able to follow simple directions and retain information. Many tools are available to a evaluate mental status. To evaluate mental status the Folstein Mini-Mental Examination can be used (see Chapter 7, Table 7-5).

If no specific evaluation tool is available, the nurse can assess mental ability by requesting that the patient repeat three unrelated words several minutes after first hearing them. This type of request is a method to determine the potential to retain information. Tell the patient that you are going to say three words and that you will ask him to repeat those words after several minutes. For example, when evaluating the potential for restorative care in a patient in a nursing facility, say the words *cake, apple,* and *scissors.* Continue talking with the

patient for a few minutes and then request that the patient repeat the words. If the words are easily remembered, the ability to retain information is most likely intact.

To determine the ability to follow directions, the patient can be asked to follow two- or three-step commands, such as "touch your elbow, then your nose, and then your ear." If the person can perform simple three-step commands, the potential for actively participating and succeeding in restorative care is probably good.

Lower-level functioning skills that are repetitive in nature require less keen mental functioning. These lower-level skills, such as brushing the teeth or self-feeding, are simply relearned and require less mental functioning than the higher-level skills such as walking, dressing, or using crutches.

Evaluation of physical needs focus on functional and self-care abilities. Activities such as feeding, bathing, hygiene, dressing, toileting, and mobility are assessed. To assess self-care, the nurse observes the elderly person doing self-care activities. Areas of importance are how independently the person performs these tasks, how much time is required to perform the tasks, and the amount of assistance needed. During ambulation, gait, mobility, and coordination are assessed. Many assessment tools can help measure functional ability. Chapter 7 offers more information on functional assessment.

Emotional responses are also important when evaluating the potential for rehabilitation. Anxiety and depression are emotions that can affect rehabilitation outcomes. Anxiety and fear can prevent an elderly adult from attempting restorative care. For example, if a hip was fractured as a result of walking down stairs, the person may fear using stairs again, or he may be so fearful of falling again that no attempts to walk at all are made. Assessment for anxiety is made by observation of several behaviors: perception of danger that is distorted or unrealistic, withdrawal, purposeless activity such as wringing of the hands, a sense of impending doom, or an inability to concentrate. Other signs may be more subtle, such as increased confusion, irritability, frequency of urination, or incontinence.

Emotional responses such as depression or anxiety affect motivation to participate in care. Motivation of the person needing restorative care is vital. If there is no desire to participate in restorative care, it is unlikely any progress can be made.

Depression can have a profound effect on rehabilitation. A patient who is depressed is unhappy, sad, and often irritable. Feelings of hopelessness and helplessness are also seen. Physiologic problems such as changes in sleeping patterns, changes in appetite, or lack of energy are common. A depressed person may have trouble thinking, concentrating, or remembering. Any of these symptoms can interfere with the patient's ability to actively participate in restorative care. Careful assessment for the symptoms of depression is vital, especially because depression can easily go undetected in the elderly and depressive behaviors may be discounted as simply "old age" or mistaken for dementia. The elderly respond well to treatment when depression is identified. As the depression lifts, the patient is able to participate in restorative care.

Role of the Nurse

Ideally, after the physical, mental, and emotional areas have been evaluated, the patient, family, and nurse develop a plan of care using the nursing process. Long- and short-term goals for rehabilitation are developed with input from all members of the multidisciplinary team. The nurse develops a therapeutic relationship with the patient through active listening, praise, and supportive care. Asking open-ended questions may also help the older adult to verbalize thoughts and feelings.

As a member of the interdisciplinary team, the nurse collaborates with other members of the team and coordinates the care. Careful observation and monitoring of the nurse aide or restorative aide is important to ensure the restorative care plan is followed. The nurse documents progress in the chart weekly or whenever there is a significant change.

RESTORATIVE CARE GUIDELINES

Assisting the Patient With Restorative Care
- Believe in the patient's potential to improve.
- Emphasize strengths and successes.
- Help the patient to make attainable short-term goals.
- Promote independence while giving necessary assistance.
- Be patient. Allow plenty of time for the patient to accomplish the activities of daily living (ADLs).
- Praise the patient and family when appropriate.

An important role for the nurse is to plan interventions that prevent secondary complications such as muscular contractures, pressure ulcers, disease, muscular atrophy, and psychological problems. The nurse is the health care professional who observes small changes in improvement or deterioration. It is important for the nurse to communicate any change to the appropriate member of the rehabilitation team and to document changes as they occur.

Custodial Versus Restorative Care

Unfortunately, ageism can affect nurses and health care workers, causing the emphasis of care to be custodial care rather than restorative care. This type of nurse views aging as a time of inevitable deterioration and disability. **Custodial care** is a low-level type of care in which the emphasis is on "doing to" the patient rather than working with the patient. In custodial care, the nurse does for the resident what needs to be done. The resident remains predominately passive.

This type of atmosphere promotes learned helplessness. **Learned helplessness** is the individual's belief that he has no control over a situation and that nothing he can do or say will change the situation. Learned helplessness develops when all control is taken away and the person lives in an environment totally controlled by others. This type of atmosphere leads to depression, passive behavior, and feelings of hopelessness.

The elderly person is prone to develop learned helplessness when strictly custodial care is given. Nurses reinforce feelings of helplessness when the person is given no opportunity to have a voice in the type of care received. These nurses do not expect the older adult to improve. Outcomes meet expectations. When expectations are low, outcomes are low as well. With this type of care, interventions that satisfy Maslow's physiologic or basic needs (see Chapter 2) provide the major source care. Although these needs are essential, the need for safety, love and belonging, and esteem cannot be neglected or ignored. Only when cognitive and functional loss is so severe that the individual is unable to function mentally or physically should custodial care be implemented. Even at this point, the nurse is alert for any signs that would indicate a possible increase in functional ability.

Unfortunately, some nursing facilities provide more custodial care than restorative care. All care of the elderly must focus on restorative care. Interventions that promote functional ability and encourage independence are emphasized. One reason custodial care is used is that less of the nurse's time is required to bathe, toilet, and dress the patient than to assist the elderly person to do these activities for himself. This is unfortunate, because by spending time encouraging and promoting self-care, the nurse assistant's job would be easier in the long run, and the patient would have greater life satisfaction.

To combat feelings of learned helplessness, provide opportunities for decision making by the patient. Even small decisions can make a difference in the person's perception of control. Choices such as whether to eat in the cafeteria or in the room, whether to take a bath or a shower, whether to take a shower today or tomorrow, and when to wake up in the morning or when go to sleep at night can increase a person's feelings of self-worth and decrease feelings of helplessness and loss of control.

PROVIDING RESTORATIVE CARE

The ultimate aim of restorative care is to assist the patient to return to independent or semi-independent living or the previous level of functioning. In nursing home patients, the goal of restorative care may not be to return the patient to independent living or even former levels of independent living. The goal for the elder patient may be improvement in self-care even if dismissal from the nursing home is not a possibility. It is important not to exclude the elderly from the rehabilitation process.

> **RESTORATIVE CARE GUIDELINES**
>
> Goals for the Elderly
> - Maintain existing abilities.
> - Strengthen functional abilities.
> - Prevent secondary complications.

To accomplish these goals, restorative nursing care focuses on promoting mobility, personal care, and home management.

Promoting Mobility

Mobility is the ability to move body parts and to move from one place to another. Some older people move well. Exercise programs that begin in early life and are continued through old age decrease problems with mobility in later life. However, many older adults have problems with mobility. Elderly patients who are totally immobile require frequent turning (a minimum of every 2 hours) and daily range-of-motion (ROM) exercises.

Range-of-Motion Exercises
ROM exercises help to maintain existing muscle tone and prevent contractures (ie, permanent shortening of muscle fibers because of muscles surrounding a joint remaining contracted for an extended time). Joints have a specific capability for movement through extension, flexion, and rotation. Range of motion exercises moves a joint through all of the movements possible for that particular joint.

Not all elderly are able to move each joint though full ROM. Sometimes, calcium deposits accumulate

---

DISPLAY 9-1. Guidelines for Performing Range-of-Motion Exercises

- Grasp the extremity firmly but without undue pressure.
- Support joints and dependent areas of each extremity when performing passive range-of-motion (ROM) exercises. For example, support the elbow with one hand and hold the wrist with the other hand when giving ROM to the elbow or shoulder joint.
- Repeat each movement at least three times.
- Use slow, gentle movements.
- Discontinue if movement causes pain, discomfort, or fatigue.
- Flex, extend, and rotate all joints (ie, neck, shoulder, elbow, wrist, each finger, hip, leg, ankle, foot, and each toe).
- Supervise the patient in active ROM.
- Assist as needed for assistive ROM.

---

in the joints that limit movement. Active ROM occurs when the movement of the joint is done by the individual. Passive ROM occurs when the nurse or other caregiver moves the patient's joint through its full range of mobility. Active ROM provides the greatest benefit to the older adult, but passive ROM is an important alternative in some situations. Guidelines for performing ROM can be found in Display 9-1. Sometimes, individuals need some assistance to complete ROM exercises but can perform some actions independently. This type of ROM is called **active assistive range of motion**. Active assistive ROM is often needed in the nursing home. It is preferable to passive in that the patient is encouraged to perform actions that he is able to do and helped to perform those actions he cannot perform. This helps prevent loss of mobility.

Assistive Devices

Some elderly people can remain mobile through the use of an assistive device. Assistive devices such as canes, walkers, crutches, and wheelchairs increase mobility and independent function (Fig. 9-1). The choice of an assistive device depends on the extent of the disability and the existing abilities. These devices can decrease the incidence of falls in the elderly. Assistive devices widen the base of support and decrease weight bearing on the lower extremities.

Using a Cane
Canes are useful for patients with hip disorders resulting from hip replacement or arthritis. A cane relieves pressure on weight-bearing joints by redistributing the

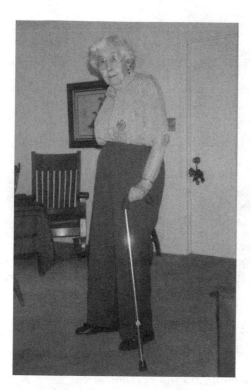

FIGURE 9-1. This 88-year-old woman uses a cane to assist in walking. The cane is placed on the stronger side of the body, and the elbow is slightly flexed.

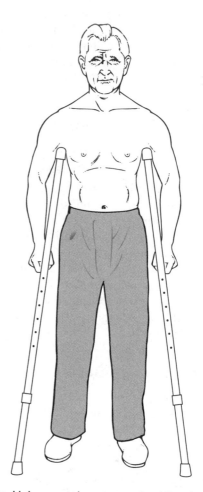

FIGURE 9-2. Using crutches correctly. All gaits begin in the tripod position. Note that the bottom of the crutch is placed aproximately 6″ to the side of the foot. The top of the crutch is two or three finger widths from the axillae when the elbows are flexed about 30 degrees.

weight. A single-point cane is inexpensive and easily managed in a nursing home or home environment. Canes are held in the opposite hand from the involved lower extremity, with the handle approximately level with the great trochanter and the tip of the cane approximately 6 inches to the side of the fifth toe. Cane length must be individually adjusted to the correct length based on height and arm length. Wooden canes are cut to the correct length, and aluminum canes are easily modified in length. Canes have rubber tips to prevent slipping. The height of the cane is cut or adjusted so that there is a 25% to 30% bend at the elbow when the patient places weight on the cane. A four-prong or quad cane is recommended when maximum support is needed. When using a cane, the opposite leg and arm are moved together as in a normal ambulation pattern. The cane is advanced at the same time the affected leg is moved forward. A gait belt can be used to provide support and stability when a patient is walking.

Using Crutches
Crutches are more difficult for the older adult because of the necessary sequencing of leg movements. Often, the physical therapist teaches crutch walking while the nurse reinforces the physical therapist's instruction and assists the patient as needed. Crutches are adjustable in height at the base and the handpiece.

The top of the crutch should rest against the chest with approximately 2 inches (two to three fingerwidths) between the crutch top and the axilla when the elbows are flexed approximately 30 degrees. Instruct the patient not to position the crutches in a way that puts pressure on the axillae (Fig. 9-2). When pressure is placed on the axilla, nerve damage can occur, resulting in numbness, tingling, weakness, and possibly paralysis. The handbars must be adjusted to a height that allows the patient to extend the arm almost completely when leaning on the palms.

The gait is selected based on the patient's weight-bearing ability. Two common gait patterns are used by the elderly:

Three-point gait is used when the patient can bear weight only on the unaffected leg.

Four-point gait is used for patients with muscular weakness, lack of balance, or lack of coordination.

Other gaits include the two-point gait, the swing to, and the swing through. The physical therapist

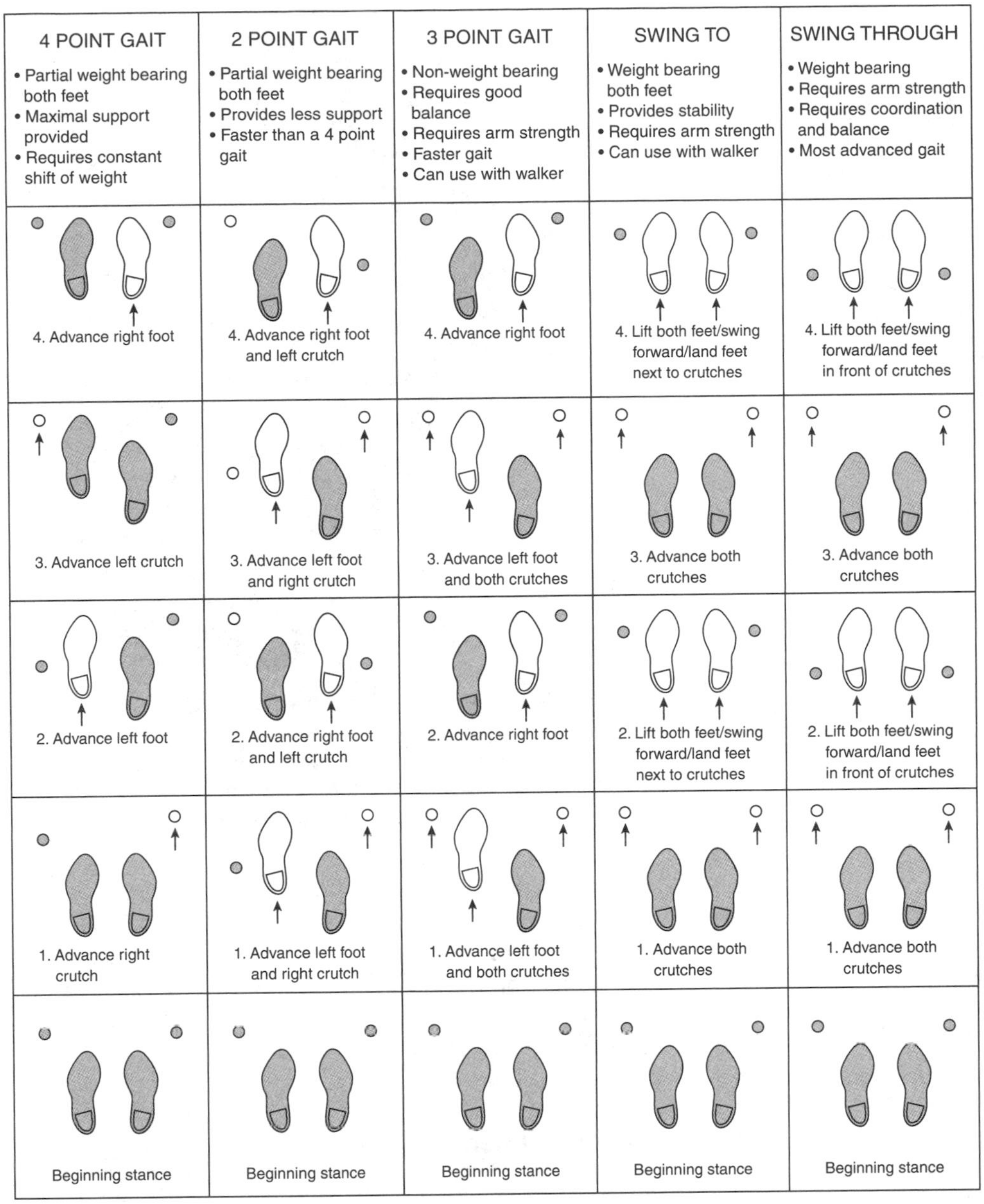

FIGURE 9-3. Gaits used for crutch walking.

4 POINT GAIT	2 POINT GAIT	3 POINT GAIT	SWING TO	SWING THROUGH
• Partial weight bearing both feet • Maximal support provided • Requires constant shift of weight	• Partial weight bearing both feet • Provides less support • Faster than a 4 point gait	• Non-weight bearing • Requires good balance • Requires arm strength • Faster gait • Can use with walker	• Weight bearing both feet • Provides stability • Requires arm strength • Can use with walker	• Weight bearing • Requires arm strength • Requires coordination and balance • Most advanced gait
4. Advance right foot	4. Advance right foot and left crutch	4. Advance right foot	4. Lift both feet/swing forward/land feet next to crutches	4. Lift both feet/swing forward/land feet in front of crutches
3. Advance left crutch	3. Advance left foot and right crutch	3. Advance left foot and both crutches	3. Advance both crutches	3. Advance both crutches
2. Advance left foot	2. Advance right foot and left crutch	2. Advance right foot	2. Lift both feet/swing forward/land feet next to crutches	2. Lift both feet/swing forward/land feet in front of crutches
1. Advance right crutch	1. Advance left foot and right crutch	1. Advance left foot and both crutches	1. Advance both crutches	1. Advance both crutches
Beginning stance	Beginning stance	Beginning stance	Beginning stance	Beginning stance

frequently instructs the patient in gait training. The nurse is responsible for reinforcing the gait training given by the physical therapist. Figure 9-3 depicts the various gaits.

Using a Walker

Walkers have a very wide base of support that provide a large amount of stability. Walkers are used by older adults with generalized weakness and those with balance problems. There are two types of walkers: the pickup walker and the rolling walker. The older adult is more stable when using the pickup walker. Walkers are adjusted so that the handgrips can be held comfortably and the arms are slightly flexed (Fig. 9-4). The arms should exhibit 20 to 30 degrees of flexion at the elbow. Less instruction is needed to use a walker. Walkers are also appropriate for older adults with cognitive impairments who have difficulty with more complex instructions. Disadvantages are that they require more space to maneuver than canes and that they cannot easily be used on stairs.

> **RESTORATIVE CARE GUIDELINES**
>
> General Instructions for the Patient Using a Walker
> - Hold the walker on the handgrips.
> - Place the walker in front of you while leaning slightly forward.
> - Using your hands for support, walk into the walker.
> - After ensuring that balance is attained, lift the walker and place it in front of you again.
> - Continue with the same pattern of walking.

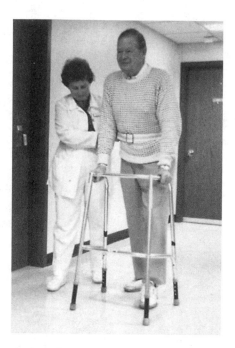

FIGURE 9-4. A walker is a molded aluminum device that functions to support the front of the body.

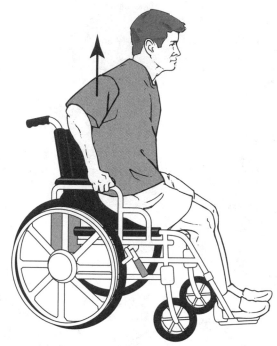

FIGURE 9-5. Shifting weight in wheelchair. Approximately every 15 minutes while sitting in a wheelchair, the patient is taught to shift weight or push the body up out of contact with the chair for several seconds. This helps prevent ischial pressure ulcers.

General Guidelines

Using the assistive device correctly is important. A device that is too low can cause flexion in the hips and trunk and forward displacement of the head. A device that is too high cannot effectively assist with balance or be used for upper body weight bearing. In general, when assisting the patient, the nurse stands on the patient's weaker side. There may be situations in which assistive devices are not recommended for patient with mobility problems. For example, if a patient uses a device to hit or strike other people or if cognitive function is not of a sufficient level to teach correct use, these devices are not recommended. There is an increased risk of falling when devices are not used properly. Patients are encouraged to wear sturdy, well-fitting shoes for extra support.

Wheelchairs

Many elderly patients who have had cerebrovascular accidents or fractures can benefit from a wheelchair. Wheelchairs range from a standard, manually propelled styles to those that are highly computerized and managed with a puff of breath. Most elderly use the standard type of chair. However, older adults with spinal cord injuries or neurologic diseases may benefit from one of the more technically advanced chairs. Selection of the chair is important and is best accomplished with the aid of a physical therapist. When using a wheelchair, the elderly person is encouraged to shift weight often and to use the arms to raise up for a few seconds every 15 minutes (Fig. 9-5).

Care must be taken not to place an older adult in a wheelchair too soon, because she can lose any remaining ambulatory ability. Assessory equipment for wheelchair use in the elderly includes elevating leg rests to help prevent edema and removable arm and foot rests for easier transfers.

Promoting Personal Care

Personal care or **self-care activities** include the activities of feeding, dressing, bathing, grooming, and toileting. Self-care activities are also called ADLs. When older adults lose the ability to care for themselves, there is also a loss of self-esteem. Whenever self-care becomes a problem, the older person faces the possibility of having to go to a nursing home or becoming increasingly dependent on family or friends. Restorative nursing care is aimed at restoring, maintaining, and when possible, increasing the ability to perform self-care activities. Some older adults need specialized assistive devices to help them perform self-care. A variety of self-care assistive devices are available (Fig. 9-6).

Feeding

Self-feeding is often a problem for patients recovering from stroke, with arthritis, or with parkinsonism. Adaptive equipment can be used to increase

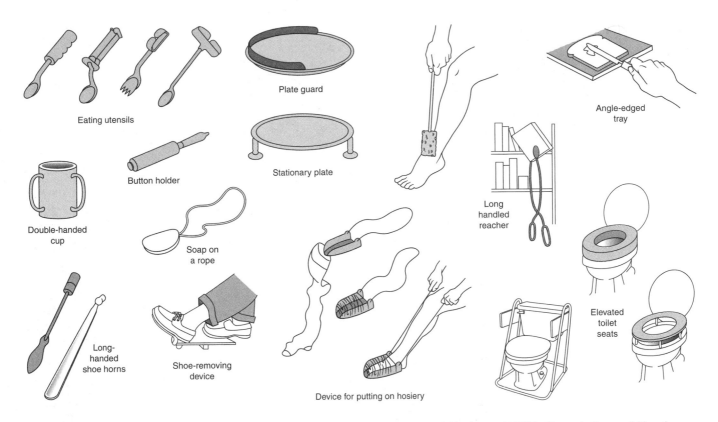

Eating utensils

Plate guard

Button holder

Stationary plate

Double-handed cup

Soap on a rope

Long handled reacher

Angle-edged tray

Long-handed shoe horns

Shoe-removing device

Device for putting on hosiery

Elevated toilet seats

FIGURE 9-6. Examples of assistive devices. Adapted from Christensen and Kockrow (1996). *Foundations of Nursing,* 2nd ed., Fig. 45-4, p. 1454.

independence. Friction mats stabilize plates and wide-rimmed dishes keep food on the plate. Utensils with specialized handles help patients who have difficulty grasping. These utensils can be curved, enlarged, or weighted according to individual needs. Arm supports are available when the shoulders and elbows are weak. The variety of tools available ranges from simple (eg, using a straw to drink) to complex (eg, mechanical devices that guide a spoon to pick up food on the plate and take it to the mouth). Diet modifications may be helpful. For example, a soft diet requires less manipulation of food (ie, chewing). For those with difficulties in handling utensils, finger foods may be appropriate.

Dressing and Grooming
Patients with pain or limited movement of the hip, knee, and shoulder have problems dressing and grooming. Evaluation and consultation by an occupational therapist is helpful. There are numerous self-help devices for dressing and grooming. Adaptive measures include the use of Velcro on closures for shoes or in place of zippers or buttons, large rings on zippers, or the use of a button hook. Dresses that open down the front or gowns that fasten at the shoulder may be helpful. Having grab rails near dressing areas and placing clothing within easy reach make dressing easier. A patient

with hemiplegia (ie, paralysis of one side of the body) is taught to dress by placing clothing on the affected arm or leg first. When undressing, the hemiplegic is instructed to undress the unaffected arm or leg first. These simple measures enable many to groom and dress themselves with greater independence.

Bathing
Bathing chairs can be used when getting in and out of the bathtub is a problem. Extended-handle brushes for bathing are also available. Use of a hand-held shower device may be helpful for showering. Placing handles in strategic locations can help prevent falls in the shower (Fig. 9-7) or the bath tub. The occupational therapist can assist the older adult in finding devices that meet individual needs.

Toileting
Mobility problems increase the potential for difficulty with toileting. Helpful devices include raised toilet seats (Fig. 9-8), grab rails in the toilet area, and long-handled toilet paper holders. Patients with arthritis and hemiplegia are particularly prone to toileting problems. A bedside commode placed for easy access may make toileting easier for those with mobility problems. Men may benefit from the use of urinals.

mBaylly

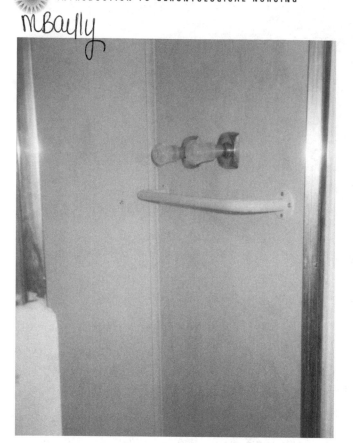

FIGURE 9-7. Handle bars placed in strategic locations in the shower or bathtub can help prevent falls for the older adult.

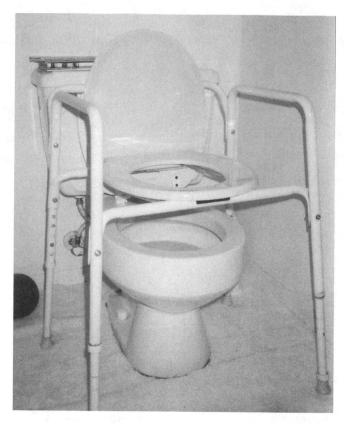

FIGURE 9-8. A raised toilet seat assists the older adult who has problems bending the knees in a sitting position or those who are too weak to rise after sitting.

HOME MANAGEMENT

Self-care is facilitated in a safe home environment. The nurse first inspects the home environment and assesses for unsafe areas or situations. The patient and family members are then taught measures to make the environment safer for the older adult. Display 9-2 identifies ways to make the home environment safer.

Roles of the Physical and Occupational Therapists

Referral to a physical therapist or an occupational therapist is helpful for training in the use of assistive devices to increase the elder's functional ability. Other conditions may indicate the need for consulting with a physical therapist or an occupational therapist:

- Problems with mobility or in performing ADLs
- Conditions such as a cerebrovascular accident, myocardial infarction, arthritis, or Alzheimer's disease

- Functional decline without apparent cause
- Environmental safety concerns in the home setting

☼ CRITICAL THINKING EXERCISES

1. Mr. Wadell, age 82 years, was recently admitted to the nursing home for rehabilitation after hip surgery. What areas would be important for you to assess to determine his potential for restorative care? How would you assess those areas?
2. A 79-year-old woman with limited mobility is to be discharged home to be cared for by her daughter. The daughter is concerned about her mother's potential for falling. What areas of assessment would be most important? What suggestions could you make to the daughter to decrease her mother's potential for falling?
3. Brainstorm with your classmates to identify at least six ways that nurses can foster learned helplessness in a nursing home environment.

DISPLAY 9-2. Guidelines for Making the Home Environment Safe

Personal Safety Practices
- Move slowly and carefully, especially on stairs.
- Avoid loose, floppy slippers without soles. Wear shoes and slippers that fit securely and have nonskid soles.
- Avoid long, flowing, loose clothing, which may cause tripping.
- Use canes and other assistive devices when feeling unsteady.
- Never hold objects in both hands when walking or climbing stairs.

Floors
- Floors should not be waxed or have a high-gloss finish.
- Do not use throw rugs.
- Clutter should be eliminated so pathways are wide.
- Light cords should not be in pathways.
- Hallways should be well lighted.

Stairways
- Stairways should be well lighted.
- A lightswitch should be located at the top and bottom of each stairway. The switch should be of a different color from that of the walls and should be about 2 feet from the first step.
- Stairways should have handrails on both sides, and if possible, the handrails should extend past the top and bottom of the steps.
- Carpeting should not be loose or torn; no nails should protrude.
- Put colored tape on the edge of the top and the bottom steps.

Bathroom
- Use nonskid mats in the tub, in the shower, and on the floor.
- Grab bars should be attached to the structural supports in the wall.

- Keep soap in a dish or on a soap rope to prevent it from falling and causing a fall.
- Hold only grab bars—never hold towel racks or other wall-attached items such as a soap dish—when getting in and out of the tub or shower.
- Never touch electrical appliances when you are wet.
- Check the temperature of the water before getting into the bathtub to avoid being burned.

Bedroom
- Keep a flashlight next to the bed, and check it frequently.
- Do not smoke in bed.
- Keep path to the bathroom clean.
- Use a nightlight.
- Have the phone next to the bed and within easy reach. Keep a list of important phone numbers such as those of the police, fire department, and close relatives in large letters near the each phone.

Kitchen
- Keep the handles of pans turned in and away from the outside edge of the stove.
- Keep flammable, combustible items, such as solvents and cleaning fluids, away from the stove.
- Keep dishtowels, potholders, and paper towels away from the burners.
- Do not wear garments with loose-fitting sleeves that can get caught on pan handles or catch fire from the burners.
- Separate all insecticide and cleaning fluids from food, and keep them out of reach of children.
- Wipe up spills from the floor immediately to avoid slipping.
- Keep the kitchen well lighted. Use at least 60-watt bulbs in ceiling light fixtures.
- Do not stand on chairs; use step stools. The object you are reaching for should be directly in front of you and not off to the side, requiring a long reach.
- Keep a fire extinguisher in the kitchen.

Adapted from Farrell, J. (1990). *Nursing care of the older adult.* 180–183. Philadelphia: J. B. Lippincott.

REFERENCES AND SUGGESTED READING

Easton, K. (Ed.). (1999). *Gerontological rehabilitation nursing.* Philadelphia: W.B. Saunders.

Rosdahl, C.B. (1995). *Textbook of basic nursing* (6th ed.). Philadelphia: J.B. Lippincott.

Schaie, K., & Pietrucha (Eds.). (2000). *Mobility and transportation in the elderly.* New York: Springer Publishing.

CHAPTER 10

CHAPTER OUTLINE

KEY TERMS
CHAPTER OBJECTIVES
DIETARY GUIDELINES
NUTRIENTS AND HEALTH
EFFECTS OF AGING ON NUTRITIONAL STATUS
CANCER PREVENTION AND DETECTION
OSTEOPOROSIS
CRITICAL THINKING EXERCISES
REFERENCES AND SUGGESTED READING

KEY TERMS

aerobic exercise
atherosclerosis
cholesterol
heat exhaustion
heat stroke
high-density lipoprotein (HDL)
lactose intolerance
lipid
lipoprotein
low-density lipoprotein (LDL)
minerals
nutrients
osteoporosis
vitamins

Promoting Physiologic Health

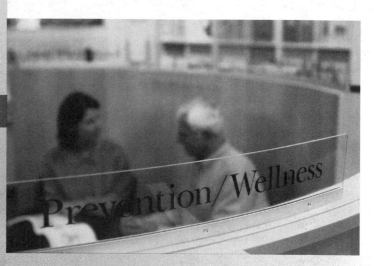

CHAPTER OBJECTIVES

At the completion of this chapter, the student will be able to

- Describe the role the seven dietary guidelines play in maintaining health

- Identify the major nutrients and their role in maintaining health

- Discuss effects of aging on nutritional status

- Describe economic and social changes that affect nutrition

- Discuss the role of exercise in promoting the health of the older adult

- Describe health promoting behaviors that affect cardiovascular health

- Discuss methods of cancer prevention and detection

- Identify important aspects of prevention and treatment of osteoporosis

More and more older adults are remaining active, self-sufficient, and relatively healthy well into old age. Positive health-promoting lifestyles play an important role maintaining a high quality of life and greater independence for the older generation. Promoting the physiologic health of older adults includes helping them to understand the importance of good nutrition and proper exercise and how to decrease their risk for certain chronic diseases such as cardiovascular disease, cancer, and osteoporosis. Despite the fact that four of five older adults have at least one chronic illness, most rate their overall health as good.

DIETARY GUIDELINES

Good nutrition is vital for a healthy lifestyle. The basics of a healthy diet are simple and relatively easy to follow. The U.S. Dietary Guidelines, published by the U.S. Department of Agriculture (USDA) and the U.S. Department of Health and Human Services, provide a sound framework to build a healthy diet.

NUTRITION ALERT

The USDA has provided the following recommendations:

- Eat a variety of foods.
- Maintain a desirable weight.
- Avoid foods high in fat, saturated fat, and cholesterol.
- Limit alcoholic beverages.
- Choose a diet high in vegetables, fruits, and grain products.
- Use sugar in moderation.
- Use salt sparingly.

Eat a Variety of Foods

There is no one perfect food. Eating a variety of foods supplies all of the necessary nutrients needed on a daily basis. Including different foods each day helps prevent boredom and ensures adequate nutrient intake. The Food Guide Pyramid was developed to help individuals make healthy food choices by eating a variety of foods. The pyramid is a guide for what to eat each day and gives approximate amounts of specific foods. The foods at the base (ie, breads, cereals, rice, and pasta) of the pyramid should provide the bulk of the diet. Grain products, beans, vegetables, fruits, and dairy products are filled with vitamins, minerals, and fiber to give the body needed nutrients. Foods at the tip of the pyramid (ie, fats, oils, and sweets) should be eaten only in limited amounts. The Good Guide Pyramid has been modified to meet the changing nutritional needs of people older than 70 years (Fig. 10-1). It differs from the pyramid for younger people in that eight 8-ounce glasses of water are added at the base of the pyramid to prevent constipation and dehydration. Additional supplementation of calcium and vitamins B_{12} and D is suggested. There are no upper limits on the number of servings of foods (except for fats and sweets) and water.

Maintain a Desirable Weight

Maintaining a desirable weight requires self-discipline and careful planning. Weight loss occurs when the number of calories consumed is less than the number of calories expended. When fewer calories are consumed, the body uses the stored fat as a source of energy. One pound of body weight is equal to 3,500 calories. To lose 1 pound of body fat, more calories must be used by the body than are ingested. The best method to rid the body of fat is through reducing the daily caloric intake and increasing the amount of exercise. A desirable weight is a weight that is appropriate for age, height (Table 10-1), body build, and health status.

Approximately 20% of adults older than 65 years of age are overweight. Being overweight increases the risk for heart disease, hypertension, cancer, and gallbladder disease. Older adults must adjust caloric intake with age. A moderately active adult between the ages of 60 and 69 requires 10% fewer calories. After the age of 70, another 10% fewer calories are needed to maintain normal weight.

Avoid Foods High in Fat

The healthiest way to lose weight is to cut calories and fat from the diet and exercise regularly. Most Americans eat a diet that is 35% to 40% fat. A diet high in fat is associated with heart disease, hypertension, and some forms of cancer. To decrease the risk of disease, it is recommended that dietary fat be less than 30% of total calories each day.

Limit Alcoholic Beverages

Older adults take longer to metabolize alcohol, making them more sensitive to the effects of alcohol and needing less alcohol to become intoxicated. Those who drink more than three alcoholic drinks per day increase their risk of destroying liver tissue. Heavy drinking can cause cirrhosis of the liver

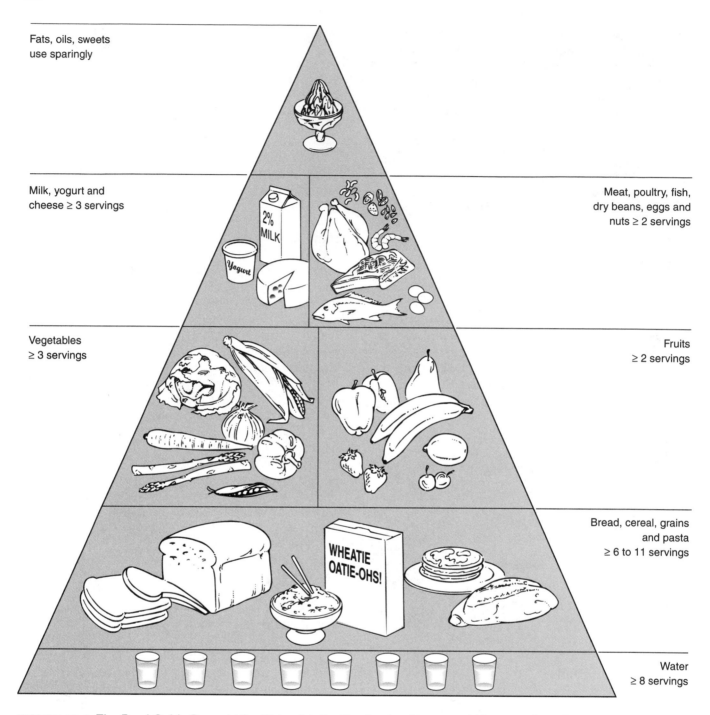

Fats, oils, sweets
use sparingly

Milk, yogurt and
cheese ≥ 3 servings

2% MILK

Yogurt

Meat, poultry, fish,
dry beans, eggs and
nuts ≥ 2 servings

Vegetables
≥ 3 servings

Fruits
≥ 2 servings

WHEATIE OATIE-OHS!

Bread, cereal, grains
and pasta
≥ 6 to 11 servings

Water
≥ 8 servings

FIGURE 10-1. The Food Guide Pyramid for Older Adults. The food guide pyramid is an outline of what to eat each day. Foods from the lower three levels of the pyramid are emphasized in daily meal planning. Eating a variety of foods will assist in obtaining the nutrients needed for optimal health.

and mental deterioration. Drinking also increases the risk of developing cancer of the mouth, esophagus, and liver. Alcohol intake should be limited to no more than two drinks per day. An alcoholic drink is defined as

- 1 ounce of hard liquor
- 5 ounces of wine
- 12 ounces of beer ("Light" beer contains fewer calories but the same amount of alcohol.)

Choose a Diet High in Vegetables, Fruits, and Grains

Foods high in complex carbohydrates, such as vegetables, grains, bread, and rice, are high in fiber and low in calories, fat, and cholesterol. A diet high in fiber reduces the risk of cancer and heart disease. Daily consumption of vegetables and fruits is associated with a decreased risk of prostate, lung, bladder,

TABLE 10-1. Recommended Weights For Men and Women

Height (ft, in)	Men		Women	
	Recommended Weight (lb)	40% Overweight Range (lb)	Recommended Weight (lb)	40% Overweight Range (lb)
4 10	—	—	92–119	129–167
4 11	—	—	94–122	132–171
5 0	—	—	95–125	133–175
5 1	—	—	99–128	139–179
5 2	112–141	157–197	102–131	143–183
5 3	115–144	161–202	105–134	147–188
5 4	118–148	165–207	108–138	151–193
5 5	121–152	169–213	111–142	155–199
5 6	124–156	174–218	114–146	160–204
5 7	128–161	179–225	118–150	165–210
5 8	132–166	185–232	122–154	171–216
5 9	136–170	190–238	126–158	176–221
5 10	140–174	196–244	130–163	182–228
5 11	144–179	202–250	134–168	188–235
6 0	148–184	207–258	138–173	193–242
6 1	152–189	213–265	—	—
6 2	156–194	218–272	—	—
6 3	160–199	224–279	—	—
6 4	164–204	230–286	—	—

From the Metropolitan Life Insurance Company

esophagus, and stomach cancer. Choose whole-grain products, such as whole wheat or cracked wheat breads, oatmeal, popcorn, or brown rice. These complex carbohydrates have more fiber than enriched products. The Food Guide Pyramid illustrates the importance of including these foods as a foundation for all meals (see Fig. 10-1).

Use Sugar and Salt in Moderation

The major hazards from eating sugar are tooth decay and weight gain. Eat fresh fruit or canned fruits packed without sugar. Consider low-calorie sweeteners instead of sugar. Sodium occurs naturally in many foods. Other foods have sodium added during processing. Sodium intake should be no more than 2,400 to 3,000 mg/day. One level teaspoon of salt contains 2,300 mg of sodium.

PATIENT TEACHING AID

Include this information when teaching the older adult about limiting the use of salt:
- **Cook without adding extra salt.**
- **Substitute lemon juice, basil, dill, or curry powder.**
- **Eat fresh or frozen vegetables.**
- **Check labels for salt or sodium content.**
- **Check with your health care provider before using a salt substitute, because it may contain potassium and may not be recommended for some individuals.**

NUTRIENTS FOR HEALTH

Nutrients are chemical substances found in foods that are needed by the body to maintain health. Proteins, carbohydrates, and fats play an important role in the health of the older adult. These nutrients are needed for energy, immunity, and maintenance and repair of body tissue. Vitamins and minerals also play an vital role in the health of the older adult.

Proteins

Protein is essential for growth, maintenance, and repair of body tissue. Every cell in the body is made of protein. Antibodies are made of proteins. Our immunity against disease depends on the production of antibodies to fight infection.

In general, the elderly person receives adequate protein. When health problems such as infection, fractures, surgery, or burns occur, increased protein is needed. Older persons on fixed incomes, those living alone, and those with limited transportation may have problems obtaining adequate protein. Protein foods are often more expensive than foods high in fat or carbohydrate and may require more preparation. Proteins such as milk, cheese, or meat also tend to spoil more easily.

Carbohydrates

Carbohydrates are the major sources of energy for the body. Carbohydrates include sugars and starches. Simple carbohydrates provide mostly empty calories and include candy, table sugar, brown sugar, honey, molasses, and sweet desserts. Complex carbohydrates (eg, starch) are the most important sources of carbohydrates in the diet. Starch is found in grains, cereals, breads, pasta, and starchy vegetables such as potatoes and legumes (ie, dried beans and peas).

Complex carbohydrates are also rich in dietary fiber, which is necessary for maintaining a healthy bowel. Dietary fiber is the skeletal portion of foods that cannot be digested by the body. These foods provide the roughage or bulk that forms normal fecal material. The recommended amount of dietary fiber in the diet is a minimum of 20 to 25 g per day. Most people ingest only about one half of the dietary fiber needed daily. Eating according to the Food Guide Pyramid and choosing whole-grain breads, cereals, fruits, and vegetables helps ensure adequate amounts of fiber.

Increasing the amount of fiber in the diet of older adults helps prevent constipation and keeps the intestine functioning properly. A diet high in fiber may protect against colon cancer. It is important for the older adult to understand that increased amounts of fluids are necessary when fiber is increased. Gas and bloating may occur as the body adjusts to increased fiber. This normal occurrence decreases as the body adapts to the increased fiber. Gradually increasing fiber in the diet while simultaneously increasing the fluid intake helps decrease bloating and gas formation.

Fats

Lipid is a term that includes all types of fats and fat-related compounds such as fats, oil, and cholesterol. Dietary fat should be limited to no more 30% of daily caloric intake. Although cholesterol is not a true fat, it is discussed with fats because it has properties similar to fat. **Cholesterol** is manufactured by all animals, including humans. It is therefore found in all foods from animal sources. An elevated blood cholesterol level (>200 mg/dL) is associated with an increased risk for coronary artery disease (CAD). Foods high in cholesterol, such as whole milk, dairy products, meat, and eggs, should be avoided. Cholesterol intake should be limited to 300 mg per day (see the High Blood Cholesterol section).

Vitamins and Minerals

Vitamins are organic compounds needed in minute amounts by the body. Although needed in small amounts, vitamins are essential for normal digestion, tissue building and repair, energy production, and normal nerve functioning. **Minerals** are inorganic substances that are found in the body that help to regulate body functions. Major minerals include calcium, chloride, magnesium, phosphorus, potassium, sodium, and sulfur. Although trace minerals are essential, they are needed only in small amounts. Some of the trace minerals include iron, iodine, selenium, and zinc. Because of problems with absorption, the older adult is at risk for decreased absorption of vitamins and minerals, particularly folic acid, calcium, iron, and vitamins C, B_6, and B_{12}. Vitamin and mineral supplements may be needed to provide adequate nutrition.

EFFECTS OF AGING ON NUTRITIONAL STATUS

Most older people lead full and productive lives, but with increased age and frailty, the risk of nutritional problems increases. Aging diminishes the ability to ingest, digest, absorb, and metabolize nutrients in food. The metabolic rate slows, and the amount of lean body mass is reduced, resulting in a decrease in caloric requirements and an increase in fatty tissue. Exercise helps to counteract these problems. Although energy needs decrease, nutrient needs remain the same as for younger adults.

Loss of teeth can decrease food choices and make eating less enjoyable. If chewing is a problem, ground or pureed meats, stewed fruits, and chopped or ground vegetables may be needed to provide adequate nutrition. Changes in the digestive system increase the risk of constipation. A diet high in fiber, increased fluids, and regular exercise is recommended to help prevent constipation. With age, digestion becomes less efficient. If digestion is a problem, six smaller meals may be preferable to three large meals.

Decreases in sensory functioning contribute to loss of appetite. For example, taste may be altered because of decreased number of taste buds as a result of the aging process. Lower food intake can result from a decreased ability to smell, or hearing difficulties may decrease the social enjoyment that occurs with eating.

Aging sometimes brings about a condition called **lactose intolerance.** With the condition, the milk sugar lactose cannot be digested because the enzyme lactase is lacking. This results in abdominal bloating, flatus, cramping, and diarrhea after the ingestion of milk or milk products. LactAid, one of several over-the-counter enzyme products, may be used to aid the digestion of milk. The liquid form of LactAid can be added to milk, or the tablet form can be chewed before ingesting milk or milk products. Milk containing LactAid is available at some grocery stores. Commercial liquid food supplements such as Ensure and Sustacal are lactose free. Instruct the patient with lactose intolerance to read all labels carefully to avoid foods containing lactose, whey, dry milk solids, and non-fat dry milk.

Nurses play an important role in helping the patient to meet nutritional needs by keeping a record of the amount and type of foods eaten, determining food preferences, and identifying any mechanical problems with eating. Referral to a dietitian is made when the elderly person is not eating an adequate diet or a weight loss of 3 pounds pounds or more occurs.

Economic and Social Changes That Affect Nutrition

Most older adults live on decreased or fixed incomes. Less money is available to purchase food. Transportation to and from the supermarket may be difficult. Protein foods may be limited because of cost and time required in preparation. Carbohydrates are less expensive, simple to prepare, and easily obtained. Poor vision and limited mobility make cooking more difficult.

Social changes occur in the older person's life that can affect the elder in meeting nutritional needs. Loss of loved ones, living alone, and lack of social interaction contribute to decreased appetite. Eating in a pleasant atmosphere and in the presence of friends stimulates the appetite. Older adults are encouraged to attend senior citizen centers, churches, or other sites where congregate meals are served and socialization is provided.

For those elderly who are homebound, many communities have programs to provide nutritionally sound meals 5 or more days each week. Meals on Wheels is a food service that delivers hot meals at noon and sometimes cold meals for the evening to those who cannot purchase their own groceries or prepare their own meals. Senior citizen centers serve hot meals daily to those at the center. Trans-

DISPLAY 10-1. Ten Benefits of Regular Exercise

- Increases energy
- Increases resistance to fatigue
- Decreases anxiety and depression
- Improves ability to rest and sleep
- Decreases risk of developing cardiovascular disease
- Tones muscles and increases strength
- Burns calories for weight control
- Builds endurance for other physical activities
- Increases the efficiency of the heart and lungs
- Helps to maintain balance and agility

portation is sometimes provided for the elderly needing that service. Churches, synagogues, or schools may also offer free or low-cost meals.

Home delivered meals and those offered to senior citizens at congregate sites are often subsidized and in many cases are free. Sometimes, a contribution is requested, but payment is often purely voluntary. Some programs use a sliding scale based on income to determine individual fees. Food stamps may also be used to pay for government-approved sites or home delivered meals.

Exercise

Most older adults do not exercise. Many individuals believe that a decline in physical ability is an inevitable consequence of aging and exercising is not profitable for older adults. Evidence suggests otherwise. All ages, even the old elderly benefit from increased physical activity. Display 10-1 identifies 10 benefits of regular exercise.

Regular exercise helps to protect against coronary heart disease, the major health threat to older Americans. Even low- to moderate-intensity exercise can be beneficial in lowering the risk for heart disease. Activities such as walking, swimming, gardening, yard work, dancing, and home exercise are beneficial. The more vigorous activities such as swimming, brisk walking, running, cycling, or rope jumping are aerobic exercises and give the most consistent benefits.

Aerobic exercise is a type of physical activity in which the body uses oxygen to produce the energy to perform the activity. For the maximum benefits in preventing cardiovascular disease, aerobic exercises must be done consistently and for at least 30 minutes, three or four times each week. For an exercise to be considered aerobic, it must work the large muscles (ie, muscles in the legs, buttocks, or arms) for an extended period. Three factors are essential for a successful exercise program:

1. Frequency: Exercise a minimum of three times per week (five to six times per week if weight loss is a goal).
2. Intensity: Aim for a target zone heart rate that is 65% to 85% of the maximum heart rate per minute (Display 10-2).
3. Time: Exercise for 20 to 30 minutes in the target zone.

In addition to its effect on the cardiovascular system, regular exercise provides some protection against certain cancers, type II diabetes, arthritis, hypertension, and osteoporosis.

Considerations Before Beginning an Exercise Program

Persons older than 50 years of age may want to consult with a health care provider before beginning any exercise program, particularly if they have been relatively inactive over the years. However, a gradual, sensible exercise program usually has minimal health risks. Conditions that require a medical consultation before beginning an exercise program include diabetes, cardiovascular diseases, bone or joint conditions, or any other medical condition that may be affected by physical activity. For those with mobility limitations, exercise programs should be monitored.

Role of the Nurse

Nurses may work in an outpatient care center, an adult day care, or a wellness center where health promotion activities are taught. It is important to be aware of the health benefits of exercise and to teach these benefits to the older adults at these facilities. Before beginning an exercise program, the older adult should be given information about hydration, warming up, and frequency of exercising.

 PATIENT TEACHING AID

Before engaging in an exercise program, the older adult should be given the following information:

- Before exercising, have a warm-up period to gradually increase heart rate.
- Start gradually (5 to 10 minutes in the beginning) and gradually increase the amount of exercise (up to 30 to 60 minutes/day).
- Drink plenty of water before, during, and after physical activity.
- Set a regular time to exercise each day.
- Breathe deeply and evenly when exercising.
- Stop if you become excessively short of breath, develop pain, or feel dizzy. Report this to your physician or health care provider.

DISPLAY 10-2. How to Determine the Target Zone

1. Subtract the age from 220.
2. Multiply the result by 0.65 to find the lower end of the target zone.
3. Multiply the result by 0.85 to find the upper target zone.

Example: Alma, age 65, wants to begin an exercise program. Her physician has determined that she is able to participate in a walking program. Alma wants to determine her target zone.

1. Subtract 65 (Alma's age) from 220 = 155.
2. To find the lower end of the target zone: 155 × 0.65 = 100.75 or 100.
3. To find the upper target zone: 155 × 0.85 = 131.75 or 131.

When exercising, Alma should keep her heart rate within the target zone of 100 to 131 beats per minute for at least 20 minutes.

- **Keep a daily written log of exercise and include type of exercise, time, and intensity of exercise.**
- **Do not stop vigorous physical activity abruptly; gradually reduce the intensity of the exercise.**
- **Many exercises, particularly arm strengthening exercises, can be performed from a wheelchair.**

Walking

One of the most beneficial overall exercises is walking. Walking improves the blood flow back to the heart by the massaging action of the leg muscles against the walls of the veins. Walking has the added benefit of strengthening the leg muscles. Walking is an activity that almost anyone can do with little preparation. It can be done almost anywhere and costs no more than the price of a good pair of shoes. Walking has the lowest rate of injury of any form of exercise. The American Association of Retired Persons has recommendations for those older adult beginning an exercise program.

 PATIENT TEACHING AID

Recommendations for older adults beginning a walking for fitness program include the following:

- Choose a comfortable time of day to walk, preferably several hours after eating and when the temperature is cooler.
- Be careful not to overexert. Stop if feelings of shortness of breath or nausea develop (breathing should return to normal within 10 minutes after exercising).

DISPLAY 10-3. Suggested Walking Program

	Warm-up	Target Zone Exercising	Cool Down	Total Time
Week 1				
Session A	Walk 5 min	Then walk briskly 5 min	Then walk more slowly 5 min	15 min
Session B	Repeat above pattern			
Session C	Repeat above pattern			
Continue with at least three exercise sessions during each week of the program.				
Week 2	Walk 5 min	Walk briskly 7 min	Walk 5 min	17 min
Week 3	Walk 5 min	Walk briskly 9 min	Walk 5 min	19 min
Week 4	Walk 5 min	Walk briskly 11 min	Walk 5 min	21 min
Week 5	Walk 5 min	Walk briskly 13 min	Walk 5 min	23 min
Week 6	Walk 5 min	Walk briskly 15 min	Walk 5 min	25 min
Week 7	Walk 5 min	Walk briskly 18 min	Walk 5 min	28 min
Week 8	Walk 5 min	Walk briskly 20 min	Walk 5 min	30 min
Week 9	Walk 5 min	Walk briskly 23 min	Walk 5 min	33 min
Week 10	Walk 5 min	Walk briskly 26 min	Walk 5 min	36 min
Week 11	Walk 5 min	Walk briskly 28 min	Walk 5 min	38 min
Week 12	Walk 5 min	Walk briskly 30 min	Walk 5 min	40 min
Week 13 on:				

Check your pulse periodically to see if you are exercising within your target zone. As you become more fit, try exercising within the upper range of your target zone. Gradually increase your brisk walking time to 30 to 60 minutes, three or four times each week. Remember that your goal is to get the benefits you are seeking and enjoy your activity.

(1993). *Exercise and your heart: A guide to physical activity.* American Heart Association.

- **If you are following a walking program and feel uncomfortable progressing at the recommended rate, spend an additional week at each level.**
- **Walk briskly enough to increase the heart rate.**
- **Hold the head erect, keep the back straight, and keep the abdomen flat.**
- **To prevent soreness, land on the heel of the foot and roll the foot forward.**
- **Take long, easy strides.**
- **Breathe deeply with your mouth slightly open.**
- **Wear comfortable shoes that provide good support.**
- **Wear light clothing in warm weather and layer clothing in cooler weather. Layered clothing can be removed if exercise generates excessive heat. In cold weather, wear gloves and a cap.**

Display 10-3 is an example of a walking program designed by the American Heart Association.

Maintaining Strength and Flexibility

Maintaining strength and flexibility is important for older adults. Flexibility is the ability to bend easily and move body parts. With age, the muscles lose elasticity, and tissues around the joints thicken, making moving through the normal range of motion more difficult. Arthritis (ie, inflammation of the joint) is a common disorder in the elderly population that stiffens the joints and decreases flexibility.

To enhance flexibility, the older adult is encouraged to keep moving, to bend, and stretch every day. Moving all joints through their normal range of motion increases flexibility. Exercises such as yoga, swimming, gardening, and housework enhance flexibility. Muscle strengthening exercises help to prevent loss of muscle tissue and can improve muscle strength at any age (Display 10-4).

Recreational activities that increase muscular strength include bicycling, swimming, hiking, shuffleboard, tennis, and golf. Strong muscles also help prevent back injury. Weight-lifting programs designed especially for older adults are a part of many community wellness programs. Joining a wellness center that is medically managed can provide the older adult with expert instruction in activities that strengthen the body.

DISPLAY 10-4. Muscle Building at Age 90 and Beyond

A dramatic example of "mutability" at almost any age is a National Institute on Aging (NIA) study that shows exercise can improve the muscle strength and mobility of people who are well into their nineties. Ten men and women (ages 86–96) exercised their legs on a weight machine, with heavier loads as the 8-week study progressed. The average gain in strength after 8 weeks was 174% in the right leg and 180% in the left. Improvement of muscle strength and size corresponded with the individuals' ability to function and with their mobility. NIA is impressed with these and other study findings that suggest physical frailty can be prevented or reversed, so much so that NIA and the National Center for Nursing Research are involved in collaborative studies on frailty intervention.

Fiatrone, M. A., & Marks, E. C., et al. (1990). High-intensity strength training in nonagenarians. *American Journal of the American Medical Association*, 262 (22), 3029–3034.

Health Risks From Exercising

Health problems can occur when exercising, especially if exercise programs are too vigorous. Problems that can occur include muscle and joint injury, heat stroke, or cardiac problems. The most common problems encountered when exercising are muscle or joint injury. This occurs from exercising too hard or for too long. If an individual has been inactive for some time and very quickly and vigorously begins an exercise program, the risks of injury are increased. To avoid injury, start slow and, gradually increase the intensity of the exercise. A gradual increase in activity levels allows muscles time to strengthen. By keeping the heart rate within the target zone, the heart muscle strengthens slowly. Occasional minor stiffness in the morning after exercise is normal. Soreness indicates that the exercise was overdone.

Heat Stroke and Heat Exhaustion
Serious problems that can occur when exercising are heat exhaustion and heat stroke. These conditions are rare but can occur when exercising in hot, humid weather or when environmental temperatures rise and the elderly, particularly the frail elderly, are not able to maintain a cool environment. Older adults are more sensitive to the effects of heat because of a decreased ability to rid the body of heat. Heat stroke has more serious consequences than heat exhaustion.

Heat exhaustion occurs when the body loses large quantities of salt and water as the result of pro-longed perspiration. Symptoms of heat exhaustion include weakness, dizziness, headache, nausea, confusion, and normal or below normal body temperature. If heat exhaustion is suspected and the person is conscious, one-half glass of water is given every 15 to 30 minutes. If the person is drowsy or vomiting, transportation to a medical facility as soon as possible is the most appropriate action.

Heat stroke is a medical emergency caused by a failure of the heat regulating mechanism of the body. The body becomes seriously overheated, but the normal cooling mechanism of perspiring does not occur. Symptoms of heat stroke include dizziness, headache, nausea, increased thirst, and muscle cramping. Serious symptoms of heat stroke occur when sweating stops, and the body temperature becomes dangerously elevated (body temperature can increase up to 106°F) Heat stroke is a medical emergency and must be treated in a medical facility. Treatment involves maintaining an airway, the use of cold packs, fans, and intravenous fluids.

The elderly are at increased risk for heat exhaustion and heat stroke because they have a diminished thirst mechanism despite dehydration. Heat exhaustion and heat stroke can be prevented by drinking adequate fluids to replace those lost from the heat and exercise.

Heat stroke and heat exhaustion can occur in the elderly during extended heat waves, especially when the humidity is also high. Older adults need to be instructed on precautions to protect themselves against heat exhaustion or heat stroke. Information to give the older adult to prevent heat stroke and heat exhaustion in a teaching plan should include information about hydration and nutrition.

 PATIENT TEACHING AID

Information for preventing heat stroke and heat exhaustion should be given to the elderly:
- **Monitor local weather forecasts to be aware of projected temperatures.**
- **Drink 2 to 4 cups of water each hour, even if not thirsty.**
- **Keep meals cool and simple.**
- **Wear loose, lightweight clothing.**
- **Keep house or apartment cool (<80°F).**
- **If living without air conditioning, use fans in living quarters and go to a shopping mall, movie theater, or senior citizen center.**

Cardiovascular Problems
Myocardial infarction can occur at any time, in any place, and during any activity. There is no evidence to suggest that exercise may cause myocardial

infarction. There is, however, a reduced risk of sudden death for those who are physically active. Warning signs often occur and should be reported, regardless of when they occur and what activity the individual is engaged in. Symptoms such as chest pain or pressure; pain in the arms, shoulders, or jaw; feeling faint; diaphoresis (ie, sweating); or loss of consciousness indicate a potential cardiac problem and should be reported to the physician immediately. For elderly individuals who have had a previous myocardial infarction, the physician is consulted before beginning an exercise program. These individuals require periodic monitoring of cardiac status.

Promoting Cardiovascular Health

CAD is a leading cause of death in the elderly. CAD develops when fatty deposits collect on the walls of the artery that supply the heart with blood. Eventually, one or more of the major coronary arteries may become blocked, resulting in myocardial infarction. Risk factors of CAD include high blood pressure, cigarette smoking, and elevated blood cholesterol levels.

Hypertension

Hypertension (ie, elevated blood pressure) is a common problem in the elderly. Blood pressure is the force exerted on the walls of the arteries by the pumping action of the heart. A blood pressure that is consistently 140/90 mmHg or greater is considered hypertension. Hypertension increases the risk of developing cardiovascular disease and stroke. Regular exercise, a diet low in sodium, and weight loss (if obesity is a problem) can help reduce high blood pressure in many people. As little as a 10-pound weight loss can lower blood pressure significantly in some individuals. Regular exercise and following the dietary guidelines can help prevent hypertension.

Cigarette Smoking

According to the American Heart Association, heavy smokers are two to four times more likely to have a myocardial infarction than nonsmokers. The nicotine in cigarettes acts as a vasoconstrictor (ie, decreases the amount of blood), impairing circulation. Smokers breathe in tar and chemicals that are unable to be expelled by the lungs. The chemicals and tar can begin the growth of cancerous cells in the lung tissue. The carbon monoxide in tobacco smoke prevents adequate amounts of oxygen from reaching the tissues of the body, particularly the brain, and can lead to headache, dizziness, and lack of energy. Although the smoker to nonsmoker mortality ratio decreases with increasing age, elderly smokers continue to experience greater death rates from coronary heart disease.

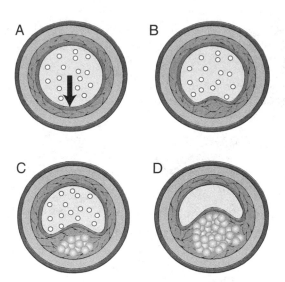

FIGURE 10-2. Progressive development of atherosclerosis. (**A**) Injury to intima (inner layer of vessel). (**B**) Lipoprotein invasion and beginning of plaque development. (**C**) Fibrous plaque hardens on intima. (**D**) Progressive blockage of lumen with plaque.

By conveying understanding and acceptance, the nurse can assist the smoker who desires to quit smoking. Referral can be made to one of several self-help programs, such as the Fresh Start Program offered through the American Cancer Society. Other methods, such as the use of nicotine gum or nicotine patches, are also beneficial to the elderly person desiring to quit smoking.

High Blood Cholesterol

High blood cholesterol levels increase the risk of developing atherosclerosis and coronary heart disease. **Atherosclerosis** is a collection of fatty deposits of cholesterol, fat, or other substances on the inside walls of the arteries. The fatty substances, called plaque, harden and decrease the lumen (opening) of the artery. The lumen through which blood flows becomes more narrow, and the artery becomes less able to dilate or constrict in response to the body's needs (Fig. 10-2).

Although this process begins early in life, symptoms may not appear until middle or old age. The person may not show any signs of atherosclerosis until the plaque causes a 70% or greater blockage of the artery.

Cholesterol and fats do not dissolve in water and must combine with a protein to travel in the bloodstream. The combination of a fat (ie, lipid) with a protein results in a substance called **lipoprotein.** The two most significant lipoproteins

---

DISPLAY 10-5. Cholesterol Levels

Total Blood Cholesterol
Desirable: <200 mg/dL
Borderline high: 200–239 mg/dL
High: ≥240 mg/dL

Low-Density Lipoprotein (LDL)
Desirable: <130 mg/dL
Borderline high: 130–159 mg/dL
High: ≥160 mg/dL

High-Density Lipoprotein (HDL)
High risk associated with >35 mg/dL

DISPLAY 10-6. Seven Warning Signals For Cancer

C A change in bowel or bladder habits
A A sore that will not heal
U Unusual bleeding or discharge
T Thickening or lump in breast or elsewhere
I Indigestion or difficulty in swallowing
O Obvious change in a wart or mole
N Nagging cough or hoarseness

---

related to cholesterol are **low-density lipoprotein** (LDL) and **high-density lipoprotein** (HDL). HDL is often called the "good" cholesterol. HDL is a plasma protein that carries fat and cholesterol from the tissues to the liver to be excreted. High levels of HDL are associated with a decreased risk of heart disease. LDL is a plasma protein that is composed mostly of cholesterol and fat. High levels of LDL are associated with increased risk of heart disease. Display 10-5 shows normal cholesterol, HDL, and LDL levels.

A diet low in cholesterol helps to control cholesterol blood levels. Foods low in cholesterol include chicken, turkey, fish, egg whites, dry beans, soybean curd, and all vegetables and fruits. Foods that are high in cholesterol and should be avoided are fatty meats, duck, goose, ham, sausage, bacon, luncheon meats, egg yolks (limit to three or four per week), butter, cream, whole milk, and milk products. A total blood cholesterol level that is less than 200 mg/dL decreases the risk of heart disease. A blood cholesterol level of 240 mg/dL or higher increases the risk of heart disease.

Physical Activity

A regular exercise program that is moderately intense, frequent (three to four times per week), and lasts for 20 to 30 minutes can help reduce the risk of heart disease. Regular physical activity helps to maintain a desirable body weight. Excess weight increases the risk of developing hypertension, elevated blood cholesterol, and diabetes.

Role of the Nurse

Maintaining cardiovascular health is an important factor in decreasing the risk of heart disease in the older adult. The older adult may be exhibiting signs of CAD. When a person has CAD, efforts are aimed at restoring the levels of cardiac functioning

as much as possible and decreasing the risk of further damage. Cardiovascular health in the elderly can be promoted by providing regular exercise programs, teaching proper dietary guidelines, weight control, monitoring blood pressure for hypertension, not smoking, and managing stress (see Chapter 11). Adult day care centers, home health agencies, and participation in health fairs and any place where older adults congregate are excellent avenues to teach aspects of health promotion to older adults.

CANCER PREVENTION AND DETECTION

Although cancer affects every age group, most cancers occur in people older than 65 years of age. Cancer is a group of diseases characterized by the uncontrolled growth of abnormal cells with the body. Cancer is a group of many different and distinct diseases. Usually, cancer does not develop quickly but results from cellular changes that occur over several decades.

The goal is to prevent cancer by adopting a lifestyle that minimizes the risk of developing cancer. Understanding the early warning signs of cancer is important because many cancers are curable by surgery or through the use of drugs if they are detected early. Seven warning signals have been developed by the American Cancer Society to aid in early detection. These warning signals spell the word CAUTION (Display 10-6).

Role of the Nurse

The major role of the nurse in early detection and prevention of cancer is that of teacher. Nurses must educate the older adult in all aspects of cancer prevention and detection. Information to include in a cancer prevention teaching plan for the older adult and family of the older adult should include information about

PATIENT AND FAMILY TEACHING AID

Information for the older adult about cancer prevention includes the following:

- See the physician immediately if any of the seven warning signals are identified.
- Increase amounts of fresh vegetables (particularly vegetables in the cabbage family) and fiber in the diet.
- Increase the intake of foods high in vitamin A (ie, dark green leafy vegetables, and carrots) and vitamin C (ie, citrus fruits, strawberries, cantaloupe, and tomatoes).
- Maintain normal weight.
- Reduce the amount of dietary fat, salt-cured, smoked, and nitrate-containing foods (eg, bacon).
- Do not smoke.
- Use alcohol in moderation.
- Avoid overexposure to the sun. Wear sunscreen and protective clothing when exposed to the sun.
- Perform monthly BSEs.

nutrition, maintaining a normal weight, and monthly breast self-examinations (BSEs).

Many cancers can be prevented if a healthy lifestyle is adopted. Diet is known to play a large role in the development of cancer. High-fiber diets reduce the risk of developing cancer of the breast, prostate, and colon. Vitamin A reduces the risk of cancer of the esophagus, larynx, and lungs. A diet high in vitamin C may provide protection against stomach and esophageal cancer.

Obesity is linked to a number of cancers, particularly cancer of the breast, colon, and uterus. Salt-cured and nitrate-cured foods are thought to increase the risk of cancer of the esophagus and stomach. Smoking increases the risk of lung cancer. Heavy drinkers who smoke have an increased incidence of cancer of the mouth, throat, larynx, and esophagus. Overexposure to the sun increases the risk of skin cancer.

Breast Cancer

Of particular importance is early detection and prevention of breast cancer. Breast cancer is a leading cause of death from cancer in women. Early detection allows treatment to begin early and is an important step in the cure. The risk factors for breast cancer include the following:

- Family history of breast cancer
- Menstrual periods beginning before the age of 12
- Menopause after the age of 50
- Being 40% overweight (see Table 10-1)

For early detection, women are encouraged to perform a thorough BSE once every month (Fig. 10-3). After menopause, it is recommended that the breast be checked on a set date each month, such as the first or last day of each month. Figure 10-4 shows a method developed by the American Cancer Society that can serve as a monthly reminder to perform a monthly BSE.

OSTEOPOROSIS

Osteoporosis is a disorder of the musculoskeletal system in which there is a reduction of total bone mass. The bones become porous, brittle, and fragile. Pathogenic or spontaneous fractures can occur. Ninety percent of the women older than age 75 have some degree of osteoporosis. A more detailed discussion of osteoporosis can be found in Chapter 19. Risk factors include a history of smoking, heavy drinking, lack of weight-bearing exercise, low calcium or low vitamin D intake, and a family history of osteoporosis.

Osteoporosis is responsible for a loss of functional ability and loss of mobility in many older women. Elderly women may need up to 1,500 mg of calcium or more daily to obtain adequate calcium. Older adults absorb calcium less efficiently and excrete it more readily through the kidney than do younger women. A teaching plan for the older adult for osteoporosis should include information about diet, exercise, and hormone replacement for female patients.

 PATIENT TEACHING AID

This information should be included in a teaching plan for osteoporosis:

- Eat a balanced diet, with emphasis on foods high in calcium and vitamin D (ie, milk, cheese, salmon, and broccoli).
- A calcium supplement may be prescribed by the physician. Take supplement with meals to reduce gastric upset.
- At menopause, the physician may prescribe hormone replacement therapy (HRT). Be sure to take the hormone exactly as prescribed, and do not stop taking the hormone unless instructed to do so by the physician.
- Regular weight-bearing exercises are needed.
- Avoid the use of caffeine, cigarettes, and alcohol.
- Plan regular exercise and physical activity.

WHY YOU SHOULD EXAMINE
YOUR BREASTS MONTHLY

Most breast cancers are first discovered by
women themselves. Since breast cancers
found early and treated promptly have
excellent chances for cure, learning how to
examine your breast properly can help save
your life.

Use the simple 3-step breast self-examination (BSE) procedure shown here.

Before a mirror:

Inspect your breasts
with arms at your
sides. Next, raise your
arms high overhead.
Look for any changes
in shape or contour of
each breast, a swelling, dimpling of skin or
changes in the skin or nipple.
  Then, rest palms on hips and press down
firmly to flex your chest muscles. Left and

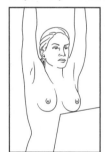

right breast will not
exactly match – few
women's breast do.
  Regular inspection
shows what is normal
for you and will give
you confidence in
your examination.

Lying down:

Lie down. Flatten your right breast by
placing a pillow under your right shoulder.
Fingers flat, use the sensitive pads of the
middle three fingers on your left hand. Feel
for lumps or changes using a rubbing
motion. Press firmly enough to feel the
different breast tissues. Completely feel all
of the breast and chest area from your
collarbone to the base of a properly fitted
bra; and from your breast bone to the
underarm. Allow enough time for a complete exam.

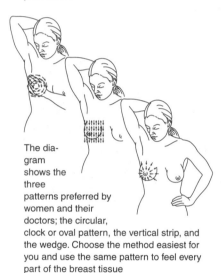

The dia-
gram
shows the
three
patterns preferred by
women and their
doctors; the circular,
clock or oval pattern, the vertical strip, and
the wedge. Choose the method easiest for
you and use the same pattern to feel every
part of the breast tissue

After you have completely examined your
right breast, then examine your left breast
using the same method. Compare what you
have felt in one breast with the other.
  Finally, squeeze the nipple of each breast
gently between the thumb and index finger.
Any discharge, clear or bloody, should be
reported to your doctor.

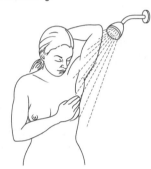

In the shower:

Examine your breasts during a bath or
shower; hands glide easier over wet skin.
Fingers flat, move gently over every part of
each breast. Check for any lump, hard knot
or thickening.

WHAT YOU SHOULD DO IF YOU
FIND A CHANGE

If you find a lump or dimple or discharge
during BSE, it is important to see your
doctor as soon as possible. Don't be frightened. Most breast lumps or changes are not
cancer, but only your doctor can make the
diagnosis.

FIGURE 10-3. How to Perform a Breast Self Examination. From "How To Do Breast Self Examination," Code 508. (1992). American Cancer Society. Used with permission.

When assisting the elderly person in selecting the best calcium supplement, suggest calcium citrate, since calcium carbonate may cause constipation in the elderly. Most physicians advise against using compounds such as dolomite or bone meal because they may contain lead and other impurities. Adequate amounts of vitamin D are needed for proper calcium absorption. When taking calcium, it is also important to supplement magnesium at a ratio of 2:1 or 3:1 (calcium to magnesium) since both minerals are necessary for bone health. Postmenopausal women, men over 65, and any person taking corticosteroids need 1,500 mg of calcium each day. Women taking hormone replacement need about 1,000 mg/day. To increase calcium absorption, instruct the older adult not to take more than 500 mg at one time.

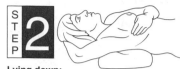

CRITICAL THINKING EXERCISES

1. Ms. Garcia, age 67, wants to begin an exercise program. She has never participated in any type of exercise program. After attending a health promotion class, she decided to make some changes in her daily routines to have a healthier lifestyle. What assessments would you perform initially for Ms. Garcia? What type of exercise program, if any, would be most beneficial. Plan an exercise program for Mr. Garcia, if appropriate.

2. Plan an inservice on "Keeping Blood Cholesterol Levels within Normal Range" for a group of

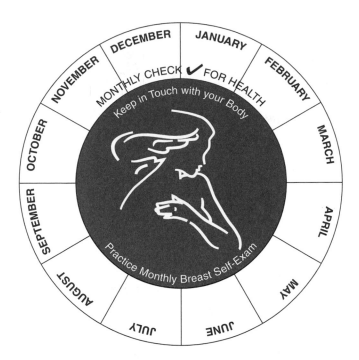

FIGURE 10-4. Monthly Reminder for Breast Self Examination. As a monthly reminder to do BSE, this illustration can be ordered from the American Cancer society as a sticker for the bathroom mirror. From "How to Do Breast Self Examination," Code 508. (1992). American Cancer Society. Reprinted by the permission of the American Cancer Society, Inc.

practical and vocational nurses working in an geriatric outpatient setting.

3. When working at a hypertension screening for older adults, one of the older participants asks you to explain exactly what hypertension is and "why is it bad for her to have high blood pressure." Detail your response. What information would you need from this person before the teaching session.

REFERENCES AND SUGGESTED READING

American Association of Retired Persons, prepared in cooperation with the President's Council on Physical Fitness and Sports. *Pep up your life: A fitness book for mid-life and older adults.* Publication no. PF 3248 (496) D549. Washington, D.C.: U.S. Government Printing Office.

Ewles, L., & Simmett, I. (1999). *Promoting health: A practical guide.* Philadelphia: W.B. Saunders.

Mahan, L., & Escott-Stump, S. (1999). *Krause's Food, nutrition and diet therapy* (10th ed.). Philadelphia: W.B. Saunders.

Pechenpaugh, N.J., & Poleman, C.M. (1995). *Nutrition: Essentials and diet therapy* (7th ed.). Philadelphia: W.B. Saunders.

CHAPTER **11**

CHAPTER OUTLINE

KEY TERMS

CHAPTER OBJECTIVES

POTENTIAL STRESSORS THAT OCCUR WITH AGE

USING THE NURSING PROCESS TO HELP THE
  ELDERLY REDUCE STRESS

PROMOTING A HEALTHY SELF-ESTEEM

USING THE NURSING PROCESS TO PROMOTE SELF-
  ESTEEM IN THE ELDERLY

PROMOTING SEXUAL HEALTH

USING THE NURSING PROCESS TO PROMOTE
  SEXUALITY IN THE ELDERLY

PROMOTING SPIRITUALITY IN THE OLDER ADULT

USING THE NURSING PROCESS TO PROMOTE
  SPIRITUALITY IN THE ELDERLY

CRITICAL THINKING EXERCISES

REFERENCES AND SUGGESTED READING

Promoting Psychosocial Health

KEY TERMS

adaptation

alarm stage

coping strategy

exhaustion stage

libido

mantra

resistance

self-esteem

stress

stressor

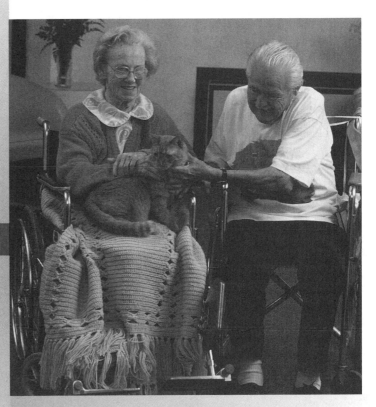

CHAPTER OBJECTIVES

At the completion of this chapter, the student will
be able to

- Identify potential stressors for the older adult

- Discuss the transactional model of stress

- Describe the three stages of the general
  adaptation syndrome

- List positive coping strategies used to manage
  stress

- Use the nursing process to manage stress and
  promote self-esteem, sexuality, and spirituality
  in the older adult

- Identify barriers to sexual activity in the
  nursing home

Promoting psychosocial health is an important aspect of caring for the older adult. This chapter focuses on four important aspects of psychosocial health: stress management, self-esteem, sexuality, and meeting the spiritual needs of the older adult. A focus on these four areas helps the older adult meet the psychosocial challenges associated with aging. In promoting psychosocial health, the nurse assists the older adult to understand the important aspects of psychosocial issues, identify coping skills, maximize strengths, and develop new coping techniques.

POTENTIAL STRESSORS THAT OCCUR WITH AGE

Each person encounters stressors (ie, agents that produce stress) that require a certain amount of adaptation and coping. For most older adults, the mere fact that they have survived for 65 or more years gives some indication that they have at least adequate coping skills. Age brings a unique set of losses that requires adaptation. Sometimes, older adults are ill prepared to meet the stressors of growing older, and assistance is needed in developing new ways of coping. Older adults deal with stress in different ways. What may cause stress in one older adult may be a welcome challenge for another adult or even a neutral issue for another older adult. Figure 11-1 identifies some of the psychosocial challenges that occur with age. Each challenge can be a stressor as the older adult attempts to adapt.

Transactional Stress Model

Lazarus and Folkman developed a model of stress called the transactional model of stress in which stress is viewed as a relationship between the person and his surroundings or environment. **Stress** is defined as a specific relationship between the person and the environment in which the person views someone, something, or some event as a threat to his or her well-being. The specific event or condition that produces stress is called a **stressor.** An event is not stressful unless an individual perceives it as stressful. Stress can occur in any one or combination of four areas: physical, psychological, social, and environmental. Examples of physical stressors in the older adult include the occurrence of acute or chronic diseases such as arthritis, diabetes, or cardiovascular disease. Psychological stressors are stressors that cause psychological dis-

tress such as fear, anger, anxiety, and frustration. Social stressors include changes, such as when the elderly person loses a part of his social network through death, retirement, or moving to a new area. Environmental stressors include moving to a new home environment, such as a nursing home or a different city, or surviving a tornado, hurricane, or other environmental disaster.

The goal with any perceived stressor is adaptation using positive coping strategies. **Adaptation** is a continuous process by which an organism adjusts to physical, emotional, and mental stressors. **Coping** strategies are methods used by individuals to adapt to stress. When stress is managed through positive coping adaptation occurs. Coping strategies focus in two areas: emotionally focused coping strategies or problem-focused coping strategies.

Emotionally focused coping strategies are coping methods designed to make the individual feel better or to boost self-esteem. Examples of emotionally oriented coping strategies include talking with friends, a clergyman, or a counselor; using social support; or positive self-talk. Emotionally focused strategies decrease the intensity of the emotions associated with stress such as fear or anger.

Problem-focused coping strategies are coping methods that are more logical and change oriented than emotionally focused coping strategies. Direct efforts to change environmental threats are considered problem oriented methods of coping. An example of problem focused coping is seen when two individuals having a conflict use the problem-solving technique (see Chapter 25) to resolve the issue or conflict. The problem solving method requires time to think through the situation to determine the most logical and effective methods of coping. Methods of coping may be to learn a new task, to change goals, or to redirect desires or feelings.

When coping strategies are successful, adaptation occurs, and life satisfaction increases. Sometimes, stressors are dealt with using a combination of emotional- and problem-focused coping strategies. Figure 11-2 depicts the transactional model of stress.

General Adaptation Syndrome

Hans Selye developed the stress theory called the general adaptation syndrome (GAS). According to Seyle, the body has a generalized physiologic (bodily) response to a stressor. This generalized response is nonspecific and any occurrence, even a positive one, can cause stress. For example, a family gathering or a vacation can be just as stressful as adjusting to the death of a loved one. The GAS has three phases: alarm, resistance, and exhaustion.

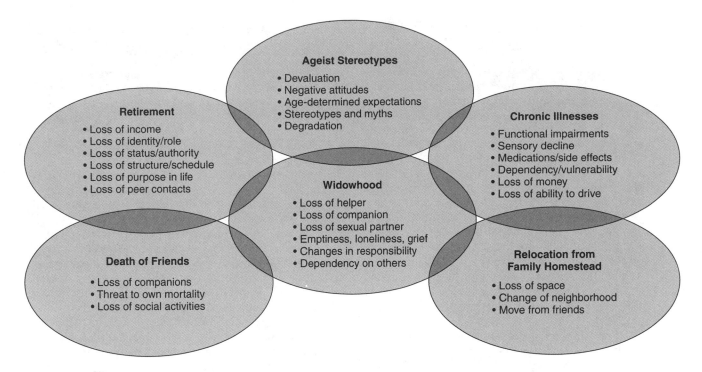

FIGURE 11-1. Psychosocial challenges of the older adult.

Alarm Stage

The first stage, the **alarm stage,** is the stage in which the body prepares itself to withstand the stressor. The body responds in the alarm stage with the fight or flight response. The fight or flight response is the manner in which all animals prepare to face danger or to flee from it. Every response of the body during the alarm stage is geared to preparing the person to have the stamina and strength to fight or flee the stressful situation. Display 11-1 identifies the physiologic changes that occur in the alarm stage of the GAS.

Figure 11-3 summarizes the physiologic changes that occur during the alarm stage of the GAS. It is impossible to maintain the alarm stage indefinitely. If the reactions that occur in the alarm stage continue, the body systems involved can be damaged, resulting in heart disease, diabetes, or hypertension.

Resistance

After some period, the second or resistance stage begins to take over. In the **resistance** stage, the person adapts to stress with increased and intensified use of coping mechanisms. If coping mechanisms are adequate during the resistance stage, adaptation to the stressor occurs. If efforts in resistance become excessive or adaptation does not occur, there is a deterioration of the areas involved in the struggle.

The first two stages, alarm and resistance, are repeated each time the person is faced with a stressor. The greater the perceived threat, the more intense is the response. Diseases associated with prolonged resistance to stress are listed in Display 11-2.

Exhaustion

If exposure to the stress continues, exhaustion occurs. In the **exhaustion stage,** all energy for adaptation is

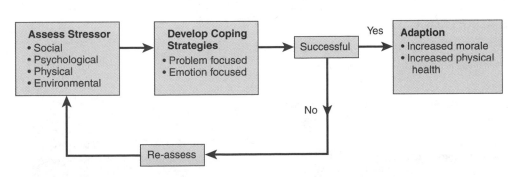

FIGURE 11-2. Transactional model of stress (adapted from Ignativicius & Bayne. (1991). *Medical-Surgical Nursing: A Nursing Process Approach,* W.B. Saunders, 93).

DISPLAY 11-1. Physiologic Changes That Occur in the Alarm Stage of the General Adaptation Syndrome

1. When faced with a stressor, the limbic system (the part of the brain that controls emotions and feelings) initiates the fight or flight response.
2. The two branches of the autonomic nervous system (ANS), the sympathetic and the parasympathetic branches, manage the physiologic reactions that occur in GAS. The sympathetic branch is responsible for preparing the body for the fight or flight response, and the parasympathetic branch works to restore the body to a normal relaxed state.
3. The adrenal medulla gland is stimulated to release norepinephrine and epinephrine. The release of epinephrine results in an increased heart rate and increased force of cardiac muscle contraction.
4. Vasodilatation occurs, resulting in an increased blood flow to areas that are active in the fight or flight response, such as the heart, muscles, and brain.
5. Vasoconstriction in areas such as the superficial vessels of the skin, the gastrointestinal tract, and the genitourinary tract result in a decreased blood flow to areas not active during the alarm reaction. This vasoconstrictive action mainly results from norepinephrine.
6. Because more oxygen is needed to sustain the alarm reaction, the bronchial tubes dilate, the respiratory rate increases, and the depth of respirations increases.
7. The pupils dilate to increase the visual field.
8. Blood clotting time decreases to prevent blood loss in case of injury.
9. The hypothalamus releases corticotropin-releasing hormone, which in turn stimulates the release of ACTH, which causes the release of the glucocorticoid cortisol from the adrenal cortex.
10. The release of cortisol from the adrenal cortex increases the available glucose needed for energy. With the release of cortisol, the spleen contracts, reducing the potential for injury and loss of blood. The contraction of the spleen results in the release of T-lymphocytes, specialized white blood cells that are needed to fight infection.
11. An increase in blood pressure results from the stimulation of the adrenal cortex to release the mineralocorticoid aldosterone.

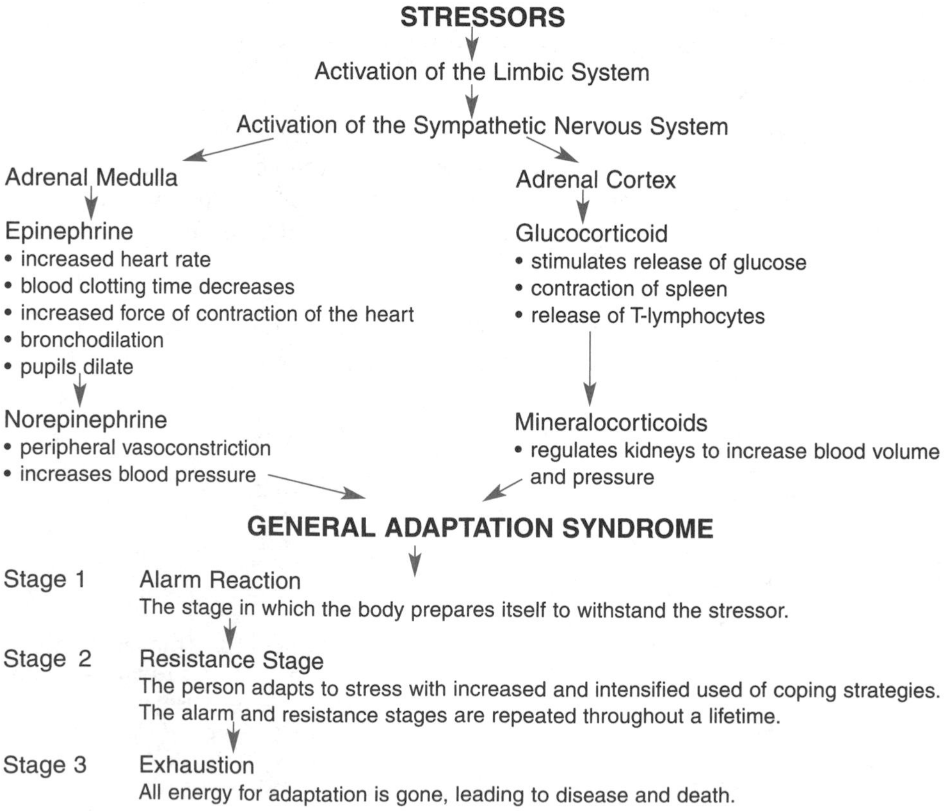

STRESSORS

Activation of the Limbic System

Activation of the Sympathetic Nervous System

Adrenal Medulla

Epinephrine
- increased heart rate
- blood clotting time decreases
- increased force of contraction of the heart
- bronchodilation
- pupils dilate

Norepinephrine
- peripheral vasoconstriction
- increases blood pressure

Adrenal Cortex

Glucocorticoid
- stimulates release of glucose
- contraction of spleen
- release of T-lymphocytes

Mineralocorticoids
- regulates kidneys to increase blood volume and pressure

GENERAL ADAPTATION SYNDROME

Stage 1   Alarm Reaction
The stage in which the body prepares itself to withstand the stressor.

Stage 2   Resistance Stage
The person adapts to stress with increased and intensified used of coping strategies.
The alarm and resistance stages are repeated throughout a lifetime.

Stage 3   Exhaustion
All energy for adaptation is gone, leading to disease and death.

FIGURE 11-3. The general adaptation syndrome.

DISPLAY 11-2. Disorders Linked to Stress

Asthma
Allergies
Atherosclerosis
Cancer
Cardiovascular disease
Connective tissue disease
Crohn's disease
Essential hypertension
Inflammatory disease
Migraine and tension headaches
Obesity
Sexual dysfunction
Ulcerative colitis

gone because of depletion of body resources. Exhaustion can cause serious adverse effects on the body systems. Exhaustion decreases the immune response, increasing susceptibility to many disorders such as infection, inflammatory diseases, allergic diseases, digestive diseases, and cancer (see Display 11-2).

With aging, the body becomes less able to adapt to stressors, and the resistance that develops in youth and middle age begins to fail. Over time, the wear and tear on the body takes its toll, resistance fails, and death occurs.

Coping Strategies to Decrease Stress

Any illness, especially chronic illness, loss, or perceived threat, can illicit a stress response. Positive coping strategies promote psychosocial health and decrease stress. Outcomes that occur as a result of positive coping include optimal health, increased life satisfaction, and supportive interpersonal relationships.

Assistance may be needed to help the elderly adult develop new copings strategies. Any time an elderly person is faced with an unfamiliar situation, such as hospitalization, illness, or moving to a nursing home, stress occurs.

PSYCHOSOCIAL ASPECTS OF NURSING: EXAMPLES OF POSITIVE COPING STRATEGIES

Problem solving
Exercise or physical activity
Relaxation techniques
Providing information
Social support systems
Faith
Denial

Past coping strategies determine how older adults will deal with current stressors. If coping strategies have been healthy and successful in the past, the older adult will more likely adapt well to the stressors of old age. However, if maladaptive coping strategies have been used, the older adult may need help to explore other alternatives.

Families are often surprised by how well older adults adapt and cope with stressful situations. They forget that for many years the older person has been bombarded with stress and that most have dealt with these stressors successfully. For example, a family may be uneasy about telling an 82-year-old parent about some tragic event such as the death of a loved one in the family. However, when told, the older adult may cope surprisingly well. Perhaps it is because she has survived the death of parents, a spouse, siblings, or even a child.

Problem Solving. In using the problem-solving technique, the problem is discussed and clearly identified. All possible coping strategies to relieve the stressor are identified. After discussion, one solution is selected and implemented. If the selected solution does not relieve the stressor, other strategies are implemented. Chapter 25 provides more information on problem solving.

Exercise and Physical Activity. Regular physical exercise decreases stress and is a good coping strategy if mobility is not a consideration. A regular exercise program consisting of activities such as walking, swimming, or aerobic exercise relieves stress, increases energy levels, and boosts self-esteem. Chapter 10 provides more information on physical activity and exercise for the older adult. However, the frail elderly, those with debilitating illnesses such as arthritis or any disorder that significantly decreases mobility, cannot easily use exercise as a coping strategy. For these individuals, alternate methods of coping must be explored.

Relaxation Techniques. Coping strategies that may be unfamiliar and need special instruction include strategies involving relaxation training, visualization, yoga, and meditation.

Progressive Muscle Relaxation and Visualization. Progressive muscle relaxation is a form of stress reduction accomplished through alternately tensing and relaxing large muscle groups of the body to produce total body relaxation. This is done by the nurse or another person giving instructions in a low, relaxed manner. Tapes or specific scripts to read are available until the nurse feels comfortable giving instructions for relaxation. The stressed individual is asked to assume a comfortable position, clear his mind of all thoughts, and focus on breathing quietly and evenly. The nurse who is guiding the relaxation response leads the individual in alternately tensing

DISPLAY 11-3. Abbreviated Script for Progressive Muscle Relaxation

Preparation
- Provide a quiet, comfortable atmosphere.
- Reinforce the reason of the session, such as to reduce tension, to help sleep, or to decrease sensation of pain.
- Have the individual sit in a chair with hands in the lap and feet flat on the floor or lie supine with hands to the sides or on the abdomen. If supine, the legs should be uncrossed.
- Have the individual begin by concentrating on taking several deep breaths.

Relaxation Script
- Now that you have taken several deep breaths, find a position that is comfortable and relax. Take one more breath, and exhale very slowly and completely. Concentrate on breathing slowly and deeply. Allow every muscle in your body to be as relaxed as possible.
- Be aware of your feet. Allow your feet to become very relaxed. Feel the tension draining from your feet. As the muscles relax, you may notice a tingly sensation in the soles and toes of the feet. This indicates that the muscles are relaxing.
- This sensation moves upward from the feet to the ankles and flows from the ankles to the calves of both legs. The muscles of the calves relax as tension is released. The calves become very heavy and relaxed.
- This comfortable, relaxed sensation moves upward from the calves to the upper legs and thighs. These muscles also relax and become very comfortable. Feel the muscles of the upper legs relax.

- This sensation of relaxation moves up toward the buttocks and toward the pelvic area. The tension of the muscles of the buttocks, the pelvic area, and the lower abdomen is released. The internal organs relax and the muscles that surround them feel completely tension free.
- Relaxation extends to the upper abdomen and chest and from the lower back to the upper back into the shoulders. The shoulders, chest, and back relax. Tension is released.
- This relaxation extends to the neck and the throat. Feel the tension draining from the back of the neck and the head. Tension flows completely out of the body and is replaced with total body relaxation.
- From the head, to the fingertips, to the feet, the entire body is completely and totally relaxed. Take some time to savor this total relaxation of body and mind. (Allow several minutes for the person to appreciate and enjoy these feelings.)

Closure
- Allow a few minutes for the client to appreciate this restful state of complete relaxation.
- When the body is totally relaxed, you may also have the person picture in her mind a restful scene such as meadow, the ocean, a waterfall, or some other scene that would promote relaxation.
- After a few minutes, bring the person's attention back to the present. One way to accomplish this is to count slowly backward from 10 to 1. Have the client progressively return to a more wakeful state as the number approaches 1.

and relaxing large muscle groups such as the muscles in legs or abdomen. The individual is asked to sense the tension and then feel the difference with relaxation. At the conclusion, the entire body is completely relaxed.

The relaxation response can also be accomplished without the sensations of tensing and relaxing. Giving the individual the suggestion to relax the muscles through a progressive systematic sequence can accomplish total body relaxation. This technique can be used in many situations, such as to reduce stress, induce sleep, decrease pain, and relieve anxiety. Many scripts are available for the nurse when using progressive relaxation as a coping strategy. Display 11-3 is an example of a modified script that can be used for helping an individual to relax using progressive muscle relaxation and visualization.

A variation of the progressive relaxation is guided imagery. In guided imagery, the individual and the nurse select an image that promotes a pleasant peaceful response. This image becomes a scene on which to focus during a relaxation session.

Yoga and Meditation. Yoga and meditation are also useful in reducing stress. Yoga is particularly suited for older adults with stiff muscles and decreased activity levels. Yoga involves breathing and stretching exercises that vary greatly in difficulty and can be enjoyed by all ages with various levels of expertise. Yoga enhances breathing capacity and reduces stress and muscle tension. Meditation is a process of focusing attention on a mantra or word for meditation. Any word can be used, and many use the word *love* or *relax* or *peace*. The word that is selected is repeated silently or aloud as a focus while remaining quiet and still.

Providing Information. Another method to help individual coping is providing information. For example, providing information on a certain diagnostic procedure decreases anxiety concerning the procedure by helping the person to know what to expect before, during, and after the procedure. This allows her to feel a sense of control over the events, maintain composure, and cooperate more during the procedure. However, not everyone wants to be informed. Although providing information may help some individuals, others do not want to know. Be alert for cues such as turning away and not listening or changing the subject. These behaviors may indicate that the information is not important to this individual and that coping is accomplished at least partially through ignorance or denial.

Social Support. Social support helps to reduce stress by providing emotional support, identity with a group, and people with whom to share information. Engaging in pleasurable activities with friends helps to relieve stress. Activities of interest range from playing cards or dominoes to playing tennis or racquetball. Religious, civic, or professional organizations provide much social support for participants.

Support groups for those who share similar stressful situations may be helpful in gaining information, insight, and sharing special burdens of a specific problem. Participants can learn from discussing the successes and failures of others in similar situations. Support groups are available for diabetes, Alzheimer's disease, cancer, and many of the chronic diseases that affect the older adult. Problems with alcohol consumption are not uncommon in the older adult (see Chapter 15). Groups such as Alcoholics Anonymous (AA) and Alanon are beneficial support networks.

Faith. Faith in God or a supreme being is an effective coping strategy for many. Believing that God will take care of the situation, praying, and increasing participation in religious activity are important in helping many individuals cope with life's stressors. Leaving life in the hands of a higher power often provides a great sense of peace and contentment.

Denial. Denial is a coping mechanism used by persons unable to directly face stressors. In situations that are extremely difficult or painful to face, denial is a normal response. Denial may persist until the person has the emotional strength to face the stressor. Although this coping strategy may work for a short time, long-term denial can have serious consequences. For example, families sometimes use denial when loved ones are deteriorating physically or mentally and the family caregivers are unable to adequately care for the person. Denial of the severity of a loved one's decreasing functional level and avoiding the decision to find alternate living arrangements can lead to serious complications for the older adult.

USING THE NURSING PROCESS TO HELP THE ELDERLY REDUCE STRESS

Assessment

Assessing for the presence of stress is an important aspect in maintaining psychosocial health. Symp-

toms associated with increased stress can be categorized into four areas: mild, moderate, severe, and panic. Mild stress generally has a positive effect by enhancing the ability to think, solve problems, and deal with the stressor. When the elderly person has mild stress, the person may be able to deal with the stressor alone or with minimal assistance from the nurse. If coping methods are ineffective, mild stress progresses to moderate levels, in which physical and mental symptoms increase.

> **PSYCHOSOCIAL ASPECTS OF NURSING: SYMPTOMS OF MODERATE STRESS**
>
> Inability to remain attentive to instruction
> Muscle tension
> Dry mouth
> Increased respiratory and heart rate, palpitations
> Restlessness
> Purposeless activity such as pacing or wringing of the hands

If appropriate coping strategies are not implemented, the individual may develop severe stress or panic. Symptoms of severe stress and panic include:
Inability to concentrate
Sweating
Tachycardia
Urinary frequency
Headache
Nausea
Shaking and trembling
Panic is the most extreme form of stress, and the affected person can experience the following symptoms:
Chest pain
Dyspnea
Feeling of choking
Inability to communicate in a meaningful way
Extreme discomfort
Fear of dying or sense of impending doom
The nurse identifies the intensity of stress by assessing the elderly for the presence of mild, moderate, or severe symptoms.

ASSESSMENT ALERT

Assessing for stress in the elderly with a cognitive loss is difficult. In the older adult, especially an older adult with a cognitive loss, stress can be manifested by increased confusion, agitation, or irritability, especially if it occurs following a known stressor such as hospitalization, moving to a nursing home, or loss of family or friends. The occurrence of any loss that could potentially produce stress necessitates careful monitoring of the older adult.

Identification of increased stress and anxiety in the elderly is suspected with the advent of any of these symptoms, especially if the person is experiencing one or more of the stressors associated with aging (see Fig. 11-1). Carefully questioning about life events, losses, and past coping strategies is necessary to identify possible stressors.

Nursing Diagnoses

Depending on the specific stressor of the older person, one or more of the following nursing diagnoses may apply:

Ineffective Individual Coping related to retirement, change of neighborhood, loss of companion, moving to a nursing home, other factors (specify stressor)

Anxiety related to hospitalization, functional impairment, dependency, or other factors (specify stressor)

Planning and Implementation

The elderly person facing stress may come in contact with the nurse in a variety of settings, such as an outpatient clinic, a wellness center, an adult day care center, a general hospital, or a nursing home. The major goals in managing stress in an older adult include examining past coping strategies, identifying new, more effective coping strategies, and supporting patients in their efforts to cope.

Ineffective Individual Coping

Nursing interventions can help older adults cope with stress.

Be nonjudgmental.

Actively listen.

Identify and alleviate the specific stressor if possible.

Encourage reminiscing of similar past experiences to help identify usual coping patterns.

Provide information when appropriate.

Assist in using the problem solving process.

Help to identify and implement positive coping strategies.

Anxiety

When the person is anxious as a result of stress the nurse can decrease anxiety by implementing the following interventions:

Talk quietly and confidentially to provide a sense of control.

Make no demands of the person who is stressed until acute anxiety has passed.

Allow the expression of thoughts, feelings, and emotions.

Teach new coping strategies, such as relaxation techniques, yoga, and meditation (see section on Coping Strategies).

Determine amount and quality of support from friends and family.

Help to identify activities that promote relaxation, such as listening to soft music, reading, and walking on the beach.

In severe stress (panic), stay with the patient, but assess the potential for injury to self or others.

Refer those with severe anxiety or panic to a physician, a geriatric nurse practitioner or clinical nurse specialist.

Anxiety in the Elderly With Cognitive Loss

When stress or anxiety is suspected in those with cognitive loss, the nurse should do the following:

Approach in an unhurried manner

Create a calm, predictable environment

Spend time with the elderly person

Focus on appropriate behavior

Speak in short, simple sentences

Reorient as needed in a positive noncritical way

Provide a familiar atmosphere (if institutionalized, have family members bring familiar and meaningful belongings such as family pictures, personal items, or even small items of furniture from home or previous living setting)

Evaluation and Expected Outcomes

The stressful situation should be reduced to a moderate level or eliminated. Effective coping strategies are identified and implemented, and anxiety is reduced.

PROMOTING A HEALTHY SELF-ESTEEM

Self-esteem is the way, positively or negatively, that a person views himself. Those with positive self-esteem have a positive view of themselves. They like and respect themselves and feel they are deserving and worthwhile. Conversely, those with negative self-esteem have a negative perception of themselves. They feel unworthy and lack confidence in their abilities. Many occurrences of aging contribute to a loss of self esteem, such as declining physical abilities, loss of significant support systems through death, and chronic illness. Maintaining self-esteem is a major task of adjusting well to aging (see Chapter 8). Self-esteem is threatened when the person lacks the economic resources to obtain adequate food or maintain adequate living quarters, when physical health declines, when functional ability is impaired, when there is a lack of a solid support system, or when coping mechanisms are not adequate to maintain psychological health. Inadequacy in any of these areas can threaten self-esteem.

USING THE NURSING PROCESS TO PROMOTE SELF-ESTEEM IN THE ELDERLY

Assessment

In assessing the person's self-esteem, be aware of negative "I" statements such as "I can't seem to do anything right!" or "I'm always getting things messed up." These statements may indicate that the person does not have a positive regard for himself. The person may have tension, anxiety, frustration, or depression. Encourage open expression of concerns such as feelings of hopelessness, helplessness, and powerlessness. Assess feelings of rejection or nonacceptance by others. Those with low self-esteem may have a lack of eye contact and express confusion about self, life issues, or purpose in life.

Nursing Diagnosis

The following nursing diagnosis is most often used for those who have a low self-esteem: Self-Esteem Disturbance related to retirement, low income, decline in functional abilities, or other factors (specify).

Planning and Implementation

Promoting healthy self-esteem is an ongoing process with the elderly. Persons with positive self-esteem have attained acceptance of the good and bad aspects of themselves. Increased self-esteem enhances a feeling of control and promotes hope. Display 11-4 describes nursing interventions that enhance self-esteem.

Evaluation and Expected Outcomes

Self-esteem should increase. The client increases the use of positive "I" statements and verbalizes increased acceptance of self.

DISPLAY 11-4. Nursing Interventions That Enhance Self-Esteem

- Treat with dignity and respect.
- Allow decision making concerning care, if possible.
- Plan short-term goals that can be accomplished.
- Praise accomplishments.
- Teach the use of positive "I" statements for self-talk.
- Encourage verbalization.
- Actively listen as the patient talks.
- Have the patient identify past successes and achievements.
- Encourage socialization with others.
- Convey confidence in the person's ability to cope.
- Encourage life review to reexamine positive past experiences.
- Assist the older adult in identifying and obtaining social services and resources necessary to maintain adequate income, food, and living arrangements.

PROMOTING SEXUAL HEALTH

Sexuality is an important component of most elderly persons' lives well into old age. Sexuality encompasses more than having the physical ability to perform sexual intercourse. It is a feeling of attractiveness and desirability to and by the opposite sex. Sexuality for most people becomes a part of their physical and emotional identity. Feelings of sexuality are enhanced by intimacy.

The elderly can meet sexuality needs by engaging in self-care activities that make them feel attractive. For example, women can go to the beauty shop weekly or dress attractively. These activities help promote self-esteem and make them feel more desirable. Companionship, touching, caressing, kissing, and sexual intercourse all contribute to meeting sexual needs. Men and women are capable of engaging in and enjoying sexual intercourse well into old age.

Contrary to popular belief, older adults remain interested in sex and engage in sexual activities. Sexual desire does not end for women with menopause. Impotence (ie, inability of the male to achieve erection of the penis) is not a natural occurrence with age. Older men are capable of fathering a child well into their nineties. The major deterrent of sexual activity is often lack of a partner.

Changes That Occur With Aging Affecting Sexual Functioning

Some changes in men and women do affect sexual activity. In men, more time is needed to become aroused, erections are less firm, and ejaculations are less forceful. Some older men report that the sensations associated with ejaculation are less intense. With age, many men experience decreased **libido** (ie, sexual desire). This decrease may result from the effects of medications, chronic disease, physiologic changes, or psychological factors. For men who are unable to have an erection because of organic reasons, surgically implanted penile prostheses are available. Some penile prosthetics are rigid, and others are inflatable. Several commercial external impotence management devices are available if surgery is not an option or an alternate method of treatment is desired.

Women also experience changes that affect their sexual activity. Menopause brings about a decrease in hormonal production, particularly estrogen. Decline in estrogen levels cause vaginal dryness and decrease in vaginal size, leading to discomfort during intercourse. These effects can largely be remedied with the use of water-based lubricants such as K-Y jelly before intercourse. Estrogen replacement therapy (ERT) may be used to decrease atrophy of the vagina and increase vaginal lubrication. ERT is accomplished through the administration of oral estrogen, estrogen patches, or a topical estrogen cream. After menopause, the freedom from the risk of pregnancy can have a positive effect on a woman's libido.

Although interest in sex remains, there is a gradual decline in the frequency of sexual activity with age. Although women may also have a decline in libido, the health and attitudes of the male partner appear to have the greatest influence on the frequency of intercourse.

Effects of Chronic Illness on Sexual Activity

Several chronic illnesses affect sexual functioning of the elderly, such as benign prostatic hypertrophy (BPH) (ie, enlargement of the prostate gland resulting in the obstruction of the release of urine), hypothyroidism, diabetes, and degenerative joint disease. BPH is common in men. The most common surgical procedure used to correct BPH is transurethral resection of the prostate (TURP). Although this procedure does not cause physical impotence, psychological impotence can result. Other prostate surgeries such as the suprapubic (ie, surgical incision is made above the pubic area)

DISPLAY 11-5. Selected Drugs That Affect Sexual Functioning

Antidepressants
imipramine (Tofranil)
amitriptyline (Elavil)
sertraline (Zoloft)

Antipsychotics
thioridazine (Mellaril)
chlorpromazine (Thorazine)
fluphenazine (Prolixin)
haloperidol (Haldol)

Antianxiety Agents
diazepam (Valium)

H$_2$ Blockers
cimetidine (Tagamet)

Antihypertensive
clonidine (Catapres)
methyldopa (Aldomet)
propranolol (Inderal)
labetalol (Normodyne)
prazosin (Minipress)

Cardiovascular Drugs
digoxin (Lanoxin)
disopyramide (Norpace)

Diuretics
spironolactone (Aldactone)
hydrochlorothiazide (Esidrix)

---

and the retropubic (ie, surgical incision is made behind the pubic area) prostatectomies can result in impotence. In these cases, a penile implant or an external device may be helpful in restoring sexual function.

Hypothyroidism most often occurs in elderly women and can cause a decrease in libido. The administration of thyroxine (ie, hormone produced by the thyroid gland that affects metabolism) may help to correct a decreased libido, although many times no improvement occurs in libido.

Diabetes can also cause impotence in the elderly. Failure to achieve an erection of the penis in the male diabetic is thought to be at least partially because of the changes in the vascular system as a result of the diabetes. Arthritic changes in the elderly that cause pain, stiffness, and deformity can affect sexual activity. It may be helpful if the older adult with arthritis plans sexual activity to coincide with administration of pain medication. Changes in position for sexual intercourse may help in decreasing physical discomfort.

Many commonly prescribed medications have a profound effect on the sexual function of the elderly. Antihypertensive agents, antianxiety agents, and antidepressants can cause impotence, decreased libido, and problems with ejaculation (ie, sudden release of semen from the male urethra). Display 11-5 lists commonly prescribed drugs for the elderly that can adversely affect sexual function.

Barriers to Sexual Activity in a Nursing Home

Many barriers exist in the nursing home setting that make sexual activity difficult and sometimes impossible. Some older adults living in nursing homes desire to continue sexual activity. However, the lack of privacy in the nursing home and negative attitudes from nurses and ancillary staff make sexual expression difficult.

Negative attitudes by nurses and ancillary staff members reinforce societal stereotypes that people somehow become sexless after 65. These negative attitudes make the older adult feel inadequate and uncomfortable in expressing sexual feelings. Although interest in sex declines with age, many men and women still desire the companionship and close association with the opposite sex. Sometimes, lack of a partner or feelings of unattractiveness keep the elderly from seeking intimate relationships. Chronic illness contributes to the problem by creating mobility problems, impotence, or confusion.

USING THE NURSING PROCESS TO PROMOTE SEXUALITY IN THE ELDERLY

Assessment

Before helping others with sexual problems, nurses must assess their own prejudices, bias, and feelings concerning sexuality in the elderly. Stereotypical attitudes and ageism can be present that cause communication barriers with the older adult. Use Display 11-6 to clarify and explore feelings about sexuality of the older adult.

It is important to establish a trusting nurse-patient relationship. There may be a reluctance to answer questions concerning sexuality unless the person feels comfortable with the nurse. Assess for the presence of any disorder or disease (acute and chronic) that may interfere with sexual function, such as arthritis, stroke, or BPH. Evaluate current medications for those that may interfere with sexual function. Assess for the presence of physiologic changes that may affect sexual function, eg vaginal dryness can cause painful intercourse. Question the patient regarding previous and current sexual patterns.

Nursing Diagnoses

Depending on the nature of the sexual problem one or more of the following nursing diagnoses may be used:

> **DISPLAY 11-6. Exploring Feelings About Sexuality in the Elderly**
>
> Nurses need to examine their own attitudes to identify biases or prejudices against the elderly. Reflect on the following questions to explore personal feelings toward sexuality in the older adult.
> - How do older people express sexuality?
> - Do I feel that being sexually active after the age of 60 is normal?
> - What would I do if I walked into a patient's room and discovered two elderly people together sexually?
> - What are societal attitudes about sexuality in the elderly that indicate ageism?
> - How can I help the elderly to express their sexuality?

Sexual Dysfunction related to decreased libido, impotence, other (specify)

Altered Sexuality Patterns related to arthritic condition, depression, other (specify)

Planning and Implementation

Creating an atmosphere of understanding, openness, and acceptance is critical to assisting the older person in meeting sexual needs. Display 11-7 lists the nursing interventions that help promote normal sexual functioning in the older adult.

Evaluation and Expected Outcomes

The client expresses the idea that sexual needs are met and verbalizes the use of alternate ways to meet sexual needs.

PROMOTING SPIRITUALITY IN THE OLDER ADULT

All individuals are spiritual beings and have spiritual needs. Spiritual fulfillment is found when individuals, young or old, find meaning in life and feel a sense of accomplishment and life satisfaction. Many seek and fulfill spiritual needs through a relationship with God. There is a basic need to feel forgiveness for misdeeds, love and acceptance as individuals, and hope for the future. Religion helps to fulfill these needs. Religion provides a value system and, through association with others of similar beliefs, a support system.

DISPLAY 11-7. Nursing Interventions that Help Promote Normal Sexual Functioning in the Older Adult

- Be sensitive to the sexual needs of the older adult.
- Look for indicators that the older adult needs to express sexual needs.
- Question the older adult about his or her sexual needs.
- Provide privacy (eg, place "do not disturb" signs on the doors, discuss privacy issues with staff, respect closed doors).
- Teach other staff members about the sexual needs of the older adult (ie, closing doors to be alone, escorting each other to the cafeteria, or masturbation).
- Discuss sexuality in the elderly with residents.
- Assess prescribed medications for the cause of sexual dysfunction. Notify the physician if any prescribed drug can cause sexual dysfunction.
- Instruct those with arthritis to take pain medication before sexual activity.
- Use praise and positive reinforcement to increase self-esteem.
- Provide information concerning sexual needs and ways to satisfy those needs.
- Provide information on external devices or penile implants if indicated.
- Discuss alternate methods of obtaining sexual satisfaction.
- Refer for further counseling if indicated.

Spirituality is a broad term; *religion* is more narrow. Spirituality can be found in the belief in a higher power, authority, or guiding spirit or in an appreciation and love for creation or in valuing the qualities of love, honesty, or wisdom. Many times, spirituality involves organized religion where the individual worships God and forms relationships with like-minded people.

Religion is a more organized form of spirituality, usually with an established system of worship. A chronic illness or disability may cause a person to question her spirituality. When faced with chronic illness, disability, and death, many reaffirm their spirituality, question their spirituality, or seek other avenues to gain spirituality. It is unlikely that many will drastically change their spirituality with age. If religion or a close relationship with God has been an important part of an older adults life since young or middle adulthood, it is likely it will continue to be an important and valued part of life. More time may be available to pursue religious interests such as more time for Bible study, association with like believers in social activities, or opportunities to help others. If religion has not been a significant area of life before old age, spirituality may be pursued in other ways.

USING THE NURSING PROCESS TO PROMOTE SPIRITUALITY

Assessment

It is helpful if the nurse has spent some time exploring her own spirituality before discussing spiritual concerns with others. A nurse who is comfortable with spiritual matters is better able to discuss spirituality with the older adults.

Do ask about spiritual needs. Unmet spiritual needs may be manifested by expressions of anger toward God, concerns about death or the meaning of life, or questions about why some illness or problem occurred. Review religious and spiritual history, such as participation in religious activities, church attendance, and importance placed on spirituality.

Assess current spiritual needs. Observe for the presence of religious literature in the immediate environment such as a Bible, a rosary, or spiritual literature on the bedside table. Be alert for statements such as "My life has no meaning anymore" or "I hate what God has allowed to happen" or "I can't seem to pray anymore." Spiritual distress occurs when the older adult feels that life no longer has meaning, that God has failed them, or there is a feeling of hopelessness with a current situation.

Nursing Diagnoses

The following nursing diagnoses may be used for patients having spiritual problems:

Spiritual Distress related to chronic disease, death of a loved one, or other (specify)

Potential for Enhanced Spiritual Well-Being

Other nursing diagnoses may be appropriate, depending on the identified needs of the older adult.

Planning and Implementation

Meeting spiritual needs can help the older adult to come to terms with life, accept death and feel that life has been worthwhile. Sometimes, the nurse is able to help meet spiritual needs. At other times, a referral may be needed to be made to the hospital chaplain, a clergyman, priest, or rabbi.

Patients in hospital settings usually do not enter the hospital because of a spiritual problem although spiritual issues may be present. The nursing home is a good place to address spiritual needs. Opportunities for the nurse to ask the resident their feelings concerning spirituality are present on a daily basis.

DISPLAY 11-8. Nursing Interventions That Help Relieve Spiritual Distress

- Develop a trusting nurse-patient relationship.
- Use self-disclosure if appropriate to meet therapeutic goals.
- Use problem-solving method to resolve conflicting feelings.
- Accept the person.
- Encourage verbalization of thoughts and feelings.
- Actively listen.
- Permit the performance of religious rituals if requested and they will not harm the patient.
- Be open to expressions of spiritual concern.
- Respect thoughts and feelings.
- Pray if the individual requests your prayers and you feel comfortable doing so.

DISPLAY 11-9. Nursing Interventions to Assist in Enhancing Spiritual Well-being

- Explore ways that faith and beliefs give meaning to life.
- Discuss the role of spirituality in one's life.
- Use problem-solving technique to resolve any conflicts that interfere with spirituality.
- Identify ways to enhance spirituality on a daily basis. Some nursing homes have daily or weekly devotional periods.
- If the individual is living in a nursing home, arrange for a pass to attend church.
- Suggest books on spirituality for personal reading and growth.

Through open ended questioning, active listening, and a nonjudgmental attitude, the nurse can assist the resident to explore spiritual matters. Adjustment depends on past coping strategies and how successful past coping strategies were.

Planning and Implementation

Spiritual Distress
A chronic illness or disability may cause a person to question his spirituality or cause spiritual distress. The nursing interventions in Display 11-8 may help in relieving the spiritual distress of patients.

Enhancing Spiritual Well-being
A useful way in which the nurse can assist with the spirituality of her patients is by enhancing their spiritual well-being. Display 11-9 describes nursing interventions that may assist in enhancing spiritual well-being.

Evaluation and Expected Outcomes

The client expresses spiritual contentment, verbalizes a sense of peace, and acknowledges an increase in spiritual well-being.

CRITICAL THINKING EXERCISES

1. Mr. Hightower, age 79, visits his 82-year-old wife, Agnes, in the nursing home daily. Although in good health, he is unable to care for all of her physical needs, and she was admitted to the nursing home 3 months ago. You notice that Mr. Hightower and Agnes frequently close the door to Agnes' room and appear to want to be alone. How would you assess this situation? What potential needs could Mr. and Mrs. Hightower have that are unmet? How could you assist the Hightowers to meet those needs.

2. Mr. Garcia is very ill and requests that the *curandero* (ie, folk healer in the Mexican-American culture) come to see him in the hospital. How would you handle this situation? Give a rationale for your response. What assessments would you make initially?

3. When entering the room of a resident at the nursing home, you discover her crying. The resident states that she does not understand why God has allowed her to remain alive so long. What would you say to the resident? How would you make her feel more comfortable?

4. Mr. Kieper requests that you work with him using the relaxation process. He has not been sleeping well and hopes that this will help him to "get a good night's sleep." Write a script for a visualization scenario to help Mr. Kieper relax his body and promote a restful night's sleep.

REFERENCES AND SUGGESTED READING

Carpenito, L. (1999). *Nursing Diagnosis: Application to Clinical Practice* (8th ed.). Philadelphia: Lippincott Williams & Wilkins.

Dossey, B., & Dossey, L. (1998). Body-mind-spirit: Attending to holistic care. *American Journal of Nursing, 98 (2),* 35–38.

Farfan, D. (1997). There's always hope. *RN, 6 (60),* 31–32.

Gorman, L., Sultan, D., & Raines, L. (1996). *Davis's Manual of Psychosocial Nursing for General Patient Care*. Philadelphia: F.A. Davis.

Ghusn, H. (1995). Sexuality in institutionalized patients. *Physical Medicine & Rehabilitation: State of the Art Reviews, 9 (2)*, 475–486.

Hicks, T. (1999). Spirituality and the elderly: Nursing implications with nursing home residents. *Geriatric Nursing, 20 (3)*, 144–146.

Lorenzi, E. (1999). Complementary/alternative therapies: So many choices. *Geriatric Nursing, 20 (3)*, 125–133.

Monea, H., & Boldi, M. (1999). Practicalities of an alternative pathway. *Geriatric Nursing, 20 (3)*, 134–138.

Roach, S., & Nieto, B. (1996). *Healing and the Grief Process*. Albany, NY: Delmar Publishing.

CHAPTER 12

Effects of Medication in the Older Adult

CHAPTER OUTLINE

KEY TERMS
CHAPTER OBJECTIVES
PHARMACOKINETICS
    Absorption
    Distribution
    Metabolism
    Excretion
DRUG REACTIONS IN THE OLDER ADULT
    Adverse Reactions
    Cumulative Drug Effect
    Toxic Drug Effect
    Drug Idiosyncrasy
    Polypharmacy
    Drug-Drug Interactions
CRITICAL THINKING EXERCISES
REFERENCES AND SUGGESTED READING

KEY TERMS

absorption
adverse reactions
distribution
drug idiosyncrasy
excretion
lipid solubility
metabolism
pharmacokinetics
polypharmacy
protein binding
therapeutic blood level

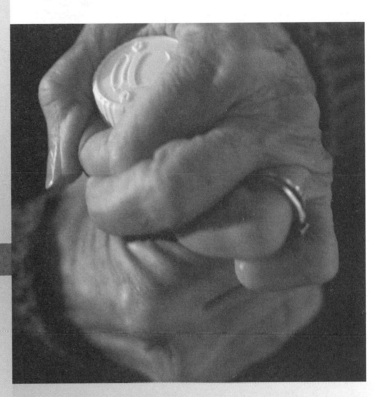

CHAPTER OBJECTIVES

At the completion of this chapter, the student will be able to

- Describe the four processes involved in pharmacokinetics

- Identify age-related changes associated with absorption, distribution, metabolism, and excretion of drugs

- Explain how protein binding and tepid solubility affects distribution of drugs

- Discuss various drug reactions in the older adults

- Explain polypharmacy and its impact on the older adult

- Discuss drug-drug interactions

Aging causes a number of physiologic changes within the body. These changes affect the activity and response of drugs within the body. A medication dosage that is appropriate for a 40- or 50-year-old may be excessive for an 80-year-old person. Another area of concern is the large number of drugs prescribed for the elderly. Twenty-five percent of all prescriptions are written for people older than age 65, making older adults users of the largest number of medications of any age group. Seventy percent of older adults use over-the-counter (OTC) drugs, but only 10% of younger adults use OTC drugs. This chapter discusses the effects of medication in the older adult.

PHARMACOKINETICS

After drugs are administered, pharmacokinetic activity begins. **Pharmacokinetics** is the movement of drugs within the body and includes the four processes of absorption, distribution, metabolism, and excretion. With age, the pharmacokinetic activity of drugs changes, increasing the risk of developing adverse reactions and toxic (harmful or poisonous) effects.

Absorption

Absorption is the process by which a drug passes into the circulatory system (ie, bloodstream or lymphatic system) for distribution throughout the body. Factors that influence absorption include the amount of blood flow to a particular area, the route of administration, and how thoroughly the drug dissolves in the blood.

Absorption is facilitated by a good blood supply to the absorption site. Poor absorption can occur if a drug is administered parenterally into tissue that has poor blood supply or circulation. The intravenous route results in the most rapid absorption with the subcutaneous and the intramuscular route having a slower absorption rate. Drugs administered topically or that are inhaled come into contact with the blood-rich mucous membranes and are absorbed rapidly. When drugs are administered orally or rectally, a slower rate of absorption occurs.

Some age-related changes may affect absorption of drugs in the older adult:

1. An increase in gastric pH caused by achlorhydria (ie, decreased production of hydrochloric acid in the stomach)
2. A decrease in gastric blood flow and in gastric motility (ie, movement)

Decreased gastric motility allows an oral drug to be exposed to the gastric mucosa for a longer period and can increase absorption of the drug. Changes in the pH can affect the absorption of some oral drugs. When the pH of the gastric contents is alkaline, drugs that are made to dissolve in an acid environment dissolve at a less efficient rate and absorption is decreased. For example, the increase in gastric pH results in a more alkaline environment in the stomach. This causes a decrease in absorption of the drug tetracycline. This same alkaline environment can cause an increase in the absorption of penicillin.

Distribution

Distribution refers to the dispersion of the drug to different parts of the body. After absorption into the circulation, drugs are distributed throughout the body by the blood and the lymphatic system. Areas with the greatest blood supply such as the heart, liver, kidney, and brain receive the drug more rapidly than areas of the body with a lesser blood supply such as muscles and adipose tissue.

Some drugs are distributed throughout the body attached to plasma proteins circulating in the blood. **Protein binding** occurs when a drug is relatively insoluble and binds (or attaches) to a plasma protein, usually albumin. A part of the drug binds with protein, and the remainder of the drug remains unbound while circulating in the blood. The unbound part of the drug can reach the receptor site and produce the desired effect, be metabolized, and then be excreted. The portion of the drug that is bound to the protein has no pharmacologic effect. Protein binding serves as a storehouse for drugs, gradually releasing the drug and prolonging the action. As the unbound drug reaches the receptor site or is excreted, the blood level of the drug decreases, allowing some of the drug to be released from the albumin. A balance of bound and unbound drug is maintained until all of the drug is released from the albumin and excreted.

Lipid solubility refers to how soluble a drug is in fatty tissue. Fat or adipose tissue attracts lipid soluble drugs that bind to the adipose tissue. Because blood supply to adipose tissue is low, lipid-soluble drugs remain in the adipose tissue. As the drug leaves the circulatory system, a decrease in the blood level of the drug occurs, causing some of the drug in the adipose tissue to be released into the bloodstream, where it can be distributed to the receptor site, metabolized, and then be excreted.

Other drugs are water soluble, and distribution occurs readily in the more fluid-filled parts of the body, particularly lean tissue. The distribution of water-soluble drugs is inhibited if the older adult is dehydrated.

The distribution of drugs is affected by several age-related changes. The following list identifies age-related changes in the older adult that affect the distribution of drugs. Compared with younger adults, the older adult has

A smaller amount of total body water

An increase in adipose tissue (fat)

A lower body weight

A decrease in cardiac output

A decrease in serum albumin

An increase in adipose tissue results in more of the lipid-soluble drug being distributed in adipose tissue. Lipid-soluble drugs tend to stay in the adipose tissue, resulting in a decrease in blood levels of the drug and a longer duration of action in the body. If this age-related change is not taken into account, the patient may have the dosage of a lipid-soluble drug incorrectly increased. This increases the risk of drug toxicity. The hangover effect of the lipid-soluble sedative phenobarbital, seen in many older adults, may be the result of the drug being released from the adipose tissue over a longer period.

Because there is a decrease in the total amount of body water in the older adult, drugs that are water-soluble may not be distributed well and may remain in the body, causing an increase in blood levels of the drug and symptoms of toxicity. This may require a dosage reduction. Dehydration can cause high drug levels in the blood and increase the risk of adverse reactions in the elderly.

Cardiac output (ie, amount of blood to leave the left ventricle with each contraction) decreases with age. This affects the distribution of water-soluble drugs. When cardiac output is decreased, an increase in blood levels of the drug occurs, increasing the risk of toxicity.

With age, blood levels of albumin decrease slightly. This decrease of albumin can cause a problem in the distribution of protein-bound drugs. Low albumin levels in the blood allow more drug to circulate unbound in the blood. This increases the risk for adverse reactions. Examples of highly protein-bound drugs are listed in Display 12-1. If more than one protein-bound drug is administered, each drug competes with the other for the same protein molecules, and blood drug levels increase. Hypoalbuminemia (ie, low blood levels of albumin) can cause high drug levels in the blood.

Metabolism

Metabolism is the chemical processes that occur within the body that transforms a drug to a form that can be used and excreted. This process occurs pri-

---

DISPLAY 12-1. Selected Highly Protein-Bound Drugs

acetazolamide (Diamox)
amitriptyline (Elavil)
chloropromazine (Thorazine)
digitoxin (Digitaline)
phenytoin (Dilantin)
haloperidol (Haldol)
propranolol (Inderal)
salicylate (aspirin)
spironolactone (Aldactone)
tolbutamide (Orinase)
warfarin (Coumadin)

---

marily in the liver. Many drugs are also detoxified (ie, made less harmful) by the liver.

Some age-related changes in the liver may affect the metabolism of drugs:

Decreased blood flow to the liver

Decreased enzyme function

Decreased liver mass

All of these age-related changes decrease the rate drugs are metabolized and increase the risk of developing high blood levels of the drug. Increased drug levels increase the risk of developing adverse or toxic reactions. Liver enzymes function in the detoxification process. With a decrease in enzyme activity, drugs are not detoxified as rapidly as normal, resulting in an increased risk for toxicity. Liver disease also decreases the liver's ability to metabolize drugs and increases the risk of adverse reactions and toxicity.

Excretion

Excretion is the elimination of waste products from the body. Excretion of drugs is accomplished by the activity of the urinary system (ie, kidney and other tissues). The drug, along with other constituents of blood, passes thorough the capillaries of the glomerulus into Bowman's capsule. The blood (containing the drug) then passes along the tubules, where beneficial substances are reabsorbed and waste materials (ie, urea and drugs) are excreted in the urine.

Aging brings about a significant decrease in renal functioning. By the age of 80 years, a person has lost 40% to 50% of renal functioning. Excretion is specifically affected by a decrease in the glomerular filtration rate (ie, amount of filtrate formed by blood moving through the glomeruli of the kidney) and renal blood flow. When the kidneys are not functioning properly, drugs are not excreted and remain in the bloodstream longer, increasing the risk of adverse reactions and drug toxicity.

Some age-related changes affect excretion:

Decreased renal blood flow

Decreased glomerular filtration rate

Many drugs affect kidney functioning. A decrease in kidney functioning can occur even when low dosages are administered to the elderly. Examples of drugs that can inhibit renal functioning include digoxin, cimetidine, lithium, and procainamide.

DRUG REACTIONS IN THE OLDER ADULT

Adverse Reactions

The older adult is particularly prone to develop adverse reactions when taking any drug. The drug response may be different in an older adult. **Adverse reactions** are undesirable drug effects, and they may be mild or severe. They may occur after the first dose, several doses, or after the drug has been discontinued. Adverse reactions may occur even when the drug has been given successfully over a long period. Certain adverse reactions are predictable. Predictable drug reactions are reactions that are seen often when the drug is administered. For example, if a sedative was administered for anxiety, drowsiness is a predictable adverse reaction. Other adverse reactions are unexpected and unpredictable. Any complaint or symptom that is unusual or different is immediately reported to the charge nurse and the primary nurse care provider.

Common adverse reactions related to drug therapy seen in the elderly include confusion, incontinence, and a decrease in mobility. Older adults take more OTC and prescription drugs than the general population. This predisposes them to an increased risk of drug-drug interactions. Confusion must always be investigated, particularly if a patient who has previously been alert and responsive suddenly becomes confused. There is a tendency to ignore or accept some confusion in the elderly, brushing it off as a natural occurrence in old age. In the absence of disease confusion is *not* normal in the elderly.

There appears to be a decrease in the perfusion (ie, passage of blood, nutrients, and fluid) to certain areas of the brain with age, and the central nervous system (CNS) loses some of its functional reserve, making the older adult more sensitive to drugs and increases the risk of changes in the CNS. Drugs that can cause confusion include antianxiety agents, analgesics, antihypertensives, anticholinergics, antipsychotics, and antidepressants. A decrease in dosage or a change to a different drug can sometimes alleviate the problem of confusion. The physician or primary care giver should be notified if confusion occurs in an otherwise alert older person. These drugs can also cause behavior changes, restlessness, irritability, anxiety, and hallucinations. These types of behaviors may go unrecognized as adverse reactions and allowed to persist because they are labeled as normal symptoms of old age.

Incontinence of urine and bowel is a functional problem that can occur as the result of drugs. Some drugs, such as cholinergics and anticholinergics, affect sphincter control. Other drugs, such as sedatives, decrease mental alertness. When mental alertness decreases, the elderly person may not be aware of the need to defecate or urinate. Mobility may be affected because of the depressant effects of the sedative. Problems with ambulation decrease the ability of some elderly to get to the bathroom before bowel or bladder elimination occurs. Other drugs promote excretion of urine (ie, diuretics) and bowel elimination (ie, laxatives), causing a shorter warning time indicating the need to urinate or defecate. All of these factors contribute to drug-induced incontinence. Placing a bedside commode near the bed may help promote continence. A decrease in dosage or a change in medication may also be required. Incontinence should always be examined in the elderly as a possible adverse reaction to the drug regimen.

A decrease in mobility can occur whenever a drug that depresses the CNS is given. Sedatives, hypnotics, antianxiety agents, and antipsychotics can sedate the older adult to a point where simply getting out of bed, performing the activities of daily living, or ambulation may be too much of a chore. The antipsychotic drugs have extrapyramidal adverse reactions resulting in irregular rhythmic motor movements, usually of the lower extremities, that can cause unsteadiness or gait problems. This causes a decrease in mobility and increases the potential for falls. Nurses must have good baseline data to evaluate the potential for falls as a result of drugs. Careful documentation and daily assessment are important in monitoring the elderly for the risk of decreased mobility because of medications.

Cumulative Drug Effect

Older adults are more likely to have a cumulative drug effect because of the age-related changes that occur in the liver and kidneys of older adults. A cumulative drug effect occurs when a second dose of the drug is administered before the previous dose has been fully metabolized and excreted. For example, if a drug has not been eliminated by the kidney as a result of a decrease in kidney function and a second dose is given, high levels of the drug can accumulate in the blood, causing serious adverse reactions.

TABLE 12-1. Examples of Selected Drugs, Therapeutic Levels, and Symptoms of Toxicity

Drug	Therapeutic Drug Levels	Symptoms of Toxicity*
digoxin (Lanoxin)	0.5–2 ng/mL	Abdominal pain, anorexia, nausea, vomiting, visual disturbances, bradycardia, arrhythmias
lithium	0.5–1.5 mEq/L	Vomiting, diarrhea, slurred speech, decreased coordination, drowsiness, muscle weakness, or twitching
phenytoin (Dilantin)	10–20 mcg/mL	Nystagmus, ataxia, confusion, nausea, slurred speech, dizziness
quinidine sulfate (Quinidex Extentabs)	2–6 µg/mL	Tinnitus, hearing loss, visual disturbances, headache, nausea, and dizziness
theophylline, theophylline extended release	10–20 µg/mL	Anorexia, nausea, vomiting, restlessness, insomnia, tachycardia, arrhythmias seizures

*Primary health care provider should be notified if any symptoms of toxicity occur.

Monitor kidney functioning when administering drugs that affect renal functioning. Any decrease in urinary output, cloudy or concentrated urine, or elevated blood urea nitrogen (BUN) or creatinine levels may indicate decreased kidney functioning and is reported immediately. However, creatinine levels may remain normal despite decreased renal clearance because the muscle mass that is the source of creatinine is decreased in the elderly.

Toxic Drug Effect

Drugs can produce toxic or dangerous reactions when blood concentrations exceed the therapeutic level. The **therapeutic blood level** is the amount of drug circulating in the blood that is able to produce the desired effect in the body. A blood drug level can be determined by drawing several milliliters of blood from a vein for laboratory analysis. The blood level of a drug is the amount of drug present in the circulating fluid at a specific time. When the blood levels of a drug exceeds the therapeutic level, toxic symptoms can occur. The elderly are at risk to develop toxic effects because of decrease in kidney function. Therapeutic drug levels and symptoms of toxicity of selected drugs commonly administered to the elderly are listed in Table 12-1. Drug levels must be carefully monitored to ensure that they are within the therapeutic range. Any increase or decrease in the therapeutic level must be reported to the physician immediately.

Drug Idiosyncrasy

Drug idiosyncrasy describes any unusual, abnormal, or exaggerated reaction to a drug. When a reaction that is different from the reaction expected occurs,

drug idiosyncrasy is suspected. An example of drug idiosyncrasy is when an elderly person is given a sedative to induce sleep, but the person sleeps all night and well into the next day. On awakening, the sedative effects continue, causing lethargy and drowsiness. This is an exaggerated response. Elderly persons may manifest a drug idiosyncrasy to any drug that is taken.

Older people may also have a paradoxical (opposite) response to a drug. In the case of the administration of a sedative, a paradoxical response is when the sedative causes the older person to become overly excited or anxious. Any unusual or exaggerated behavior or symptom observed in an elderly person is reported. A thorough assessment is made to determine possible causes of these reactions.

Polypharmacy

Polypharmacy is the use of an excessive number of prescribed and OTC drugs that are often unnecessary and can interact within the body to cause a number of adverse reactions. The presence of one or more chronic illnesses, each with several drugs prescribed, contributes to the problem of polypharmacy in the elderly. The drugs are usually taken several times each day, and the prescriptions may be obtained from more than one physician and filled at more than one pharmacy. The phrase "over four, give no more" is applicable in medication administration for older adults. Taking more than four prescription drugs necessitates evaluation by the primary health care provider to determine the need and the effectiveness of each drug. The more drugs being taken, the greater is the risk for adverse reactions. Sometimes, having several chronic illnesses means the elderly person must take a large number of drugs.

TABLE 12-2. Examples of Potential Drug–Drug Interactions

Drug	Interacting Agent(s)	Potential Reaction
amitriptyline (Elavil)	MAO inhibitors	Hypotension, tachycardia, and death can occur
	antihypertensives	May prevent therapeutic response
	clonidine	Severe hypertension
	antihistamines, opioid analgesics, sedatives	Additive CNS depression
lorazepam (Ativan)	alcohol, antihistamines, antidepressants, opioid analgesics	Additive CNS depression
flurazepam (Dalmane)	alcohol, antidepressants, antihistamines, opioid analgesics	Additive CNS depression
	cimetidine, isoniazid, ketoconazole, propranolol	Enhances action of flurazepam
	theophylline	Sedative effects decreased
	rifampin	Decreases effects of flurazepam
furosemide (Lasix)	antihypertensives, nitrates	Severe hypotension
	cardiac glycosides	Electrolyte imbalance and digitalis toxicity
	other diuretics, amphotericin B, glucocorticoids	Additive hypokalemia
	lithium	Decreases excretion of lithium
	aminoglycosides	Increases risk of ototoxicity
haloperidol (Haldol)	anticholinergics	Additive anticholinergic effects
	tricyclic antidepressants	Increases effects of antidepressants
	barbiturates	Decreases effects of haloperidol
	phenytoin	Decreases effects of haloperidol
propranolol (Inderal)	digoxin	Additive bradycardia
	antihypertensive agents	Additive hypotensive effects
	epinephrine, norepinephrine, or pseudoephedrine	Hypertension bradycardia
	insulin	Prolonged hypoglycemia
	MAO inhibitors	Hypertension
	cimetidine	Increases effects of propranolol
	theophylline	Increases theophylline blood levels

From Deglin, J.H. & Vallerand, A.H. (1997). *Davis Drug Guide for Nurses* (5th ed.). Philadelphia: F.A. Davis.

Drug-Drug Interactions

Because the elderly often take four or more prescription drugs, the danger of drug-drug interactions increases. The more drugs taken, the greater is the risk for interactions among the various drugs. The risks are compounded when kidney and liver function is compromised as a result of aging. Table 12-2 identifies examples of potential drug-drug interactions in selected drugs often prescribed for the elderly.

CRITICAL THINKING EXERCISES

1. Mrs. Gibbins, age 73, informs you that she has been experiencing some "weird" feelings lately. She states that she is dizzy, walks in a very unsteady gait, and is nauseated. In doing a medication review, you notice that Mrs. Gibbins is taking Humulin insulin (60 units) subcutaneously daily in the morning, Tylenol grains V orally daily, and phenytoin (300 mg/day) orally. Given this information, what additional assessments would you make? What problem would you suspect? What action would you take first?

2. A nurse assistant reports to you that Mr. Hartsel, age 69, has developed a problem with mobility over the past several days. You suspect an adverse reaction to his medications. What types of drugs would be most likely to cause Mr. Hartsel's mobility problems? How would you assess this problem?

3. Use the nursing process to develop a teaching plan for other nurses concerning the pharmacokinetic effects of drugs in the elderly.

4. The physician writes an order to monitor the patient closely for signs of digoxin toxicity. What

symptoms would you expect the patient with digoxin toxicity to exhibit? How would you expect toxicity to be confirmed?

REFERENCES AND SUGGESTED READING

Edwards, J. (1997). Guarding against adverse drug events. *American Journal of Nursing, 97 (5),* 26–31.

Lee, M. (1996). Drugs and the elderly: Do you know the risks? *American Journal of Nursing, 96 (7),* 25–32.

Kidder, S., & Kalachnik, J. (1999). Regulation of inappropriate psychopharmacologic medication use in U.S. nursing homes from 1954–1997. *Annals of Long-Term Care, 7 (2),* 56–62.

Miller, C. (1999). Drug/food/food supplements. *Geriatric Nursing, 20 (3),* 164.

Roach, S., & Scherer, J. (2000). *Introductory Clinical Pharmacology* (6th ed.). Philadelphia: Lippincott Williams & Wilkins.

White, C. P. (1993). Medications and the elderly. In: Carnevali, D. L., & Patrick, M. (Eds.). *Nursing Management for the Elderly.* Philadelphia: J. B. Lippincott, 171–191.

Walker, M., & Foreman, M. (1999). Medication safety: A protocol for nursing action. *Geriatric Nursing, 20 (1),* 34–39.

CHAPTER 13

Medication Administration Considerations

CHAPTER OUTLINE

KEY TERMS

CHAPTER OBJECTIVES

USING THE NURSING PROCESS IN THE
ADMINISTRATION OF MEDICATIONS

  Assessment

  Nursing Diagnoses

  Planning

  Implementation

  Evaluation

  Polypharmacy

HELPING OLDER ADULTS ADMINISTER THEIR OWN
MEDICATION

  Visual Disturbances

  Monitoring Systems for Self-Medication

  General Guidelines for Patient and Family
    Teaching

NONCOMPLIANCE WITH THE MEDICATION
REGIMEN

CRITICAL THINKING EXERCISES

REFERENCES AND SUGGESTED READING

KEY TERMS

generic drug

Medication Administration Record (MAR)

polypharmacy

Six Rights

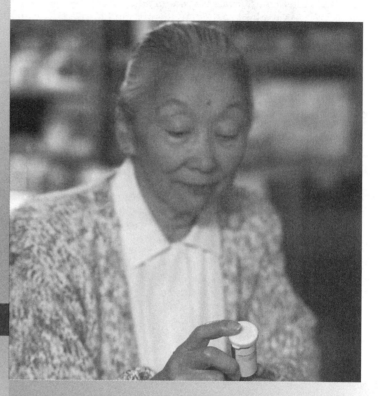

CHAPTER OBJECTIVES

At the completion of this chapter, the student will
be able to

- Use the nursing process in the administration
  of medications to the elderly

- Discuss the Six Rights of medication
  administration

- Describe three methods to teach older adults
  how to monitor a medication regimen

- Describe ways to assist the visually impaired in
  medication administration

- Identify general guidelines for teaching the
  patient and family how to self-administer drugs

- Discuss noncompliance with the medication
  regimen in the elderly

Medication administration is an important nursing responsibility at anytime, but it is particularly important when drugs are administered to older adults. Because of the increased risk of adverse reactions, toxic effects, and drug-drug interactions, careful assessment and evaluation must occur on a continuous basis. Nurses must be knowledgeable about how to safely administer medications and monitor patients for adverse reactions.

USING THE NURSING PROCESS IN ADMINISTRATION OF MEDICATIONS

The nursing process is provides a practical framework to discuss the administration of medications.

Assessment

Before the administration of any medication, the nurse must review the patient's chart and general health history. The health history reveals all medical and surgical treatments, a drug history, and the current symptoms. Identification of all drugs being taken, including prescription and over-the-counter (OTC) medications, is essential.

Check the health history to determine whether the patient has any allergies. Explore any drug allergies thoroughly. Question the patient regarding the symptoms experienced with the allergy. Determine the reason the medication is ordered. Verify the amount to be administered, the times the drug is to be administered, and the route of administration.

Establish a baseline assessment, including vital signs (eg, temperature, pulse, respirations, blood pressure). Identify signs or symptoms that will be relieved after administration of the medication to evaluate effectiveness of the drug regimen.

It is especially important to determine the elderly patient's ability to swallow if an oral drug is ordered. Assess all drugs currently prescribed for possible drug-drug interactions (see Chapter 12). Determine the patient's understanding of why the drug is prescribed.

Nursing Diagnoses

Nursing diagnoses associated with administration of medication are most often aimed at monitoring for effects of adverse reactions, patient and family teaching, or to address potential problems associated with a particular drug. When administering a narcotic analgesic for pain, a nursing diagnosis to monitor for a potential problem may be Risk for Injury related to effect of the narcotic on the central nervous system. Another diagnosis may be Knowledge Deficit or Risk for Ineffective Management of Therapeutic Regimen related to adverse drug effects or lack of knowledge of the medication regimen. Placement of the actual intervention of administering the drug is under the appropriate nursing diagnosis. For example, the intervention "administer indomethacin (Indocin), 25 mg, qid" would be placed under the nursing diagnosis of Pain, related to inflammation of the joints.

Planning

Planning is an important aspect of medication administration. Improper planning leads to incorrect administration and medication errors. It is helpful to discuss planning from the viewpoint of the **Six Rights:** the right patient, the right drug, the right dosage, the right route, the right time, and the right documentation. All medications are given using the Six Rights. Consistent use of these "rights" decreases medication errors.

Right Patient

A drug must be administered to the right patient. Sometimes, administering a drug to the right patient can be a problem. In a hospital or acute care setting, patients have identification bracelets or bands worn on the wrist with their name, hospital number, and other information such as allergies. However, in nursing facilities such as nursing homes, long-term care facilities, and adult day care centers, individuals may not have identification bracelets. This complicates safe medication administration. The nurse must properly identify the patient before administering medications. Simply asking "Are you Juan Garcia?" is not sufficient for patient identification. A confused patient may not remember his name and may answer to any name.

Many nursing facilities have the resident's picture attached to the chart or the **Medication Administration Record** (MAR), a form on which the patient's medications are recorded or documented. Pictures are current and not torn, blurred, or outdated. Clear pictures that without question resemble the resident are critical. A resident can be identified by the nurse requesting that he state his name. For example, the nurse may ask "Can you tell me your name please?"

Identification bracelets or pictures are the best form of identification and must always be used to determine if the right patient is receiving the medication, particularly with patients who are confused

TABLE 13-1. Undesirable Drugs for Older Patients

Drug	Problem
Long-acting benzodiazepines: diazepam (Valium), chlordiazepoxide (Librium), furazepam (Dalmane)	Produces daytime hangover-like effect due to prolonged duration of action; shorter-acting benzodiazepines are considered safer
meprobamate (Equanil, Miltown)	Accumulates with repeated dosing; shorter-acting benzodiazepines are considered safer
pentobarbital (Nembutal), secobarbital (Seconal)	Accumulate with repeated dosing; shorter-acting benzodiazepines are considered safer
amitriptryline (Elavil)	Has potent anticholinergic side effects
indomethacin (Indocin)	Headaches are more common than with other nonsteroidal anti-inflammatory agents; may also worsen depression
chlorpropamide (Diabinese)	Causes prolonged hypoglycemia
propoxyphene (Darvon)	Metabolite, norpropoxyphene, can cause arrhythmias, particularly in patients with impaired renal function
pentazocine (Talwin)	Can cause seizures, hallucinations, or arrhythmias when taken in large doses
cyclandelate (Cyclospasmol)	Ineffective as dementia treatment
isoxsuprine (Vasodilan)	Ineffective as dementia treatment
Muscle relaxants: cyclobenzaprine (Flexeril), orphenadrine (Norflex), methocarbamol (Robaxin), carisoprodol (Soma)	Potential for central nervous system toxicity is greater than potential benefit
trimethobenzamide (Tigan)	Less effective than alternative agents; may cause drowsiness and other adverse effects
dipyridamole (Persantine)	Efficacy unproven

From Lee, M. (1996). Drugs and the elderly: Do you know the risks? *American Journal of Nursing, 96 (7)*, 30.

or comatose. The nurse never assumes to know the patient, regardless of how many times or how long medication has been administered to that particular patient.

Right Drug
Before drug administration, the nurse verifies the medication to be given with the MAR and with the physician's order. A **generic drug** is the common name for a drug or a name that can be used in any country by any manufacturer. Generic drugs are less expensive and may be used unless the physician specifies that only a certain brand name be used. The names of drugs are verified as well. Drugs may have similar spellings and can easily be confused, such as Levoxine (for low thyroid) can be mistaken for Lanoxin (for heart failure), or Prilosec (for duodenal ulcer) can be mistaken for Prozac (for depression).

Certain drugs are undesirable drugs for older patients (Table 13-1). When the nurse observes that any of these drugs are prescribed for an elderly patient, the primary health care provider is notified. In some situations, the health care provider may elect to continued the medication. In this case, the patient is monitored closely for any evidence of adverse reactions or problems associated with the

drug. If any problems are observed, the health care provider is notified immediately.

Right Dosage
It is essential to check the dosage when administering drugs to older adults. The smallest dose that produces a therapeutic effect is considered the correct dosage. The elderly may require a smaller dose than the normal adult dose. In elderly patients, drug therapy may be begin with lower doses. If a therapeutic effect does not occur, the dosage is gradually increased.

Right Route
Many drugs can be given by several routes. Call the physician to specify a route if no route is written on the physician order sheet or if the order is illegible.

Right Time
Check the times of administration on the MAR, and give the medication at the specified times. If a dose is missed, an extra dose is *not* given to "catch up." When administering as-needed medications, the last time the drug was administered is checked before administering another dose of the drug.

Drugs must not be given to the elderly too close together because the potential for adverse reactions, toxic effects, and cumulative effects is great. If the physician order reads "every 4 hours prn," be careful not to administer a second dose within 4 hours of the first dose.

Right Documentation

Documentation is never done before administration of the medication. Proper documentation immediately after the medication is given, including the exact time of administration, is critical. If a nurse fails to document the administration of the medication, the patient is in danger of receiving an additional dose from another nurse, who thinks that the patient has not received any medication. An additional notation is made by the nurse 30 to 45 minutes after administration to document the patient's response to the medication.

Implementation

Administer the drug using the Six Rights. Before administration of any drug, explain to the patient the name of the drug, why the drug was prescribed, and how the drug is to be given. Answer the patient's questions.

Medication administration may be more difficult in the elderly because of physiologic changes such as dysphagia (ie, difficulty swallowing), hand tremors, or poor tissue perfusion (ie, movement of fluids through an area or the body). A tremor may make it difficult for the elderly to maneuver the medication container or the tablet for self-administration. Poor tissue perfusion interferes with absorption of drugs. If dysphasia is a problem, the nurse may request that the physician order a liquid form of the drug. If the patient is unable to swallow, a feeding tube may be inserted in order for the patient to receive adequate nutrition. The feeding tube can be used for medication administration.

When administering oral tablets or capsules, allow the patient to choose which method is best for that individual. Some patients take one capsule or tablet at a time and followed by water, and others prefer to take several or all of the tablets at the same time. Remember that the elderly may loose some sensitivity in their fingers. This can cause them (without their awareness) to pick up more than one tablet at a time or not feel a tablet in the medication cup and neglect to take that tablet. Be certain that all tablets are taken. Always administer oral tablets with a full glass of water unless instructed otherwise. If the patient's mouth is dry, a few sips of water before taking a tablet can facilitate swallowing.

Some tablets may be crushed (check appropriate sources for suitability to be crushed) and mixed with a small amount of food (eg, Jell-O, ice cream, jelly). If this method is approved by the physician, it is important that the patient take the entire mixture to obtain the correct dosage.

When administering medications by the intramuscular (IM) or subcutaneous (SC) route, the site should be assessed. The elderly have less muscle mass. The length of the needle may need to be shorter to prevent contact with the bone during an injection in a very thin person. For example, a 1-inch needle may be better than a 1.5-inch needle. The ventrogluteal site is preferred for the elderly. The ventrogluteal area has the most consistent depth of subcutaneous tissue, and fatty tissue usually is less than 1.5 inches.

During therapy, compare baseline data obtained during the assessment with the patient's current condition. Note any changes or adverse reactions. Pay close attention to any changes in the level of consciousness (LOC). A change in the LOC, such as confusion, may indicate adverse or toxic effects. After administration of the drug, document in the chart or in the MAR according to agency policy.

Some nursing facilities use a "punch card" for administering medications. As the medication is given, it is "punched out" from bubble containers that house the tablets. This type of system provides a method to check if a dosage was administered and helps to prevent medication errors.

Monitor for adverse reactions and toxic effects associated with each drug administered. Drugs with high potential for toxicity must be monitored closely. Report any signs or symptoms of toxicity immediately, because the physician may need to reduce the dosage or discontinue the drug. Report any behavior change, change in the LOC, or sudden confusion immediately, because this may indicate an adverse reaction.

Nurses must be aware of any special concerns when administering medication to the elderly. Table 13-2 lists selected drug classifications, drug names, their use, and implications for the elderly patient.

Evaluation

Evaluation of the patient's response to drug therapy is ongoing to determine if the patient is experiencing a therapeutic drug effect, adverse reactions, or toxic effects. The impact of the drug on self-care abilities is evaluated as well. For example, drugs that cause excessive drowsiness or gait problems interfere with self-care. Self-care is an important functional ability in the elderly patient, and every effort is made to preserve that function. To prevent deterioration of self-care ability, the dosage of the drug may need to be decreased or another drug prescribed.

Table 13-2. Special Considerations for the Elderly When Administering Commonly Prescribed Medications

Classification & Examples	Use	Implications for the Elderly

SEDATIVE/HYPNOTICS
Nonbarbiturates
  chloral hydrate
Benzodiazepines
  flurazepam (Dalmane)
  temazepam (Restoril)
  triazolam (Halcion)
	Short-term treatment of insomnia	Attempt to use other methods rather than sedative/hypnotics to induce sleep because idiosyncrasy reactions can occur in the elderly.
		If a sedative is necessary, the short-acting drugs are recommended because they are eliminated quickly and less likely to cause adverse reactions.
		Smaller dosages are required than for younger adults.
		Do not use longer than 3–4 nights consecutively.
		Monitor closely for excessive sedation, dizziness, ataxia (unsteady gait), and confusion.
		Do not discontinue abruptly. Discontinue over a period of several days.
		Can cause paradoxical reactions, respiratory distress, agitation, and psychoses.

ANTIANXIETY DRUGS
Benzodiazepines
  alprazolam (Xanax)
  clorazepate (Tranxene)
  oxazepam (Serax)
Nonbenzodiazepines
  buspirone (BuSpar)
	Management of anxiety states or for short-term relief of symptoms of anxiety	Antianxiety agents are metabolized and excreted more slowly in older adults causing the effects to last longer.
		These drugs may have a cumulative effect, increasing the risk of adverse reactions.
		Initial dosages are small and increased gradually to minimize the risk of adverse reactions.
		Monitor closely for hypotension, oversedation, confusion, dizziness, and decreased mobility.
		Potential for falls is increased.
		Taper drugs when discontinuing. Abrupt discontinuation may cause withdrawal symptoms.
		The benzodiazepines may cause short periods of memory loss, which aggravates any already existing cognitive problem.
		BuSpar does not cause cognitive impairment.

ANTIPSYCHOTIC DRUGS chlorpromazine (Thorazine) prochlorperazine (Compazine) haloperidol (Haldol) perphenazine (Trilafon) thioridazine (Mellaril)	Schizophrenia, in chronic brain syndrome to control hyperactivity, delusions, agitation	Use cautiously in the elderly. Dosage is reduced by 30% to 50% of normal adult dosage and increased gradually if needed. Reduce dosage to the lowest effective level. Drug metabolism is slowed, resulting in an increased risk for adverse reactions (eg, hypotension, arrhythmias, sedation). Immediately report any signs of tardive dyskinesia (abnormal rigidity and muscle movements such as sucking, smacking of the lips, protrusion of the tongue, and facial grimaces) because these symptoms are irreversible. Contraindicated in patients with severe cardiovascular disease, parkinsonism, liver damage Use cautiously in patients with diabetes mellitus, glaucoma, prostatic hypertrophy, peptic ulcer disease, or chronic respiratory disorders. Potential for overuse when used to control agitated or unruly behavior. These behaviors may respond better to other forms of treatment. Adverse reactions, such as inability to speak or swallow and decrease in ambulation, have been reported in the elderly.

Table 13-2. Special Considerations for the Elderly When Administering Commonly Prescribed Medications *continued*

Classification & Examples	Use	Implications for the Elderly

ANTIDEPRESSANTS
Tricyclic antidepressants
  imipramine (Tofranil)
Miscellaneous
  sertraline (Zoloft)
  bupropion
    (Wellbutrin)
Monoamine oxidase
    (MAO) inhibitors
  phenelzine (Nardil)
  tranylcypromide
    (Parnate)
	Depression	Give in small dosages initially, and gradually increase dosage over several weeks, if necessary.
		Use the smallest dose possible to achieve therapeutic results.
		Dosages are decreased by 30% to 50% to avoid serious adverse reactions.
		Increased risk of developing confusion anticholinergic effects, hypotension, and sedation
		Increased risk for hypertensive crisis when using MAO inhibitors.
		May cause paradoxical effect and deepen depression
		Contraindicated in patients with narrow-angle glaucoma (tricyclics).

ANTIPARKINSON DRUGS
levodopa (Larodopa)
carbidopa (Lodosyn)
bromocriptine (Parlodel)
amantadine (Symmetrel)
Anticholinergic drugs
  benztropine (Cogentin)
  trihexyphenidyl
    (Artane)
	Parkinsonism symptoms: tremors, bradykinesia, joint and muscular rigidity	Reduce dosage of amantadine.
		Amantadine is excreted unchanged in the kidney. If kidney function is decreased in older aldults, accumulation of the drug and toxicity can occur.
		Anticholinergic drugs cause dry mouth, tachycardia, urinary retention, blurred vision, confusion, and decreased sweating (leading to fever or heat stroke).
		With benztropine, there is an increased risk of mental confusion, agitation, hallucination, and psychotic symptoms in the elderly.

LAXATIVES
Stimulant
  bisacodyl (Dulcolax)
Stool softeners
  docusate sodium
    (Colace)
  psyllium preparations
    (Metamucil)
	Constipation	Tendency to overuse in older adults because constipation is a common complaint.
		Preferred methods to treat constipation are nondrug measures (ie, increase fluids, increase fiber in the diet, and exercise).
		Preferred laxative for the elderly is psyllium.
		Avoid stimulant laxatives.

ANTI-INFECTIVES
Penicillins
  penicillin G
    benzathine (Bicillin)
  cloxacillin (Tegopen)
  ampicillin (Omnipen)
Cephalosporins
  cephalexin (Keflex)
  cefaclor (Ceclor)
	Treatment and prophylaxis of susceptible bacterial infections	Penicillins are generally safe.
		Impaired renal function in older adults could cause hyperkalemia.
		In older adults, there is an increased risk of superinfection (eg, black, furry overgrowth on the tongue, vaginal itching or discharge, loose or foul-smelling stools).
		May cause renal impairment
		Reduce dosage if renal impairment occurs.
		Monitor CBC, BUN, creatinine, and liver function tests periodically during therapy.

CARDIAC GLYCOSIDES digoxin (Lanoxin)	Heart failure, atrial arrhythmias (eg, artrial fibrillation, atrial flutter)	Increased risk for adverse and toxic reactions May require reduced dosages if liver or kidney functions decreased Impaired renal function increases risk of cumulative effects and adverse reactions. Dosage reduced by 50% in patients with renal failure or when quinidine, nifedipine, or verapamil are given with digoxin. Withhold the drug and report immediately symptoms of toxicity such as abdominal pain, anorexia, nausea, vomiting, visual disturbances, bradycardia, or other arrhythmias.

Continued

Table 13-2. Special Considerations for the Elderly When Administering Commonly Prescribed Medications *continued*

Classification & Examples	Use	Implications for the Elderly
CARDIAC GLYCOSIDES *CONTINUED*		Withhold drug and notify the physician if any changes in rate, rhythm, or pulse occur. Auscultate lungs for rales or crackles at least every 8 hours. Check apical pulse before administration. If rate is >100 or <60, withhold drug and notify the physician.
DIURETICS chlorothiazide (Diuril) furosemide (Lasix) hydrochlorothiazide (HydroDIURIL, Esidrix) **POTASSIUM-SPARING DIURETICS** amiloride (Midamor) spironolactone (Aldactone)	Edema, heart failure	Older adults have an increased risk for adverse reactions, especially hypotension, dehydration, electrolyte imbalance (hypokalemia), and impaired mental functioning. Administer the smallest effective dose. Rapid diuresis may cause urinary incontinence. With potassium-sparing diuretics, elderly are at increased risk for hyperkalemia. Monitor blood pressure, intake and output, and daily weight. Assess feet, legs, and sacrum for edema daily. Patients taking cardiac glycosides with a diuretic are at increased risk for digitalis toxicity (except when taking potassium-sparing diuretics). Rapid effects may cause incontinence.
BETA-ADRENERGIC BLOCKING DRUGS labetalol, propranolol, timolol, atenolol, esmolol, metoprolol	Hypertension, angina pectoris, tachyarrhythmias, prevention of myocardial infarction	Elderly are more likely to experience orthostatic hypotension, hypoglycemia, thyroid dysfunction, depression, and arthritis. Take apical pulse before administration. Withhold medication and notify the physician if rate is <50 bpm or systolic B/P <90. Do not administer in patients with bradyarrhythmias, heart failure, or heart block.
NONSTEROIDAL ANTI-INFLAMMATORY DRUGS (NSAIDS) fenoprofen, ibuprofen, naproxen, phenylbutazone, aspirin, indomethacin, sulindac	Can potentiate effects of oral hypoglycemics and warfarin	Give with a full glass of water and with the body in the upright position. With aspirin, tinnitus occurs quickly with large doses. Increased risk of bleeding Should not be given to elderly with ulcer or with liver or kidney disease. Aspirin interferes with pain-relieving effects of other NSAIDs. Can be taken with food, milk, or antacids if gastrointestinal upset occurs. Report any bleeding, blurred vision, tinnitus, rashes, weight gain, easy bruising, or edema.

Polypharmacy

Another aspect of evaluation is observation of the number and types of drugs administered. The tendency for **polypharmacy** (ie, prescription and administration of many drugs) in the elderly is a common problem. The older adult takes an average of 5 to 12 medications per day. The potential for adverse reactions and drug-drug interactions increases dramatically with the increased number of medications

taken. The nurse is the member of the health care team who is most likely to identify the problem of polypharmacy. When the patient is taking a large number of drugs, the nurse may choose to refer this to the primary health care provider for further evaluation. Some of the drugs may be discontinued or the dosage reduced. However, patients with multiple health problems sometimes require large numbers of prescription drugs, and all of the drugs are necessary.

DISPLAY 13-1. Guide for Obtaining Important Drug Information

Question	Drug A	Drug B
What is the name of the drug?		
Why am I taking it? What's it for?		
How often should I take it?		
How long must I take it?		
Will there be side effects? What are they?		
Are there any side effects I should report to the doctor immediately?		
Is there anything special I should know about in taking this drug? (For example, take with meals; other drugs I shouldn't take with it; driving restrictions.)		

From Department of Health and Human Services, Publication no. (ADM)90-705. Distributed by the National Clearinghouse for Alcohol and Drug Information, P.O. Box 2345, Rockville, MD 20852, 1-800-729-6686 or 1-800-SAY-NO-TO(DRUGS).

HELPING OLDER ADULTS ADMINISTER THEIR OWN MEDICATION

Most older adults are capable of managing their health care with only minimal assistance from family and friends. Generally, only those who are hospitalized, living in nursing facilities, or incapacitated need assistance. When the older adult is able to manage the medication regimen, the role of the nurse is that of educator to provide information about the specific medications such as how and when to administer the drug, adverse reactions, and any special instructions.

Older adults sometimes have trouble keeping track of what drug to take and when to take it or remembering if they took a drug or not. Because elderly people usually take more medications than individuals in the general population, they are at greater risk for problems with administration. Medication errors are common among older adults. Potential errors include taking drugs at the wrong times, omitting certain prescribed drugs, and taking drugs without understanding why they are prescribed. The elderly who are at increased risk for errors in self-medication are those who are confused, less educated, live alone, take many drugs, or have visual disturbances.

When an older adult is prescribed a medication, information is provided about the name of the drug, why the drug is prescribed, how the drug is taken, what reactions they should expect, and what reactions should they report. Sometimes, the nurse gives the necessary information, but the patient does not fully understand. The patient may be anxious, too

embarrassed to ask questions, or feel that the nurse does not have time to answer questions. There may be an uncertainty about what questions to ask. Nurses must be aware that patients may have feelings of uncertainty and take measures to ensure that the information about medications is thoroughly understood.

Encourage the older adult to prepare a written list of all medications she is taking, including all prescription drugs and OTC (eg, laxatives, antacids, aspirin) drugs. The amount and times these drugs are taken and the existence of allergies to drugs or foods are included. Instruct the person to keep a list of questions to ask and things to tell the health care provider at the next appointment. Explain that one drug could decrease or increase the effect of another or that the combination of two drugs may cause dangerous reactions. Display 13-1 gives an example of a chart that can be given to the older adult to use as a guide for the information needed about each drug. This information is filled out every time a new medication is prescribed and kept in a convenient place at home. Emphasize that it is important to write the information about the drugs down so they do not forget.

Visual Disturbances

Visual disturbances are of special concern for the elderly living alone and requiring several medications at different times of the day. Older adults are often prescribed several prescription drugs. In addition to prescription drugs, individuals older than 65 years take approximately 40% of the OTC drugs.

DISPLAY 13-2. Guidelines for Medication Usage for the Visually Impaired

1. Carefully evaluate the patient's capacity to follow the medication instructions accurately. Can the patient read the instructions? Can he open the drug container? Can the patient differentiate one drug from another? If there is a problem, assess the patient's needs, and find out what help is available.
2. Position medications in the client's visual field.
   a. Simplify the visual field.
   b. Keep the area clean of clutter.
3. Maintain adequate illumination in the drug preparation area.
   a. Try different rooms with different lamps.
   b. Light should be placed on the side of the eye capable of best near vision.
4. If needed, teach the patient to use an optical device such as a magnifying glass.
5. Improve signage.
   a. Large print directions, enlarge on a photocopier or computer
   b. Color coding
   c. Multiple colored bands around bottles
   d. Colored caps or a piece of sandpaper on the cap to identify a certain drug
   e. Color contrast (Typically there is a diminished ability to differentiate between pastel colors or dark tones. Reds and yellows can be discrimi-

nated most readily. Place dark equipment on a white background and vice versa.)
6. Instruct the patient in the safe and proper instillation of eye drops and ointment, a critical factor in the treatment of ocular disease. Wash hands thoroughly, and wipe eye clean with a moist tissue or cotton ball before instilling the medication. Patient should be warned not to touch the dropper tip to any surface because this may contaminate the solution.
7. Listen to the patient. The complaints may be caused by a drug the patient is taking. Is the syncope caused by an ophthalmic beta-blocker preparation, such as timolol eye drops used in the treatment of glaucoma? Are topical beta-blocking agents being added to systemic beta blockers, causing episodes of bradycardia and hypotension? Epinephrine drops may exacerbate hypertension.
8. Periodically assess the patient's ability to take their drugs. Changes in visual acuity occur over time.
9. Investigate the possibility of referring your patient to a low vision specialist.
10. Remind patients to discard any obsolete or outdated medicines.
    Remember, your goal is to keep patients at home; therefore, if possible, observe patients in their home environment.

From Lee, M. (1996). Drugs and the elderly: Do you know the risks? *American Journal of Nursing, 96 (7)*, 30.

Of the more than 3 million older adults who are visually impaired, at least 1 million are legally blind. These individuals may have difficulty reading drug labels, physician's printed instructions, or the printed material given by the pharmacist. Many of these individuals are living at home and many live alone. The safe administration of medication to those with visual impairment is a significant problem. Display 13-2 provides guidelines for medication usage for the visually impaired.

Monitoring Systems for Self-Administration

Older adults have three major problems when self-administering drugs: knowing which drugs are prescribed, knowing at what times the various drugs are to be taken, and remembering whether a drug has been taken.

Many older adults take several drugs on a regular basis. If several drugs are taken each day and at different times it is difficult to remember whether or not a drug was taken. Several systems assist the elderly in taking medications correctly. The first system is a chart listing the prescribed medications (Display 13-3). The chart provides space for the names of each drug and what the drug is for, what the drug looks like, directions for taking the drug, and the specific times the drug is taken. Suggest that the chart be posted in a convenient place for reference.

An alternate system is a check-off chart (Display 13-4). This is particularly appropriate to keep track of when a drug should be taken and to check off after the drug has been taken. To use the chart, write the name of the drug and any special directions needed for administration. Under the days of the week, write in the times to take the drug each day. Every time a drug is taken, cross out that time.

Some older adults use a color coding system to quickly identify their medications. This may be used in combination with the other systems mentioned previously. A color coding system is good for elderly patients who have problems reading the fine print of the labels on prescription containers. The chart and the medication container are color coded. Gummed labels in several colors are needed. After the chart listing all the drugs being taken is completed, place a different color on the label of each container. On the chart place the gummed color tag that matches the color on the medication container for each drug listed. After the

DISPLAY 13-3. Patient Drug Monitoring System

Name of Drug and What It Is For	Color/Shape	Directions and Cautions	Times

From Department of Health and Human Services, Publication no. (ADM)90-705. Distributed by the National Clearinghouse for Alcohol and Drug Information, P.O. Box 2345, Rockville, MD 20852, 1-800-729-6686 or 1-800-SAY-NO-TO(DRUGS).

color coding is completed, the label on the container does not need to be read each time the drug is taken. The chart can be used instead. The patient can determine at a glance what medication to take by looking at the chart and matching the color with the color on the medication container.

Colors should be visibly different so that no mistakes are made. When prescriptions are refilled, the new bottle must be coded with the correct color. The lens of the eye yellows with age, causing difficulty in distinguishing colors. The colors most often causing difficulty are blue and green. When using gummed-label color coding for medication containers, be certain that the colors are distinguishable by the older adult. Have them demonstrate the ability to identify and match these colors. An alternate method for labeling the containers if color vision is a problem is to use large letters of the alphabet or numbers as codes.

The last system is a daily or weekly container (Fig. 13-1). Some pharmaceutical companies produce small medication holders with a different compartment for each day of the week. These are useful for daily medications or drugs that are to be taken every other day or in different dosages on different days. When using any container, be certain to keep it out of the reach of children. Some medications lose their strength when exposed to air, and others

DISPLAY 13-4. Self-Monitoring Check-Off Chart

Name of Drug/Directions	Sun	Mon	Tue	Wed	Thu	Fri	Sat

Name of Drug/Directions	Sun	Mon	Tue	Wed	Thu	Fri	Sat
Drug A—3 times/day	8̶ 12̶ 8̶	8̶ 12̶ 8̶	8̶ 12̶ 5	8 12 5	8 12 5	8 12 5	8 12 5
Drug B—once a day in AM	8̶	8̶	8̶	8	8	8	8
Drug C—3 times/day	8̶ 12̶ 8̶	8̶ 12̶ 8̶	8̶ 12̶ 5	8 12 5	8 12 5	8 12 5	8 12 5

From Department of Health and Human Services, Publication no. (ADM)90-705. Distributed by the National Clearinghouse for Alcohol and Drug Information, P.O. Box 2345, Rockville, MD 20852, 1-800-729-6686 or 1-800-SAY-NO-TO(DRUGS).

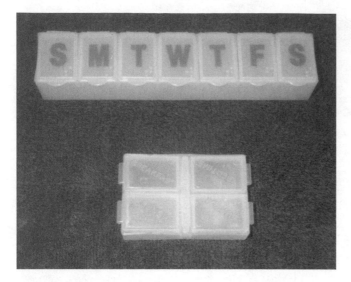

FIGURE 13-1. Examples of containers used to assist in self-medication administration. The top container is labeled for the 7 days of the week, while the bottom container is used for daily medicaions and is labeled "breakfast, lunch, supper, and bedtime."

must be refrigerated. Be certain that drugs will not deteriorate or lose potency if a daily or weekly medication container is used.

General Guidelines for Patient and Family Teaching

When taking medications at home, the patient and family members are instructed to follow these general guidelines:

Inform all health care providers about all the medicines you are taking and any allergies you have to any drug.

Make certain that you understand all instructions before using a new drug.

Take medications exactly as prescribed. Do not take more or less than the prescribed amount of any drug.

Request non–child-proof containers if you have difficulty opening medication containers because of arthritis or other medical conditions.

Use a system for keeping track of what drugs you are supposed to take and what drugs you have taken each day.

If a dose is missed, take it as soon as possible. If it is almost time for the next dose, skip the missed dose. Do not take two doses at once.

Keep drugs in airtight containers, and store them properly.

Keep a record of all allergies and the symptoms you experienced with the allergies.

Do not stop taking a drug without checking with your physician, even if you feel better.

Do not mix alcohol with any medication without your doctor's approval.

Do not take any drug prescribed for someone else or give your prescription to someone else.

Throw out old or expired medicine. Check expiratory dates and throw any leftover drug away when the course of therapy is completed.

Know what reactions to report for each drug you are taking.

Assume any new symptom that develops after starting a new drug may be caused by the drug. Report any unusual or unexpected effects.

Know the telephone numbers of your physician, nurse practitioner, and pharmacist in case you have questions concerning your medications.

NONCOMPLIANCE WITH THE MEDICATION REGIMEN

Noncompliance with the medication regimen is a potential problem in the older adult. There are many reasons the drug therapy regimen is not followed:

There may be too many medications for the elderly person to keep up with.

Adverse reactions may be too bothersome.

The regimens are complicated, or doses are required several times each day.

The medications are too expensive.

There may be a lack of understanding of rationale or purpose of the therapeutic regimen.

The entire medication dosage regimen may need to be reviewed by the primary heath care provider with the intent to discontinue some of the medications if possible. For example, if a diuretic must be taken, perhaps the potassium supplement can be discontinued if the patient will eat foods high in potassium on a daily basis. Nursing interventions are used instead of the drug therapy if possible. For example, to induce sleep, back rubs, a relaxing atmosphere, warm milk, and stress reductions techniques may prove just as effective as medication. For complicated drug regimens, teach patients to use the monitoring methods suggested in the previous sections.

If a patient lives on a fixed income or has financial problems, drugs may become an expendable item within the budget. Suggest the use of generic drugs rather than brand names or contact the social services department. To combat a lack of understanding of the therapeutic regimen, give a thorough explanation of the drug regimen, have them write the dosage regimen and answer the questions listed on Table 13-2. Explain the importance of the drug therapy and why it is essential. Allow ample time for questions and feedback.

Decreased ability to hear may cause problems with patient teaching and compliance. The older adult may not hear the instructions, or sounds may be muffled, and the person may not fully understand the instructions. Admitting to a hearing problem is sometimes difficult, and the older adult may not ask for clarification. Have the person repeat the instructions in his own words, and provide written information as well. Having a family member present also increases the likelihood of compliance, because someone besides the patient receives the instructions.

CRITICAL THINKING EXERCISES

1. Ms. Carter, age 92, lives at home alone. She manages well with the help of a home health aid three times each week to help her with self-care and to do light house work and shopping. Ms. Carter's vision is deteriorating, and you are concerned that she will not be able to take her medications safely. She is taking the following oral medications: Sinemet, 10/100 tid; Cardene SR (nicardipine) 30 mg tid; and Prilosec (omeprazole), 20 mg daily. What assessment would be the most important to make? What suggestions would you make to Ms. Carter to assist her in taking her medications safely?

2. Ms. Walters, age 77, was recently prescribed 2 mg of haloperidol (Haldol) three times a day. After several doses, Ms. Walters begins to make sucking and smacking movements with her mouth. Would you suspect a problem at this time? If yes, what additional assessments would you make? What do you suspect is causing Ms. Walters' facial movements? What action would you take first?

3. Mr. Watson is complaining of constipation. You note in the chart that he had a bowel movement 2 days ago. What assessments would you make concerning this complaint? What action, if any, would you take?

REFERENCES AND SUGGESTED READING

Berthelot, K. (1999). Collaborative home practice: Nursing and occupational therapy ensure appropriate medication administration. *Home Healthcare, 17 (1),* 45.

Lee, M. (1996). Drugs and the elderly: Do you know the risks? *American Journal of Nursing, 96 (7),* 25–31.

Planchock, N.Y., & Slay, L.E. (1996). Pharmacokinetic and pharmacodynamic monitoring of the elderly in critical care. *Critical Care Nursing Clinics of North America, 8 (1),* 79–89.

Salom, I.L., & Davis, K. (1995). Prescribing for older patients: How to avoid toxic drug reactions. *Geriatrics, 50 (10),* 37–43.

Roach, S., & Scherer, J. (2000). *Introductory clinical pharmacology.* Philadelphia: Lippincott Williams & Wilkins.

Walker. M., & Foreman, M. (1999). Medication safety: A protocol for nursing action. *Geriatric Nursing, 20 (1),* 34–39.

CHAPTER 14

Managing Common Physiologic Problems

CHAPTER OUTLINE

KEY TERMS
CHAPTER OBJECTIVES
URINARY INCONTINENCE
SLEEP DISTURBANCES
PAIN
ACUTE CONFUSION
FALLS
UNDERNUTRITION
CRITICAL THINKING EXERCISES
REFERENCES AND SUGGESTED READING

KEY TERMS

acute pain
chronic pain
chronic insomnia
confusion
delirium
dementia
endorphins
enkephalins
functional incontinence
Kegel exercises
pain
postfall syndrome
reality orientation
rebound insomnia
reflux incontinence
residual volume
stress incontinence
total incontinence
transient insomnia
urge incontinence
urinary incontinence

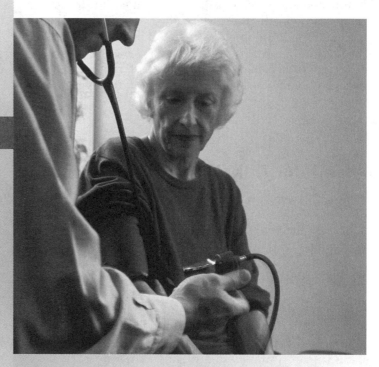

CHAPTER OBJECTIVES

At the completion of this chapter, the student will be able to

- Identify common physiologic problems that occur with aging

- Discuss the physiologic changes that contribute to urinary incontinence, sleep disturbances, pain, acute confusion, falls, undernutrition, and dehydration in the older adult

- Discuss the distinguishing characteristics of delirium, dementia, and depression

- Discuss important aspects of caring for patients with urinary incontinence, sleep disturbances, pain, acute confusion, undernutrition, and dehydration

- Identify important aspects of care in patients who are at risk for falling

Although older adults cannot be grouped together and stereotyped as all having the same needs or problems, certain physiologic problems occur more often in the older population. Although this chapter by no means covers all problems common to the older adult, it does explore some of the more common physiologic problems that occur with aging such as urinary incontinence, sleep disturbances, pain, acute confusion, nutritional deficits, falls, and dehydration.

URINARY INCONTINENCE

Urinary incontinence is the inability to control excretion of urine from the bladder. Although urinary incontinence is not a natural consequence of aging, a significant number of older adults face this problem. Approximately 1 in 10 people who are 65 years of age or older have some form of incontinence ranging from mild to severe. Urinary incontinence affects up to 50% of older adults in nursing homes, 30% of those in acute care settings (eg, hospitals), and 15% to 30% of elders in the community. Psychological effects of urinary incontinence include social isolation, embarrassment, and depression. Physical problems such as perineal rash, decubitus ulcer, urinary tract infections, falls, and fractures can occur as a result of urinary incontinence. It is a significant and common health problem among the elderly. Too often, however, it is ignored or dismissed as a normal consequence of aging and not adequately treated. Regardless of the cause, urinary incontinence is treatable and often curable.

Physiologic Changes That Affect Continence

Age-related changes occur in the lower urinary tract of men and women. With age, bladder capacity decreases, and the bladder is able to hold a smaller amount of urine. Decreased muscle tone reduces the ability to postpone voiding. A weakness in the urethral sphincter causes urine to leak. Certain drugs such as beta blockers may worsen incontinence because they act to relax the smooth muscles of the urinary sphincter. **Residual volume,** the amount of urine remaining in the bladder after voiding, increases from a normal value of about 50 mL to as much as 100 mL. There also appears to be a delayed perception to the sensation of needing to void.

The pattern of urination also changes with age. Younger people excrete most of their urine in the waking hours, and many older adults tend to excrete much of their urine during the night. For many, this results in at least one or two episodes of nocturia (ie, nighttime voiding) each night. None of these age-related changes cause incontinence. They do, along with disease processes or medication, increase the risk of the older adult becoming incontinent.

Types of Urinary Incontinence

Incontinence is classified according to duration of symptoms, the presence of specific symptoms, or by physiologic abnormalities. Some episodes of incontinence are of recent onset and transient, but in others, episodes of incontinence are chronic. Some individuals cannot control the external urethral sphincter, causing a loss of urine that may be continual or intermittent. There are five basic types of urinary incontinence common in the older adult: functional, urge, stress, reflux, and total incontinence.

Functional incontinence occurs as a result of mobility impairment, cognitive changes, or environmental barriers. With functional incontinence, the urge to urinate is strong, but the individual is unable to reach the toileting facilities before urine is excreted. **Urge incontinence** is the inability to voluntarily hold the urine after feeling a strong urge to void. Urge incontinence can be caused by bladder contractions that occur as a result of a disease process such as a urinary tract infection. **Stress incontinence** is a leakage of urine resulting from weakened perineal muscles combined with increased intra-abdominal pressure. For example, in persons with weakened perineal muscles, coughing, sneezing, laughing, or even picking up a bag of groceries can result in leakage of urine. **Reflux incontinence,** also called neurogenic bladder, is the type of incontinence associated with a spinal cord injury causing a lack of awareness of bladder fullness and involuntary urination. **Total incontinence** is total uncontrolled and continuous loss of urine due to multiple causes such as urinary tract infection, detrusor instability, or neurogenic impairment.

Using the Nursing Process to Manage Urinary Incontinence

Assessment
In assessing urinary incontinence, it is necessary to obtain an accurate voiding pattern. The chart on Display 14-1 provides an excellent method for evaluating voiding patterns and incontinent episodes. Compare the amount of urine excreted with the amount

DISPLAY 14-1. Voiding and Incontinence Record

INSTRUCTIONS: EACH TIME THE PATIENT IS CHECKED:
1) Mark one of the circles in the BLADDER section at the hour closest to the time the patient is checked.
2) Make an X in the BOWEL section if the patient has had an incontinent or normal bowel movement.

⌀ = Incontinent, small amount   ⌀ = Dry   X = Incontinence BOWEL
● = Incontinent, large amount   Δ = Voided correctly   X = Normal BOWEL

PATIENT NAME _____ ROOM # _____ DATE _____

| | **BLADDER** | | | | **BOWEL** | | | |
	INCONTINENCE OF URINE	DRY	VOIDED CORRECTLY	INCONTINENCE X	NORMAL X	INITIALS	COMMENTS
12 am	• ●	○	Δ cc ___				
1	• ●	○	Δ cc ___				
2	• ●	○	Δ cc ___				
3	• ●	○	Δ cc ___				
4	• ●	○	Δ cc ___				
5	• ●	○	Δ cc ___				
6	• ●	○	Δ cc ___				
7	• ●	○	Δ cc ___				
8	• ●	○	Δ cc ___				
9	• ●	○	Δ cc ___				
10	• ●	○	Δ cc ___				
11	• ●	○	Δ cc ___				
12 pm	• ●	○	Δ cc ___				
1	• ●	○	Δ cc ___				
2	• ●	○	Δ cc ___				
3	• ●	○	Δ cc ___				
4	• ●	○	Δ cc ___				
5	• ●	○	Δ cc ___				
6	• ●	○	Δ cc ___				
7	• ●	○	Δ cc ___				
8	• ●	○	Δ cc ___				
9	• ●	○	Δ cc ___				
10	• ●	○	Δ cc ___				
11	• ●	○	Δ cc ___				
TOTALS:							

From Urinary Incontinence Guideline Panel. *Incontinence in adults: Clinical practice guideline.* AHCPR Pub. No. 92-0038, Rockville, MD: Agency for Health Care Policy and Research, Public Health Service, US Department of Health and Human Services, March 1992.

of fluid taken in. Ask the individual to discuss voiding patterns. Display 14-2 identifies questions that may be helpful in determining the type of incontinent episodes.

Underlying pathology such as delirium or infection can also contribute to incontinence. Incontinence associated with delirium usually reverses when the delirium is treated. The presence of a urinary tract infection in the elderly predisposes the elderly to incontinence.

NURSING ALERT

Always assess mobility and mental status in the older adult with incontinence. The nurse must determine whether the patient is alert and able to understand a treatment plan or where the bathroom is located. A patient who cannot ambulate well enough to get to the toilet or one who is so confused that he or she does not know where the toilet is located may develop functional incontinence.

- Do you experience the need to void more frequently than usual?
- Do you have to get up in the night to void?
- How often do you void during the day?
- Can you hold urine in the bladder after you feel the urge to void?
- Do you have a constant flow of urine, flow of urine at unpredictable times, or dribbling of urine?
- Can you hold your urine when you cough or sneeze?
- After you have the urge to void, can you get to the toilet in time?
- Do you void in small amounts?

Assess the medication regimen. Certain medications can affect urinary excretion. For example, diuretics cause increased urine volume, sedatives alter sensitivity to bladder cues, and anticholinergic agents cause urinary retention. Table 14-1 lists drugs that affect continence.

Nursing Diagnosis

The following nursing diagnosis may be used when a patient is incontinent: Altered Elimination Patterns related to urinary incontinence. Other nursing diagnoses may be appropriate for individual patients with specific problems.

Planning and Implementation

After identifying the type of incontinence, a care plan is developed. There are numerous approaches to control urinary incontinence. Perhaps the most important component in implementation is the cooperation of the patient and the patient's determination to regain control. Involving the patient and family in devising an individualized care plan can be the difference in the success or failure of regaining continence. Display 14-3 identified general nursing interventions to use in caring for a patient with urinary incontinence.

Methods to Promote Urinary Continence

Specific methods used to promote continence include Kegel exercises, bladder training, increased environment access, and habit training. Indwelling catheters are not recommended. Short-term use may be necessary during the treatment of severe skin breakdown resulting from the acidity of the urine.

Kegel Exercises. Kegel exercises are exercises that strengthen the pelvic floor muscles. It is the pelvic floor muscles that are tightened to keep urine from escaping or to hold back a bowel movement. These

TABLE 14-1. **Drugs That Affect Continence**

Medication	Potential Effect
Alcohol	Urinary frequency, sedation, or delirium leading to decreased mobility, urgency
Anticholinergics	Urinary retention
Antihypertensives	Bladder outlet relaxation
Antipsychotics	Sedation leading to decreased mobility, urinary retention
Antidepressants	Constipation, fecal impaction, or sedation leading to decreased mobility, urinary retention
Calcium channel blockers	Urinary retention, frequency
Diuretics	Urinary frequency, urgency
Narcotics	Constipation, bladder relaxation, or sedation leading to decreased mobility, urinary retention
Sedatives/hypnotics	Sedation leading to decreased mobility, urinary sphincter relaxation

From Catanzaro, J. (1996). Managing Incontinence: An Update: *RN, 56* (10), 44.

DISPLAY 14-3. **Nursing Interventions for a Patient with Urinary Incontinence.**

- Provide frequent opportunities for voiding (at least every 2 hours).
- Assist the patient to the bathroom or place a bedpan or bedside commode within easy reach of the patient.
- Keep a record of bladder function (see Display 14-1).
- Check frequently for wetting and for redness or excoriation in the perineal area.
- Clean skin in perineal area thoroughly after each incontinent episode.
- Protective barriers such as ointment may be applied to skin if constant leakage occurs.
- Keep an intake and output record. Do not limit fluids. Keep intake to approximately 2,000 mL/day.
- Consume most of the daily fluid before evening to minimize nocturia.
- Monitor for and report any signs of urinary infection such as discomfort on urination, scant or cloudy urination, or elevated temperature. However, temperature elevation is not always a good indicator of infection in the elderly. A serious infection can develop without significant temperature elevation.
- Encourage the retention of urine for at least 2 hours, if possible.
- Use normal posture for voiding (eg, allow men to stand), if possible.

exercises are particularly important for women who experience stress incontinence. To increase control stopping and starting the steam during urination, these exercises should be practiced.

PATIENT TEACHING AID

Instructions for teaching Kegel exercises:
• **The purpose for performing the exercise is to strengthen the pelvic floor muscles.**
• **Identify the pelvic floor muscles.**
• **Squeeze the pelvic floor muscles 6 to 10 times for 5 to 10 seconds. This tightening and relaxing is done 4 to 6 times per day. The patient should work up to 20 repetitions (or tightening and relaxing) at each session, if possible.**
• **Improvement should be observed in 2 to 4 weeks if the exercises are performed consistently each day.**

Bladder Training. Bladder training is used to aid in restoring normal urination. It is effective with older adults who are alert and experience urge incontinence. Display 14-4 identifies nursing interventions for a bladder training program.

Increased Environmental Access. Creating an environment with easier access is helpful for older adults with functional incontinence. The environment can be modified to promote ease in toileting, such as relocating furniture, obtaining a portable toilet, or installing an elevated toilet seat or grab rails in the bathroom. A portable toilet placed at a convenient location may provide easier access. Velcro fasteners can replace buttons and hooks on the patient's clothing, if this is a problem. It is important to provide easy access to toileting even with decreased mental status. A trend toward incontinence in older patients can be reversed by encouraging them to dress, be up and about, and offering assistance with toileting.

Habit Training. Habit training is a method of strict adherence to a toileting schedule to keep a patient dry. A confused person with stress, urge, or functional incontinence may benefit from habit training. This system is based on maintaining consistency and praising the person for continence. The nurse or caregiver takes the person to the toilet at scheduled times. Methods to encourage voiding may be used such as running water from a faucet, placing a hand in warm water, suprapubic tapping, or stroking the inner thigh. Positive feedback and praise is given when voiding occurs at the correct times. The nurse expresses no negative response when incontinent episodes occur.

Total Incontinence. External catheters or condom catheters are useful for male patients with total incontinence. They are nonintrusive and fairly easy

---

DISPLAY 14-4. Nursing Interventions for a Bladder Training Program

• Explain the procedure to the patient and enlist her cooperation.
• Allow the patient to assist with record keeping and in planning scheduled voidings.
• Analyze data from voiding pattern record (see Display 14-1) to develop a toileting schedule.
• Set specific times to try to void.
• Maintain privacy during toileting sessions.
• Allow no more than 1.5 to 2 hours between scheduled voiding sessions.
• Record continent and incontinent episodes and results of scheduled toileting.
• Encourage the patient to try to hold urine until scheduled toileting time.
• Increase time between scheduled toileting as control and bladder capacity increases.

---

to manage. The appropriate size is selected, and the patient or caregiver can be taught to apply the condom and provide daily skin care to reduce the risk of infection. Incontinence pads (ie, diapers) are used only as a last resort. Their use is discouraged because of the negative effect on the self-esteem of adults. If used, incontinence pads are changed promptly to prevent skin breakdown. When changing, the skin is cleaned and inspected, and a moisture barrier is applied for protection.

Catheter Care. Sometimes, a catheter is used when the patient or resident is totally incontinent and all other methods of bladder training have failed. These individuals are at increased risk for urinary tract infection. The following actions by the nurse can minimize the risk for infection:

Use the smallest catheter size possible (14 or 16 French).
Provide routine catheter and meatal care once each day.
Keep catheters in place for as short a time as possible.

Ointments or lubricating agents are not recommended for use around the meatus. The catheter is changed only when it is no longer patent to reduce the chance of introducing bacteria into the bladder.

Before discontinuing the catheter, a bladder rehabilitation program may be initiated to encourage the return of normal bladder functioning. The physician usually orders a clamp and release system before the removal of the catheter to help restore normal functioning. With this type of system, the catheter is clamped for a specified period and then released for a short time (usually 15 to 20 minutes) to empty the bladder. Initially, the catheter is clamped for 30 minutes at a time or until the patient complains of feelings of fullness or slight cramping. The timeframe for clamping the catheter is gradually increased as tolerance increases until the patient is able to tolerate having the catheter clamped for 2 hours.

If the patient is unconscious or unable to communicate discomfort when the catheter is clamped, the nurse must be alert for cues such as restlessness or agitation that may indicate discomfort from a full bladder. For unconscious patients, begin the clamping routine at 30 minutes, and gradually increase the time the catheter is clamped. After the catheter is removed, continue with a bladder training program as discussed previously.

Evaluation and Expected Outcomes
Using the methods previously described can effect certain outcomes:

No episodes of incontinence occur.
Independent toileting is achieved.

SLEEP DISTURBANCES

Many older adults complain of sleep pattern disturbances. There is no clear indication about whether these disturbances are a part of the aging process or simply normal individual differences. Sleep disturbances are associated with depression, grief, anxiety, and losses that occur with aging.

Environmental factors influence sleep patterns. For example, the noises and activity of shift changes in nursing homes and hospitals affect sleeping in these facilities. When patients are awakened throughout the night for periodic checks, vital signs, or medication administration these individuals complain about sleep difficulties. Comfort factors such as uncomfortable beds or room temperatures that are too hot or too cold also affect sleep.

Two types of sleep disturbances occur in the older adult: transient insomnia and chronic insomnia. **Transient insomnia** is the inability to sleep as the result of a stressful situation such as hospitalization, grief, or a significant loss. Transient insomnia is typically self-limiting and resolves in 5 to 7 days. No treatment is normally required. If sedatives are used, the physician prescribes the drug for no more than 2 to 3 days and at the lowest effective dosage. **Chronic insomnia** is disturbance in sleep patterns for longer than 1 month. This type of insomnia can cause symptoms such as anxiety, irritability, fatigue, and impaired mental functioning. Habitual use of a sedative or hypnotic complicates the problem because adverse reactions of the drug can mimic the sleep disorder.

Physiologic Changes That Affect Sleep

Older adults are less tolerant to shifts of the sleep–wake cycle (eg, jet lag). Sleep patterns of older adults change, although older adults need as much sleep as their younger counterparts. In some cases, sleep needs increase with age. Although many older adults report poor nighttime sleep, the daytime napping pattern of many older adults redistributes sleep throughout a 24-hour timeframe. This seems to compensate for nighttime sleep disturbances. The quality of nighttime sleep diminishes, and sleep may be 70% to 80% less effective than in younger adults.

With age, there are changes in the stages of sleep. Normal sleep progresses through four stages. Stage 1 is the lightest level of sleep, from which a person can easily be awakened. Older adults spend more time in the lighter stages of sleep (stages 1 and 2), resulting in more nighttime sleep disturbances. Stages 3 and 4 are the deeper levels of sleep. The older adult spends substantially less time in stages 3 and 4. Some studies indicate that in extreme old age stages 3 and 4 may disappear completely.

Sleep is divided into rapid eye movement (REM) sleep and non–rapid eye movement (NREM) sleep. Throughout the sleep cycle, NREM sleep alternates with REM sleep. REM sleep is characterized by rapid eye movements that can be observed though closed eyelids and by complete relaxation of the lower jaw. REM sleep occurs in several cycles during a normal sleeping pattern. Five or six cycles of NREM sleep are followed by REM sleep. Most dreams occur during REM sleep. Some studies indicate that there is a reduction in the amount of REM sleep with age. Other studies indicate that REM sleep remains relatively constant throughout the life cycle.

Assessing Sleep Patterns

When assessing sleep pattern disturbances, determine normal sleep patterns. Question the older adult for the presence of any physical symptom that disturbs sleep (eg, dyspnea, chest pain, anxiety). Obtain a history of the medication regimen. Many drugs interfere with sleep, particularly antianxiety agents or narcotics. Question family members or nursing assistants about sleep patterns. Residents in nursing homes or hospitals sometimes report insomnia, but direct observation during the night by the nurse indicates that they are sleeping. Display 14-5 identifies questions to use when assessing sleep patterns.

> ## DISPLAY 14-5. Questions to Ask the Patient When Assessing Sleep Patterns
>
> - Describe your sleeping habits.
> - How would you describe your sleeping patterns over the last several years?
> - What time do you go to sleep? Get up?
> - Do you experience any problems in staying asleep?
> - Rate your quality of sleep.
> - How does the environment affect your sleep?
> - Do you drink caffeine-containing beverages in the evening?
> - Do you have a nighttime ritual before going to sleep?

Caring for a Patient With a Sleep Pattern Disturbance

After a careful assessment, an individualized plan of care is developed. Input from the patient is helpful to determine ways to normalize sleep patterns. Avoid the use of sedatives, hypnotics, or over-the-counter sleeping aids. These drugs can cause **rebound insomnia,** an increase in insomnia that occurs as an abrupt withdrawal of the drug. If the individual is taking any drug to assist in sleeping, it is necessary to taper the drug dosage slowly to decrease the potential for rebound insomnia. Display 14-6 identifies nursing interventions that may be included in a care plan to promote sleep.

In most nursing homes, nursing assistants make rounds every hour to observe immobile residents. If the resident is found awake, the nursing assistant can perform the necessary tasks such as repositioning and incontinence care. However, if the resident is asleep, no action may be taken on that hourly round. If the resident remains asleep through three consecutive rounds, the resident must be awakened for care.

PAIN

Because of the high incidence of chronic disease in the elderly, pain often becomes a constant companion. Many older adults feel that with age pain is inevitable and must be endured. Because of this misconception, there is often an underreporting of pain by the elderly. Pain contributes to depression, anxiety, decreased functional ability, and decreased socialization. The occurrence of pain in nursing homes is as high as 85%. Chronic conditions such

> ## DISPLAY 14-6. Nursing Interventions That Promote Sleep
>
> - Inform the patient of normal sleep-related changes. For example, tell the patient that sleep can be less restful at age 70 than it was at age 30 without indicating a serious medical problem.
> - Modify the environment to provide a more restful atmosphere.
> - Advise the patient to avoid daytime naps.
> - Advise the patient not to eat caffeine-containing foods after 5 PM.
> - Instruct the patient to develop a bedtime ritual. Do not perform activities other than sleeping and sex in the bedroom.
> - Advise the patient to avoid the use of alcohol, because this drug can cause sleep disturbances.
> - A bedtime snack of warm milk may be beneficial for some. (Tryptophan, a natural sedative, is found in milk.)
> - Encourage the use of relaxation strategies such as back rubs, meditation, visualization, music, a bedtime snack, or reading.
> - Have a set sleep routine. Go to bed at the same time, follow the same nighttime routine, and awaken at approximately the same time each day.
> - Use sedatives or hypnotics only as a last resort and for no more than 2 to 3 days.
> - Plan to have minimal or no (if possible) interruption of sleep at night by nursing home or hospital staff.
> - Exercise regularly, preferably in the morning or early evening, if mobility permits.

as arthritis, gout, rheumatism, peripheral vascular disease, and cardiovascular disorders predispose the elderly to pain. The presence of pain can contribute to a decline in functional ability of an older person.

Pain can be defined as a subjective experience that causes moderate to extreme discomfort. Pain can be categorized as acute or chronic. **Acute pain** is moderate to severe discomfort of sudden onset. Immediate treatment is necessary to relieve acute pain. **Chronic pain** is moderate to extreme discomfort of more than 6 months' duration and is more difficult to manage. The causes of pain are complex, particularly in the elderly.

Physiologic Aspects of Pain

The gate control theory of pain offers an explanation of the role of the nervous system in response to pain. The gate control theory posits that pain signals reach a specific group of nerve cells that form a "pain center." As excitement or stimulation of this pain center reaches a certain level, a theoretical gate opens, allowing the pain signals to stimulate higher centers of the brain and spinal cord.

The body has an internal system that helps to control pain. This internal system involves the production of morphine-like substances called endorphins and enkephalins. **Endorphins** are naturally occurring chemicals that inhibit the transmission of pain impulses. These morphine-like chemicals are found in the nerve cells of the brain, spinal cord, and gastrointestinal tract. **Enkephalins** are a type of endorphins found in the brain and spinal cord that appear to be more potent and longer lasting than morphine. All endorphins attach to opiate receptors, inhibiting the release of the neurotransmitter and blocking the transmission of a painful stimulus. Stress and physical activity are two factors that naturally increase the levels of endorphins, raising the pain threshold.

Elderly adults appear to have similar pain tolerances to that of younger adults. Some authorities believe that, at least in some older adults, pain tolerance increases with age. For others, particularly women, there may be a decrease in pain tolerance. Because pain is a subjective symptom, it is important not to make any assumptions about pain and the elderly. The nurse should instead carefully assess and document any indication of pain.

Assessment of Pain

The older adult may not report pain as readily as a younger adult. The older adult may have lived with chronic pain and come to believe that it is a normal consequence of aging, or the older adult may not report pain for fear of being labeled as cranky, a complainer, or a hypochondriac. During the assessment, ask the person what methods are used to manage pain at home. Determine the effectiveness of the home management. Incorporate effective measures into the care plan.

ASSESSMENT ALERT

Do not assume that an elderly patient who appears to be busy, asleep, or functioning does not have pain. The older adult may not exhibit outward signs of pain even when experiencing pain.

In assessing pain, question the patient about the character of the pain, the location, the severity, the onset, and the duration. Determine if there are any factors that tend to increase the pain or alleviate the

---

DISPLAY 14-7. Nursing Interventions That Help to Alleviate Pain

- Establish a therapeutic relationship with the patient.
- Accept the patient's description of the pain.
- Observe nonverbal cues of pain such as body posture and facial expression.
- Use the Pain Management Flow Sheet (see Table 14-2) to monitor effectiveness of pain management plan.
- Use comfort measures such as back rubs, position changes, music, and relaxation techniques.
- Use diversionary activities such as TV, radio, games, or books.
- Encourage verbalization about pain and pain management.
- Administer analgesics as ordered.
- Notify the physician if pain management techniques are unsuccessful.

---

pain. Request a description of the effect of pain on daily living (eating, sleeping, social interaction). Asking the individual to rate the pain on a scale of 0 to 10, with 10 being the most severe pain and 0 being no feelings of pain, may be helpful.

ASSESSMENT ALERT

Patients with dementia or cognitive impairment may be unable to verbally express pain. For these patients, monitor for an increase in behavioral symptoms such as agitation, aggression, or wandering. Other expressions of pain in a patient with dementia include groaning, irritability, grimacing, and fetal positioning.

Management of Pain

In planning the care for the elderly experiencing pain, it is crucial to take all complaints of pain seriously and to act as quickly as possible to alleviate the pain. Some patients exhibit overt signs of pain such as changes in vital signs, facial gestures, or other nonverbal expressions. Others do not report any pain. Consult with the patient about the method of choice for pain control. Common options include medication, relaxation techniques, and imagery. Less common pain management practices include the use of herbs, yoga, therapeutic touch, or music. Be open to alternate methods of pain relief. Display 14-7 identifies nursing interventions that help to alleviate pain.

TABLE 14-2. **Pain Management Flow Sheet**				
Pain Location	Intensity 0–10	Therapeutic Intervention	Response	Time Pain Recurs*

*The Pain Mangement Flow Sheet can be used to monitor the effectiveness of pain management strategies.

Pharmacologic Aspects of Pain Management

Acute and chronic pain in older adults must be quickly and adequately treated. Analgesics are the first choice of treatment and are used in conjunction with nonpharmacologic interventions. In older adults, pain is particularly debilitating and can result in loss of functional ability. Particular attention should be given to managing pain in several conditions: musculoskeletal arthritis, lower back pain, leg cramping, diabetic neuropathy, headaches, and herpes zoster.

Narcotic analgesics (eg, morphine, codeine, meperidine hydrochloride) are indicated for severe acute pain in older adults. Because the elderly have an increased sensitivity and a slower clearance of narcotic analgesics, the dosage should be lower than dosages for younger adults. Narcotics and nonnarcotic analgesics sometimes are used in combination, allowing a reduction in the dosage of the narcotic. Although care should be given to administration of narcotics within guidelines prescribed by the physician, there is little evidence to support excessive concern for the development of addiction. Analgesics are to be given to, not withheld from, patients in pain. In general, when giving narcotic analgesics to the elderly, the medication is withheld and the physician notified if respirations are less than 12 to 14 breaths per minute.

The nonsteroidal antiinflammatory drugs (NSAIDs) and aspirin have analgesic, antiinflammatory, and antipyretic activity. These drugs cause gastric irritation and are not given when active ulcer disease is suspected. Aspirin interferes with analgesia of other NSAIDs. Acetaminophen is used as an analgesic but has minimal anti-inflammatory action. Table 14-3 identifies common analgesics used to treat pain in the elderly.

Potential therapies to use in conjunction with analgesics include: physical therapy transcutaneous electrical nerve stimulation (TENS), relaxation, and hypnosis. The TENS unit is a device that provides mild electrical stimuli from elec-

trodes placed on the skin over the painful area. This stimuli interferes with the transmission of pain signals, thereby decreasing the sensation of pain in a particular area. The TENS unit is not used in a patient with a demand-type cardiac pacemaker.

ACUTE CONFUSION

Confusion is an altered mental state characterized by decreased mental alertness and attention deficit. Confusion can result from three states: delirium, dementia, and depression.

Delirium is a term that describes a temporary, acute confusional state that is a symptom of a variety of treatable medical conditions such as infection, dehydration, electrolyte imbalance, or hypoxia. Delirium is never a symptom of normal aging. Acute confusion or delirium predisposes the elderly to experience falls, develop pressure ulcers, and infection. Acute confusion develops suddenly and tends to fluctuate during the day. Characteristically, the confusion worsens during the evening hours. Along with the confusion symptoms of memory deficit, illusions, hallucinations, and inattentiveness may occur.

Dementia is a permanent and often progressive loss of cognitive function that affects memory, the ability to learn new information, and intellectual function (see Chapter 17). Common causes of dementia include Alzheimer's disease and vascular dementia. Delirium and dementia are often confused in the clinical setting. Depression (see Chapter 15) can also be confused with delirium and dementia.

Table 14-4 compares depression, dementia, and delirium. These three confusional conditions can occur simultaneously or alone. Determining the exact cause of the confusion is sometimes difficult. Because treatment of each of these conditions is

TABLE 14-3. Analgesics Commonly Used for Mild to Moderate Pain in the Elderly

Drug	Recommended Oral Dosages for the Elderly	Nursing Considerations
NONNARCOTICS		
aspirin (Empirin)	325–500 mg q 3 hr 325–650 mg q 4 hr 650–1000 mg q 6 hr	Do not exceed 4 g/day. Decreases platelet aggregation. Decreases incidence of transient ischemic attack. Use cautiously in elderly patient with GI bleeding or ulcer disease. Monitor serum salicylate levels when administering prolonged therapy. Report symptoms of toxicity (tinnitus, headache hyperventilation, mental confusion). Administer with meals or with food.
acetaminophen (Tylenol)	325–1000 mg/day	Do not exceed 2.6 g/day. Has minimal anti-inflammatory properties Well absorbed orally Use cautiously in patients with liver damage. Do not take concurrently with the salicylates for more than a few days.
ibuprofen (Advil, Motrin)	200–400 mg q 4–6 hr	Higher analgesic properties than aspirin Increased risk of side effects in geriatric patients (headaches, drowsiness, nausea, dyspepsia, constipation) Do not exceed 1200 mg/day. Administering with a narcotic analgesic may permit lower narcotic dosage.
fenoprofen (Nalfon)	200–400 mg q 4–6 hr	Same as ibuprofen Use cautiously in patient with peptic ulcer disease or GI bleeding.
diflunisal (Dolobid)	250–500 mg bid	Patients with asthma and nasal polyps are at increased risk for hypersensitivity. Longer duration than ibuprofen. Higher analgesic potential than aspirin Inform patient to wear sunscreen and protective clothing to prevent photosensitivity reaction.
naproxen (Naprosyn)	200–400 mg initially, followed by 200 mg q 12 hr	In geriatric patients, do not exceed 200 mg in 12 hr. Same as diflunisal
ketorolac (Toradol)	10 mg q 4–6 hr prn	In geriatric patients, do not exceed 40 mg/day. Do not use for more than 5 days. Administration with narcotics may permit administration of lower narcotic dosages.
NARCOTICS		
codeine	15–60 mg q 3–6 hr as needed	A weak morphine derivative, it may cause drowsiness. Call for assistance when ambulating or performing activities that require mental alertness. Assess blood pressure, pulse, and respiration frequently. May cause dry mouth
oxycodone (Oxycontin)	5–10 mg q 3–4 hr	Used in combination with nonnarcotics Regularly administered dosages are more effective than prn dosages. May cause sedation or confusion Same as codeine
merperidine (Demerol)	50–100 mg	Same as codeine and oxycodone If respiratory rate is less than 12, assess level of sedation. Assess bowel function. Can cause constipation.
propoxyphene (Darvon)	65 mg q 4 hr	A weak opioid, it may be used in combination with nonnarcotic analgesics. It may cause drowsiness or dizziness. Use caution in activities that require mental alertness. Advise patient to make position changes slowly to minimize postural hypotension.
pentazocine (Talwin)	50–100 mg q 3–4 hr	Do not exceed 600 mg/day. May cause sedation, headache, euphoria, hallucination, dizziness, and nausea Assistance may be needed when ambulating. Use caution in performing activities that require mental alertness.

TABLE 14-4. Comparison of Depression, Dementia, and Delirium

Characteristic	Delirium	Depression	Dementia
Onset	Rapid (hours to days)	Rapid (weeks to months)	Gradual (years)
Course	Wide fluctuations; may continue for weeks if cause not found	May be self-limited or may become chronic without treatment	Chronic; slow but continuous decline
Level of consciousness	Fluctuates	Normal	Normal
Orientation	Patient is disoriented, confused	Patient may seem disoriented	Patient is disoriented, confused
Affect	Fluctuating	Sad, depressed, worried, guilty	Labile; apathy in later stages
Attention	Always impaired	Difficulty concentrating	May be intact; may focus on one thing for long periods
Sleep	Always disturbed	Disturbed; excess sleeping or insomnia, especially early-morning waking	Usually normal
Behavior	Agitated, restless	May be fatigued, apathetic; may occasionally be agitated	May be agitated or apathetic; may wander
Speech	Sparse or rapid; may be incoherent	Flat, sparse; understands	Sparse or rapid; repetitive; may be incoherent
Memory	Impaired, especially for recent events	Varies day to day; slow recall; often short-term deficit	Impaired, especially for recent events
Cognition	Disordered reasoning	May seem impaired	Disordered reasoning and calculation
Thought content	Incoherent, confused, delusions, stereotyped	Negative, hypochondriac, thoughts of death, paranoid	Disorganized, rich content, delusional, paranoid
Perception	Misinterpretations, illusions, hallucinations	Distorted; patient may have auditory hallucinations; negative interpretation of people and events	No change
Judgment	Poor	Poor	Poor; socially inappropriate behavior
Insight	May be present in lucid moments	May be impaired	Absent
Performance on mental status examinations	Generally poor; improves during lucid moments and with recovery	Memory impaired; calculation, drawing, following directions usually not impaired; frequent "I don't know" answers	Consistently poor; progressively worsens;

Adapted from Holt, J. (1993). Causes of confusion: Comparing the three D's in how to help confused patients. *American Journal of Nursing, 93* (8), 34.

different, identifying the condition causing the confusion is important.

Physiologic Aspects of Confusion

Several physiologic factors occur with aging that increase the risk of confusion in the older adult. Older adults have less physiologic reserve and are less able to maintain homeostasis when stressed physically or mentally. Illness is a stressor that can quickly lead to delirium. Many older adults, who in their home environment are oriented and able to function, develop acute confusion (ie, delirium)

when admitted to the hospital. Older adults are particularly susceptible to delirium postoperatively because of the effects of the anesthetics and narcotic analgesics.

Sensory overload or sensory deficits can cause acute confusion. Sensory deficits in hearing and vision that accompany aging make orientation to new surroundings more difficult. If glasses or hearing aids are not used, confusion can develop. The noises of the intensive care unit made by monitors, intravenous pumps, and ventilators may not distract the nurse who works in that unit on a daily basis, but to the older adult, these noises cause a sensory overload that leads to confusion. Sleep deprivation also contributes to the development of acute confusion.

Certain drugs also cause confusion as an adverse reaction. The drugs most likely to cause confusion include anticholinergic drugs, analgesics, histamine (H_2)-blocking agents, cardiovascular drugs, and sedatives or hypnotics. Older adults who take several different drugs are more prone to delirium as a result of drug-drug interactions.

Using the Nursing Process to Decrease Confusion in the Older Adult

Assessment
When assessing confusion, it is important to determine the underlying cause of the confusion. Assessment for the cause of delirium is sometimes hampered because of the difficulty distinguishing delirium, dementia, and depression (see Table 14-4). Delirium develops suddenly, worsens at night, and lasts less than 1 month. Dementia develops slowly and lasts months to years. The onset of depression coincides with major life changes and lasts 2 weeks or longer.

Identify factors that could cause the confusion, such as a urinary tract infection or other infections, medication side effects, and drug-drug interactions. Delirium can be caused by electrolyte imbalances resulting in hypokalemia or hyponatremia. Assess serum potassium levels. Blood levels of potassium that are less than 3.5 mEq/L indicate hypokalemia. Serum sodium levels should be 136 to 145 mEq/L.

ASSESSMENT ALERT
Confusion can be the result of infection. Suspect infection in the elderly adult when a sudden change in mental status occurs. If an infection is suspected, further assessment is indicated to determine the type of infection.

Assess sleep patterns and note any periods of sleep deprivation, sensory overload, or deprivation. Evaluate the extent of cognitive loss, ability to follow directions, and presence of hallucinations, illusions, or delusions.

Nursing Diagnosis
The following nursing diagnosis is used for patients with confusion: Acute Confusion related to hypokalemia, hyponatremia, hypoxia, dehydration, medication, or other (specify). Other nursing diagnoses may be appropriate for individual patients with specific needs.

Planning and Implementation
To plan individualized care, the cause of the confusion (eg, depression, delirium, dementia) must be identified correctly. After the cause is identified, nursing interventions are planned to correct the cause of the delirium. Table 14-5 gives nursing strategies for specific causes of delirium. Monitor for adverse reactions to medications, and eliminate nonessential medications. Display 14-8 identifies general nursing interventions to use for patients with delirium.

Reality Orientation
Reality orientation is an intervention used to continually reorient those with dementia or confusion. Reality orientation requires a 24 hour per day focus on orientation. For example, the day of the week, the season, and the month are reinforced by all nurses and staff members. Calendars, pictures depicting weather conditions, large-face clocks, and signs with days of the week printed on them all help to reinforce the components of orientation. Refocusing on reality is done by all health care providers that come in contact with the person with dementia. In some institutions, reality orientation sessions are held daily with groups of three or four residents. These daily sessions are usually led by nurses or an activity director. Beginning sessions focus on the resident's name, location, and the date. New facts, such as age, home town, family names, and relationships, are introduced slowly as the resident's orientation improves. The confused person responds best to consistency, set routines, and genuine interest by the nurse. The staff focuses on the "here and now" for 24 hours each day, 7 days per week.

Not all residents respond to reality orientation. For some, especially those with Alzheimer's disease, reality remains a fog that never lifts. For these patients, whose cognitive decline is irreversible, another form of therapy, called validation therapy, may be appropriate. This type of therapy validates the patient's feelings rather than trying to focus the patient on the facts of a situation. Validation therapy is discussed in more detail in Chapter 17.

Evaluation and Expected Outcomes
The previously described approaches can achieve certain outcomes:
    Improved orientation
    Less confusion
    Appropriate responses

TABLE 14-5. Nursing Strategies for Acute Confusion

Cause	Physical Findings	Nursing Actions*
Medications	Variable, depending on the specific medication, the potential for drug-drug interactions, and the patient's underlying health problems and health status	Monitor the effects (intended and adverse) of medications. Be especially vigilant for drug interactions. With the onset of any new symptom, first rule out an adverse reaction to a medication. Encourage prescribing of and administer only those medications indicated by the patient's condition, keeping medication to a minimum. Relieve pain through adequate and appropriate administration of analgesia and alternative therapies.
Infection (urinary tract, respiratory)	Urinary tract: dysuria is frequently absent; frequency, urgency, nocturia, incontinence, or anorexia; cultures may be negative. Respiratory: cough may be dry, productive, or absent; slight cyanosis; anorexia; nausea or vomiting; tachycardia; chills, fever, and elevated WBC count may not be present; cultures may be negative; breath sounds may include wheezes, crackles, or gurgles	Determine source and site of infection. Provide adequate fluids, 2,000 mL per day, unless otherwise contraindicated. Apply cooling techniques as needed for fever. Monitor for flushed hot skin, tachycardia, seizures, changes in body temperature, and breath sounds every 2 hours or as indicated by patient condition. Monitor intake and output. Provide humidified air; cough and deep breathing therapy prn. Provide frequent oral hygiene and chest physiotherapy to mobilize secretions as ordered.
Dehydration	Hypotension with orthostatic evident, tachycardia, hyperthermia, weakness, nausea, anorexia, oliguria, dry mucous membranes and skin, poor skin turgor, increased thirst	Determine source of dehydration (eg, decreased fluid intake or increased fluid output). Check medications as a possible cause for increased loss of fluids (eg, diuretics). Assess the patient's ability to swallow, and check for any extrinsic problems preventing fluid intake (eg, patient unable to reach fluids from bed). Continue monitoring of patient every 2 to 6 hours, as indicated by patient condition. Prepare for fluid replacement and additional diagnostic and therapeutic actions.
Hypokalemia	Hypotension, tachycardia, weakness, apathy, constipation, fatigue, lethargy, tachyarrhythmias, low serum potassium levels	Determine the source of hypokalemia, such as inadequate intake of potassium-rich foods, excessive loss due to the effects of medications (such as non–potassium-sparing diuretics).
Hyponatremia	Hypotension, tachycardia, hyperthermia, nausea, malaise, lethargy, or somnolence, poor skin turgor, increased thirst, decreased serum sodium and urine osmolality, elevated BUN, hematocrit, and serum proteins	Determine the cause of hyponatremia, such as inadequate intake of sodium, renal disease, or fluid restriction. Prepare for electrolyte and possibly fluid replacement. Restrict activity to maintain energy balance. Continue to monitor assessment parameters every 2 hours or as indicated by the patient's condition.
Hypoxia	Hypertension, tachycardia, tachypnea, cyanosis, agitation, increased depth of respirations, decreased PaO_2	Determine source of hypoxia (for example, apnea, decreased respiratory muscle tone, or congestion). Position patient to facilitate air exchange (high Fowler's position as tolerated). Restrict or pace activity to reduce additional oxygen requirements. Monitor blood gas or pulse oximetry results. Administer oxygen as ordered. Continue to monitor parameters every 2 hours or as indicated by the patient's condition.

Continued

TABLE 14-5. **Nursing Strategies for Acute Confusion** *continued*

Cause	Physical Findings	Nursing Actions*
Sensory impairment	Misperceptions of visual and auditory stimuli, such as hallucinations, illusions; misidentifying objects and persons	Assist patient in accurately interpreting environmental stimuli by having patient use appropriate sensory aids (eyeglasses or hearing aids). Ensure that aids are in proper working condition. Eliminate sources of distraction (auditory and visual). Speak clearly and slowly; do not shout; repeat key phrases as necessary. Speak directly into the patient's "best" ear. Face the patient when speaking so that he can use lip-reading to facilitate understanding as necessary. With written materials, choose large print with lighter colored objects on darker backgrounds; place them directly in front of the patient; and use indirect lighting to reduce or eliminate glare.
Environmental challenge	Variable, depending on whether the environmental challenge presents as sensory overload or sensory deprivation	Provide explanations of nursing care and all diagnostic and therapeutic activities. Minimize abrupt relocations. When relocation is necessary, provide explanations of the planned change to prepare the patient, and send a health care provider or family member to accompany the patient during the move. Provide orienting stimuli: clock, watch, calendar, radio, television, newspapers, personal items from home. Encourage social interaction with friends and family. To maintain continuity of care, assign the same caregivers as often as possible. Limit the number of staff involved in the care of the patient. Eliminate meaningless and unnecessary stimuli (eg, remove unneeded equipment and supplies; turn the television off when not desired). Alternate periods of rest and activity. Communicate clearly and simply.

*In using this guide for managing common causes and risk factors for acute confusion, notify the physician of any change in the patient's status, and document interventions and responses in the medical records.
From Foreman, M. & Zane, D. (1996). Nursing strategies for acute confusion in elders. *American Journal of Nursing 96* (4), 46. Used with permission.

DISPLAY 14-8. **Nursing Interventions to Use for Patients With Delirium**

- Maintain a calm, consistent environment.
- Orient the patient to surroundings and staff members.
- Reintroduce yourself each time you have contact with the patient.
- Encourage the use of eyeglasses to correct visual defects and hearing aids to correct hearing deficits.
- Gently reorient the patient on a regular basis.

- Give simple brief instructions and allow plenty of time to complete requests.
- Avoid the use of restraints.
- Provide a safe environment (eg, use side rails, place call light within easy reach, provide supervision).
- Assess mental status every 4 hours or as needed.
- Use reality orientation techniques if indicated.

FALLS

Falls are the leading cause of accidental death of persons older than 65 years. Even a relatively minor fall by an elderly person can cause severe damage, especially if the person has osteoporosis or other age-related illnesses. Falls can lead to hospitalization for the older population. Approximately 50% of older adults who are hospitalized because of a fall die within 1 year of the hospitalization.

The most common types of fractures resulting from a fall are fractures of the humerus, the wrist, the pelvis, and the hip. Hip fractures are the most devastating of all fractures. Many who suffer a hip fracture are unable to walk again even if they were independent before the fracture.

Lifestyle is often altered drastically after a fall. Some older adults develop a condition called post-fall syndrome. **Postfall syndrome** is a decrease in mobility after a fall caused by a fear of falling again. In an effort to be safe, some elderly limit activity to prevent falling. Some even avoid leaving home and become physically and socially isolated. This lifestyle contributes to functional decline, loss of self-esteem, decreased mobility, and loss of independence. Because falling can have a devastating effect on an older adult's life, prevention of falls is important.

Physiologic Changes That Increase the Risk of Falling

Several physiologic factors associated with aging, such as a decrease in cognition, problems with coordination, and sensory deficits, place the elderly at an increased risk for falling. Reflexes are slowed with age, causing older adults to have a greater propensity for falling. The use of psychotropic drugs for certain medical conditions causes dizziness, confusion, and unsteady gait as side effects. These side effects can increase the risk of falling.

Using the Nursing Process to Prevent Falls

Assessment
When assessing for an increased risk of falling, three areas are important: mobility, sensory deficient, and cognition. Assess mobility by observing gait, steadiness during ambulation, and stability within the environment. Sensory deficits such as difficulty seeing or hearing increases the risk for falling. Assess for a decrease in cognition by checking the level of consciousness, orientation to person, place, and time, and whether the older adult has the ability to make sound decisions. If a deficit is found in any one of these areas, the individual is at risk for a fall, and interventions to address that particular deficit are planned. If the individual is deficient in two or more areas, fall prevention precautions must be implemented (Display 14-9.)

The elderly frequently do not report falls. Because of the failure to report falls, older adults must be questioned about falls as a routine part of health screening. The individual is questioned about frequency of falls, where and when the falls occurred, and any injuries as a result of a fall. Determine whether the patient had

DISPLAY 14-9. **Fall Prevention Precautions**

- Place several brightly colored (yellow, blue, or green) signs that read "FALL PREVENTION PRECAUTIONS" in various locations such as over the bed or outside the door. This serves as a reminder to the staff that the patient is at risk for falling.
- Alert all staff that the patient is on Fall Prevention Precautions.
- Place a call light within easy reach. Answer the call light within 1 minute.
- Keep the bed in a low position.
- Assess cognition, mobility, and sensory deficits every half hour.
- Provide assistance for the patient when ambulating and for toileting.

episodes of syncope (ie, fainting) or vertigo (ie, dizziness) that resulted in a fall.

When a fall does occur, the individual is assessed for injury before placing him back in bed or assisting to stand. Moving the patient before assessing for injury may result in further injury. Examine the patient from head to toe for evidence of injury, and take and record the vital signs. Notify the physician when a fall occurs because radiographs, laboratory tests, electrocardiograms, Holter monitoring, or other diagnostic tests may be needed. If the patient is in the home setting, assessment of the home environment is necessary. Evaluate the home environment for factors that increase the risk of falling. Note problems such as slippery floors, inadequate lighting, or a lack of handrails.

Nursing Diagnosis
The following nursing diagnosis is appropriate for patients who are at risk for falling: Risk for Injury related to frequent falls, unsteady gait, sensory deficit, or other (specify). Other nursing diagnoses may be appropriate for individual patients with specific problems.

Planning and Implementation
In planning the care of an individual at risk for falling, plan specific interventions that address the identified risk factor or disease process. For example, falls related to Parkinson disease may decrease when the disease is treated with dopaminergic drugs. Falls as a result of osteoarthritis may improve with adequate pain management. Glasses to correct a vision problem or a hearing aid to correct a hearing deficit may reduce risks of falling associated with sensory deficits. For the elderly with an unsteady gait, an assistive device such as a

DISPLAY 14-10. Nursing Interventions to Use If Physical Restraints Are Used

- Notify the family of the need to restrain.
- Check restraints every 30 minutes or every hour.
- Release the restraints at least every 2 hours and move restrained body parts through a full range of motion. Check for circulatory impairment (eg, pulses, color of skin, skin temperature).
- Document why restraints are ordered, how they will be evaluated, and when they should be discontinued. Document a minimum of every hour.
- Discontinue restraints as soon as possible.

cane or walker can provide additional stability. Fall prevention precautions must be taken when an individual is considered at risk for falling (see Display 14-9).

The use of restraints to prevent falls is questionable. Restraining increases confusion in already confused patients. In general, studies indicate that restraints do not lower the risk of falls or injuries in confused residents. There may be times when the physician orders physical restraints to prevent falls. Display 14-10 identifies interventions to use when physical restraints are necessary.

Having sitters to observe patients is an alternative to the use of restraints. Sitters can keep the patient from pulling out intravenous lines, nasogastric tubes, and central lines. If sitters are not an option because of cost or unavailability, place high-risk patients in rooms near the nurses station, and institute fall precautions.

Evaluation and Expected Outcomes

The previously described approaches can achieve certain outcomes:

No falls

Walking with a steady gait

Assistive devices used when ambulating

UNDERNUTRITION

Nutritional problems are not a normal response to aging. Undernutrition can be a serious problem and increases the risk of a decline in mental and physical function. Nurses must be alert to even subtle changes that indicate an increased risk for nutrition problems. Early recognition and intervention of potential problems related to nutrition can ensure adequate nutritional intake.

Physiologic Factors That Contribute to Undernutrition

Factors that contribute to nutritional problems in the older adult include sensory losses, functional problems, disease conditions, cognitive or behavioral problems, and communication problems.

Sensory decline, particularly in the areas of taste and smell, affects nutrition. Although most people enjoy eating, as the sense of taste diminishes in later years, eating is no longer the pleasurable experience that it once was. Taste buds decrease in number.

Functional problems can contribute to nutritional problems. Limited or decreased ability of upper extremities can contribute to feeding problems. For example, an elderly patient with arthritis may have limited hand grips and be unable to hold feeding utensils. An elderly person may have weakness of the dominant hand as a result of a stroke. Ill-fitting dentures, loss of teeth, broken teeth, or stomatitis may cause problems in mastication (ie, chewing food).

Certain disease conditions such as chronic obstructive pulmonary disease (COPD) or heart failure (HF) can cause shortness of breath. The older adult does not eat or eats inadequate amounts for fear of chocking. Other diseases result in increased nutrient needs which the older adult is unable to meet. Cancer, pneumonia, pressure ulcers, and Alzheimer's disease are examples of conditions that increase nutrient needs.

Conditions that affect the thinking process can also affect the older adult's food intake. An older adult with paranoid feelings (eg, "the food is poisoned") does not eat and can become malnourished. Depression and dementia can cause a decrease in appetite and a lack of desire to eat. Individuals who wander, are anxious, or are fearful or withdrawn are likely to have a decreased food intake.

Communication plays an important role in the older adult's ability to discuss food preferences and to interact during mealtime. Eating is a time for socializing in most individual's lives. Without the ability to socialize, mealtime becomes lonely and uninteresting. Difficulty making food preferences known paves the way for undernutrition.

Potential Nutrient Deficiencies

Older adults can be deficient in any of the nutrients. Riboflavin, pyridoxine, cobalamin, ascorbic acid, iron, and protein are among the most likely deficient nutrients. Table 14-6 provides the clinical signs of vitamin and mineral deficiency.

Riboflavin. Older adults may exhibit a deficiency in riboflavin (vitamin B_2). Signs of vitamin B_2

TABLE 14-6. Clinical Signs of Vitamin and Mineral Deficiency

Clinical Signs by Site*	Deficiencies
ORAL CAVITY	
Cheilosis and angular stomatitis	Vitamin B$_2$
Glossitis (ie, pink or magenta discoloration with loss of villi)	Multiple B vitamins
EYES	
Scleral changes	Vitamin A
Bitot's spots	Vitamin A
FACE	
Seborrhea-like dryness and redness of nasolabial fold and eyebrows	Zinc
UPPER EXTREMITIES	
Purplish blotches on lightly traumatized areas (due to capillary fragility and subepithelial hemorrhages)	Vitamin C
Extreme transparency of skin of hands ("cellophane skin")	Vitamin C
ABDOMEN OR BUTTOCKS	
Waxy, perifollicular hyperkeratosis	Vitamin A
LOWER EXTREMITIES	
Superficial flaking of epidermis, large flakes of dandruff	Essential fatty acids
Cracks in skin between islands of hyperkeratosis	
Pigmented	Nicotinamide (niacinamide)
Nonpigmented	Vitamin A

*These manifestations may be seen in disease processes other than vitamin deficiencies. If the cause is a deficiency, clinical improvement should be evident 4 weeks after supplementation is begun.
From Bergstrom, N., Bennett, M.A., Carlson, C.E., et al. *Treatment of pressure ulcers.* Clinical practice guideline. no. 15. AHCPR publication no. 95-0652. Rockville, MD: U.S. Department of Health and Human Services. Public Health Service Agency for Health Care Policy and Research.

deficiency include cheilosis (ie, reddened and irritated areas at the angles of the lips), glossitis (ie, inflammation of the tongue), angular stomatitis (ie, inflammation of the mouth, especially the corners of the mouth), seborrheic dermatitis (ie, condition of the skin causing scaliness, crusting, and inflammation), and a beefy red tongue. The symptoms of riboflavin deficiency relate to tissue breakdown and poor wound healing in even minor injuries. Riboflavin deficiency rarely occurs alone and most often occur with other B vitamins. When these signs are observed, a vitamin B complex supplement may be ordered.

Pyridoxine. Pyridoxine (vitamin B$_6$) deficiency may also be observed. Signs of vitamin B$_6$ deficiency include dermatitis around eyes and mouth, neuritis, anorexia, nausea, and vomiting. A supplement of pyridoxine is indicated when the older adult exhibits signs of deficiency. Older adults taking isoniazid for tuberculosis also need a pyridoxine supplement. Take this vitamin only on the advice of a physician because pyridoxine toxicity can occur. The most significant signs of toxicity include sensory losses and numbness of the hands and feet.

Cobalamin. Cobalamin (vitamin B$_{12}$) deficiency can lead to dementia, megaloblastic anemia, incontinence, or orthostatic hypotension. Up to 5% of adults older than 80 years have vitamin B$_{12}$ deficiency. Vitamin B$_{12}$ deficiency is most often the result of a lack of the intrinsic factor in the gastric secretions. The intrinsic factor is necessary for vitamin B$_{12}$ to be absorbed. Absence of the intrinsic factor leads to the development of pernicious anemia because vitamin B$_{12}$ cannot be absorbed. Treatment is monthly cobalamin injections. The Schilling test, which is used to diagnose pernicious anemia in younger adults, is not recommended for older adults. The decreased production of hydrochloric acid in the gastric mucosa of older adults gives inaccurate results for the Schilling test.

Ascorbic Acid. A vitamin C (ascorbic acid) deficiency is associated with easy bruising due to fragile capillaries, poor wound healing, and the development of pressure ulcers. Vitamin C functions to produce a special substance that cements cells together, particularly cells in connective tissue, blood vessels, and capillary walls.

Iron. Iron deficiency anemia can occur in the elderly. Symptoms of iron deficiency anemia include pallor, weakness, fatigue, angular stomatitis.

NUTRITION ALERT

There are several indicators of iron deficiency:
- Hemoglobin levels below 14 g/dL in males and below 12 g/dL in females
- Hematocrit levels below 41 g/dL in males and 36 g/dL in females
- Transferrin saturation levels below 30%

Serum transferrin is a protein found in small amounts in the blood that is necessary for the transport of iron from the small intestine to the plasma. Transferrin saturation levels decrease in iron deficiency anemia. Normal transferrin saturation value is 30% to 40%.

Protein. Protein-energy undernutrition (ie, malnutrition) is the inadequate intake of protein and calories resulting in loss of body mass and fat. Two indicators for protein-energy malnutrition are serum albumin levels and weight loss. Albumin is a protein that makes up about 60% of the total body protein. Serum albumin is used to measure nutritional status. Serum albumin levels of 3.5 to 4.8 g/dL in the elderly indicate marginal protein levels. Levels below 3.5 g/dL indicate undernutrition. Lack of adequate protein increases the risk of infection, delays in wound healing, increases the risk of pressure ulcers, and can increase the risk of developing disease.

Nutritional Assessment in the Older Adult

Nutritional assessment begins with the height and weight. The baseline height and weight are used for future comparisons to determine weight loss or gains. Report the following:

Weight loss of 5% or more of normal or baseline body weight in 1 month

Weight loss of 10% or more in 6 months

Weight 20% below ideal weight for weight and height

Laboratory tests such as those for hemoglobin, hematocrit, serum albumin, and serum transferrin are monitored.

To assess weight loss, consider the individual's usual weight throughout adult life. Obtain a diet history. Determine if the person has been on a special diet such as a calorie-restricted diet or a mechanical soft diet. Monitor food intake over 5 to 7 days. Keep a diary of food eaten, caloric intake, patterns of eating, time of day, and mood when eating. Note the percentage of uneaten food. Consistently leaving one third to one fourth of food on the plate increases the risk of malnutrition. Note the person's likes and dislikes.

Carefully assess for pale skin, dull eyes, swollen lips, dry swollen or bright red tongue, poor skin turgor, extreme thinness, edema, or muscle wasting. Examine the mouth and oral cavity for the presence of broken or loose teeth, mouth pain or sensitivity, ulcerations, and inflamed gums. Assess for protein-energy undernutrition. Check weight and serum albumin levels. Nutritional support depends on the reason for the protein-energy undernutrition.

Assess the medication regimen for drugs that can cause nutritional problems. For example, the cardiac glucoside digoxin (Lanoxin) can cause anorexia (ie, loss of appetite). Other drugs that can contribute to nutritional deficiencies include diuretics, psychotropic drugs, anticonvulsants, or overuse of the antacids or laxatives.

For the elderly person who is living at home, question about who prepares the meals and whether there is there adequate money to buy food. How do you obtain your groceries? What do you eat at home? Do you live alone? The Determine Your Nutritional Health checklist from the Nutrition Screening Initiative is an excellent tool to give to older adults for assessing their nutritional needs (Display 14-11). The nutrition checklist is based on the warning signs described in Display 14-12. The nurse discusses the checklist with the patient, provides further instruction, and answers any questions the older adult may have concerning nutrition needs.

Managing Nutritional Problems in the Older Adult

Consultation with the dietitian is usually indicated for undernutrition. Dietary instruction with the dietitian, the patient, and the caregiver is necessary. Instruct the elderly person or the caregiver on special nutritional needs. Identify food preferences or patterns. Promote a pleasant relaxing atmosphere at mealtimes. Encourage socialization when eating. Provide any assistive devices that make self-feeding easier. Weigh weekly and as needed. Refer to dental hygienist or dentist if dental care is needed. For protein-energy malnutrition, depending on the severity of the condition, oral protein supplements or intravenous albumin may be ordered.

Suggest congregate meals at community centers or senior citizen centers. For the elderly who are homebound, arrange for delivered meals for at least one meal each day. Arrange for community service organizations to assist older adults with grocery shopping. Encourage family members to be aware of food intake and to be available during mealtime. Provide access to culturally acceptable foods. Residents of nursing homes should get out of bed to eat. Brush dentures or teeth in the morning and after meals. Allow slow eaters to finish without rushing. Display 14-13 lists ways to boost caloric intake. Provide a well-balanced diet using the patient's stated food preferences.

Enteral Feedings

When an individual is unable to take adequate nutrition by eating, administration of nutrients through feeding tubes may be necessary. Enteral feedings can be accomplished by the insertion of feeding tubes directly into the stomach, duodenum, or jejunum. Enteral feedings are administered by intermittent or continuous feedings using gravity or a feeding pump that allows uniform flow. Intermittent feedings are accomplished by pouring the feeding solution into the barrel of a large syringe attached to a feeding tube and infusing by gravity.

A nasogastric (NG) tube is inserted through the nose and into the stomach. A nasointestinal (NI) tube

DISPLAY 14-11. Determine Your Nutritional Health Checklist

Read the statements below. Circle the number in the YES column for those that apply to you or someone you know. For each yes answer, score the number in the box. Total your nutritional score.

	Yes
I have an illness or condition that made me change the kind and/or amount of food I eat.	2
I eat fewer than 2 meals per day.	3
I eat few fruits or vegetables, or milk products.	2
I have 3 or more drinks of beer, liquor or wine almost every day.	2
I have tooth or mouth problems that make it hard for me to eat.	2
I don't always have enough money to buy the food I need.	4
I eat alone most of the time.	1
I take 3 or more different prescribed or over-the-counter drugs a day.	1
Without wanting to, I have lost or gained 10 pounds in the last 6 months.	2
I am not always physically able to shop, cook and/or feed myself.	2
TOTAL	

0–2 **Good!** Recheck your nutritional score in 6 months.

3–5 **You are at moderate nutritional risk.** See what can be done to improve your eating habits and lifestyle. Your office on aging, senior nutrition program, senior citizens center or health department can help. Recheck your nutritional score in 3 months.

6 or more **You are at high nutritional risk.** Bring this checklist the next time you see your doctor, dietitian or other qualified health or social service professional. Talk with them about any problems you may have. Ask for help to improve your nutritional health. Although warning signs suggest risk, they do not represent a diagnosis.

Reprinted with permission by the Nutrition Screening Initiative, a project of the American Academy of Family Physicians, the American Dietetic Association and the National Council on the Aging, Inc., and funded in part by a grant from Ross Products Division, Abbott Laboratories.

extends into the distal duodenum or proximal jejunum. NG or NI tubes may be used for short-term nutritional support. Nasogastric tubes are prone to complications and are uncomfortable for the patient. Patients requiring long-term enteral feedings usually have a gastrostomy tube or a jejunostomy tube. A percutaneous endoscopic gastrostomy (PEG) tube is often used for long-term nutritional support. Gastrostomy tubes are better tolerated by agitated patients and those requiring nutritional support for more than 2 weeks. The type, amount, and strength of the enteral feeding is determined by the physician with input from the registered dietitian. While administering enteral feedings continually, assess for any indication that oral feeding may be resumed, such as a strong cough reflex or the ability to swallow saliva.

Dehydration

Dehydration is a condition in which there is excessive water loss from the body tissues. In dehydration, fluid loss (output) exceeds fluid intake. This fluid imbalance causes an imbalance of fluids and electrolytes particularly sodium, potassium, and chloride. Other conditions, such as prolonged fever, diarrhea, and vomiting, may result in dehydration. Any condition that causes a loss of fluid or a decrease in ingestion of fluid can quickly result in dehydration in an older adult.

Physiologic Changes That Affect Hydration

Water is essential for proper functioning of all body systems. The sensation of thirst diminishes with age. As a result of diminished thirst, many older adults do not drink enough fluids and are continually in a state of mild dehydration. In normal aging, there is a decline in total body water. This places the older adult at increased risk for dehydration.

Assessing for Dehydration

When caring for the older adult, the nurse continually assesses for signs and symptoms of dehydration. Symptoms that indicate dehydration include

DISPLAY 14-12. DETERMINE Guidelines

The nutrition checklist is based on the warning signs described below. Use the word DETERMINE to remind you of the warning signs.

Disease

Any disease, illness, or chronic condition that causes you to change the way you eat or makes it hard for you to eat puts your nutritional health at risk. Four of five adults have chronic diseases that are affected by diet. Confusion or memory loss that keeps getting worse is estimated to affect one of five or more of older adults. This can make it hard to remember what, when, or if you've eaten. Feeling sad or depressed, which happens to about one in eight older adults, can cause big changes in appetite, digestion, energy level, weight, and well-being.

Eating poorly

Eating too little and eating too much lead to poor health. Eating the same foods day after day or not eating fruit, vegetables, and milk products daily also causes poor nutritional health. One in five adults skips meals daily. Only 13% of adults eat the minimum amount of fruit and vegetables needed. One in four older adults drinks too much alcohol. Many health problems become worse if you drink more than one or two alcoholic beverages per day.

Tooth loss/mouth pain

A healthy mouth, teeth, and gums are needed to eat. Missing, loose, or rotten teeth or dentures that do not fit well or cause mouth sores make it hard to eat.

Economic hardship

As many as 40% of older Americans have incomes of less than $6,000 per year. Having less—or choosing to spend less—than $25–30 per week for food makes it very hard to get the foods you need to stay healthy.

Reduced social contact

One third of all older people live alone. Being with people daily has a positive effect on morale, well-being, and eating.

Multiple medicines

Many older Americans must take medicines for health problems. Almost half of older Americans take multiple medicines daily. Growing old may change the way we respond to drugs. The more medicines you take, the greater the chance for side effects such as increased or decreased appetite, change in taste, constipation, weakness, drowsiness, diarrhea, nausea, and others. Vitamins or minerals, when taken in large doses, act like drugs and can cause harm. Alert your doctor to everything you take.

Involuntary weight loss/gain

Losing or gaining a lot of weight when you are not trying to do so is an important warning sign that must not be ignored. Being overweight or underweight also increases your chance of poor health.

Needs assistance in self care

Although most older people are able to eat, one of five has trouble walking, shopping, buying, and cooking food.

Elder years above age 80

Most older people lead full and productive lives, but as age increases, the risks of frailty and health problems increase. Checking your nutritional health regularly makes good sense.

Reprinted with permission by the Nutrition Screening Initiative, a project of the American Academy of Family Physicians, the American Dietetic Association and the National Council on the Aging, Inc., and funded in part by a grant from Ross Products Division, Abbott Laboratories.

dizziness while sitting or standing, confusion or a change in mental status, oliguria, irritability, poor skin turgor, dry mucous membranes, or a coated or furrowed tongue. Severe dehydration is exhibited by signs of shock such as low blood pressure; a rapid, thready pulse; cold extremities; rapid breathing; or lethargy that can progress to coma.

ASSESSMENT ALERT

Age-related skin changes that result in a decrease in skin elasticity makes assessment of skin turgor difficult in older adults. The use of skin turgor for assessing dehydration is not accurate in an older adult because turgor may be decreased in an adequately hydrated older adult. If assessed, skin turgor is checked on the sternum or forehead of an older adult.

When examination of the tongue reveals a dry, furrowed appearance, dehydration is suspected. Monitor laboratory values of the electrolytes sodium (Na), potassium (K), and chloride (Cl).

Managing Dehydration

Many symptoms of dehydration are not apparent until a significant fluid deficit has occurred. Because dehydration is difficult to detect, all elderly should be considered at high risk for dehydration. Treatment is aimed at restoring fluid balance orally or parenterally. For moderate to severe dehydration, the physician may order intravenous fluid replacement. Nursing interventions focus on prevention of further dehydration and restoring adequate hydration. Most older adults can be rehydrated using oral therapy. Display 14-14 identifies nursing interventions that help to restore hydration.

DISPLAY 14-13. Boosting Intake When Appetite is Poor

- Add nonfat dry milk powder to just about anything with liquid in it—sauces, cooked cereal, yogurt, mashed potatoes, desserts, and gravy. Just 1/3 cup adds 81 kcal, 8 g of protein, almost 300 mg of calcium, and 1 mg of zinc, which is 8% of an older woman's recommended dietary allowance for this important nutrient.
- Vary nourishments taken between meals so they are not all liquid and not all sweet, and make them part of routine care, like medications.
- Offer the most food at the time of day when the patient is most hungry; for most people, this is in the morning.
- Emphasize taste and eye appeal. Elders have a decreased taste and smell acuity: stronger flavors may heighten appetite.
- Offer finger foods, and encourage patients to eat any food with fingers if it will encourage eating.
- Add some fat. Low-calorie intakes are usually low-fat intakes, and adding fat boosts kilocalories without overdoing fat intake. Add margarine to vegetables, creamed foods and sauces, and cooked cereal.
- Use fortified milk to make foods that are often made with water, such as soup and cooked cereal.
- Liquid supplements are easy to use but are also easy to waste. Leaving a full can of supplement at the bedside for hours means opening a new can at the next feeding or risking bacterial contamination. Commercial formulas should not be routinely prescribed without considering other methods of increasing intake. Although some elders tolerate liquid feedings well for a while, many become quickly bored with their sameness, which affects intake.
- Calorie counts are useful indicators to show that progress is being made. Besides showing an increase in calorie intake, they can show which foods are tolerated and which should be altered.

From Yen, P. (1994). Boosting intake when appetite is poor. *Geriatric Nursing, 15,* 284. Used with permission.

DISPLAY 14-14. Nursing Interventions to Help Restore Hydration

- Unless contraindicated by a disease process, increase fluid intake to 2,000 to 2,500 mL per day.
- Keep water or other fluids within easy reach.
- Offer fluids regularly every 1 to 2 hours. Although fluids should be within easy reach, offering fluids frequently is more effective than simply having fluids available. Some older adults never experience thirst and therefore do not think to drink, but when fluids are offered, they will drink a significant amount.
- Monitor laboratory values of electrolytes (NA, K, CI) daily. Report any abnormalities.
- Keep an accurate record of intake and output. When hydration is adequate, intake should equal output.
- Weigh daily in the same clothing, at the same time, and with the same scale.
- Observe and report signs of further dehydration such as dry mucous membranes, poor skin turgor, or concentrated urine.
- Provide frequent oral care.
- Provide safety measures if the patient is confused.
- Administer and monitor intravenous fluids if indicated.

CRITICAL THINKING EXERCISES

1. Ms. Langley is a 66-year-old woman with four grown children and six grandchildren. She tells you that she lives a very active life but is sometime embarrassed by the leakage of urine that she has when she is playing with her grandchildren. This leakage occurs when she laughs, coughs, or sneezes. What information can you give Ms. Langley about this situation? Suggest three additional questions that would provide additional beneficial information. What suggestions can you make to help her with this problem?

2. Mr. Fiest, age 82, lives alone in a two-story home that he has lived in for more than 30 years. He has fallen three times in the last 2 months. Fortunately, he has not been injured as a result of these falls. His daughter is concerned that if he falls again he may be injured. What is the first action you should take? What assessments would you make? Use the nursing process to develop an individualized care plan for Mr. Fiest.

3. Ms. Prock has lost 6 pounds in the past 2 weeks. Her normal weight is 116 pounds. In reviewing her record, you notice this weight loss. What is the first action you would take? How could you use the nursing assistants to gain more information about Ms. Prock's weight loss? Select a nursing diagnosis for Ms. Prock's problem and suggest at least five nursing interventions to help alleviate the problem.

REFERENCES AND SUGGESTED READING

All, A., & LaRae, I. (1999). Pain, cancer and older adults. *Geriatric Nursing, 20 (5),* 241.

Amella, E., et al. (1998). Assessment and management of eating and feeding difficulties for older people: A NICHE protocol. *Geriatric Nursing, 19* (5), 269–274.

Boska, R., & Maloney, C. (1998). Current thinking in incontinence care. *The Annals of Long-Term Care, 6 (6),* 64–70.

Dexter, D. (1999). Sleep disorders in the elderly. *The Annals of Long-Term Care, 7* (Special Issue, Meeting Highlights), 33–36.

Feil, N. (1996). *The validation breakthrough.* Baltimore, MD: Health Professions Press.

Gordon, D., & Ward, S. (1995). Correcting patient misconceptions about pain. *American Journal of Nursing, July,* 43–45.

Johnson, E. (1999). Evaluation and management of urinary incontinence among long-term care facility residents. *The Annals of Long-Term Care, 7* (Special Issue, Meeting Highlights), 25–26.

Lawhorne, L., & Stein, W. (1999). Guidelines for pain management. *The Annals of Long-Term Care, 7* (Special Issue, Meeting Highlights), 27–29.

Luft, J., & Vriheas-Nichols, A. (1998). Identifying risk factors for developing incontinence: Can we modify the risk? *Geriatric Nursing, 19 (2),* 66–70.

Matteson, M., McConnell, E., & Linton, A. (1996). *Gerontological nursing.* Philadelphia: W.B. Saunders.

Miller, C. (2000). Advising older adults about pain remedies. *Geriatric Nursing, 21 (1),* 55.

Morley, J., Thomas, D., & Kamel, H. (1998). Nutritional deficiencies in long-term care: Part I detection and diagnosis. *The Annals of Long-Term Care, 6 (5),* 183–190.

Smith, D. (1998). A continence care approach for long-term care facilities. *Geriatric Nursing, 19 (2),* 81–86.

Smith, D. (1998). Sleep disorders in the elderly. *The Annals of Long-Term Care, 6 (6),* 36–42.

Steinberg, M., et al. (1998). Falls in the institutionalized elderly with dementia: A pilot study. *The Annals of Long-Term Care, 6 (5),* 153–162.

U.S. Department of Health and Human Services. (1996). *Urinary incontinence in adults: Acute and chronic management agency for health care policy and research.* AHCPR Publication no. 96-0682. Rockville, MD: U.S. Department of Health and Human Services.

CHAPTER 15

CHAPTER OUTLINE

KEY TERMS

CHAPTER OBJECTIVES

DEPRESSION

USING THE NURSING PROCESS IN THE CARE OF THE PATIENT WITH DEPRESSION

SUICIDE

GRIEF

SUBSTANCE ABUSE

ELDER ABUSE AND NEGLECT

CRITICAL THINKING EXERCISES

REFERENCES AND SUGGESTED READING

Managing Psychosocial Problems

KEY TERMS

abuse

active neglect

anticipatory grief

bipolar disorder

dysfunctional grief

dysthymia

financial abuse

grief

hopelessness

Korsakoff syndrome

major depression

neglect

passive neglect

passive suicide

physical abuse

psychological abuse

psychomotor agitation

psychomotor retardation

reactive drinker

self-neglect

sexual abuse

suicidal ideation

Wernicke encephalopathy

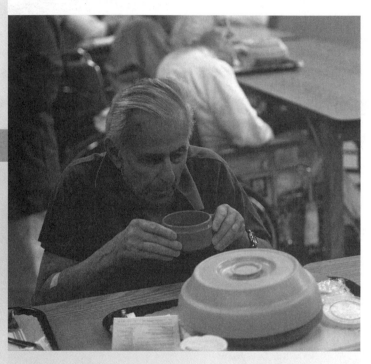

CHAPTER OBJECTIVES

At the completion of this chapter, the student will be able to

○ Describe the various types of depression found in the older adult

○ Identify common misunderstandings about suicide

○ Describe two conditions that develop in later life as a result of excessive alcohol consumption

○ Identify risk factors for elder abuse

○ Identify the various types of abuse

○ Discuss institutional abuse

○ Discuss important aspects of assessment and care for an older adult who is depressed, suicidal, grieving, or abuses alcohol or who is abused

Nurses are challenged daily to assist the elderly in meeting psychosocial needs. Psychosocial needs affect every area of an older adult's life. However, in the elderly patient psychosocial needs may be masked behind physical problems. The nurse who sees the older adult as a holistic being is better prepared to detect psychosocial needs and to assist the older adult toward optimum health. Examining physical, psychological, social, and emotional aspects of the older adult's life can result in correctly identifying psychosocial problems.

Psychosocial problems discussed in this chapter include depression, suicide, grief, alcohol abuse, and elder abuse. Although these psychosocial problems are not all inclusive, they do represent some of the more common psychosocial problems that the older adult faces. Chapters 8 and 11 also deal with psychosocial issues and the reader is encouraged to refer to those chapters for more information.

DEPRESSION

Depression is not a part of normal aging. It is, however, the most common psychiatric disorder in older adults. As many as 3 of 100 people who are age 65 or older suffer from depression. There is an increased rate of depression for those older than 80 years. Even the most severe forms of depression can be successfully treated with the proper medication, psychotherapy, or a combination of medication and psychotherapy.

Why Depression Occurs in the Elderly

Depression occurs for a combination of reasons such as a result of illness or as a side effect of medication. Certain personality types are more prone to depression. Certain illnesses common to older adults such as stroke, diabetes, or Parkinson disease can aggravate or precipitate a depressive episode. Certain medications cause depression as a side effect (Display 15-1). Individuals with a low self-esteem, the frail elderly, or those with high dependency needs are at greater risk for depression. Loss is one of the major risk factors leading to depression in older adults. Loss of a mate, friends, or functional abilities; retirement; or any other loss experienced by the elderly can result in a depressive episode.

DISPLAY 15-1. Drugs That May Precipitate Depression

Anti-inflammatory agents and analgesics
  indomethacin
  phenacetin
  phenylbutazone
  pentazocine
Antimicrobials
  sulfonamides
  ethambutol
  cycloserine
  selected Gram-negative
    antibiotics
Cardiovascular antihypertensive agents
  digitalis
  clonidine
  guanethidine
  methyldopa
  reserpine
  hydralazine
  propranolol
  indapamide
  prazosin
  procainamide
Central nervous system agents
  amantadine
  L-dopa
  barbiturates
  chloral hydrate
  succinimide derivatives
  diazepam and other
    benzodiazepines
  haloperidol
  phenothiazines
  alcohol
  amphetamines
Hormones
  corticosteroid
  estrogen
  progesterone
Others
  disulfiram
  physostigmine
  antineoplastic agents
  organic pesticides

Types of Depression in Older Adults

Three types of depression seen in older adults are discussed in this chapter: major depression, dysthymia, and bipolar disorder. Depression usually is described as feeling blue, hopeless, worthless, or down in the dumps. Sometimes, the depressed person may withdraw from family, friends, and activities. With treatment, these depressive episodes last approximately 3 months. Without treatment, they can last for as long as a year. Most depressive episodes recur if untreated. Sometimes, depression in the elderly is treated as an ongoing illness, much like diabetes. In this case, antidepressant medications are given for extended periods.

According to the American Psychiatric Association's *Diagnostic and Statistical Manual of Mental Disorders (DSM-IV-R)* (1994), major depressive disorders are identified in patients when they exhibit a depressed mood, diminished pleasure in life, and four or more of the following symptoms:
- Significant weight loss (loss of 5% of body weight within 1 month) or a decrease or increase in appetite
- Insomnia (a common symptom of depression in the older adult)

- **Psychomotor agitation** (ie, restlessness or rapid purposeless movements such as pacing or wringing hands) or **psychomotor retardation** (ie, slow movements and speech)
- Fatigue
- Inappropriate guilt or feelings of worthlessness
- Decrease in ability to think, concentrate, or make decisions
- Recurrent thoughts of death

If these symptoms are present almost daily for 2 or more weeks, **major depression** should be suspected.

Another type of depression called **dysthymia** is a moderate form of chronic depression that lasts 2 or more years. Dysthymia is difficult to detect because the symptoms occur insidiously and continue for a significant period.

Bipolar disorder is a disorder characterized by two different emotional states. Emotional states range from that of extreme highs (ie, mania) with the person exhibiting seemingly unlimited energy and elation to extreme lows and deep depression. Although bipolar disorder usually begins in young adulthood, it may be a part of the health history of an older adult's life. In these cases, it requires continuous medical treatment. The most common medication used in the treatment for mania is lithium.

USING THE NURSING PROCESS IN THE CARE OF THE PATIENT WITH DEPRESSION

Assessment

Identifying depression in the older adult requires careful assessment. Although depression is common in the elderly, it often goes undetected. Depression can be superimposed on dementia or confused with dementia. Common symptoms of depression in the older adult include anxiety, agitation, confusion, decrease in mental functioning, and memory loss. These symptoms are also commonly seen with dementia. Table 14-5 in Chapter 14 compares dementia and depression. If agitation is present with depression the symptom may be labeled as a behavior problem and the depression goes untreated. Symptoms of depression in the elderly can be confused with physical illness, medication interactions, substance abuse, or "old age." Residents in nursing facilities are at high risk for depression, particularly within the first several months after admission.

ASSESSMENT ALERT

Suspect depression when an older person becomes agitated or anxious but has no cognitive impairment. Most older adults do not verbalize feelings of depression but do complain of bodily aches and pains such as generalized fatigue or gastrointestinal complaints or exhibit a lack of interest in their surroundings. Careful assessment of all bodily complaints is done to determine whether a physical problem exists. Symptoms in some disorders such as Alzheimer's disease, heart failure, cerebrovascular accident, or malnutrition can mimic depression in the elderly.

Assess interest in self-care activities. Older adults who are physically able to perform activities of daily living but who lose interest in self-care and refuse to perform self-care activities such as dressing, bathing, or grooming may be depressed.

Certain medications can cause depression as an adverse reaction (see Display 15-1). Antihypertensive medications, antiparkinsonian medications, narcotic analgesics, and sedatives are among the most likely medications to cause depression. The nurse needs to be aware of the medications that can cause depression and assess for any signs of depression in elderly patients prescribed these drugs. A careful assessment of the medication regimen is needed to identify drugs that can cause depression.

The Geriatric Depression Scale (Display 15-2) may be used to assess depression. Asking about the presence of symptoms may be all that is necessary to provide the encouragement the older adult needs to verbalize feelings associated with depression.

PSYCHOSOCIAL ASPECTS OF NURSING: ADDITIONAL ASSESSMENTS WHEN DEPRESSION IS SUSPECTED

- **Recent weight loss or gain**
- **Recent losses or changes in life patterns**
- **Feelings of anxiety or fatigue**
- **Insomnia or other sleep disturbances**
- **Feelings of hopelessness or worthlessness**
- **Inability to concentrate or make decisions**
- **Thoughts of death or dying**

Involvement of the family is an important factor in assessing depression. Carefully question family members about the presence of the symptoms of depression in the loved one. Accurately document and report any symptoms of depression to the physician. Note any observations of psychomotor excitation or retardation.

DISPLAY 15-2. Geriatric Depression Scale

Choose the best answer for how you felt over the past week.

1. Are you basically satisfied with your life? yes/no
2. Have you dropped many of your activities and interests? yes/no
3. Do you feel that your life is empty? yes/no
4. Do you often get bored? yes/no
5. Are you hopeful about the future? yes/no
6. Are you bothered by thoughts you can't get out of your head? yes/no
7. Are you in good spirits most of the time? yes/no
8. Are you afraid that something bad is going to happen to you? yes/no
9. Do you feel happy most of the time? yes/no
10. Do you often feel helpless? yes/no
11. Do you often get restless and fidgety? yes/no
12. Do you prefer to stay at home, rather than going out and doing new things? yes/no
13. Do you frequently worry about the future? yes/no
14. Do you feel you have more problems with memory than most? yes/no
15. Do you think it is wonderful to be alive now? yes/no
16. Do you often feel downhearted and blue? yes/no
17. Do you feel pretty worthless the way you are now? yes/no
18. Do you worry a lot about the past? yes/no
19. Do you find life very exciting? yes/no
20. Is it hard for you to get started on new projects? yes/no
21. Do you feel full of energy? yes/no
22. Do you feel that your situation is hopeless? yes/no
23. Do you think that most people are better off than you are? yes/no
24. Do you frequently get upset over little things? yes/no
25. Do you frequently feel like crying? yes/no
26. Do you have trouble concentrating? yes/no
27. Do you enjoy getting up in the morning? yes/no
28. Do you prefer to avoid social gatherings? yes/no
29. Is it easy for you to make decisions? yes/no
30. Is your mind as clear as it used to be? yes/no

From Yesavage, J.A., Brink, T.L., Rose, T.L., et al. (1983). The Geriatric Depression Scale. *Journal Psychiatric Research, 17*, 37–49.

With dysthymia, the depression may be difficult to detect. Suspect dysthymia when the patient expresses symptoms of low self-esteem, poor concentration, decreased energy, and feelings of hopelessness that have continued for the past 2 years or longer. Mania is an indication of bipolar disorder.

> **PSYCHOSOCIAL ASPECTS OF NURSING: COMMON SIGNS AND SYMPTOMS OF THE MANIC PHASE OF THE BIPOLAR PERSONALITY**
>
> • Irritability
> • Decreased need for sleep
> • Increased energy
> • Excessive talking and moving, and sexual activity
> • Grandiose (exaggerated) thoughts
> • Easily distracted
> • Inflated self-esteem
> • Excessively high moods
> • Decreased ability to make rational decisions

Nursing Diagnoses

One or more of the following nursing diagnoses may be used for an individual with depression:

Hopelessness related to depressed mood, stress, loss of spouse, other (specify)

Impaired Social Interaction related to withdrawal from family, friends, depressed mood, other (specify)

Self-Care Deficit related to grooming, feeding, hygiene, lack of energy, or other (specify)

Other nursing diagnoses may also be appropriate for an individual with depression.

Planning and Implementation

In planning the care of a depressed individual take into consideration the specific symptoms exhibited. For example, many older adults with depression exhibit agitation and psychomotor excitement. These individuals require a different plan of care from that for the individual with psychomotor retardation. The care plan is individualized to meet specific needs. If the older adult has a low self-esteem, specific interventions are planned to increase self-esteem (see Chapter 11). General nursing interventions when caring for a depressed individual are listed in Display 15-3.

Mania is the hyperactive mood of the bipolar disorder. The individual suffering form this disorder can have depressive episodes alternating with manic episodes. This manic episode may begin suddenly and last days to months. Nursing interventions when caring for a patient in the manic phase of the bipolar disorder are identified in Display 15-4.

DISPLAY 15-3. Nursing Interventions When Caring for a Depressed Individual

- Develop a trusting relationship.
- Provide a nurturing environment by empathetic listening.
- Promote expression of feeling (eg, talking, crying, laughing).
- Encourage participation in a life review and reminiscence therapy (see Chapter 11).
- Encourage participation in an exercise program or social activities with others.
- Review medication regimen for possible drugs that cause depression.
- Develop ability to engage in positive self-talk.
- Identify possible losses contributing to the depression, and discuss these losses and possible coping mechanisms.

DISPLAY 15-4. Nursing Interventions for a Patient in the Manic Phase of Bipolar Disorder

- Approach the patient in a calm but firm manner.
- Set limits.
- Be consistent.
- Use short and concise statements when conversing.
- Calmly and quietly deal with loud or vulgar speech or behavior.
- Keep environmental stimuli to a minimum.
- Provide solitary activities until becomes less manic.
- Protect the person from engaging in grandiose activities (eg, spending sprees, giving away money).
- Provide snacks such as finger foods or high-protein drinks frequently.
- Observe and report any signs of lithium toxicity (see Table 15-1).

Antidepressant Medications

Antidepressants are the drugs most often used to treat depression. Commonly used antidepressants for the elderly include desipramine (Norpramin), doxepin (Sinequan) and nortriptyline (Aventyl, Pamelor). These antidepressants cause less hypotension in the elderly than other antidepressants. Nortriptyline is well tolerated in the elderly and is considered by some physicians to be the drug of choice for depression in the older adult. Desipramine causes fewer anticholinergic effects than other antidepressants. Older adults are particularly sensitive to anticholinergic effects such as dry mouth, difficulty in urinating, constipation, postural hypotension, and blurred vision. Fluoxetine (Prozac) is also used for depression in the elderly because it is well tolerated and has relatively few side effects. Common side effects of the antidepressants include sedation, anticholinergic effects, confusion (especially in older adults), diminished concentration, dry mouth, constipation, nausea, and orthostatic hypotension.

Antidepressants are given in small dosages and gradually increased according to the patient's response. Allow 3 to 4 weeks before expecting a response to drug therapy; the response may be delayed for up to 4 to 6 weeks in the elderly. Treatment must be given for a minimum of 4 to 6 weeks in older adults before determining the drug is ineffective. In conjunction with the administration of antidepressants, psychotherapy and group therapy may be used. The complete dosage regimen usually lasts up to 6 months after the depression subsides to prevent recurrence. Some clinicians view depression in the elderly as a chronic illness and treat it with long-term use of antidepressants.

Lithium

Lithium is used to treat the manic phase of bipolar disorder. Carefully monitor lithium blood levels in the elderly because a reduced renal clearance increases the risk for lithium toxicity. Lithium levels should be between 0.4 and 1.0 mEq/L. Signs and symptoms of lithium toxicity are listed on Table 15-1. Toxic symptoms may be seen with levels of 1.5 mEq/L or greater.

Lithium levels are monitored weekly for the first month of treatment, then every other week for 2 months, and then every 2 months. After stabilization, lithium levels are monitored three or four times per year or whenever signs or symptoms of toxicity are observed. If any signs or symptoms of toxicity are observed the lithium is discontinued and the physician is notified immediately.

Hopelessness

Hopelessness is a negative feeling or view about the future. The individual sees few or no alternatives or choices that cause optimism concerning the future. Display 15-5 identifies nursing interventions that foster hope.

Self-Care Deficit

Psychomotor retardation, lack of energy or lack of motivation brought on by depression causes the older adult to become passive and nonparticipative in daily self-care activities. Display 15-6 identifies nursing interventions that encourage self-care.

Impaired Social Interaction

With depression, there is a withdrawal from family, friends, or spouse. Failure to participate in social

TABLE 15-1. Signs of Lithium Toxicity

Lithium Level	Signs of Toxicity
1.5–2 mEq/L	Diarrhea, vomiting, nausea, drowsiness, muscular weakness, lack of coordination (early signs of toxicity)
2–3 mEq/L	Giddiness, ataxia, blurred vision, tinnitus, vertigo, increasing confusion, slurred speech, blackouts, myoclonic twitching or movement of entire limbs, choreo-athetoid movements, urinary or fecal incontinence, agitation or manic-like behavior, hyperreflexia, hypertonia, dysarthria
> 3 mEq/L	May produce a complex clinical picture involving multiple organs and organ systems, including seizures (generalized and focal), arrhythmias, hypotension, peripheral vascular collapse, stupor, muscle group twitching, spasticity, coma

From Scherer, J., & Roach, S. (1996). *Introductory clinical pharmacology.* Philadelphia: Lippincott-Raven, 213.

DISPLAY 15-5. Nursing Interventions That Foster Hope

- Encourage verbalization of thoughts and feelings.
- Actively listen.
- Use open-ended questions or statements such as "Tell me more about your feelings. . ." "Do you feel there is no hope that the future will improve?"
- Develop attainable goals.
- Correct incorrect beliefs about self or situations.
- Encourage a regular schedule of activity.
- Involve a chaplain or clergy, if requested.

DISPLAY 15-6. Nursing Interventions That Encourage Self-Care

- Initially, feed, bathe, and dress the patient. As improvement occurs, encourage more independence.
- Allow plenty of time for the performance of self-care activities. Do not hurry or rush the patient.
- Present tasks in small, achievable steps.
- Provide a supportive environment.
- Give encouragement when tasks are performed successfully.

DISPLAY 15-7. Nursing Interventions to Promote Social Interaction

- Identify support systems.
- Encourage visits from family members or friends, even if the patient does not seem to respond.
- Encourage verbalization with the nurse and others.
- Allow family members and friends to vent frustration.
- Encourage participation in social activities.
- Identify past interests and activities.
- Discuss new ways with the patient to form social relations.

activities leads to further depression, the depression leads to withdrawal, and a vicious cycle develops that must be broken to restore normal social interaction. Display 15-7 identifies nursing interventions to promote social interaction.

Evaluation and Expected Outcomes

Successful treatment may produce the following responses by the elderly person:
Expression of hope for the future
Engagement in social activities
Performance of self-care activities

SUICIDE

Older people are at increased risk for suicide. Even though older adults represent only 13% of the population, approximately 20% of suicides are attempted by those older than 65. More people older than age 65 commit suicide than any other age group. It is estimated that approximately 20,000 to 24,000 people age 65 or older attempt suicide each year. Older men, especially those older than 80 years have the highest risk for suicide. Factors that increase the risk of an elderly person committing suicide include loneliness, loss of a spouse, poverty or near poverty, poor health, and social isolation. Older adults may fear death, a prolonged death, becoming dependent, or cognitive loss. Depressed individuals and those who abuse alcohol and drugs are also at high risk for suicide. Individuals who feel hopeless about the future, live with physical or emotional pain, or who dwell on past failures may develop a suicidal ideation.

DISPLAY 15-8. Common Misunderstandings About Suicide

Myth	Truth
Asking people about their suicide thoughts makes them more likely to act on them.	Most patients are not afraid to talk about their thoughts of committing suicide and are usually grateful that someone is available and cares. Talking can reduce the sense of isolation.
All people who attempt suicide have a psychiatric disorder.	People can become overwhelmed with life circumstances without having a psychiatric disorder.
A person who talks about suicide won't do it.	Approximately 80% of individuals who attempt or complete suicide give some definite verbal or indirect clues. As many as 50% have seen their physician within the previous month, often with vague somatic complaints.
A person who attempts suicide won't try again.	Almost 75% of individuals who complete suicide have attempted it at least once before.
People who attempt suicide are always determined to die.	Many individuals are ambivalent and are using the suicide as a cry for help.
People who attempt suicide just want attention.	Even if the suicide attempt is manipulative, the individual may go on to complete the suicide.
As the person becomes less depressed, the risk of suicide decreases.	As the depression lifts, the individual's energy level can increase before feelings of hopelessness are relieved. Once the individual makes the decision that suicide is an effective solution to the problems, his or her mood may even elevate.

From Gorman, L., Sultan, D., & Raines, M. (1996). *Davis's manual of psychosocial nursing in general patient care.* Philadelphia: F.A. Davis, 133.

Suicidal ideation is persistent or recurring thoughts about harming oneself. Older adults suffering from depression or chronic illness, those with family history of suicide, those with patterns of impulsive behavior, and those with poor social support networks are at risk for suicide.

Older individuals do not verbalize the intent to commit suicide as often as younger adults, but they are more likely to be successful if suicide is attempted. Older adults also are at increased risk for passive suicide. **Passive suicide** occurs when an individual participates in activities that hasten death, such as noncompliance with medical treatments, refusal to eat, or self-neglect. Many misconceptions persist, even by nurses, concerning suicide. Display 15-8 clarifies the common misunderstandings about suicide.

Surviving family members and friends often feel great guilt along with the pain and anguish that accompanies any death. They feel guilty because they failed to observe the clues given by the victim before the suicide or because they were not available to prevent the suicide. This guilt can lead to complications in the grieving process. Dysfunctional grieving is discussed in a later section.

Assessing an Older Adult's Suicide Potential

In assessing for suicidal potential, question the individual about the desire to do self-harm. Be alert for statements such as "I won't be around much longer to cause problems" or "You can have my bracelet; I won't be needing it any more." Display 15-9 discusses suicide lethality.

PSYCHOSOCIAL ASPECTS OF NURSING: CLUES THAT AN INDIVIDUAL CONTEMPLATES SUICIDE

- Giving away personal items or prized possessions
- Any changes in sleeping or eating habits
- Expressing feelings of depression, hopelessness, or anxiety
- Irrational thinking
- Poor judgment
- Recent loss
- Social withdrawal
- Previous unsuccessful suicide attempts
- Discussing a specific method of suicide
- Having a chronic or terminal illness

ASSESSMENT ALERT

Frequently assess suicide potential in all patients who are depressed or anxious. Depression and anxiety increase the risk for suicide. Take any indication of not wanting to live or intention to do bodily harm seriously.

DISPLAY 15-9. **Suicide Lethality**

1. Do you think about hurting or killing yourself? If *yes:*
2. Do you have a plan? If *yes:* How have you considered doing it?
3. Do you think you may or will do something to act on your thoughts? If *yes:* Where and when? Do you feel you have control over your own behavior?
4. Do you have the means available (eg, rope, rolled-up sheet, gun, saved-up pills).
5. Have you ever tried to harm yourself in the past? If *yes:* How? Did you expect to survive?
6. Are you willing to contract or notify staff whenever you feel you may act on these thoughts?

   Our side of the contract is to be available and actively help during these times. **If the patient denies having a suicide plan, ask about other plans for the future and the support system.**

1. What do you see yourself doing in a week, in a month, a year from now?
2. Do you feel optimistic or pessimistic about the future?
3. Do you have family members or friends with whom you can freely discuss your problems?

From Gorman, L., Sultan, D., & Raines, M. (1996). *Davis's manual of phychosocial nursing in general patient care.* Philadelphia: FA Davis, 141.

DISPLAY 15-10. **Nursing Interventions for a Patient Considering Suicide and for Those at High Risk for Suicide**

- Establish a trusting relationship.
- Determine whether the patient thinks about suicide or has plan for suicide.
- Explore past methods of coping.
- Assist the patient in selecting alternate methods of coping.
- Actively listen as the patient expresses concerns, fears, and stresses.
- Encourage the expression of feelings such as anger, sadness, or disappointment.
- Refer to a support group such as Alcoholics Anonymous or Widow-to-Widow, if indicated.
- When caring for a patient at a high risk for suicide
  - Provide a supportive, nonthreatening atmosphere.
  - Determine the seriousness of the intent to commit suicide.
  - Write a No Suicide Contract in which the patient agrees to not attempt suicide without talking to a designated health care provider such as a nurse, counselor, or physician.
  - Remove all objects from the environment by which the patient can harm himself (eg, sharp objects, belts, razors, guns, medications).
  - Ascertain that the patient is not hoarding medication to be taken at a later date. Direct observation and inspection of the oral mucosa of the mouth may be necessary.
  - Provide frequent observation at unpredictable intervals.
  - Encourage social interaction with family and friends.
  - Follow agency policy for continuous supervision.

Assess all depressed individuals for the seriousness of their intent to commit suicide. Asking the older adult or any depressed individual if she has contemplated suicide does not increase the risk of her committing the act. It is particularly important for nurses working in outpatient clinics, adult day care centers, and other outpatient settings to be alert for suicidal clues.

Caring for an Older Adult At Risk for Suicide

Nursing care for the patient who is at risk for suicide requires constant monitoring and care. These patients are most often under the care of a psychiatrist. Frequent contact with health care provider is important and transfer to a psychiatric facility is usually indicated. Display 15-10 identifies nursing interventions that are appropriate for a patient considering suicide as a coping mechanism.

GRIEF

Grief is intense feelings or emotions experienced as the result of a loss. Older adults face multiple losses. The more years they live, the more losses they must face. Examples of losses that may occur in an older person's life includes loss of a parent, a mate, siblings, or personal health. Grief is highly individualized, and people pass through grief at their own pace. At times, grief may be intense but short lived. At other times, the grief is intense and extremely painful.

When a person loses someone or something he has an emotional attachment to, feelings of grief result. Grief is characterized by intense emotional pain, sorrow, weeping, and despair. Although grief is most often associated with the death of a loved one, intense grief can occur after retirement, a move to another home, a chronic illness, or any change in a life situation. The loss of a spouse has the most profound effect on an older adult's life. An older adult must also find meaning in life and accept the reality of his own death.

Anticipatory grief is a type of grief that occurs with the expectation of a significant loss. The individual sees the loss as inevitable and begins to grieve before the loss actually occurs.

Normal grief generally lasts from 6 months to 2 years. During normal grief, the individual must accept the reality of the loss, experience the pain of the loss, adjust to an environment without the lost object, and reinvest in life. Grief is not a series of well-organized steps, with one phase following another. Rather, the individual goes in and out of the different phases of grief and emotions ebb and flow. Reinvesting in life is the last phase and must be accomplished for the grieving process to be complete. For some older adults, the pain of the loss of a spouse is so great reinvesting in life is difficult and sometimes does not occur at all. The nurse's responsibility is to assist the person through the grieving process without the development of dysfunctional grief.

Dysfunctional grief refers to grief that is delayed, prolonged, or inappropriate. Grief that completely absorbs an individual, resulting in the inability to reinvest in life, is dysfunctional. Dysfunctional grief can result in self-destructive behavior, social isolation, extreme physiologic distress, or severe depression.

Assessment of an Older Adult Experiencing Grief

When assessing an individual who is experiencing a loss expect feelings of sadness, anxiety, numbness, shock, and helplessness. Physical symptoms such as fatigue, tightness in the chest or throat, or muscular weakness may be present. The individual may cry, have difficulty sleeping, or have a lack of appetite. In the elderly, grief can be hidden by alcohol, substance abuse, or dementia. Question the individuals about the death, how long ago it occurred, the relationship with the deceased, and physical and emotional symptoms experienced. Grief that is prolonged or so intense that it interferes with daily life may require intervention.

DISPLAY 15-11. What to Say to Someone Who is Grieving

When caring for someone who has lost a loved one, specific questions and phrases can help him express his feelings:

- "I'm sorry for your loss."
- "Tell me how you're feeling."
- "Were you there when _____ (name of loved one) died? What was that like for you?"
- "Tell me about _____ (name of loved one) and your life with her."
- "What special memories do you have?"

Keep in mind that you do not always have to say something. Sometimes, your presence alone can be as therapeutic as verbal communication. Crying with the family member and touching him on the hand, arm, shoulder, or back is also acceptable, when appropriate, and shows your compassion.

Do not say things just to make yourself feel better or more comfortable around the bereaved. Avoid using clichés and other common phrases that may not be true or appropriate:

- "I know just how you feel."
- "Her death was for the best."
- "It was God's will. He never gives us more than we can handle."
- "Things will get better."
- "Time heals all wounds."
- "Now you have an angel in heaven watching over you."

From Wheeler, S.R. (1996). Helping families cope with death and dying. *Nursing 96, 26 (7)*, 28. Used with permission.

Caring for the Older Adult Experiencing Grief

People often need only to have reassurance that the emotions and thoughts they are experiencing are normal expressions of grief that will pass in time. Display 15-11 describes what to do for someone who is grieving. This can alleviate any anxiety, allowing the full expression of grief. When the grief is freely expressed, readjustment to life as it is now, without the loved one, occurs. However, if reinvestment in life does not occur, if loneliness is severe, or if grief becomes dysfunctional, intervention by a geriatric clinical nurse specialist or psychiatric nurse may be necessary.

Loneliness

It is natural to be lonely after the loss of a loved one or when adjusting to the loss of a particular life situation. Sometimes, the individual needs encouragement to

DISPLAY 15-12. Interventions That Help Overcome Loneliness

- Develop a trusting nurse-patient relationship.
- Recognize that it takes time to adjust to loss.
- Use supportive comments to encourage verbalization.
- Acknowledge the loneliness.
- Encourage involvement in social activity.
- Help to develop new social support systems.
- Capitalize on support systems (family members and friends) already in place.
- Identify interests and give encouragement to try new activities.

DISPLAY 15-14. Nursing Interventions for a Patient With Dysfunctional Grief

- Develop a trusting relationship.
- Encourage the individual to confront the loss.
- Ask open-ended questions to allow the expression of feelings.
- Encourage the individual to relive past memories and discuss the loss.
- Involve clergy, chaplain, or other spiritual leaders if requested.
- Report any unusual or disturbing behavior such as hallucinations, delusions, or illusions.
- Report any suspicions of alcohol or drug abuse.
- Encourage attendance at a bereavement support group.

overcome the loneliness and reinvest in life. Interventions that help to overcome loneliness are identified in Display 15-12.

Anticipatory Grief

The older adult may experience anticipatory grief when a loved one is faced with a terminal illness or even when faced with the inevitability of his own death. With anticipatory grief, the individual acknowledges the potential loss and expresses those feelings associated with the loss. Display 15-13 identifies nursing interventions that assist the individual with anticipatory grief.

Dysfunctional Grief

Because the grief process is individualistic, dysfunctional grief is sometimes difficult to detect. With

DISPLAY 15-13. Nursing Interventions for Anticipatory Grief

- Encourage the individual to discuss the positive and negative feelings about the anticipated loss.
- Be supportive.
- Actively listen as the patient discusses feelings.
- Use open-ended questions to encourage verbalization.
- Allow the expression of sadness, anger, or intense pain.
- Recognize that some hope may be needed. Do not foster inappropriate hope. Discuss normal grief response.
- Encourage the use of a life review.
- Discuss what to expect when the loss occurs.

dysfunctional grief, the grief is more intense or prolonged. In certain situations, the grief may be denied. When dysfunctional grief is suspected, the nurse should notify the physician or primary care provider. Display 15-14 identifies nursing interventions for a patient with dysfunctional grief.

SUBSTANCE ABUSE

The elderly, like any other age group, engage in substance abuse. Substance abuse can result from the use of alcohol, prescribed medications, over-the-counter (OTC) medications or illicit drug use. Substance abuse occurs when the individual develops recurrent and significant adverse reactions related to the use of the substance. Adverse reactions may be related to alcohol-drug interactions or may be of a social nature. Problems of a social nature include failure to maintain role obligations, interpersonal or family problems, social isolation, or repeated episodes of intoxication. Alcohol abuse is of particular concern in the older adult.

Alcohol Abuse

Although most elderly people cope well with the stresses brought about as a result of aging, a significant number are using alcohol as a coping mechanism. Approximately one third of older alcoholics begin drinking heavily after the age of 60. Some of the elderly population have abused alcohol for many years, and their problem with alcohol is known.

However, many elderly are reactive drinkers. **Reactive drinkers** are those who begin heavy drinking as a reaction to a specific stressor that occurs with age, such as the death of a spouse, retirement, or health problems. These abusers may be more difficult to detect. Reactive drinkers are usually not working, live alone, have few social contacts, and most often have infrequent contact with family members. Alcoholism that occurs in this manner may go undetected. However, once detected, this type of drinker usually responds well to therapy.

Alcohol is a central nervous system depressant that is mind altering and mood altering. Symptoms of alcohol abuse include mood swings, anxiety, depression, social withdrawal, sleep disturbances, gait disturbances, frequent nausea and vomiting, or tremors of the hands, trunk, or head. These symptoms may be attributed to medical problems (eg, dementia, parkinsonism, electrolyte imbalance) or to "old age."

Effects of Alcohol in the Aging Adult

The older adult has an increased sensitivity to the effects of alcohol resulting in decreased tolerance for alcohol. This means lower levels of alcohol consumption can result in intoxication. With age, the metabolic rate usually slows down, causing alcohol and other drugs to remain in the body longer. This increases the risk of alcohol intoxication. Alcohol's effects on the brain can mimic the cognitive changes that occur with some of the more common disorders of aging. Because alcoholism can be mistaken for dementia, alcoholism can be difficult to detect. Even a moderate intake of alcohol can cause gait problems, forgetfulness, disorientation, and frequent falls. Depression is also associated with increased use of alcohol. Another significant problem can occur as the result of combining alcohol with prescription and OTC drugs.

Most older adults regularly take one or more prescription drugs along with OTC drugs, increasing the potential for an alcohol-drug interaction. For example, sedatives, hypnotics, antidepressants, or antianxiety drugs combined with alcohol result in additive central nervous system depressant effects.

Two conditions can develop in later life as a result of excessive alcohol consumption: Korsakoff syndrome and Wernicke encephalopathy. **Korsakoff syndrome** is a type of amnesia seen in chronic alcoholics. The individual with Korsakoff syndrome has a loss of short-term memory and has difficulty learning new information or skills. This individual is disoriented and confabulates (ie, fills in memory gaps with inappropriate words). **Wernicke encephalopathy** is an inflammatory degenerative condition of the brain resulting in double vision, poor muscle coordination, and decreased mental functioning. Wernicke encephalopathy and Korsakoff syndrome are associated with a thiamine (vitamin B_1) deficiency and with chronic alcoholism.

Assessing for Alcohol Abuse in the Older Adult

A careful and thoughtful nursing assessment is vital when working with geriatric patients to correctly identify the problem of alcohol abuse. Question the older adult and family members about alcohol consumption, amount of alcohol consumed, and where consumption occurs (ie, alone, socially, or with certain individuals). Assess gait, level of consciousness, unexplained bruises or burns, sleep disturbances, or any alteration of mood. Note any trembling of the hand, trunk, or head. Appearance may be unkempt, sloppy, or normal.

Be alert for any family member who wants to ignore the problem. Sometimes, family members or friends want to ignore alcohol abuse in the older adult. They may say, "It's her only pleasure in life; why take it away?" or "He has been drinking for years; he won't give it up." These individuals can sabotage any efforts by health care providers to curb the abuse. Discuss the need for intervention and assure the family that it is not too late to deal with abusive behaviors. Reactive drinkers respond particularly well to intervention.

Assess the individual for other symptoms of alcohol abuse such as anxiety, depression, low self-esteem, unhappiness, anger, hurt, guilt, hostility, or loneliness. Assess for signs of intoxication (eg, smell of alcohol, slurred speech, poor judgment, unsteady gait). Of particular importance in dealing with the older adult is to question about recent losses or changes in lifestyle.

Caring for the Older Adult Who Abuses Alcohol

In planning the care of those who abuse alcohol, avoid a judgmental attitude that adds to the abuser's guilt and shame. Do not discuss issues if the individual is intoxicated, sedated, or confused. Avoid using the word *addict* or *alcoholic* when talking to the resident or the patient. Treatment options to maintain abstinence include Alcoholics Anonymous (AA), behavioral therapy, support groups, and disulfiram (Antabuse) therapy. AA is a self-help group that is beneficial in assisting the individual to deal with the problem of alcohol abuse, abstain from alcohol, and obtain support. AA has an effective 12-step program that can provide a framework for personal change. Display 15-15 identifies interventions for

---

DISPLAY 15-15. Nursing Interventions to Assist the Patient Abusing Alcohol to Cope More Effectively

- Explore the reasons for drinking.
- Discuss the negative effects of the drinking.
- Encourage the use of stress management techniques such as relaxation, imagery, and meditation (see Chapter 11).
- Discuss alternate methods of coping.
- Determine the availability of support systems.
- Provide factual information regarding the effects of alcohol.
- Encourage attendance at Alcoholic Anonymous meetings or other appropriate support groups.
- Refer to a physician or a chemical dependency counselor.

---

the nurse in assisting a patient who is abusing alcohol to cope more effectively.

Altered Family Process: Alcoholism

The entire family is usually involved in the development and continuation of alcoholism, particularly if the drinking has been going on for some time. Older adults may have had a lifetime of alcohol abuse or may begin drinking intemperately with age. The reactive drinker may be drinking only as a coping mechanism for a specific loss associated with age such as retirement, loss of a spouse, loneliness, or chronic illness. For example, the older adult may be caring for a mate who has a chronic disease such as Alzheimer's disease. Alcohol may be a means of coping with a difficult situation. If the person began drinking late in life and is a reactive drinker, the family may not be involved. Nursing care may involve determining individual strengths and weakness. Individuals can be helped to identify ways to cope in a more positive manner. Attendance at self-help groups such as AA and Al-Anon should be encouraged.

ELDER ABUSE AND NEGLECT

Elder abuse is neither rare nor isolated. It is relatively widespread and takes several forms. The incidence of elder abuse appears to have risen within the past several years. This increase is thought to be due partially to the increase in the number of elderly people, particularly the frail elderly. More attention has been given to the problem of elder abuse than in

past years. The stress of caring for older parents falls on fewer children than in past generations, and these children are busy with their own lives and personal stresses.

Risk Factors

The following acronym has been suggested to detect certain behaviors in individuals that are at increased risk for elder abuse:

S (stress)
A (alcohol or other substance of abuse)
V (violence)
E (emotion and family dynamics)
D (dependency)

Abusers are usually family members and often live with the elderly person. The abuser is frequently under stress, has financial problems, or is an alcoholic or drug abuser. Most abusers have been the recipients of violent acts themselves. Abused at an earlier point in their lives, the abuser deals with stress and the dependency needs of the older adult by inflicting abuse.

Dependency of the older adult on the abuser increases the risk for abuse, particularly if the family members have inappropriate coping methods. Family dynamics may be dysfunctional with a history of maladaptive coping. Social isolation makes it more difficult to observe the abuse or observe the effects of the abuse. With social isolation, the older adult is less likely to have someone with whom to reveal the abuse.

The elderly person may not be able to face the fact that a family member is abusive and may deny the problem. For example, an elderly woman whose grandson regularly took her social security check for alcohol and drugs refused to acknowledge the occurrence. She continually blamed a neighbor for "stealing that check out of my mailbox."

Caregivers of the elderly needing physical care sometimes do not know how to care for the elderly person. For example, a granddaughter caring for her aging grandmother who was unable to get out of bed did not turn her or reposition her regularly because her grandmother did not want to move. As a result, the grandmother developed large pressure ulcers on both hips. The granddaughter did not want Granny to have "to move if she did not want to."

Types of Abuse

Abuse is defined as *willfully* inflicting physical or mental pain, unjustifiable confinement or deliberately withholding care to an elderly person. **Neglect**

refers to an elderly person who is not able to provide for himself the services necessary to maintain health or is not receiving these services from the caregiver. The distinction is the lack of desire or intent (ie, willingness) of the caregiver to provide care to the individual.

Elder abuse or neglect takes at least seven forms:

Self-neglect: neglecting to care for self, most often because of depression, dementia, or lack of resources

Passive neglect: caregiver not providing adequate care because of lack of knowledge, skills, or physical ability

Active neglect: deliberately not caring for an elderly person

Financial abuse: unauthorized use of money or property of an elderly person

Physical abuse: inflicting physical pain or injury (eg, physical restraints, hitting, slapping, kicking, biting, pinching)

Psychological abuse: emotional or mental abuse, including belittling, ridiculing, name calling, isolating, and saying things to frighten an older adult

Sexual abuse: abuse of a sexual nature including sexual harassment, sexual coercion, or sexual assault

The problem of elder abuse is complicated by lack of a consensus on the definition of abuse and laws that vary from state to state. Depending on the laws of a given state, elder abuse may or may not be considered a crime. Most states consider physical, sexual, and financial abuse crimes. However, emotional abuse and self-neglect may or may not be a crime. Most instances of reported abuse are in the area of self-neglect.

Institutional Abuse

Another tragic form of abuse occurs in nursing homes, long-term care facilities, or any institutions entrusted with the care of the older adult. Nurses or nurse assistants may neglect elderly residents, speak in an abusive manner, or steal belongings or money from the elderly. This is abuse and this type of behavior must not be tolerated under any circumstance. Any suspicion of abuse or neglect from a health care worker must be reported and investigated thoroughly. The elderly are one of our most fragile populations, and nurses working with the elderly must have a commitment to care and protect these individuals.

Residents at the greatest risk for institutional abuse or neglect include residents with dementia, residents who seldom have visitors, terminally ill residents, residents who cannot communicate (eg, those who are aphasic or speak a different language), and residents who require total care.

Nurses working in institutions responsible for caring for the elderly must provide nursing assistants and other ancillary staff in close contact with the older adult with information and training to deal with any inclination toward abuse. Nursing assistants must be encouraged to report any instances of abuse witnessed. The nurse assistant has the most direct contact with the resident and is the health care worker with the greatest opportunity to engage in abusive behaviors. Through care conferences, inservice education, or staff development, nursing assistants can be given information on what types of behaviors constitute abuse and how to handle stressful situations with residents.

Using the Nursing Process in Caring for an Abused Elderly Person

Assessment

Regardless of the form of abuse, nurses must be knowledgeable about the signs of abuse to detect its occurrence. This is not an easy task, because neither the abuser nor the one abused wishes to discuss the problem. More often than not, the nurse must look for subtle clues that indicate the abuse. Abuse may be suspected if any of the following indicators are present. The elderly person may be abused if she is

Excessively compliant or exhibits fear of the caregiver

Malnourished

Bruised (especially trunk, buttocks, or upper arms), burned, or has pressure sores

Found to have multiple bruises in various stages of healing

Unkempt (eg, is unclean, has body odor, shows signs of poor hygiene, has inadequate clothing)

Lacking medical attention

Verbalizing the lack of care

The abuser may live with the victim, may have a problem with alcohol, or speak with disrespect. An unusual or strange explanation for injuries may be offered. There may be a history of repeated visits to the hospital or the emergency department for unexplained injuries.

Nursing Diagnoses

The following nursing diagnoses may be appropriate for a situation in which an elderly person is being abused or there is suspicion of abuse:

Caregiver Role Strain related to financial siltation, loss of job, other (specify)

Ineffective Family Coping related to abuse of parent or other family member, other (specify)

DISPLAY 15-16. Nursing Interventions When Elder Abuse is Suspected

- Develop a trusting relationship with the elderly person.
- Examine patient for unexplained bruises, burns, or other injuries.
- Identify alternate support systems.
- Carefully document and consider taking pictures of wounds or injuries.
- Observe and document inappropriate family interactions, such as avoidance or fear of family members and expression of concern when family members or the caregiver takes money or property.
- Document any evidence of malnutrition, inadequate care, poor hygiene, etc.
- Make appropriate community referrals to support services, such as day care or home health.
- Report suspected abuse to a supervisor, physician, and social service agencies such as Adult Protective Service or police or sheriff's department (if indicated).

Other nursing diagnoses may be appropriate for specific abusive situations.

Planning and Implementation

Implementing a plan of care may be difficult because of the resistance of the abuser and the abused. The person abused is reluctant to cooperate with health care providers and to confirm the abuse because of fear of reprisal or abandonment. Reporting the abuse to the appropriate agency is sometimes the only option. Specific nursing interventions depend on the type of abuse, the victim's response, and individual characteristics of the abuser. In situations where the victim refuses assistance the only recourse may be to document the incident, report the suspected abuse, and, if possible, monitor the situation. Display 15-16 identifies nursing interventions when elder abuse is suspected.

When families are unable to cope in appropriate ways or to handle the stresses brought on by a current situation, the older adult may become the target for abuse. Family members may feel guilt, anger, or hostility that causes them to act out toward the victim. In abusive situations, family coping mechanisms are ineffective. The caregiver may have an extremely low self-esteem and seek to enhance his feelings of power and control by abusive behavior. The nurse can assist in the development of alternate coping mechanism by using the interventions identified in Display 15-17.

DISPLAY 15-17. Nursing Interventions to Assist the Patient in Developing Alternate Coping Mechanisms

- Establish a trusting relationship with the abuser and the victim.
- Talk with the suspected abuser and the victim separately.
- Talk with other family members, if possible.
- Determine the ability of the abuser to act as a caregiver.
- If a situation is out of control or the environment is unsafe, remove the older adult from the situation.
- Recognize that altered mental status on the part of the older adult can result in false accusations.
- Explore ways that the older adult can be more independent.
- Explore alternate methods of coping.
- Suggest the use of the problem-solving technique to find solutions (see Chapter 25).

The caregiver may not have enough resources to provide the needed care, or he may resent the care needed by the older adult and see it as an intrusion in his life. In addition to the interventions suggested in the previous section, the interventions identified in Display 15-18 may be helpful for caregiver role strain. Determine the need for additional resources such as counseling or psychotherapy.

Evaluation and Expected Outcomes

Successful treatment can be gauged by the following responses:

Abuser seeks professional help.
More effective coping techniques are demonstrated.
Abuse is no longer occurring.

DISPLAY 15-18. Nursing Interventions for Caregiver Role Strain

- Acknowledge positive accomplishments of the caregivers.
- Assess stress level of caregiver.
- Determine if alcohol is used to handle stress.
- Encourage expressions of feelings, especially anger and hostility.
- Explore stress reduction techniques.
- Provide respite care, if available and if indicated.
- Suggest ways to manage stressful situations such as referral to a financial planning service if money management is a problem or referral to social services for help in finding alternate ways to care for the older adult.

CRITICAL THINKING EXERCISES

1. As a nurse working in a nursing facility, you are asked to plan an in-service education program for the nursing assistants. The topic is elder abuse. What information would be most important to include? What are six examples of elder abuse you could give the nurse assistants?

2. Mr. Whitmore, age 75, is a resident in the nursing facility where you work. His wife of 40 years died 2 months ago. Since that time, he has been moody and easily irritated. Other nurses and some of the residents have tried to comfort him, but he avoids them and spends as much time as possible in his room. What assessments would be most important for you to make? What interventions would be most helpful for Mr. Whitmore?

3. Mr. Carpenter, age 80, has not been to the senior citizen's center all week. He was recently diagnosed with prostate cancer. He gave one of the men at the center his watch and said, "I will not be needing it anymore." As a nurse, what is your responsibility to Mr. Carpenter? What additional information would you need to know? What would you do to help Mr. Carpenter?

4. Ms. Parker, age 78, came to the emergency department with her son. She is wearing soiled clothing and appears malnourished. X-ray films reveal that Ms. Parker has a fracture of the right ulna. An assessment reveals multiple bruises on her trunk and upper arms that her son attributes to frequent falls. What additional assessments should you, as a nurse, make? Would you talk with Ms. Parker's son? If so, what should you ask? How could this situation be handled?

REFERENCES AND SUGGESTED READING

Antai-Otong, D. (1995). Helping the alcoholic patient recover. *American Journal of Nursing, 95 (8),* 22–30.

Arino-Norris, N. (1997). Nursing rounds: Sexual concerns after an MI. *American Journal of Nursing, 97 (8),* 48–49.

American Psychiatric Association. (1994). *Diagnostic and statistical manual of mental disorders* (4th ed.). Washington DC: American Psychiatric Association.

Ellner, L. (1997). Reflections: What grandma Clara wanted. *American Journal of Nursing, 97 (8),* 51.

Gorman, L.M., Sultan, D.F., & Raines, M.L. (1996). *Davis's manual of psychosocial nursing for general patient care.* Philadelphia: F.A. Davis.

Isaacs, A. (1998). Depression and your patient. *American Journal of Nursing, 98 (7),* 255.

Reynolds, C.F. (1995). Recognition and differentiation of elderly depression in the clinical setting. *Geriatrics, 50* (Suppl 1), S6–15.

Roach, S., & Nieto, B. (1996). *Healing and the grief process.* Albany, NY: Delmar Publishers.

Robie, D. (1999). Suicide prevention protocol. *American Journal of Nursing, 99 (12),* 53.

Smith-Stoner, M., & Frost, A. (1998). Coping with grief and loss: Bringing your shadow self into the light. *Nursing 98, 28 (2),* 48–50.

CHAPTER **16**

The Integumentary System

CHAPTER OUTLINE

KEY TERMS
CHAPTER OBJECTIVES
AGE-RELATED CHANGES IN THE INTEGUMENTARY
    SYSTEM
PRESSURE ULCERS
SKIN CANCER
COMMON DISORDERS AFFECTING THE SKIN
CRITICAL THINKING EXERCISES
REFERENCES AND SUGGESTED READING

KEY TERMS

actinic keratosis

autolytic débridement

basal cell carcinoma

débridement

dermatitis

dextranomers

epithelization

herpes zoster

integumentary system

intertrigo

lentigo senilis

malignant melanoma

melanin

pressure ulcer

psoriasis

scabies

seborrheic dermatitis

senilis purpura

squamous cell carcinoma

stasis ulcer

stasis dermatitis

xerosis

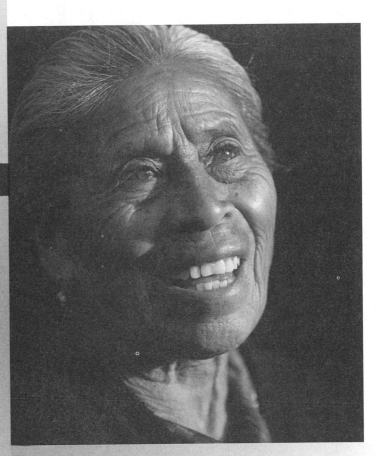

CHAPTER OBJECTIVES

At the completion of this chapter, the student will
be able to

- Discuss age-related changes to the
  integumentary system

- Identify the four stages of a pressure ulcer

- Discuss ways to prevent pressure ulcers

- Discuss ways to assess, manage, and evaluate
  pressure ulcers

- Discuss the three basic types of skin cancer

- Identify nursing interventions for protection
  and detection of skin cancer

- Identify common skin lesions and disorders
  affecting the skin

The **integumentary system** includes the skin and its appendages such as hair, nails, sweat glands, and sebaceous glands. Although age-related changes occur in almost every body system, the changes that occur in the integumentary are often the most apparent because they affect the individual's outward appearance.

The skin is the largest organ of the body and consists of two layers, the epidermis (outermost layer) and the dermis (fibrous inner layer). The dermis is the true skin and is well supplied with blood vessels and nerves. The thickness of the dermis and epidermis varies. For example, thick layers of skin cover the soles of the feet and the palms of the hands, but the eyelids are covered with exceptionally thin layers of skin. Under the dermis lies the subcutaneous layer that consists of connective tissue and adipose (fat) tissue. The subcutaneous layer is composed of an outer fatty layer and an inner elastic layer. Between the two layers are the superficial blood vessels, nerves, and sweat glands. Appendages of the skin include the hair, nails, sweat glands, and sebaceous glands. Figure 16-1 shows a cross section of the skin.

Melanin is the major pigment of the skin and is found in the hair, skin, and eye. Melanin is a black or brown pigment and is responsible for the darker coloring found in some individuals. For example, dark-skinned people have more melanin than fair-skinned people.

AGE-RELATED CHANGES IN THE INTEGUMENTARY SYSTEM

Changes to the integumentary system related to aging are often dramatic and easily identified. Other changes are subtle and go largely unrecognized. Age-related changes are found in all parts of the integumentary system—the skin, hair, nails, sweat glands, and sebaceous glands.

Skin

With age, the skin loses the ability to retain moisture and becomes dry and scaly. This condition is called **xerosis**. Xerosis is often accompanied by itching (ie, pruritus) and flaking of the skin. A decrease in production of certain hormones such as estrogen and progesterone contributes to drying and thinning of the skin.

The epidermis thins with age, causing the appearance of the skin to be pale and somewhat translucent.

The melanocytes (ie, cells that produce melanin) decrease in number, reducing the amount of melanin in the skin and contributing to the increased paleness of the skin. Localized areas of extra pigmentation result in the formation of brown spots called age spots, liver spots, or **lentigo senilis.** Lentigo senilis occurs most often on the dorsal portion of the hands, the face, arms, and legs. The most significant skin changes are found in the areas exposed to ultraviolet light on a regular basis. There is a generalized increase in the occurrence of benign (noncancerous) and malignant (cancerous) skin lesions with age.

Age decreases the number of blood vessels available to supply the skin with needed nutrients. Vessels are more fragile, resulting in the occurrence of **senilis purpura** (ie, hemorrhagic areas under the skin) and other vascular lesions such as cherry angiomas.

Subcutaneous tissue decreases, contributing to wrinkling. This wrinkling is particularly noticeable on the face. Creases and lines appear on the face in areas of expression and use. Frown lines and crow's feet (ie, fan-shaped wrinkles at the corners of the eye) appear as well. Ptosis (ie, drooping of the eyelids) can occur as the result of weakened musculature and loss of subcutaneous tissue around the eyes.

Hair and Nails

Hair follicles become less active and do not replace themselves as efficiently as when younger, causing hair to thin. The hair in the axilla and pubic area also thin. Women, however, may develop facial hair on the chin or above the lip because of hormonal changes. Hair loss occurs in an orderly fashion from the peripheral part of the body to the center of the body. Hair thickens in the nose and ears. Balding patterns in men develop from the center of the scalp to the sides. Women also may develop male-pattern baldness. Decreased production of melanin causes the hair to become gray.

Decreased vascular access causes nails to become brittle and thick. Longitudinal lines may appear, and growth of the nails is slower. Toenails become particularly thickened, and debris can accumulate under the nail, leading to fungal infections.

Sweat and Sebaceous Glands

The sweat and sebaceous glands atrophy, decreasing the skin's ability to provide lubrication. Sweat glands decrease in number, reducing the amount of perspiration. Lack of sweating under the arms (ie, axillae) and in the groin area is a normal finding in

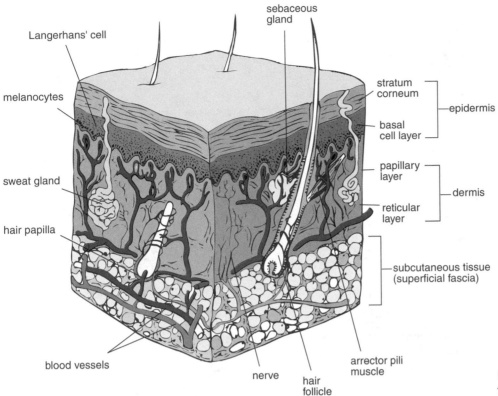

FIGURE 16-1. Cross section of the skin.

aging persons and does not indicate dehydration. The sebaceous glands secrete sebum through the hair follicles. Although the sebaceous glands increase in size with age, their functional ability decreases, and less sebum is secreted. The decreased production of sebum contributes to the generalized drying of the skin.

PRESSURE ULCERS

Pressure ulcers are areas of unrelieved pressure that result in damage to the underlying tissue and the development of skin lesions. Other commonly used terms include decubitus ulcer, pressure sore, and bed sore. All elderly patients, particularly those who are immobile, are at risk for pressure ulcers. This type of ulcer can develop on any area of unrelieved pressure, but bony prominences are at greater risk. Figure 16-2 illustrates areas at greatest risk for developing a pressure ulcer. Pressure ulcers require careful assessment and diligent care for healing to occur.

Staging

A system of staging is used to classify the extent of tissue damage in pressure ulcers. The following staging system is recommended by the National Pressure Ulcer Advisory Panel Consensus Development Conference (NPUAP) for pressure ulcers:

Stage I: Skin remains intact, but nonblanchable erythema (ie, redness) is evident. Other indications are warmth, edema, and induration (ie, hardness). Discoloration of the skin is found in persons with darker skin.

Stage II: A superficial ulcer is present that can be described as an abrasion, blister, or shallow crater. There is partial-thickness skin loss of the epidermis, dermis, or both.

Stage III: Full-thickness skin loss with damage to the subcutaneous tissue up to the underlying fascia. Necrosis may occur. The ulcer may appear as a deep crater with or without damage to the underlying tissue.

Stage IV: Ulcers exhibit full-thickness skin loss with extensive damage to muscle, bone, or support structures such as tendons. Sinus tract involvement may occur. Tissue necrosis may also be evident.

Staging is useful in the identification and treatment of pressure ulcers.

Preventing Pressure Ulcers

When body tissue is exposed to pressure, friction, or shear (ie, force on the skin parallel to the body's sur-

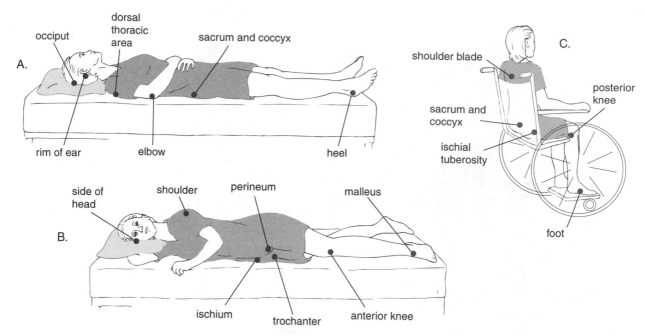

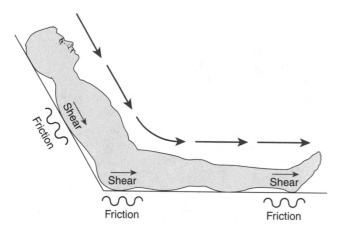

FIGURE 16-2. Areas of greatest risk for developing pressure ulcers. From Craven R.F. & Hirnle C.J. *Fundamentals of Nursing: Human Health and Function.* Philadelphia: J.B. Lippincott, 1992. Used with permission.

FIGURE 16-3. Example of shear and friction. As the individual slides or slips down in bed, the body resists this movement, resulting in *friction. Shearing* occurs when one layer of tissue slides over another layer of skin, disrupting the microcirculation of the skin and subcutaneous tissue.

face), tissue health is compromised, and a pressure ulcer can develop (Fig. 16-3). To prevent pressure ulcers, interventions are planned that decrease pressure on the underlying tissue and support a good blood supply to the area. Display 16-1 identifies interventions to prevent pressure ulcers.

Assessing Pressure Ulcers

Careful assessment of the pressure ulcer is critical to plan care of the ulcer. Determine the stage of the

---

DISPLAY 16-1. Nursing Interventions for Prevention of Pressure Ulcers

- Do not position immobile individuals directly on the trochanter (ie, bony process at the upper end of the femur).
- Use pillows or foam wedges to raise the heels off the bed.
- Keep the head of the bed at the lowest elevation for the shortest period.
- Avoid direct pressure on bony prominences.
- Check areas at risk every 2 to 3 hours for redness that does not subside within 30 minutes after repositioning.
- Use seat cushions instead of donut-type devices. Avoid the use of donut-type cushions (ring cushions), because these cushions cause venous congestion and edema, increasing the risk of developing pressure ulcers.
- Reposition sitting individuals at a minimum of every hour.
- Instruct patients who sit to shift their weight every 15 to 20 minutes (see Chapter 4) or if adequate upper body strength is present have them do wheelchair push-ups every 15 to 20 minutes.
- Use pillows or foam to prevent contact between the bony prominences of the knees or ankles.
- Do not position on the great trochanter. Position with patient in a side-lying position at approximately a 30-degree angle using a foam wedge for support.
- Turn and reposition every 1 to 1.5 hours.
- Monitor all patients with pressure ulcers for the development of additional pressure ulcers.

Sample Pressure Ulcer Assessment Guide

Patient Name: _____   Date: _____   Time: _____

Ulcer 1:			Ulcer 2:		
Site _____			Site _____		
Stage[a] _____			Stage[a] _____		
Size (cm)			Size (cm)		
Length _____			Length _____		
Width _____			Width _____		
Depth _____	No	Yes	Depth _____	No	Yes
Sinus Tract	☐	☐	Sinus Tract	☐	☐
Tunneling	☐	☐	Tunneling	☐	☐
Undermining	☐	☐	Undermining	☐	☐
Necrotic Tissue	☐	☐	Necrotic Tissue	☐	☐
Slough	☐	☐	Slough	☐	☐
Eschar	☐	☐	Eschar	☐	☐
Exudate	☐	☐	Exudate	☐	☐
Serous	☐	☐	Serous	☐	☐
Serosanuineous	☐	☐	Serosanuineous	☐	☐
Purulent	☐	☐	Purulent	☐	☐
Granulation	☐	☐	Granulation	☐	☐
Epithelialization	☐	☐	Epithelialization	☐	☐
Pain	☐	☐	Pain	☐	☐

Surrounding Skin:					
Erythema	☐	☐	Erythema	☐	☐
Maceration	☐	☐	Maceration	☐	☐
Induration	☐	☐	Induration	☐	☐
Description of Ulcer(s):					

Indicate Ulcer Sites:

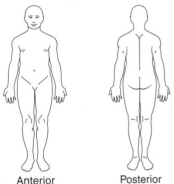

Anterior   Posterior

(Attach a color photo of the pressure ulcer(s) (Optional)

[a]Classification of pressure ulcers:

Stage I: Nonblanchable erythema of intact skin, the heralding lesion of skin ulceration. In individuals with darker skin, discoloration of the skin, warmth, edema, induration, or hardness may also be indicators.

Stage II: Partial thickness skin loss involving epidermis, dermis or both.

Stage III: Full thickness skin loss involving damage to or necrosis of subcutaneous tissue that may extend down to, but not through, underlying fascia. The ulcer presents clinically as a deep crater with or without undermining adjacent tissue.

Stage IV: Full thickness skin loss with extensive destruction, tissue necrosis, or damage to muscle, bone, or supporting structures (*e.g.*, tendon or joint capsule).

FIGURE 16-4. Sample pressure ulcer assessment guide. Bertstrom, N., Bennett, M.A., Carlson, C.E. et al. *Treatment of Pressure Ulcers.* Clinical Practice Guideline No. 15. Rockville, MD: U.S. Department of Health and Human Services Public Health Service Agency for Health Care Policy and Research. AHCPR Publication No. 95–0652, December 1994.

ulcer using the staging method discussed in the previous section. In addition to staging, the ulcer is assessed for size (ie, length, width, and depth), tunneling (ie, passageways under the skin), drainage (ie, color and odor), and the presence of necrotic tissue. Figure 16-4 illustrates a sample pressure

ulcer assessment guide. Whenever possible, take a color photo of the pressure ulcer, and place it in the chart to monitor progress.

A nutritional assessment is important in managing pressure ulcers. Dietary intake, weight, hydration, and laboratory results are used to assess

Patient Name: _____ Date: _____ Time: _____

To be filled out for all patients at risk on initial evaluation and every 12 weeks thereafter, as indicated. Trends will document the efficacy of nutritional support therapy.

Protein Compartments

Somatic:
Current Weight (kg)   _____
Previous Weight (kg)   _____ (_____ date)
Percent Change in Weight   _____

Height (cm)
Height/Weight
Current Body Mass Index (BMI)   _____ [wt/(ht)^2]
Previous BMI   _____ (_____ date)
Percent Change in BMI   _____

Visceral:
Serum Albumin   _____
    (Normal ≥ 3.5 mg/dL)
Total Lymphocyte Count (TLC)   _____ (optional)
    (White Blood Cell count × percent Lymphocytes/100)

Guide to TLC:
• Immune competence   ≥1,800 mm3
• Immunity partly impaired   <1,800 but ≥900 mm^3
• Anergy   <900 mm^3

State of Hydration

24-Hour Intake _____ mL   24-Hour Output _____ mL

Note: Thirst, tongue dryness in non-mouth-breathers and tenting or cervical skin may indicate dehydration. Jugular vein distension may indicate overhydration.

Estimated Nutritional Requirement

Estimated Nonprotein Calories (NPC) _____ /kg   Estimated Protein _____ (g/kg)

Actual NPC   _____ /kg   Actual Protein   _____ (g/kg)

Recommendations/Plan
1.
2.
3.
4.

FIGURE 16-5. Sample nutritional assessment guide for patients with pressure ulcers. Bergstrom, N., Bennett, M.A., Carlson, C.E., et al. *Treatment of Pressure Ulcers.* Clinical Practice Guideline No. 15. Rockville, MD: U.S. Department of health and Human Services. Public Health Service Agency for Health Care Policy and Research. AHCPR Publication No. 95–0652 December 1994.

nutritional status. Protein is important for healing. A serum albumin level of less than 3.5 mg/dL indicates protein deficiency. Dry mucous membranes of the mouth, increased thirst, and decreased urine output may indicated dehydration. Figure 16-5 is a sample nutritional assessment guide for patient with pressure ulcers. A registered dietitian may be consulted for guidance with protein requirements. Weight loss of 20% or more of ideal body weight or weight loss of 10% of body weight within 1 month requires close monitoring and careful dietary planning to prevent skin breakdown.

Nursing Care for Patients With Pressure Ulcers

All pressure ulcers require diligent care, regardless of the stage of the ulcer. Although in stage I the skin is not broken, diligent care is necessary to prevent a stage II or III ulcer from developing. The section on Preventing Pressure Ulcers offers suggestions to help prevent stage I ulcers from progressing to a higher-stage lesion. Additional measures include application of a thin layer of liquid copolymer skin sealant and covering the area with a moisture permeable dressing. Dressing may be left untouched several days, depending on the physician's orders and dressing manufacturer's directions. Most authorities suggest keeping the ulcer covered with a dressing to promote healing.

Débridement

In managing pressure ulcers, three areas are of particular importance; débridement, wound care, and prevention of infection. Débridement is removal of dead tissue and foreign matter from a wound. It is necessary before wound healing can occur. Débridement can be accomplished in any one of four ways:

Mechanical débridement
Autolytic débridement
Chemical (enzymatic) débridement
Sharp débridement

Mechanical débridement is accomplished by mechanical means such as wet-to-dry dressings, whirlpool, or dextranomers. Wet-to-dry dressing débridement is a method by which gauze moistened with normal saline is applied to the ulcer. When the gauze dries, it adheres to the wound. Débridement occurs when the dressing is removed by pulling the dead tissue off with the dressing. A problem develops when damage occurs to the granulation and epithelial tissue as the dry dressing is removed. Débridement is not accomplished if the dry dressing is moistened before its removal. Analgesics may be necessary when this type of débridement is done because dressing removal may be painful.

Whirlpool or hydrotherapy is an effective method of débridement. Wound irrigation with a syringe can provide the pressure necessary to remove eschar and debris from pressure ulcers. Care must be taken to not damage healthy tissue. **Dextranomers** are dextran-polymer beads that are applied to the wound to débride and absorb wound secretions.

In **autolytic débridement,** a synthetic dressing is applied to the wound to allow eschar to self-digest by the contents of the wound exudate. The body's own enzymes in the exudate are able to break down the dead tissue. Autolytic débridement requires a longer period for healing. For autolytic débridement to be effective, no infection should be present.

Enzymatic or chemical débridement is used for the chronically ill or for the elderly who cannot tolerate surgery. Collagenase is an example of an enzyme used for débridement. The enzyme collagenase is able to digest necrotic tissue remains, resulting in effective débridement. With collagenase, complete débridement occurs within 10 to 14 days. The collagen in healthy tissue is not affected. Display 16-2 provides information on the administration of collagenase.

Sharp débridement is done when cellulitis (ie, inflammation of the underlying tissue) or sepsis (ie,

---

DISPLAY 16-2. Administering Collagenase Correctly

Collagenase is an enzymatic ointment used to débride (ie, remove dead or damaged tissue) a pressure ulcer. This enzyme has the unique ability to digest the necrotic tissue, leaving healthy tissue to continue its growth.

- Apply ointment once daily.
- Apply sterile dressing after applying collagenase.
- Clean the lesion by gently rubbing with a gauze pad saturated with sterile normal saline.
- Apply directly on the lesion using a wooden tongue depressor or on sterile gauze applied to the wound.
- Remove as much necrotic tissue and debris as possible before administering the cream.
- Remove excess ointment at each dressing change.
- Discontinue when débridement of necrotic tissue is complete and granulation tissue forms.
- If infection occurs, apply topical antibacterial agent such as neomycin-bacitracin-polymyxin B (apply before collagenase is applied). If infection does not subside, discontinue therapy.

---

pathogenic microorganisms or toxins in the blood) is present and rapid débridement is necessary. For sharp débridement, a sharp instrument such as a scalpel or scissors is used to remove necrotic tissue. Sharp débridement of stage IV pressure ulcers is usually done in the operating room, but débridement of small ulcers can be done at the bedside.

Wound Care

Wound cleaning is done each time the dressing is changed, using only enough force to remove debris without damaging granulation tissue. Decubitus ulcers should not be cleaned with antiseptic solutions such as povidone iodine, sodium hypochlorite solution (Dakin's solution), or hydrogen peroxide. These solutions damage new granulation tissue and inhibit epithelialization. Normal saline is the solution of choice for cleaning most pressure ulcers. Cleaning can be done using a 35-mL syringe with a 19-gauge needle to remove most debris from pressure ulcers. Care is taken not to traumatize the wound with too much force. Wound cavities may be packed loosely to fill in gaps in the wound area and prevent an abscess. Overpacking a wound increases internal pressure on the underlying tissue and retards new tissue growth.

Choosing the Correct Dressing

Evidence indicates that pressure ulcers heal most effectively when covered with a dressing that keeps the ulcer wet and the surrounding skin dry. Dressings that support moist wound healing are transparent films, hydrocolloids, hydrogels, alginates, foams, and continuously moist saline gauze dressings. For stage I and stage II pressure ulcers, transparent dressings such as Op-Site or Bioclusive are appropriate. Transparent dressings are waterproof but permeable to moisture vapor, allowing for oxygen exchange. They may be left in place for up to 7 days. If the drainage in stage II pressure ulcers is moderate, transparent dressings are not effective. For moderate drainage, a transparent pouch dressing is more effective.

Hydrocolloids, hydrogels, and polyurethane foams are useful for partial- and full-thickness ulcers with minimal drainage. A hydrocolloid dressing such as Duoderm interacts with the exudate, forming a hydrated gel over the ulcer. The gel protects the new tissue from damage when the dressing is removed. The dressing may be left in place up to 7 days unless leakage occurs or the dressing come lose. If the wound produces large amounts of exudate, the dressing may need to be changed more often. A hydrocolloid dressing is impermeable to odor. A yellow malodorous fluid may form in the ulcer. This does not necessarily indicate infection. After removing the dressing, clean the ulcer with normal saline, and reassess the site for signs of infection. Often, the yellowish gel can be removed when the wound is irrigated leaving granulation tissue. Alginates are suitable for ulcers that produce large amounts of exudate. Follow the manufacturer's directions when using any of these dressing products.

Although it is important to maintain a moist healing environment, research has not proven that one dressing material is superior to another. Selection is based on the patient's needs and the type of pressure ulcer to be treated.

Preventing Infection
All stage II, III, and IV pressure ulcers are contaminated with bacteria. This does not mean that all ulcers are infected. Careful cleansing and débridement prevent infection in most wounds. Clean gloves are recommended for each patient. When treating multiple ulcers on the same patient, treat the least contaminated ulcer first, and care for the most contaminated ulcer last. Protect ulcers from fecal contamination. The presence of a foul odor does not always indicate an infection in a pressure ulcer that has an occlusive dressing. Reassess for infection after cleaning and débriding the ulcer. Whirlpool equipment must be disinfected between patients. Topical antiseptics are not routinely used to reduce bacteria in pressure ulcers.

Promoting Adequate Nutrition
To promote adequate nutrition and promote healing provide a well-balanced, high-protein diet with extra protein supplements. A consultation with the dietitian may be necessary to ensure adequate nutrition. Weigh the patient daily, if possible. Monitor serum albumin levels, and report levels below 3.5 mg/dL. Encourage fluids to prevent dehydration. Monitor intake and output. Provide a pleasant atmosphere for meals. Note total daily intake. Monitor for adequate protein intake. Take likes and dislikes into account when planning meals.

Evaluating Pressure Ulcer Healing
Evaluate all pressure ulcers at least weekly if an occlusive dressing is used or daily if possible. In an open ulcer the presence of pink moist tissue with a good blood supply indicates the presence of granulation tissue and that healing is occurring. When cells move across the wound, giving the appearance of ground glass, this is a sign of healing called **epithelization.** When epithelization occurs and granulation tissue develops, healing is usually seen within 2 to 4 weeks. If no evidence of healing is seen within 4 weeks, reevaluation of the treatment regimen is necessary so that changes can be made to facilitate healing. Continue daily to weekly evaluation to monitor for redevelopment of the ulcer after healing has occurred.

SKIN CANCER

Cancer of the skin is the most common type of cancer. Older, fair-skinned people are those who are most at risk for developing skin cancer. Skin cancer is rare among black people. Melanin helps to prevent burning. Dark-skinned people have more melanin in their skin and more protection against skin cancer than fair-skinned individuals with less melanin. Most skin cancer is related to overexposure to the ultraviolet rays of the sun.

Cancer is caused by the abnormal growth of cells. Cells normally function in a well-organized manner, reproducing and replacing worn out body tissue. In normal cell growth, cell birth approximates cell death. When exposed to a carcinogen (ie, agent that is capable of changing the genetic makeup of a cell), cells can with time transform, resulting in uncontrolled cell proliferation and tumors. Some tumors interfere with body function and need to be removed but do not spread to other parts of the body. This type of tumor is benign. Malignant or cancerous tumors invade and destroy normal body tissue. Malignant tumors can metastasize (ie, break away from the original tumor and spread to other parts of the body).

Types of Skin Cancer

The three most common types of skin cancer are basal cell carcinoma, squamous cell carcinoma, and malignant melanoma.

Basal Cell Cancer

Basal cell carcinoma is the most commonly occurring malignant tumor found in humans. This type of cancer develops in the cells at the base of the epidermis. Older adults with a history of sun exposure are at greatest risk. Basal cell carcinoma is characteristically slow growing and does not usually spread to other parts of the body. However, if untreated, basal cell cancer can invade the bone or other tissues beneath the skin.

This tumor is usually seen as a small fleshy bump or nodule on the head, neck, or hands. The tumors are slow growing, and it may take months to years to reach a diameter of one-half inch (1 cm). If a basal cell tumor is left untreated, it will bleed and crust over. Within 5 years, 35% of patients diagnosed with basal cell cancer develop another basal cell tumor elsewhere in the body.

Squamous Cell Carcinoma

Squamous cell carcinoma is the second most common skin cancer and arises from the epidermis layer of the skin. This type of carcinoma can most often be found on sun exposed areas on the face, ears, neck, lips, and hands. This cancer sometimes develops in other skin lesions, such as scars or ulcers. Squamous cell carcinoma typically appears as red, scaly patches but can appear as opaque, elevated nodules. Squamous cell cancer grows more rapidly than basal cell cancer and can develop into a large mass that metastasizes to other areas of the body. If detected early and treated properly, 95% of basal cell and squamous cell carcinomas can be cured.

Malignant Melanoma

Although the least common, **malignant melanoma** is the most deadly of all skin cancers. Melanoma develops from melanocytes (ie, cells that produce melanin). Normally, the melanocytes produce more melanin to cause the body to tan and help protect the skin from sun burn. A melanoma may continue to produce melanin, giving the tumor the characteristic black or brown color. Melanin typically begins in or near a nevi (mole) or dark spot in the skin. Melanoma may develop on the trunk, lower leg, or face. In dark-skinned people, the palms and the soles of the feet

are common areas of melanoma. Melanoma may also appear without warning. Any changes that occur on the skin should be reported to the physician immediately. Individuals should be taught to perform a regular monthly skin self-assessment to monitor for lesions. Figure 16-6 offers an example of a skin assessment guide.

One of the most dangerous aspects of melanoma is its tendency to spread to other parts of the body by metastasis. Excessive exposure to the sun is the most important risk factor associated with melanoma. Heredity may also play a role. Early detection and prompt treatment are essential. Warning signs that indicate a mole could be developing cancerous changes can be assessed by using the ABCDs of melanoma.

ASSESSMENT ALERT

The ABCDs of melanoma are

Asymmetry: One half of the lesion does not match the other half of the lesion.

Border irregularity: The edges of the mole are irregular (eg, ragged, notched, blurred).

Color: The color or pigmentation is not uniform. There may be colors of tan, brown, and black intermingled with red, white, and blue. The mole may have a mottled appearance.

Diameter: Any increase in the size of a mole or a mole that is larger than the size of a pencil eraser (about 6 mm) is considered suspicious.

Other symptoms include scaliness, oozing, bleeding, appearance of a bump or nodule, and spreading of the pigment from the border to the surrounding skin. Itching, tenderness, or pain are also warning signs of melanoma.

Diagnosis and Treatment

Diagnosis begins with a complete medical history and a thorough assessment to identify all suspicious lesions. A biopsy is taken of any suspicious areas. For a biopsy, the physician removes a small sample of tissue from the area for microscopic examination. If the tumor is very small, the entire tumor may be removed during the biopsy. If the results of the biopsy reveal that the outer edges contain cancer cells, additional treatment is needed, and larger and deeper biopsies may be needed to diagnose melanoma.

Treatment is accomplished by excisional surgery (ie, surgically removing the tumor) electrodesiccation (ie, using heat to destroy the tissue), cryosurgery

MONTHLY SELF-EXAMINATION

Prevention of melanoma/skin cancer is obviously the most desirable weapon against this disease. But if a lesion should develop, it is almost always totally curable if caught in the early stages. To ensure that any developing lesion is caught in the early stage, a regular program of monthly self-examinations should be followed. The following is a suggested method of self-examination that will ensure that no area of the body is neglected in a regular program of self-examination.

To perform your examination you wil need a full-length mirror, a hand mirror and a brightly lit room where you can study your skin in privacy. This step-by-step method, if done monthly, will provide you with an "early warning system" against melanoma/skin cancer:

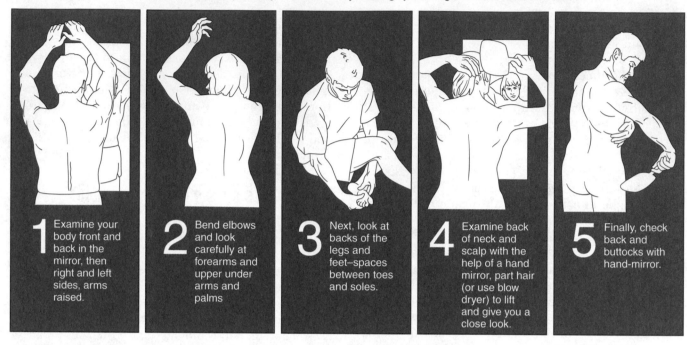

1 Examine your body front and back in the mirror, then right and left sides, arms raised.

2 Bend elbows and look carefully at forearms and upper under arms and palms

3 Next, look at backs of the legs and feet–spaces between toes and soles.

4 Examine back of neck and scalp with the help of a hand mirror, part hair (or use blow dryer) to lift and give you a close look.

5 Finally, check back and buttocks with hand-mirror.

FIGURE 16-6. Skin self assessment guide. From Melanoma/Skin Cancer. You Can Recognize the Signs. Code 904. American Cancer Society, 1990. Used with permission.

(ie, tissue destruction by freezing), and radiation therapy. Radiation may be used in the elderly who are unable to tolerate a surgical procedure. A combination of treatments may be indicated. For example, some squamous cell carcinoma may be followed by radiation if metastasis is suspected.

Surgical excision is the only method that cures melanoma. Areas of metastasis are located and if possible these tumors are surgically excised as well. Malignant melanoma may spread to any organ. Common sites of metastasis include the skin, bone, brain, and lung. With metastasis, the cure rate is decreased, but surgical excision can help relieve the pain and increase survival time. Chemotherapy (ie, anticancer drugs) has produced only limited success in the treatment of melanoma.

Nursing Interventions for Preventing and Detecting Skin Cancer

Nursing interventions focus on prevention and detection of skin cancer. Patients and family members should be instructed on the importance of periodic skin self-examination. Older adults with visual problems or limited mobility may be unable

---

DISPLAY 16-3. Instructing the Older Adult to Guard Against Skin Cancer

- Avoid exposure to the sun when the rays are the strongest (between 10 AM and 3 PM).
- Cover up as much of the skin as possible by wearing long-sleeved shirts and hats with wide brims.
- Apply a sunscreen with a sun protection factor (SPF) of at least 15 to exposed areas.
- Avoid the use of sunlamps at tanning salons.
- Report any unusual blemish, mole, or marking of the skin, especially one that changes in size or color, to the physician immediately.

---

to perform self-examination. When physical problems or chronic disease prevents self-examination, family members may perform the examination periodically, usually every 6 to 8 weeks. By becoming familiar with their own skin lesions (eg, moles, freckles, birthmarks), they are better able to identify changes when they occur. If changes are found, the physician or dermatologist is notified.

Patient teaching is an important aspect of preventing and detecting skin cancer. Display 16-3

DISPLAY 16-4. Descriptive Terms for Skin Lesions

Term	Description
Macule	Small, nonpalpable spot or discoloration
Papule	Discoloration <0.5 cm in diameter with palpable elevation
Plaque	Group of papules
Nodule	Lesion 0.5 to 1 cm in diameter with palpable elevation
Tumor	Lesion >1 cm with palpable elevation
Wheal	Red or white, palpable elevation that may occur in various sizes
Vesicle	Lesion <0.5 cm that contains fluid and is palpable
Bulla	Lesion >0.5 cm that contains fluid and has a palpable elevation
Pustule	Palpable lesion containing purulent fluid (variable sizes)
Fissure	Groove in the skin
Ulcer	Open depression in the skin, various sizes
Cyst	Capsule containing semi-solid or liquid substance

TABLE 16-1. Common Skin Lesions Found in the Elderly

Term	Description
Lentigos	Small, brown macules or brown-pigmented areas on the skin, sometimes called liver spots
Ichthyosis	Dry, scaly, fish scale appearance of the skin
Acrochordons	Soft, flesh-colored lesions of epidermal tissue occurring most often on the eyelids, neck, and axillae
Senile keratosis	Precancerous lesions found in the head, neck, and trunk that develop as small, reddened areas that change to rough, yellow to brown or black lesions also called actinic keratosis
Seborrheic keratosis	Pigmented, raised, warty, and sometimes slightly greasy lesions that develop on the trunk, face, and hands
Cherry angiomas	Bright or ruby red, round sometimes raised lesions 1–3 mm in diameter. Usually found on the trunk
Senile purpura	Large bruised areas caused by blood extravasating outside the vessels secondary to trauma
Nevi (plural), nevus (singular)	Brown, black, or flesh colored mole; circumscribed malformation of the skin
Senile papillomas	Small, yellow-brown or black warts found on chest, limbs, and face

identifies information the older adult needs to protect the skin and help prevent skin cancer.

COMMON DISORDERS AFFECTING THE SKIN

More than 90% of older adults have some type of skin disorder, ranging from a simple nevi to psoriasis. Display 16-4 identifies common terms used to identify skin lesions. Some lesions common in older adults include keratosis, cherry angiomas, nevi, skin tags, and lentigo.

Senile purpura is particularly common in the aging adult. Senile purpura is hemorrhagic areas or bruising under the skin of older adults. This bruising is largely caused by the loss of subcutaneous tissue and increased fragility of the vessels, which rupture as a result of minimal trauma. Even minor injury can traumatize the skin and cause these ecchymotic (bruised) areas. The most common site is the forearms. Table 16-1 identifies skin lesions common in the older adult. Most of the lesions associated with aging are considered normal and are nonpathogenic.

Actinic Keratosis

Actinic keratosis (ie, solar keratosis) are small flat, scaly, reddish patches associated with excessive exposure to the sun. These are precancerous lesions that are closely monitored for change leading to skin cancer. They may also appear yellow to brown with a rough surface. Actinic keratosis are slow growing and can, but usually do not, progress to squamous cell carcinoma. They are treated with chemical peels, freezing, and topical creams (eg, Curaderm).

Xerosis

Xerosis is excessive dryness of the skin, causing the skin to have a scaly fishlike appearance. This dryness in part results from decreased activity of the sebaceous glands and occurs most often on the lower legs, hands, arms, and feet. Xerosis causes intense itching (ie, pruritus) in these areas and in the genitalia and anal areas. If pruritus is ignored, the skin can become traumatized, and infection occurs. Several methods can help alleviate dry skin:

Apply a moisturizing lotion to the skin daily or as needed.

Use Vaseline or petroleum jelly as a lubricant for very dry areas.

Bathe every other day rather than daily, and use a mild soap.

Keep nails well trimmed to minimize infection from scratching.

Antihistamines can be used to relieve the itching if nursing measures are unsuccessful. If an oil-based bath oil is used, the bathtub may become slippery. Care must be taken to ensure the older adult does not fall when getting out of the bathtub or shower.

Stasis Dermatitis

Stasis dermatitis is a condition of the lower extremities caused by poor venous return in which the leg's skin becomes pigmented and cracked. A leg ulcer can easily form in response to scratching because of dry skin, poor venous return, and skin breakdown. This type of ulcer is called a **stasis ulcer.** The legs become swollen and edematous, and the patient complains of aching, stinging, and burning from exposed nerves endings. Although pulses are present, they may be difficult to palpate when edema is present. Ulcers develop in any area on the leg but most often are found on the ankle. Stasis ulcers often have copious drainage that decreases as the ulcer heals. The ulcer is covered with an occlusive dressing such as a hydrocolloid to maintain a moist environment and promote healing. A moist environment encourages granulation and epithelization. Hydrocolloids, foams, gels and other moist dressings do not need to be changed daily and provide a healing environment. Venous return can be enhanced by elevating the legs during the day. The patient is instructed to avoid standing for long periods, sitting with the legs crossed, or wearing garters.

Dermatitis

Dermatitis (ie, eczema) is inflammation of the skin with itching, redness, edema, heat, and pain. Dermatitis may be caused by disease, skin irritants (eg, soaps, plants, clothing), or hypersensitivity (allergic) reactions.

Seborrheic dermatitis is chronic inflammatory skin diseases with greasy scales and yellowish crusts. The scalp, eyelids, face, and external surfaces of the ears, axillae, breasts, and groin are common sites. Seborrheic dermatitis requires scrupulous care with emphasis on good skin hygiene, keeping the skin dry, and treatment with selenium-containing shampoos and topical anti-inflammatory creams.

Intertrigo is a form of seborrheic dermatitis that results when opposing skin surfaces rub together and cause irritation. The elderly are often affected by this condition, particularly in the skin folds of the breast, in the axillae, inner aspects of the thighs, and in transverse abdominal folds. The condition is more common in the obese. Treatment is weight reduction, powdering, cleaning, and topical hydrocortisone cream. If a monilial (fungal) infection develops, Nystatin topical cream is used.

Psoriasis

Psoriasis can appear at any age, but there is an increased incidence in older adults in their sixties. This chronic skin condition is characterized by red patches covered with silvery dry scales caused by excessive growth of epithelial cells. The most commonly affected areas are the scalp, ears, face, trunk, genitalia, hands, and feet. Although not contagious, the disorder is chronic and requires lifelong treatment. Emphasis is placed on maintaining a healthy lifestyle and stress management techniques. Psoriasis exacerbates as the result of emotional stress, exposure to the sun, and when taking certain medications such as lithium and certain beta blockers. Several topical drugs such as the corticosteroids and dithranol are used to decrease the rapid growth of epidermal cells. Ultraviolet radiation is also used as a treatment for psoriasis.

Herpes Zoster

Herpes zoster, commonly known as shingles, most often affects older adults between 50 to 75 years of age. Herpes zoster is caused by the varicella-zoster virus. The disorder is characterized by painful vesicular eruptions occurring along the nerve route and is almost always unilateral. Pain occurs and may be constant or intermittent. Intense itching may also occur. The symptoms continue for 3 to 5 weeks. Older adults are more likely to develop complications such as neuralgia that can persist for several months.

The most effective treatment is the antiviral drug acyclovir (Zovirax). The drug does not cure herpes zoster but does lessen the severity of the attack by relieving pain and promoting healing. Acyclovir must be used within 48 to 72 hours after the onset of the rash for the greatest benefit.

Scabies

Scabies is a contagious disease caused by the itch mite, resulting in intense itching of the skin and excoriation from scratching. The mite lays its eggs in the outer layers of the skin. Scabies appear as discolored lines several millimeters to several centimeters long on the outer surface of the skin. Within several weeks, papules, vesicles, and pustules develop, causing intense itching and the potential for infection. Common sites include areas between the fingers, wrists, axillae, genitalia, and on the inner thighs. All contacts are treated with a scabicide such as lindane (G-well). Display 16-5 offers general guidelines on administering lindane.

CRITICAL THINKING EXERCISES

1. Mr. Herford, age 69, states that as a farmer he was exposed to a great amount of sun over the past 30 years. He wore sun screen only in the last several years. He is concerned about developing skin cancer. How would you discuss this topic with Mr. Herford? What would be the most effective method to help Mr. Herford detect any cancerous lesions?
2. The physician prescribes collagenase for débridement of a Stage III decubitus ulcer on the sacrum of an elderly nursing home patient. How would you administer the drug? What would be the most important assessment before administering the drug? Why is this assessment important?

DISPLAY 16-5. Using Lindane Correctly

- Apply a thin layer of lindane lotion to dry skin and rub thoroughly.
- Do not use on open wounds, cuts, or sores.
- Trim nails and apply under nails with a toothbrush (dispose of the toothbrush after use).
- Cover all body parts from the neck to the soles of the feet.
- Allow the cream to remain for 8 to 12 hours (overnight) and then remove by thorough washing. One application is usually sufficient.
- Inform the patient of the following points:
  - Wash clothing, underwear, pajamas, gowns, towels, and all linen in very hot water.
  - Itching will continue for several weeks.
  - A repeat application is usually unnecessary.
  - This drug is not used to ward off a possible infestation.
  - Itching after treatment does not indicate need for reapplication unless living mites are apparent.

---

3. Ms. Taylor, age 82, is unable to care for herself and has gone to live with her daughter. She is confined to the bed or the wheelchair most of the day. Her daughter is concerned about the development of pressure ulcers. Drawing from your knowledge of the elderly what assessments would you make? What suggestions could you give the daughter to help prevent Ms. Taylor from developing pressure ulcers?

REFERENCES AND SUGGESTED READING

American Cancer Society and the American Academy of Dermatology. (1995). *Why you should know about melanoma.* Publication No. 2619.

Bergstrom, N., Bennett, M., Carlson, D., et al. (1994). *Treatment of pressure ulcers: Clinical practice guideline,* no. 15. AHCPR Publication no. 95-0652. Rockville, MD: Agency for Health Care Policy and Research, Public Health Service, U.S. Department of Health and Human Services.

Maklebust, J. (1999). Treating pressure ulcers in the home. *Home Health Nurse, 17*(5) 307–315.

Maklebust, J. (1999). Interrupting the pressure ulcer cycle. *Nursing Clinics of North America, 34*(4), 861–871.

CHAPTER 17

The Neurologic System

CHAPTER OUTLINE

KEY TERMS

CHAPTER OBJECTIVES

AGE-RELATED CHANGES IN THE NERVOUS SYSTEM

COMMON AGE-RELATED DISORDERS OF THE NERVOUS SYSTEM

PARKINSONISM

SEIZURE DISORDERS IN THE ELDERLY

CRITICAL THINKING EXERCISES

REFERENCES AND SUGGESTED READING

KEY TERMS

agnosia

Alzheimer's disease

aphasia

apraxia

behavioral symptoms

benign essential tremor

bradykinesia

delirium

dementia

epilepsy

multi-infarct dementia

myoclonic seizure

neurons

normal pressure hydrocephalus

parkinsonism

partial seizure

respite care

seizure disorder

sundown syndrome

tonic-clonic seizure

transient ischemic attack

wandering

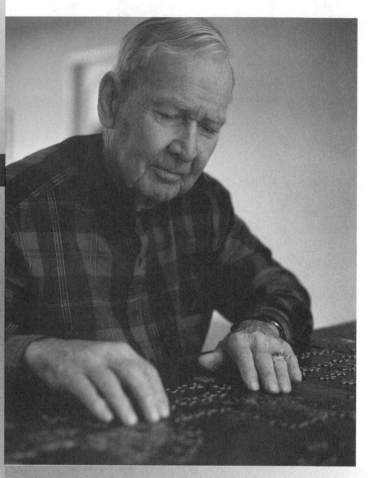

CHAPTER OBJECTIVES

At the completion of this chapter, the student will be able to

- Discuss age-related changes in the nervous system

- Distinguish between dementia and delirium

- Discuss signs and symptoms, diagnosis, etiology and stages, treatment, and nursing management of Alzheimer's disease

- Discuss important aspects in caring for the caregiver

- Identify ways to evaluate a nursing home

- Discuss important aspects in the care of patients with multi-infarct dementia and normal pressure hydrocephalus

● **Use the nursing process to care for a patient with dementia**

● **Discuss signs and symptoms, physiologic changes, diagnosis, treatment, and nursing management of patients with parkinsonism**

● **Use the nursing process to care for patients with parkinsonism**

● **Describe the various types of seizures**

● **Discuss assessment and nursing care of patients with a seizure disorder**

The nervous system is composed of two separate but interrelated parts: the central nervous system (CNS) and the peripheral nervous system (PNS). The CNS consists of the brain and spinal cord. The function of the CNS is to process and coordinate information to and from the PNS. The PNS consists of the cranial, spinal, and peripheral nerves. Twelve pair of cranial nerves, 31 pairs of spinal nerves, and the various branches of these nerves that spread throughout the body make up the PNS. These nerves form communicating networks between the CNS and PNS.

The nervous system functions to maintain homeostasis, (eg, body temperature, fluid balance, and heart rate), promote body functions (eg, digestion, excretion), and in the regulation of the body's reaction to stress. Neurons are basic nerve cells that conduct nervous impulses from one area in the body to another area in the body.

Many individuals assume that loss of the neurologic function is a natural consequence of aging, but this assumption is not true. Impaired neurologic function in the elderly is a result of a disease process and is not part of the normal aging process.

AGE-RELATED CHANGES IN THE NERVOUS SYSTEM

Aging brings about a steady loss of **neurons** (ie, nerve cells) in the brain and spinal cord. At age 75, the loss of neurons is estimated to be about 10%. However, because of the massive numbers of neurons present in the brain of most adults, this progressive loss of neurons does not result in a significant loss of mental functioning. There is no noticeable loss of cognition in most older adults who do not have a neurologic disease. The body does, however, lose some sensory function because of the loss of some sensory neurons. This loss of

sensory neurons results in most older adults exhibiting some degree of impairment in hearing, vision, smelling, temperature regulation, and pain sensation.

With age, there is a generalized decrease in the number of nerve conduction fibers resulting in slower reflexes and delayed response to stimuli. There is also a loss of postural control (ie, balance) in part because of the loss of sensory cues, especially visual, tactile, and hearing cues. The loss of sensory cues places the older adult at an increased risk for falling.

Decreased sensory perception also contributes to vertigo (ie, dizziness). Orthostatic or postural hypotension is also more common in the elderly. Orthostatic hypotension occurs when there is a decrease in the systolic blood pressure of 20 mmHg or more when a person moves from a reclining to an upright position. This condition is aggravated by age-related changes such as decreased cerebral blood flow and decreased cardiac output (see Chapter 18). Drugs commonly prescribed for the elderly such as vasodilators, psychotropic drugs, and antihypertensives also contribute to the possibility of hypotension.

Reaction time (ie, time between stimulation of the neuron to the beginning of a response) is slowed with aging. Older adults are generally aware of this delayed reaction time and seem to compensate for this delay with an increase in accuracy or appropriateness of response. Although older adults may be slower, as a result of the ability to compensate for decreased reaction time, they usually perform equally as well as younger adults.

Posture, movement, and reflexes change with age. Reflexes decrease, movement slows, and joints become more rigid and flexed. Posture and gait changes result in a shorter stride and decrease in arm swing resulting in what is sometimes called a shuffling gait.

Benign essential tremor is common in older adults. This tremor most often affects the hands and head. This type of tremor is not associated with disease and does not significantly interfere with the ability of the older adult to function normally. With benign essential tremor, the tremor is usually absent at rest but noticeable when performing voluntary tasks that require precision.

Thermoregulation (ie, regulation of body temperature) is more difficult with age. Hypothermia (ie, state in which the body temperature is below 95°F) occurs as a result of loss of subcutaneous tissue, decreased ability to sense the feeling of coldness, and decline in the ability to produce heat (ie, shiver). Display 17-1 lists the symptoms and treatment of hypothermia in the elderly. The older

DISPLAY 17-1. Hypothermia

Definition. Hypothermia is a condition in which body temperature falls to below normal. The condition becomes extremely serious if the temperature falls below 95° F. This condition is usually the result of exposure to cold weather. Older adults have decreased thermoregulation functioning, predisposing them to this condition.

Symptoms
- Drowsiness
- Grayish cast to the skin
- Cool to cold skin temperature
- Decreased ability to concentrate (slowed thinking)
- Decreased consciousness leading to coma
- Initial tachypnea followed by slow and shallow respirations
- Heart rate decreases
- Shivering ceases
- Face appears puffy
- Decreased temperature (below 95°F)

Treatment and Management. Treatment requires careful monitoring and gradual rewarming of the body without causing cardiac arrhythmias.
- Monitor temperature, blood pressure, and pulse.
- Handle the person gently and carefully.
- Gradually warm the body by wrapping the individual in blankets.
- Keep the room temperature warm.
- Avoid too rapid warming, because it can initiate cardiac arrhythmias.
- Body temperature below 86°F may be treated with peritoneal dialysis and inhalation warming. Antibiotics may be used to prevent sepsis. Dehydration and acidosis are corrected.

adult is also more prone to hyperthermia or heat stroke. Chapter 10 offers more information on heat stroke.

COMMON AGE-RELATED DISORDERS OF THE NERVOUS SYSTEM

Dementia versus Delirium

Delirium and dementia are common disorders found in the elderly. It is important to distinguish between delirium and dementia in order for the older adult to obtain the most effective treatment. Chapter 14, Table 14-5, compares depression, dementia, and delirium.

Delirium is impairment of intellectual functioning that occurs rapidly, lasts several hours to several weeks, and is reversible. Although the intensity of delirium fluctuates, it increases in severity during the night. With delirium, thinking is disorganized, and orientation is impaired. Illusions (ie, false interpretation of an external stimulus) and hallucinations (ie, sensory perception without any external stimulus) commonly occur. Delirium is usually the result of stress, drug intoxication, sensory overload or deprivation, or a medical condition.

Dementia is a decrease in mental or cognitive functioning characterized by one or more of the following symptoms: **aphasia** (ie, language disturbance), **apraxia** (ie, impaired ability to perform purposeful acts), **agnosia** (ie, impaired ability to recognize objects or persons), or progressive difficulty functioning in a social or occupational environment. With dementia, there is a progressive decline in memory. Individuals with dementia have difficulty learning new material, they forget previously learned material, or both.

In the early stages of dementia, the individual may lose items such as keys, wallets, or other personal belongings. They may forget to turn water faucets off or forget food cooking on the stove. As the dementia progresses, they may forget personal information such as their own birthday or wedding anniversary. They may be unable to work, balance a checkbook, pay bills, or find their way home. They may be unable to recognize their children or their own face in a mirror. Language function declines causing an inability to recall names of people and objects.

Diagnosis of dementia may be complicated because dementia can coexist with delirium. Most often, dementia is chronic and progressive, but in certain situations, the condition may remain relatively constant or even be reversed. For example, dementia caused by normal pressure hydrocephalus is reversible if properly treated.

In older adults, the most common cause of dementia is Alzheimer's disease (AD). AD accounts for approximately 50% of dementia in older adults. The second most prevalent cause of dementia in the elderly is multi-infarct dementia (MID) or vascular dementia. MID occurs as the result of hypertension or atherosclerosis. AD and MID may coexist.

Dementia may also occur as the result of normal-pressure hydrocephalus, long-term alcohol abuse, hypothyroidism, vitamin B_{12} deficiency, brain tumor, Parkinson disease, Huntington disease, or untreated syphilis.

Alzheimer's Disease

Approximately 4 million Americans have AD, and it is estimated that this number will grow to 14 million by the year 2050. One of 10 individuals older than age 65 and nearly half of those older than 85 years have AD. At least one half of all nursing home residents have AD or another form of dementia. The average lifetime cost of care for an individual with AD is $174,000. With a rapidly increasing older population, AD presents a significant health care concern for the present and future generations.

AD is a chronic condition resulting in progressive loss of neurologic functioning. The onset is gradual and characterized by progressive cognitive decline and dementia. The disease has a gradual onset and progresses slowly. The average length of the illness from the onset of symptoms until death is approximately 8 to 10 years (some have lived up to 20 years).

The disease begins with generalized forgetfulness and progresses to the point of the individual becoming mute and totally dependent on others for physical care. Early-onset AD occurs in middle age (<65 years), and late-onset AD affects those 65 years of age or older. Early-onset AD usually has a more malignant course. With late-onset AD, especially if it occurs after age 80, there is little reduction of life expectancy.

Diagnosis

There is no single or simple test to diagnose AD. When AD is suspected, it is important to have a thorough medical and neurologic evaluation to identify treatable disorders with Alzheimer-like symptoms (eg, depression, hypothyroidism, vitamin B_{12} deficiency, hydrocephalus, stroke). The comprehensive evaluation necessary to rule out these causes and to make a probable diagnosis of AD includes a complete health history, physical examination, neurologic and mental status assessment, and other tests, including blood and urine analysis, electrocardiogram, and chest radiographs. The physician may order a computed tomography (CT) scan or magnetic resonance imaging (MRI). The American Psychiatric Association's *Diagnostic and Statistical Manual of Mental Disorders* diagnostic criteria for dementia associated with AD can also be used to help establish a diagnose of AD (Display 17-2). Combining physical and neuropsychological testing, along with caregiver input, results in about 90% accuracy in diagnosing AD.

A definitive diagnosis can be made only on autopsy. The autopsy reveals senile plaques, neurofibrillary tangles, and granulovascular bodies present in the brain tissue. The senile plaques and neurofibrillary tangles are lesions in the brain consisting of coarse fibers that run throughout the cerebral cortex. Although these plaques and tangles are present in the brain of older adults without AD, they

---

DISPLAY 17-2. **Criteria for Diagnosing Alzheimer's Disease**
1. Cognitive deficits, including memory impairment
2. One or more of the following symptoms:
a. Language disturbance
b. Impairment in ability to perform motor activities
c. Inability to name objects
d. Problems with planning, organizing, or thinking abstractly
3. Significant decline in former level of functioning, including social or occupational
4. Gradual onset and progressive cognitive decline
5. Cognitive deficits are unrelated to other physical or mental conditions.

Adapted from American Psychiatric Association. (1994). *Diagnostic and statistical manual of mental disorders* (4th ed.). Washington, DC: American Psychiatric Association, 142.

---

are more prevalent in the cerebral cortex of patients with AD. Granulovascular bodies are not commonly found in the brains of those who age normally, but are present in the brain of patients with AD.

The cells most affected by AD are those that use the neurotransmitter acetylcholine. The enzyme active in producing acetylcholine is decreased in the brain of Alzheimer's victims. Acetylcholine is necessary for memory processing.

Etiology

Although the exact cause of AD is unknown several possible causes are under investigation. Possible causes include a decrease in acetylcholine, the beta-amyloid protein, genetic factors, and viral infection.

Acetylcholine is a neurotransmitter widely distributed in body tissues, particularly the brain. This chemical substance is involved in correctly processing information regarding thought, behavior, and memory. This theory postulates that a decrease of acetylcholine actively occurs in the brains of patients with AD, causing memory loss and other cognitive deficits associated with AD.

Beta-amyloid protein deposits, known as plaques, are found in the brains of those diagnosed with AD. Some researchers feel that this protein is a necessary component in the development of AD and may trigger the degeneration of brain cells. Other researchers believe that the beta-amyloid protein is a result of the disease not a trigger for the development of the disease.

Genetic factors have been linked to early-onset AD. A great deal of research has been done concerning the relationship between genetics and AD. This research links three different genes observed in only 120 families worldwide with the development of the

DISPLAY 17-3. Stages of Alzheimer's Disease

Stage I: Early Stage (Forgetfulness and Uncertainty Phase). In this stage, the individual has difficulty remembering recent events or facts associated with these events. They may forget where objects are placed (eg, keys, purse) and have more difficulty remembering names than in the past. Lists are made to aid the memory. The spouse or other family members may be the only ones to notice this decline besides the individual experiencing the memory loss.

Anxiety over the forgetfulness causes irritation and withdrawal. These individuals may withdraw from social activities and avoid new experiences. Language difficulty, such as the inability to remember certain nouns, develops. This stage is not to be confused with nonpathologic forgetfulness, which occurs as a normal process of aging in some elderly. Nonpathologic forgetfulness in aging is characterized by the inability to remember certain relatively unimportant details of an event or a past experience. With Alzheimer's disease, the individual is unable to remember the details of the experience and is unable to remember the experience itself.

Stage II: Middle Stage (Confusional Stage). In this stage, a significant decline in cognitive functioning occurs. This stage is marked by increased confusion affecting all areas of life. Family, friends, and others observe the decline, especially in work-related activities. There is increasing difficulty in making decisions and in the ability to concentrate. Declining work skills, such as in mathematical ability, writing, spelling, and problem solving, may be the most obvious. There may be gait changes resulting in unsteadiness or loss of coordination.

Stage III: Later Stage (Dementia Phase). In this stage, there is even greater cognitive loss. The individual becomes severely disoriented, with behavior and personality changes. Remembering family members or friends may be problematic. Some even lose the ability to recognize themselves. For example, they may become frightened of their own image in a mirror, thinking the reflection is a stranger or someone who will hurt them. Psychotic symptoms such as hallucinations, delusions, or paranoid thinking may develop.

Stage IV: Final Stage (Terminal Stage). In the final stage, the individual loses the ability to function mentally and physically. There is total inability to remember the family, friends, and the caregiver. The individual becomes incontinent, mute, and totally dependent on others for care.

early-onset form of the disease. This early-onset form of AD affects people in their thirties, forties, and fifties and is rare. Individuals who carry one of the early-onset genes will most likely develop AD. Much more common is the late-onset form of the disease, which occurs after age 65 and accounts for more than 90% of all cases of AD. It is unclear if a genetic abnormality causes this form of AD. What is known is that a person's risk of developing AD at any given age is slightly increased if the individual has a first-degree relative (parent, brother or sister) with the disease.

Some researchers postulate that AD is the result of a slow-growing virus that attacks brain cells. According to these theorists, the virus changes the brain chemistry and causes brain cell changes that result in AD.

Stages

Four stages have been identified for AD. The individual's decline is progressive, although highly individualized. The stages are predictable and continue until the person is totally unable to provide self-care.

    I. Early stage (forgetfulness and uncertainty phase)
    II. Middle stage (confusional phase)
    III. Later stage (dementia phase)
    IV. Final stage (terminal phase)

Display 17-3 describes the various stages of AD.

Treatment

There is no specific treatment for AD. Instead, management is aimed at

    Enhancing remaining cognitive and functional abilities
    Treating problems created by the progression of the disease (eg, dementia, incontinence, wandering, agitation)
    Providing support to the patient and the family

Drug Therapy. Several drugs are currently used to treat mild to moderate dementia associated with AD. These drugs include tacrine hydrochloride (Cognex), donepezil (Aricept), and rivastigmine tartrate (Exelon). These drugs act by enhancing the action of acetylcholine in the brain. A deficiency of acetylcholine may cause some of the symptoms associated with AD. These drugs do not cure the disease, but appear to slow the degenerative process in the brain.

Tacrine (Cognex) is best given on an empty stomach, but may be given with meals if gastric upset occurs. The most common side effects include nausea, vomiting, diarrhea, dyspepsia, anorexia, and ataxia (unsteady gait). Patients taking tacrine must be monitored closely for liver toxicity. If side effects become severe, the dosage is decreased and the drug is discontinued slowly.

Donepezil (Aricept) is administered once a day, preferably in the evening before retiring. It may be given with or without food. Side effects include nausea, vomiting, insomnia, fatigue, confusion, and changes in neurologic functioning.

Rivastigmine (Exelon) is administered with food in divided doses (AM and PM). Drug dosages may be increased at intervals to obtain maximum effect. If side effects such as nausea, vomiting, abdominal pain, and loss of appetite become intolerable, the drug is discontinued for several doses, then restarted at the same or lower dose. The drug is given as an oral solution, using the dosing syringe provided in the protective case. The correct amount of the drug is withdrawn from the container. The dose may be swallowed directly from the syringe or mixed with a small glass of water, cold fruit juice, or soda. Rivastigmine is also available in capsule form.

Other drugs such as antidepressants, antihistamines, and antipsychotics should be avoided or prescribed cautiously because their anticholinergic activity can worsen the symptoms of AD.

Donepezil hydrochloride (Aricept) is a new drug for the treatment of mild to moderate AD. This drug is effective in improving cognition and functional ability in mild to moderate AD. Functional ability improves in cognition, behavior, and performance of the activities of daily living (ADLs). Although some patients did not exhibit improvement, they showed no significant decline in cognition or functional ability. For Alzheimer's patients, showing no decline while taking donepezil is viewed as beneficial. The drug acts to inhibit the breakdown of acetylcholine in the brain. Acetylcholine is a brain chemical that helps nerve cells to communicate with each other. Fewer adverse reactions are associated with donepezil than with tacrine because tacrine has greater systemic action but donepezil acts mainly in the brain. In general, donepezil is well tolerated. Adverse reactions include nausea, diarrhea, vomiting, insomnia, fatigue, and loss of appetite. Most adverse reactions are mild and transient. Unlike tacrine, there is no need to monitor liver function while on donepezil. Dosage is 5 to 10 mg of the drug taken orally once each day.

Behavioral Symptoms

Behavioral symptoms are common as AD progresses. **Behavioral symptoms** are actions such as wandering, verbal, or physical abuse, refusal of care that are repetitive, disruptive, or generally considered as socially inappropriate. Display 17-4 gives some examples of behavioral symptoms.

Because the world is frightening to Alzheimer's patients, they may act out with unacceptable behaviors. Because they are unable to express their needs in a verbal manner, they express needs in unacceptable behaviors. These behaviors may be attempts to communicate needs.

As cognitive ability decreases, there is a decreased ability to think in an organized, coherent manner and

---

DISPLAY 17-4. Behavioral Symptoms Exhibited by Alzheimer Patients

- Paranoia
- Delusions
- Hallucinations
- Harming self
- Hitting others
- Inappropriate sexual activity or sexual remarks
- Insomnia
- Repeated questioning
- Throwing things
- Uncooperative behavior
- Undressing
- Wandering
- Yelling or screaming

---

to make sound judgments. An important aspect of care is the continuing need of the Alzheimer's patient for a kind compassionate nurse who provides a caring environment, regardless of the response of the patient.

Wandering. Wandering is persistent aimless walking often on the same pathway or route. The Alzheimer's patient can walk up to 10 miles each day, even to the point of neglecting to eat or sleep. Wandering can cause additional problems if an individual in a nursing home wanders outside the facility and is unable to find the way back. Some facilities have alarms for residents who are prone to wander. These alarms are worn on the arm or leg and alert the staff if the individual leaves the facility. For those who wander, it is important to ensure that some form of identification is worn at all times. Suitable times for supervised walking can be arranged. Additional safety precautions, such as requiring codes to gain access to outside, may be needed as well.

An effort is made to determine the reason for the wandering. Although the resident may be unable to identify why the walking is occurring, there is often a fairly logical reason. To determine the reason requires careful assessment by the nurse. For example Mr. Porter, age 72, has stage III AD. He wanders in and out of every resident's room several times each day, causing many of the other residents great distress. At a care plan conference with Mr. Porter's daughter present, the nursing staff learned that Mr. Porter was a mail carrier for 35 years. In planning his care, the staff decided that perhaps Mr. Porter's behavior was done in an effort to "deliver the mail" as he had done in the past. The nurse suggested that Mr. Porter help the volunteer who delivered the morning paper to the various rooms of the nursing home. After 2 days of delivering papers, Mr. Porter's wandering decreased significantly.

Although it is not always easy to identify a reason for wandering, an effort must always be made.

DISPLAY 17-5. Nursing Interventions for Patients Who Wander

- Use commercial alarms that alert the staff when the resident leaves the facility.
- Place a rope or a barrier across a doorway to prevent a confused patient from entering.
- Use volunteers to assist the resident or provide company.
- Use validation therapy or reality therapy as appropriate (see Display 17-11).
- Keep the bed in a low position.
- Avoid the use of restraints.
- Keep a recent photograph of the resident in the chart.
- Calmly guide the wanderer back. Be careful not to startle the wanderer.
- Place alarms on doorways.
- Use distraction such as offering food or an activity.
- Identify the need the person is seeking to meet through wandering.
- Provide a safe, secured pathway for wandering.

DISPLAY 17-6. Nursing Interventions to Manage Sundown Syndrome

- Turning the lights on before dark and keeping them on during the evening
- Using night lights
- Keeping stimulating activities (eg, social and family gatherings, exercise, television) to a minimum in the evening
- Avoiding caffeine-containing foods and beverages (eg, chocolate, cola drinks, tea, coffee) after 5 PM
- Encouraging quiet activities in the evening
- Playing soft, relaxing, soothing music
- Offering a stuffed animal or doll for comfort

DISPLAY 17-7. Nursing Interventions for Abusive Behavior by the Resident

- Avoid situations that may provoke abusive behavior.
- Speak in a calm, quiet voice.
- Continually assess for warning signs of abusive behavior (eg, cursing, pacing, speaking in an increasingly louder voice).
- Keep the resident away from other people.
- Do not react negatively or positively to comments.
- Use positive reinforcement.
- Encourage decision making in situations when possible.
- Learn individual cues that indicate that abusive behaviors are likely to occur.
- Maintain a calm, consistent environment.
- Reduce situations that may increase stress or anxiety or that may provoke fear.

Sometimes slight changes in daily routines can significantly decrease problem behaviors. Display 17-5 provides nursing interventions for patients who wander.

Sundown Syndrome. Sundown syndrome is another problem seen in the elderly. **Sundown syndrome** is an increase in behavior problems such as wandering, agitation, and disorientation after the sun goes down. This type of behavior occurs most often in residents with dementia or declining mental functioning and can be quite problematic. Display 17-6 offers nursing interventions to manage sundown syndrome.

Verbal or Physical Abuse. The elderly can be verbally and physically abusive toward other residents or staff members. Feelings of helplessness, anger, fatigue, or anxiety can result in the elderly person "acting out" with abusive behavior. Physical abuse includes such actions as biting, hitting, or kicking other residents or staff. Verbal abuse includes insulting, accusing, or threatening other residents or staff. Some residents are prone to abusive outbursts without any apparent provocation. Display 17-7 offers nursing interventions to manage abusive behavior.

Resisting Care. Resisting care is also considered a behavior problem. Resisting care includes actions by the elderly person such as refusing to take medications, to bathe, or to eat and refusing assistance with ADLs. When providing care for those who are resisting care, the nurse should try the following:

Avoid arguing or trying to reason with resident.

Give one-step simple directions.

Try various alternatives. For example, if a resident is afraid of a shower, provide a tub bath; if a tub bath causes anxiety, try a sponge bath. If the resident refuses a meal, provide finger foods or food supplement drinks.

Crush tablets and mix with food if the older adult resists taking medications.

Follow medications with a fruit drink if desired.

Socially Inappropriate or Disruptive Behavioral Symptoms. Socially inappropriate or disruptive behavioral symptoms may stem from some unmet need such as anxiety, pain, hunger, a desire to urinate, or constipation. When the need is identified and met, the behavioral symptoms decrease. Socially inappropriate and disruptive behavior includes nosiness, screaming, sexually explicit behavior, smearing or throwing food or fecal material, and hoarding or rummaging through other people's belongings. Display 17-8 identifies general nursing interventions to manage socially inappropriate behavior.

Other behaviors such as hoarding certain items, hiding their own belongings, or taking things

---

DISPLAY 17-8. Nursing Interventions for Socially Inappropriate Disruptive Behaviors

- Move resident to a more private area.
- Use distraction to avert disruptive behavior.
- Use positive reinforcement.
- Set limits for unacceptable behavior.
- Provide a calm, quiet environment.
- Protect other residents from patients with behavioral problems.
- Assess for the cause of the behavior.
- Avoid the use of restraining devices.

---

belonging to others are common. Alzheimer's patients may forget that they took articles, forget where they put them, and become angry and defensive when confronted.

Inappropriate sexual behaviors are also common. Examples include undressing in public, masturbation, urinating in public, repeating vulgar words, or making inappropriate sexual comments.

Medications Used to Manage Behavioral Symptoms. Although it is best to avoid drugs to manage behavioral symptoms major tranquilizers such as chlorpromazine, thioridazine (beginning at 25-mg doses), or haloperidol (beginning with 1.5-mg doses) may be helpful to reduce aggression or wandering. However, the drugs may cause increased confusion, excessive sedation, and extrapyramidal effects (eg, parkinsonian symptoms, akathisia, dystonia).

Any drug used for the elderly should be administered at the lowest effective dosage and the medication regimen reviewed frequently. Polypharmacy is a common problem in older adults that leads to an increased incidence of adverse reactions in patients with AD and should be avoided.

For the depression that sometimes accompanies AD, especially in the early stages, antidepressants may be used. If used, antidepressants without anticholinergic activity are most effective (eg, trazodone, fluoxetine, sertraline).

Caring For the Caregiver

Caregivers of patients with AD are faced with the difficult task of providing the day to day care to loved ones suffering from an incurable disease. These patients remain at home, particularly in the early phases of the disease, and require various levels of care in feeding, bathing, toileting, dressing, cleaning, and paying bills. The progressive nature of AD is depressing to the caregiver who sees his loved one physically and mentally deteriorating and is unable to alter the process. The reality of the situation is often difficult to accept.

Nurses must allow time to nurture the caregiver. Listening to concerns and allowing caregivers to express emotions such as anger is an important part of care. The patient's unpredictability and loss of abilities can make life increasing difficult for the caregiver. The following suggestions may be given to caregivers:

Take time for yourself. Do something enjoyable. Be social. Maintain friendships.

Realize that anger and guilt are normal emotions. Find a support network to help deal with these emotions. Family and friends are often the most supportive.

Stay physically fit. Exercise and eat a well-balanced diet.

Maintain a sense of humor.

Realize that patients cannot control their behavior.

Recognize that the grieving process may begin long before the patient dies. This is a normal process that will assist in adjusting to the loved one's eventual death.

Seek respite care if available.

Consider nursing home care if necessary.

Respite care is a service provided in many areas and allows the caregiver a temporary break in the daily care and responsibility for the Alzheimer's patient. Respite care is a form of short-term care that allows the family some relief from the stress involved in the patient's care. Specialized care and supervision that is normally given by the caregiver is given in a home or in an institutional setting.

Support groups are also available for caregivers, family, and friends of AD patients. Many support groups provide education on the disease, transportation for patients to and from appointments, discussion, and support. The local AD association chapter can provide information concerning support groups that are available. Display 17-9 lists resources for families and patients with AD.

Some communities have adult day care centers that accept AD patients. These adult day care centers provide a supervised environment with stimulating activities, regular meals, and nutritious snacks. These centers can provide relief to the caregiver in the daytime hours.

Evaluating a Nursing Home

Placing a loved one in a nursing home is a difficult decision for most caregivers. It is important for the caregiver to remember that nursing home care may improve the care and safety of the patient. Most families place AD patients in the nursing home when safety issues become insurmountable in the home environment or when providing the personal care is too demanding. Selecting the right home is often a difficult and painful process. Investigation of various nursing homes should begin several months before actual placement in a nursing home. Visiting several nursing homes is important for making an informed decision. Before the visit, the caregiver should make a list of questions to ask during the visit. Suggestions for questions to ask when evaluating a nursing home are found is Display 17-10. Other questions may come to mind for specific needs.

Taking a tour of the nursing home is important before making a decision. While touring, notice the general cleanliness of the facility, the staff, and the patient rooms. Note any odors. Observe the residents. Are they well groomed? Do they appear happy? Are any residents restrained? Tour the kitchen and dining areas during mealtimes if possible. Although there is no foolproof way to select a good nursing home, using the previous suggestions is helpful.

Multi-Infarct Dementia

MID also known as vascular dementia, is the second leading cause of dementia in the elderly. MID occurs as the result of the occlusion of blood vessels in the brain. These occlusions destroy areas of brain tissue, resulting in impaired functioning. There is often a history of hypertension and **transient ischemic attacks** (TIAs). TIAs are episodes of cerebrovascular insufficiency usually caused by atherosclerotic

changes in the arteries of the brain. Symptoms depend on the area of the brain affected and include visual disturbances, dizziness, weakness, dysphasia, numbness, and unconsciousness. The attacks are episodic and usually brief, lasting from a few minutes to several hours after which the individual seemingly recovers. Multiple TIAs over time can lead to MID.

Neurologic symptoms associated with MID include symptoms such as weakness of an extremity, dysarthria (ie, difficulty with speech), or gait changes. As with TIAs, specific symptoms are related to the area of the brain affected. Changes in mental status include cognitive decline, with difficulty concentrating, learning, and making judgments. Poor impulse control and behavior changes may also be present. Depression is common. This disorder occurs more often in men.

The symptoms of MID are similar to those of AD making diagnosis more difficult. A history of hypertension, TIAs, cardiovascular disease, or cigarette smoking can help establish a diagnosis of MID. Although the onset of AD is a slowly progressive deterioration of cognitive functioning, the onset of MID usually is abrupt, with rapid or fluctuating changes in functioning rather than slow progression.

Management is aimed at treating underlying vascular disorder, such as treating the hypertension. Symptoms of dementia are treated similar to those of the dementia associated with AD.

Normal-Pressure Hydrocephalus

Normal-pressure hydrocephalus is a form of dementia that, unlike AD and MID, is reversible. Although responsible for only approximately 2% of all dementias, normal-pressure hydrocephalus most often affects those older than age 50. Three symptoms are commonly found in this disorder: dementia, gait disturbances, and urinary incontinence. Symptoms involving dementia include loss of cognitive functioning such as difficulty concentrating, forgetfulness, and decreased spontaneity. Gait disturbances are often described as "having feet that are stuck to the floor." The patient typically has a wide stance and takes short, slow, shuffling steps. Urinary incontinence, a later sign, may or may not develop.

Diagnosis is made on the presence of the signs and symptoms, a CT scan, MRI, and a lumbar puncture. CT or MRI reveals enlarged ventricles, and the lumbar puncture most often shows normal cerebral spinal fluid (CSF) pressure. In a few atypical cases, the CSF may be abnormal (ie, increased or decreased).

Treatment involves the insertion of a ventriculoperitoneal shunt. The shunt is inserted surgically in the lateral ventricle on the nondominant side of the brain. This is done to minimize any adverse effects caused by damage to the dominant side of the brain during surgery. The shunt allows cerebrospinal fluid to flow into the peritoneal cavity. Gait and cognition improve slowly over a period of months. Results of the treatment are variable, with substantial improvement occurring in approximately one half of the patients.

Using the Nursing Process in Caring for a Patient With Dementia

Assessment
When assessing an individual for dementia, it is important to determine the extent of cognitive loss. Assess for aphasia, apraxia, agnosia, and agraphia (loss of ability to express thoughts in writing). Assess for orientation to person, time, and place. Assess problem solving ability by asking questions such as "What would you do if you had no groceries in the house?" or "What would you do if you were alone at home and became ill?"

Language ability can be assessed by asking the patient to name common items such as a watch, paper clip, or pencil. Assess memory by asking questions such as "Who is the president?" or repeat the three names of three items previously mentioned. Observe the general appearance (ie, facial expression, dress, and behavior) and ability to communicate. Determine the ability to perform ADLs and amount of assistance needed. Obtain weight, and assess nutritional status (ie, eating patterns and appetite). Assess sleep-wake patterns such as the presence of sundown syndrome, insomnia, or early wakefulness. Gait and coordination must be assessed to help identify the risk for falls and the amount of assistance needed. Determine the presence of any behavioral symptoms. A thorough neu-

rologic assessment is time consuming but important to establish a baseline and monitor care. It is also important to distinguish between delirium and dementia (see Chapter 14, Table 14-5) and assess the cause of dementia. Adequate treatment for the cause of the dementia can reverse it. If the older adult becomes fatigued during the assessment, it may be completed at a later date. Fatigue may cause the assessment to be inaccurate.

Nursing Diagnoses
The following nursing diagnoses may be appropriate for a patient with dementia:

Altered Thought Processes related to memory loss, cognitive decline, other (specify)

Self-Care Deficit related to cognitive decline and functional decline, other (specify)

Risk for Injury related to disorientation, confusion, impaired judgment, uncoordinated gait

Caregiver Role Strain related to disruptive behavior of patient, the need for prolonged care, other (specify)

Additional nursing diagnosis may be appropriate for individual patients.

Planning and Intervention
After a thorough assessment and specific nursing diagnoses are determined, the plan of care must be individualized. Interventions are aimed at maintaining functional and cognitive ability, preventing injury, and supporting the caregiver. Every effort is made to determine the contributing factors to any behavioral symptoms. Interventions to manage behavioral symptoms are specific to the problem exhibited.

Altered Thought Processes. When the thought process is altered, the individual experiences various degrees of confusion and cognitive loss. It is important to create a quiet, pleasant, predictable environment. Adapt communication to the ability level of the individual. When talking to the patient, use a slow, quiet voice. Use short sentences and simple words. Repeat instructions, giving only one step at a time and using the same words. Avoid open-ended questions. Avoid negative confrontation or remarks. Use positive reinforcement to encourage desired behavior. Maintain eye contact and a calm quiet manner. Eliminate extraneous distractors or noise, such as overhead paging systems, television, and large crowds. Use music therapy to create a soothing atmosphere. Use reminiscence therapy if cognitive ability permits. In early stages, reality orientation may prove helpful. As cognitive ability declines, validation therapy is more appropriate. Display 17-11 offers information on reality orientation and validation therapy.

DISPLAY 17-11. Understanding Validation Therapy and Reality Therapy

Validation Therapy. Validation therapy may be helpful with elderly, confused patients, particularly those with dementia who are experiencing permanent cognitive loss. The idea behind validation therapy is that the nurse seeks to validate the patient's feelings to give a sense of dignity and self-worth. Because all behavior has meaning, any behavior, even negative or regressive behavior, has meaning to the patient. By establishing trust, the nurse can explore through body language, gestures, and expressions the meaning of the patient's behavior. Those who practice validation techniques use supportive behavior and encouraging words to validate the patient's feelings. Validation therapy is not simply "going along with the patient" or "agreeing to keep peace." It is a method to provide *comfort* to the patient while allowing the nurse to explore the reason for the behavior.

Example of validation therapy: One elderly Alzheimer's patient, Ms. Trotter, had episodes of calling for "Nana." The call for Nana was painfully loud and disruptive to others. After talking with her son, the nurse discovered that Nana was Ms. Trotter's grandmother who had raised her. Rather than explain to Ms. Trotter that Nana was dead or gone, the nurses tried to discover what need she had that could possibly be met by Nana. The nurses gave her extra nurturing, sat with her, and sometimes even rocked her. After a time, the nurses discovered that Ms. Trotter cried for Nana when she was uncomfortable or in pain.

Reality Orientation. Reality orientation is best suited for those in the early stages of dementia and for those who are disoriented and slightly confused. When reality orientation is used, the entire staff in the nursing home participates. The nursing facility usually has a large calendar with the date, day of the week, the season, and perhaps the weather for that particular day. All staff reinforce these reality-based facts throughout the entire 24-hour period. Every effort is aimed at orienting the patient to the "here and now." Patients are also reminded of their names, where they are, and the nurses' names. In some facilities, group meetings of 8 to 10 residents are held to reinforce reality. The nurse facilitates these meetings.

Self-Care Deficit. Impaired ability to perform ADLs occurs with loss of cognitive and motor functioning. Although these abilities continue to decline, efforts are made to maintain these abilities as long as possible. Maintain consistency in daily routine. Encourage as much self-care as possible, assisting only when necessary. Allow plenty of time to perform ADLs. When feeding, use assistive devices if needed. Feed one food at a time, taking the patient's likes and dislikes into consideration. When assisting with dressing, offer one item of clothing at a time. If necessary, gently coax the patient when he is attempting ADLs. Do not rush, but allow sufficient time to accomplish task. Use assistive devices such as modified eating utensils, button hooks, raised toilet seats, and grab bars to increase ability to perform ADLs.

Risk for Injury. The patient may be at increased risk for injury because of a behavior problem or gait and coordination disturbances. Gait disturbances may necessitate an assistive device such as a cane or walker. Assistance may be needed when walking, getting out of bed, or when toileting. Avoid the use of restraints because their use tends to increase the risk of injury. If restraints must be used, use the least restrictive restraint possible.

Enlist the aid of family or assistive personnel to watch the patient. Modify environment to increase safety. Keep surroundings uncluttered, and provide a clear path for walking. Keep harmful substances such as cleaning supplies, toxic chemicals, and medications in inaccessible places. Use childproof locks for cabinets or drawers. If wandering is a problem, use an electronic monitoring system. Ensure that the patient is wearing a form of identification.

Evaluate medication regimen. Some medications cause gait disturbances, visual disturbances, or orthostatic hypotension that could result in the falls and injury.

Caregiver Role Strain. The 24-hour care required by patients with dementia places the caregiver at increased risk for stress. The nurse must establish a therapeutic relationship with the caregiver and encourage the caregiver to pursue activities of interest. The nurse allows sufficient time to listen to the caregiver express feelings of anxiety, fear, grief, and anger. It is important to be supportive and nonjudgmental. The nurse acknowledges the difficulty of the situation and offers support. It is important to identify and focus on strengths of the caregiver and the patient. The nurse answer questions, provides information, assesses the need for additional resources, and provides suggestions to deal with problems (eg, behavior problems, physical problems, cognitive decline).

The nurse may refer caregivers to support groups or national organizations. The caregiver may need help to identify sources to provide relief (see Display 17-9). TriAD is a support program for the caregivers, those with AD, and the health care provider. Services includes videos, newsletters, and brochures. The program provides tools to help handle the day to day reality of AD. TriAD is an educational service sponsored by Pfizer, Inc., and Eisai, Inc., in collaboration with the Alzheimer's Association and the National Council on the Aging.

Evaluation and Expected Outcomes

Successful care can produce the following outcomes:

No injury occurs.

Environment is made safer.

Self-care performed within individual
limitations.

Decreased incidence of undesired behaviors.

Caregiver expresses less stress.

Evaluation is based on maintaining as much functional ability as possible for as long as possible and not on restoring functional or mental ability.

PARKINSONISM

Parkinsonism is a slowly progressive neurologic disorder most often affecting the elderly. The incidence of parkinsonism increases with age, peaking at 75 years of age. About 1 million people in the United States have Parkinson disease. The most prominent symptoms include **bradykinesia** (ie, slowness of movement), resting tremor, muscular stiffness, and rigidity (ie, state of involuntary contraction of all skeletal muscles). Sometimes the disorder progresses rapidly, but at other times, the course is slower, with the individual remaining functional for many years.

Signs and Symptoms

There are four major symptoms of Parkinson disease:

Rigidity: stiffness when the arm, leg, or neck is
moved

Resting tremor: tremor most prominent at rest

Bradykinesia: slowness in initiating movement
resulting in decreased facial expression,
change in speech patterns, shuffling gait,
smaller-lettered handwriting, and trouble with
fine finger movements

Loss of postural reflexes: poor balance and
coordination

Early symptoms include infrequent blinking, lack of facial expression, and stiffening of the extremities. A characteristic tremor occurs as the disease progresses. This resting tremor occurs in approximately 60% of people with Parkinson's disease. The tremor usually begins in one hand and arm and later extends to the head. Although the tremor may remain on only one side, it frequently progresses to involve both upper extremities. Although present at rest, it disappears briefly when the individual performs purposeful movement and then reappears when the extremity becomes stationary. The tremor appears as a regular, rhythmic, low-amplitude

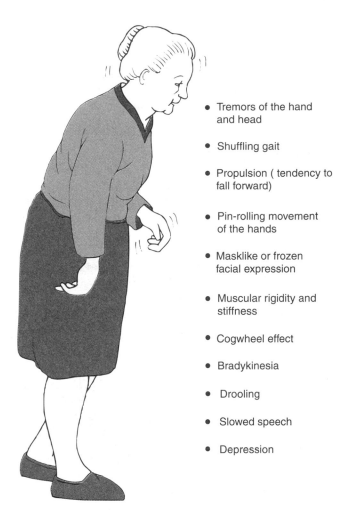

FIGURE 17-1. Summary of symptoms with parkinsonism.

- Tremors of the hand and head
- Shuffling gait
- Propulsion (tendency to fall forward)
- Pin-rolling movement of the hands
- Masklike or frozen facial expression
- Muscular rigidity and stiffness
- Cogwheel effect
- Bradykinesia
- Drooling
- Slowed speech
- Depression

tremor. There is a pin-rolling motion of the thumb against the fingers (so named because it appears as if the person is rolling a pin between the fingers).

The rigidity and muscular stiffness leads to the characteristic gait and loss of facial expression. The gait is described as "shuffling," with the body appearing to move as a unit rather than with the weight shifting from side to side. Movement occurs in a series of tiny shuffling steps with the head bent forward. There is a loss of normal arm movement. A cogwheel effect (ie, ratchet-like jerk) in movement results from the rigidity of the muscles. The problems with movement and gait increases the risk of falling. Because of the limited movement of facial muscles and infrequency of blinking, the face appears masklike.

Other symptoms include increased salivation leading to drooling, constipation, urinary incontinence, and decreased sexual function. Speech becomes slow, monotonous, and difficult. Problems with movement causes difficulty in swallowing, dressing, and self-feeding. Depression is common. Figure 17-1 provides a summary of symptoms.

No one person has all the symptoms of parkinsonism, but each has a unique combination of symptoms.

About 25% of the patients with parkinsonism develop dementia. Parkinson's disease affects more men than women and typically is seen in those over 60 years of age. The disease progresses for about 10 years, at which time death occurs, generally from pneumonia or other infection.

Physiologic Changes

The major physiologic abnormality in parkinsonism is related to the loss of cells in the substantia nigra (ie, structure in the basal ganglia of the brain). The cells in the substantia nigra normally produce high concentrations of the neurotransmitter dopamine (Fig. 17-2). With parkinsonism, dopamine levels are significantly decreased. When the neurons that produce dopamine are lost, symptoms associated with bradykinesia, rigidity, and tremors develop.

Diagnosis

Early diagnosis may be difficult. As the disease progresses, the diagnosis is made on the basis of the signs and symptoms. No laboratory test is available to confirm the diagnosis of parkinsonism. Progression of the disease varies among patient. For some, the disease progresses slowly over 20 to 30 years, but it progresses much faster in others. Without treatment, pronounced disability occurs in about 9 years.

Therapy

Drug Therapy

There is no cure for parkinsonism, but certain drugs are used to relieve the symptoms and assist in maintaining the patient's mobility and functioning capability as long as possible. Treatment is individualized, using the type and severity of symptoms as a guide. The most common drugs used to manage parkinsonism are amantadine, selegiline, levodopa-carbidopa combinations, and the anticholinergic drugs. These drugs help to replenish the diminishing dopamine. Newer drugs, such as tolcapone (Tasmar) and pramipexole dihydrochloride (Mirapex), may also be used to treat Parkinson disease.

Levodopa crosses the blood–brain barrier and is converted to dopamine in the brain. The blood–brain barrier is a term used to describe the ability of the CNS to prohibit large and potentially harmful molecules from crossing through walls of the capillaries into the brain. Levodopa may be

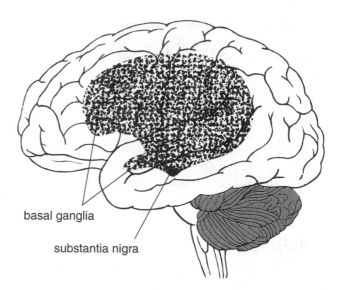

basal ganglia

substantia nigra

FIGURE 17-2. In parkinsonism there is a severe deficit of the neurotransmitter dopamine in the basal ganglia deep within the brain. The loss of dopamine results from the loss of nerve cells in the substantia nigra, where dopamine is made before being transported to the basal ganglia.

given alone or in combination with carbidopa. When given alone, levodopa causes nausea, vomiting, insomnia, orthostatic hypotension, and mental confusion. The most serious and frequent adverse reactions of levodopa include choreiform movements (ie, involuntary muscular twitching of the limbs or facial muscles), dystonic movements (ie, muscular spasms affecting the tongue, jaw, and neck), and mental changes such as depression and psychotic episodes.

Carbidopa is used in combination with levodopa to make more levodopa available to cross the blood–brain barrier, reducing the dosage of levodopa needed. By reducing the dosage, the incidence of adverse reactions also declines.

Amantadine (Symmetrel) is an antiviral drug with antiparkinsonism activity. This drug is used to treat the early symptoms of Parkinson to decrease rigidity, tremor, and bradykinesia. Adverse reactions include depression, confusion, nausea, dizziness, visual disturbance, and headache. Amantadine may be used with levodopa for a rapid therapeutic effect and maintenance therapy.

Selegiline (Eldepryl) may be used in the early stages to slow progression of the disease. The drug is generally well tolerated, with few adverse reactions. The patient's response to drug therapy requires careful monitoring to adjust the dosage of the drug upward or downward to obtain the desired therapeutic effect.

Catechol-O-methyltransferase (COMT) inhibitors block the enzyme, preventing the breakdown of levodopa in the intestinal tract. Patients then receive more levodopa from the bloodstream into the brain. Tolcapone, a COMT inhibitor, is used in conjunction with levodopa. Its used is limited because of cases of liver damage attributed to its use. Liver enzymes are monitored monthly during the first 3 months of the treatment and every 6 weeks thereafter for the next 3 months. If elevations occur in liver function test results, the physician usually discontinues the drug. However, if the physician elects to continue the drug, more frequent liver functions tests are required. Side effects (when administered with levodopa) include diarrhea, nausea, orthostatic hypotension, syncope, sleep disorder, anorexia, dyskinesia, dystonia, headache, and confusion.

Non-ergot dopamine agonists are thought to stimulate the dopamine receptors in the brain. Examples of this category of drugs include pramipexole (Mirapex) and ropinirole (Requip). Most patients taking pramipexole or ropinirole experience improvement in symptoms and overall function. Improvement may be gradual, and continued treatment is recommended for several months. It may be given with carbidopa-levodopa (Sinemet). The dosage of Sinemet may be decreased. Side effects of the nonergot dopamine agonists include nausea, dizziness, sleepiness, postural hypotension, impaired voluntary movements, and hallucinations. Older adults are at higher risk for hallucinations. Taking the drug with food may decrease the nausea.

Anticholinergic drugs such as benztropine mesylate (Cogentin), trihexyphenidyl (Artane), or procyclidine (Kemadrin) may also be used. Anticholinergic drugs are contraindicated in patients with glaucoma. Drugs with anticholinergic activity inhibit acetylcholine (ie, neurohormone produced in excess in parkinsonism). Anticholinergic drugs are generally less effective than levodopa. The anticholinergic drugs are often poorly tolerated by the elderly, causing confusion, sedation, orthostatic hypotension, urinary retention or frequency, hypotension, blurred vision, dry mouth, constipation, mental disturbances, or ataxia. The high incidence of adverse reactions makes the anticholinergic drugs a poor choice for the elderly.

Transplantation of Fetal Nigra

A new method of replenishing the dopamine in parkinsonism is by obtaining nigra cells from aborted fetuses and transplanting the cells into the brain of patients with Parkinson disease. These cells form neural connections and produce dopamine. Selection of patients to undergo this treatment is strict, and its usefulness is still under investigation and controversial.

Using the Nursing Process in Caring for a Patient With Parkinsonism

Assessment

Assessment focuses on the effects of the disease on the patient. Patients are questioned concerning what activities they can do and how the disease is affecting functional ability. Because memory impairment and alterations in thinking occur in some patients, a history from the patient may be unreliable. When necessary obtain the history from a family member or relative. Obtain information regarding the symptoms the patient is experiencing, the length of time the symptoms have been present, the ability of the patient to carry on activities of daily living, and the patient's mental condition. For patients experiencing behavioral problems, assess for the presence of pain, constipation, hunger, or other causes of the disruptive behavior.

ASSESSMENT ALERT

When assessing the tremor, it is important to distinguish between essential tremor (a normal occurrence) and the tremor associated with Parkinson disease. The parkinson tremor occurs at rest and with purposeful movement. An essential tremor occurs only with action and is not seen when the limb is at rest. Patients with essential tremor do not exhibit other symptoms associated with parkinsonism, such as a masklike expression and bradykinesia. In contrast, they have animated faces and normal rates of movement.

People with this disease may exhibit problems with dressing, handling eating utensils, and with personal hygiene. The may also have difficulty rising from chairs, turning over in bed, or getting in or out of cars. A careful assessment of the ability to perform ADLs is important in planning care. It is also important to assess the gait. Posture may appear flexed, with the feet appearing or feeling as though they are "sticking" to the ground. This may contribute to unstable and uncoordinated movements.

Nursing Diagnoses

Depending on the severity of the disease process and the symptoms the individual is experiencing, one or more of the following nursing diagnoses may be appropriate:

Impaired Physical Mobility related to weakness, muscle rigidity, other (specify)

Self-Care Deficit (eating, drinking, dressing) related to tremor, muscular weakness, other (specify)

Risk for Injury related to functional disability, muscular weakness, gait disturbance, other (specify)

Impaired Swallowing related to excessive saliva, muscular weakness, other (specify)

Ineffective Individual Coping related to the progressive nature of the disease, the inability to perform self-care, other (specify)

Other nursing diagnoses may be used to meet individual needs.

Planning and Implementation

Planning the care of the patient with parkinsonism requires careful analysis of the limitations and signs and symptoms noted during the assessment. Interventions are aimed at improving mobility, maintaining independent function, and assisting the patient in coping with the disease.

Impaired Physical Mobility. Muscular rigidity and gait disturbance leads to impaired mobility. The physical therapist may assist in planning a program of daily exercise to increase or maintain muscle strength and improve coordination. Exercises such as walking, riding a stationary bike, or swimming may be used. Special emphasis is placed on proper walking technique. The patient is encouraged to walk erect, use a long stride, and consciously swing the arms when walking. A heel-toe gait is used. Sometimes, walking to music helps to obtain the appropriate gait. Allow frequent rest periods because fatigue may occur. Passive and active range-of-motion exercises are encouraged.

Self-Care Deficit. Self-care includes ADLs such as feeding, dressing, toileting, and bathing. Bradykinesia and muscle rigidity result in limitations in self-care. These symptoms result in problems with drinking from a glass, bringing utensils to the mouth for feeding, getting out of a chair, turning in bed, shaving, and combing hair. Assistive devices may be helpful to maintain self-care (see Chapter 9). Teach the proper use of assistive devices. Give positive feedback. Allow sufficient time for performance of the self-care activity. Offer choices in planning self-care. Repeat instructions if necessary. Allow the individual the maximum amount of independence and participation. Treat the person with dignity and respect.

Risk for Injury. The patient with parkinsonism may have trouble walking. The individuals are especially prone to falls and other accidents because of their disease process. Identify safety devices to promote a safe physical environment and individual safety. Refer to a physical therapist and occupational therapist as needed. Assist with ambulation, getting out of bed or a chair, and other self-care activities. Identify community resources to assist patients still in the home setting. Educate caregivers on techniques to assist the patient and make the environment safe.

Impaired Swallowing. Patients with parkinsonism may have difficulty swallowing because of excessive salivation, muscle rigidity, or other factors related to the disease process. For patients with difficulty swallowing, plan to serve meals when the patient is rested. Keep suction equipment within easy reach. Keep in a seated position when eating or raise the head to a 90-degree angle. Keep the bed elevated at least 30 minutes after feeding. Provide food in a consistency that is most easily swallowed such as thickened liquids (using less water in preparation of foods such as Jell-O), thick drinks, scrambled eggs, or soft cooked foods. Others may prefer thinned purees rather than thickened food. Place food midway on tongue in approximately 5- to 10-mL bites. Remain with patient during mealtime or have a family member present. Consult with dietitian to assist in meal planning.

Ineffective Individual Coping. The patient with parkinsonism may have difficulty coping, particularly in the early stages. Allow patients ample time to discuss the disease and its expected progression. Carefully explain the medication regimen and answer any questions. The medication regimen is sometimes difficult to regulate and the patient may have problems coping with this aspect of care. For example, the on-off phenomenon may occur in patients taking levodopa. In this condition, the patient alternates between improved clinical status (on) and loss of therapeutic effect (off). If this occurs, the physician may order withdrawal of levodopa for 5 to 14 days, followed by gradual restarting of the drug. Another, sometimes difficult, consideration is the need for frequent dosage adjustments until maximum therapeutic response is obtained.

The nurse should assist the patient to identify problems that are most difficult to cope with and discuss possible alternatives. Actively listening and showing support will encourage the patient and family members to open up and communicate with the nurse. The nurse should facilitate emotional support from significant others. The patient may need assistance in setting realistic goals. Sometimes, ineffective coping leads to depression (see Chapter 15). The nurse may refer the patient and family members to resources that may offer information and support (Display 17-12).

Evaluation and Expected Outcomes

Successful treatment can be gauged by the following responses of the patient:

Walks with wide base of support using normal arm movement

Participates in self-care (eg, feeding, dressing, toileting, and bathing)

Copes with individual symptoms and disabilities of parkinsonism
Follows appropriate feeding methods
Has no difficulty swallowing

SEIZURE DISORDERS IN THE ELDERLY

Seizure disorders are sudden episodes of repeated electronic discharges from cerebral neurons (ie, nerves). These neural discharges result in abnormal motor, sensory, or psychic activity. The terms *seizure* and *convulsion* are used interchangeably. The exact cause of a seizure is not totally understood but seems to be related to metabolic and electro-chemical activity at the cellular level. Certain conditions can increase the probability of seizure activity (Display 17-13). Seizures are generally classified as generalized or partial, depending on the origin of the seizure activity and the symptoms exhibited.

Partial Seizures

Focal or **partial seizures** begin in a specific area of the brain. A partial seizure can spread to the entire brain, causing a generalized seizure. There are two types of partial seizures: simple partial seizures and complex partial seizures. Simple partial seizures usually last no more than 60 seconds and result in no loss of consciousness. Symptoms of simple partial seizures include uncontrolled jerking movements of a body part (eg, finger, mouth, hand, foot), mumbling, and hallucinatory symptoms that may manifest themselves as visual, auditory, or olfactory experiences.

Complex partial seizures manifest a greater variety of sensory and motor symptoms, result in some alteration of consciousness, and like the partial seizure, usually lasts no longer than 1 minute. In addition to the symptoms seen with partial seizures, inappropriate repetitive movements such as lip smacking, picking at clothes, and distorted visual and auditory sensations may be exhibited.

Generalized Seizures

Generalized seizures affect the entire brain, resulting in a loss of consciousness and lasting from several seconds to several minutes. Two types of generalized seizures affecting older adults include myoclonic seizures, and tonic-clonic seizures. **Myoclonic seizures** are manifested by sudden, excessive jerking of the arms, legs, or entire body. Although lasting only a short time, myoclonic seizures can be so forceful that the person falls to the ground.

Tonic-clonic seizures are also called grand mal seizures. This type of seizure is often preceded by a preictal phase in which they experience vague symptoms such as depression, anxiety, and nervousness for several minutes or hours before the seizure.

An aura generally occurs immediately before the beginning of the seizure. An aura is a feeling (ie, weakness or numbness) or sense (ie, odor or sound) experienced by the patient that is related to the affected area of the brain. Manifestations of a generalized tonic-clonic seizure include alternate contraction (ie, tonic phase) and relaxation (ie, clonic phase), resulting in jerking movements and thrashing of the arms and legs. The skin becomes cyanotic, and jaws are clenched causing the inner cheek and tongue to be bitten. Urinary or fecal incontinence may occur. As the excessive saliva mixes with air, frothing at the mouth can occur. The clonic phase gradually subsides and is followed by a postictal phase with symptoms of headaches, fatigue, confusion, deep sleep, and possibly muscle soreness. Some individuals sleep deeply for several hours after a tonic-clonic seizure.

Epilepsy is a term used for a permanent, recurrent seizure disorder. Most often the cause of epilepsy is unknown, but it can be caused by any of the conditions listed in Display 17-13. Status epilepticus is an emergency situation characterized by continuous seizure activity. Status epilepticus may occur spontaneously, or it may be caused by the abrupt withdrawal of anticonvulsant medication.

Diagnosis of Seizure Activity

Diagnosis is made by a neurologic examination and electroencephalogram (EEG). Although an EEG is used for diagnosis, a series of EEGs may be needed to confirm the diagnosis. Other diagnostic examinations such as CT, MRI, and serology studies may be performed for additional confirmation of the diagnosis or to identify the cause of the seizure disorder. An accurate description of the seizure given by a reliable observer can help establish the diagnosis as well.

Drug Therapy for Seizures

Anticonvulsant drugs are used to manage seizure disorders. The anticonvulsants act to reduce the excitability of the nerve cells in the brain. When the neuron excitability is decreased, the seizures are reduced in intensity and frequency. In some cases, the seizures are virtually eliminated, but in other cases, only partial control of the seizure disorder is obtained. The most commonly prescribed anticonvulsants include the barbiturates (phenobarbital), the benzodiazepenes (Valium and Klonopin), the hydantoins (Dilantin), the succinimides (Zarotin), and valproic acid. Anticonvulsants control but do not cure epilepsy. The objectives of the medication regimen is to control seizures with minimal side effects. The medication is selected on the basis of the type of seizure and the safety of the medication. Because phenobarbital and phenytoin cause sedation, dizziness, and impaired coordination, other drugs such as carbamazepine and valproic acid may be more effective in the elderly.

All anticonvulsants should be used cautiously in older adults because of the potential decrease in the ability of the liver and kidney to sufficiently metabolize and excrete the drugs. With impaired elimination, toxic effects can occur. In general starting dosages of the drugs should be the lowest possible dose, with dosages increasing slowly until a therapeutic response occurs. Serum concentration levels of the anticonvulsant are monitored on a regular basis to detect signs of toxicity. Intravenous diazepam is most often the drug given initially for status epilepticus.

DISPLAY 17-13. Factors That Increase the Probability of Seizure Disorders

- Drug toxicity
- Electrolyte imbalances (eg, hypoglycemia, hyperglycemia, hypocalcemia, hyponatremia)
- Hypoxia
- Head trauma
- Brain tumors
- Cranial surgery
- Uremia
- Central nervous system infection
- Drug withdrawal (eg, alcohol, barbiturates)

DRUG ALERT

Intravenous diazepam is given with extreme care to the elderly with limited pulmonary reserve or unstable cardiovascular status because cardiac arrest can occur.

After seizures are controlled, other anticonvulsants are used for long-term control.

Assessing a Patient With a Seizure Disorder

A thorough history is necessary to identify the type of seizure disorder. Information obtained from those who have observed the seizure should include the following:

Description of the seizure including all motor and sensory symptoms experienced

Frequency of the seizures

Average length of the seizures

Description of the preictal phase and aura, if applicable

Degrees of unconsciousness

Presence of urinary or bladder incontinence

Additional information includes a family history of seizures (if any), recent drug therapy, and if seizure activity is new, a history of recent illness or head injury. An elderly patient may not be able to give an accurate description of the seizure or seizure activity. Confirm information with family members or caregivers if possible.

Caring for a Patient With a Seizure Disorder

In caring for a patient with a seizure disorder every effort is made to prevent injury during the seizure. If a preictal phase or aura is present, instruct the patient to take precautions at that time by lying down or going to a safe place. If driving, stop the car, and turn off the ignition. If a seizure is witnessed in the hospital or nursing home, call for help, using the call bell, and stay with the patient to observe the seizure activity (eg, where the seizure began, amount of time the seizure lasted, body part involved, incontinence, unconsciousness). Provide privacy. If the patient is in a chair, ease him to the floor. Do not attempt to place anything in the mouth such as a tongue blade or airway. Loosen clothing, and remove objects that could obstruct breathing. Pad side rails if seizures are frequent.

Do not attempt to restrict movement during seizure activity. Place the patient on the side to prevent aspiration. Note the time the seizure ended and the presence of sedation or drowsiness in the postictal period. Inspect lips and oral cavity for evidence of injury. Take vital signs every 30 minutes. Notify the physician. Keep the bed flat and the patient on his side. Room lighting is kept dim, and noise is kept to a minimum to avoid stimulation and precipitation of another seizure.

For continuous seizures (ie, status epilepticus), establish an airway, notify the physician, and administer oxygen. Oral suctioning may be necessary to remove oral secretions and prevent aspiration. In addition to oxygen, the physician may order an intravenous line with the administration of intravenous diazepam.

CRITICAL THINKING EXERCISES

1. Mrs. Patterson is becoming increasingly unable to care for herself at home. Her daughter is coming to her home each day but is fearful that she will hurt herself. The home health nurse suggested placing Mrs. Patterson in a nursing home. What suggestions should the home health nurse make about selecting a nursing home? How could Mrs. Patterson's daughter prepare her mother to go into the nursing home?

2. Ms. James, age 69, has parkinsonism. She was recently admitted into the nursing home because she had fallen three times at home during the past several weeks. Identify three potential nursing diagnoses that would most probably be included in Mrs. James' care plan. Plan at least five nursing interventions for each nursing diagnosis. Include a rationale for each intervention.

3. Mr. Kilmore, age 78, is a resident at the nursing home where you work. He has begun wandering in and out of other resident's rooms. His symptoms seem to get worse in the evening. What nursing interventions would be most appropriate for Mr. Kilmore's wandering? What interventions would help with the increase in wandering in the evening? Give a rationale for each intervention.

4. While you are administering medications, you find an elderly patient on the floor who is seizuring. What action would you take first? What other actions would be important for you to take? What information would you need before notifying the physician?

REFERENCES AND SUGGESTED READING

American Psychiatric Association. (1994). *Diagnostic and statistical manual of mental disorders* (4th ed.). Washington, DC: American Psychiatric Association.

Crigger, N., & Forbes, W. (1997). Assessing neurologic function in older patients. *American Journal of Nursing, 97 (3),* 37.

Fazio, S., Seman, D., & Stansell, J. (1999). *Rethinking Alzheimer's care.* Baltimore, MD: Health Professions Press.

Fraser, C. (1996). This dementia patient can be helped. *RN, January,* 38–44.

Kaplan, M., & Hoffman, M. (Eds). (1998). *Behaviors in dementia—Best practices for successful management.* Baltimore, MD: Health Professions Press.

Kovach, C., & Wessel-Krejci, J. (1998). Facilitating change in dementia. *Journal of Nursing Administration, 28 (5),* 17.

Matteson, M.A., McConnell, E., & Linton, A. (1997). *Gerontological nursing* (2nd ed.). Philadelphia: W.B. Saunders.

Roach, S., & Scherer, J. (2000). *Introductory clinical pharmacology* (6th ed.). Philadelphia: Lippincott Williams & Wilkins.

Smeltzer, S., & Bare, B. (1996). *Textbook of medical-surgical nursing* (8th ed.). Philadelphia: Lippincott Williams & Wilkins.

Tappen, R. (1997). *Interventions for Alzheimer's disease—A caregiver's complete reference.* Baltimore, MD: Health Professions Press.

CHAPTER 18

The Cardiovascular System

CHAPTER OUTLINE

KEY TERMS

CHAPTER OBJECTIVES

NORMAL HEART FUNCTION

AGE-RELATED CHANGES OF THE CARDIOVASCULAR
   SYSTEM

HEART FAILURE

CORONARY ARTERY DISEASE

HYPERTENSION

CEREBROVASCULAR ACCIDENT

PERIPHERAL VASCULAR DISEASE

CRITICAL THINKING EXERCISES

REFERENCES AND SUGGESTED READING

KEY TERMS

angina

aphasia

atherosclerosis

cerebrovascular accident

collateral circulation

heart failure

hypertension

intermittent claudication

isolated systolic hypertension

pacemaker

thrombophlebitis

varicose veins

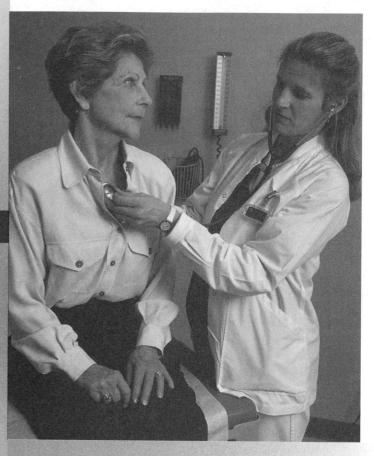

CHAPTER OBJECTIVES

**At the completion of this chapter, the student will
be able to**

- **Identify age-related changes that occur within
  the cardiovascular system**

- **Discuss the signs and symptoms, treatment,
  and nursing care of an older adult with heart
  failure, coronary artery disease, a pacemaker,
  hypertension, cerebrovascular accident, and
  peripheral vascular disease**

Cardiovascular disease is a leading cause of death in
the elderly population. Evidence of heart disease
is found in approximately 50% of those between 65
and 74 years of age and in 60% of individuals older
than age 75. With more of the population reaching

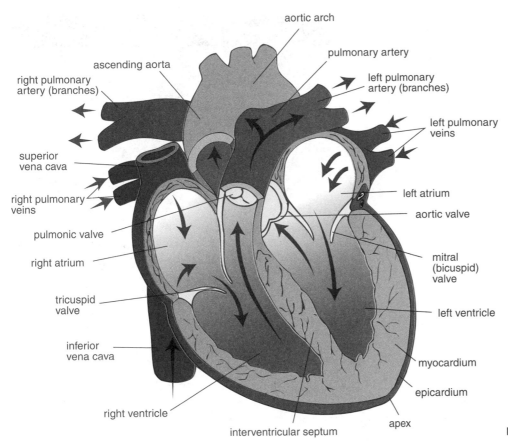

aortic arch

pulmonary artery

ascending aorta

left pulmonary artery (branches)

right pulmonary artery (branches)

left pulmonary veins

superior vena cava

left atrium

right pulmonary veins

aortic valve

pulmonic valve

mitral (bicuspid) valve

right atrium

tricuspid valve

left ventricle

inferior vena cava

myocardium

epicardium

right ventricle

apex

interventricular septum

FIGURE 18-1. Normal heart.

advanced age, cardiovascular disease will continue to be a significant threat to the health and well-being of the elderly population.

NORMAL HEART FUNCTION

Normally, the cardiovascular system serves as a closed system for the flow of blood. This system functions to deliver oxygen, nutrients, and other substances to all body cells and to remove the waste products of cellular metabolism. The heart weighs less than 1 pound and is about the size of a fist. Functioning as a muscular pump, the heart drives blood through the blood vessels through two separate, but interrelated systems. The right side of the heart is concerned with pulmonary circulation and pumps blood to the lungs. The left side of the heart pumps blood to the systemic circulation through the aorta, supplying blood to all areas of the body except the lungs. The right and left sides of the heart are interrelated; as the blood from the right side returns from the lungs, it passes into the left ventricle, where it is pumped into the systemic circulation through the aorta (Fig. 18-1). The interventricular septum separates the two sides of the heart.

AGE-RELATED CHANGES OF THE CARDIOVASCULAR SYSTEM

The most significant change in the aging heart occurs in the myocardium (ie, muscular layer). The muscular layer of the left ventricle becomes 25% thicker, myocardial elasticity decreases, and there is an increase in rigidity of the heart muscle. This results in a decrease of the contractile force of the ventricles. As muscle fibers decrease, they are replaced by fibrous tissue. With age, cardiac output (ie, volume of blood pumped by the ventricles) decreases by 25%. The aorta and other large arteries lose elasticity. The ability of the vessels to stretch decreases approximately 50% by the age of 80. The valves of the veins become less efficient, increasing the risk of varicose veins or stasis ulcers.

In general, blood vessels become less elastic and more narrow, in part because of calcium deposits that accumulate on the vessel walls. A gradual rise in blood pressure occurs with age. The increase in blood pressure is a result of a decline in arterial elasticity and an increase in peripheral resistance. Blood flow through the kidneys also decreases. These changes in vessel arterial elasticity and blood flow to the kidney account for the gradual increase in blood pressure with age.

The yellow-brown pigment, lipofuscin, increases in the aging heart. Lipofuscin found in the myocardial fibers produces a brownish color to the heart tissue. Some theorists link lipofuscin to the aging process, but its exact role in aging remains unclear.

The coronary arteries supply blood to the heart muscle. These vessels have a 35% decrease in blood flow between the ages of 20 and 60. Because the blood flow to coronary arteries decreases slowly over a number of years, collateral circulation develops. **Collateral circulation** is a method by which the heart compensates for atherosclerosis by developing alternate pathways of vessels to provide blood to the upper part of the heart muscle.

The heart valves, which prevent backflow of blood in the heart, stiffen and become thicker as collagen degenerates and fat accumulates. The two valves most affected are the mitral and aortic values (see Fig. 18-1).

The sinoatrial (SA) node, located in the upper portion of the right atrium, is made up of specialized cells called pacemaker cells. Normally, approximately 50% of the SA node's mass is composed of pacemaker cells. In the elderly, the mass of the SA node contains only about 10% pacemaker cells. This decrease in pacemaker cells may contribute to pulse irregularities such as arrhythmias or bradycardia seen in older adults.

Even with the numerous changes that occur within the cardiovascular system with age, the heart is remarkably able to adapt. It may be impossible to determine whether individual changes in the cardiovascular system are the result of normal physiologic changes or of pathologic changes due to atherosclerosis. The changes in the cardiovascular system result in a decreased ability of the aging heart to return quickly to a normal resting rate after exercise.

HEART FAILURE

Heart failure is the most common discharge diagnosis for hospitalized Medicare patients. It affects an estimated 2 million people per year in the United States. In addition to causing death, heart failure can significantly decrease quality of life and functional ability. **Heart failure** is a condition that occurs when the heart is unable to pump enough blood to meet the body's demands. Symptoms are identified in Display 18-1.

For many patients, dyspnea on exertion is the earliest symptom. Dyspnea on exertion may result in a change in functional status of the older adults. Older adults may also experience a change in mental status, especially confusion.

DISPLAY 18-1. Symptoms of Heart Failure

- Edema (general or dependent)
- Fatigue
- Poor exercise tolerance
- Dyspnea on exertion
- Paroxysmal nocturnal dyspnea
- Orthopnea
- Altered mental status (eg, confusion, especially in the elderly)

This condition is also known as congestive heart failure (CHF). Guidelines established by a multidisciplinary panel of clinicians by the Area for Health Care Policy and Research suggest using the term heart failure rather than CHF because many patients do not exhibit the classic symptoms or systemic congestion associated with the term CHF.

Heart function can be divided into two parts: systole and diastole. Systole is defined as the contraction phase of the heart cycle, and diastole is the relaxation phase (Fig. 18-2). Heart failure can occur as the result of systolic or diastolic failure. Systolic failure occurs when the heart, particularly the left ventricle, is unable to contract effectively. The heart is unable to pump forcefully enough for adequate amounts of blood to reach the systemic circulation. This reduces cardiac output (ie, amount of blood that leaves the ventricle with each contraction). As the contractibility declines, pressure builds in the pulmonary venous system, resulting in pulmonary congestion and dyspnea. The patient does not get enough oxygen to the body tissues and organs and begins to feel weak. Patients with myocardial infarction (MI) are at increased risk for systolic heart failure.

Diastolic failure occurs less frequently than systolic failure. During diastolic failure, the relaxation phase of heart function decreases, causing the left ventricle to become "stiff" and unable to fill adequately. Pulmonary congestion and a decrease in cardiac output can result. Hypertension is a common cause of diastolic dysfunction. Disorders that increase the risk of developing heart failure include

- Angina
- MI
- Diabetes (uncontrolled)
- Hypertension
- Coronary artery disease

Diagnostic Tests

Patients who exhibit symptoms of volume overload (eg, orthopnea, dyspnea on exertion, paroxysmal nocturnal dyspnea, peripheral edema) should have an echocardiogram or a radionuclide ventriculography

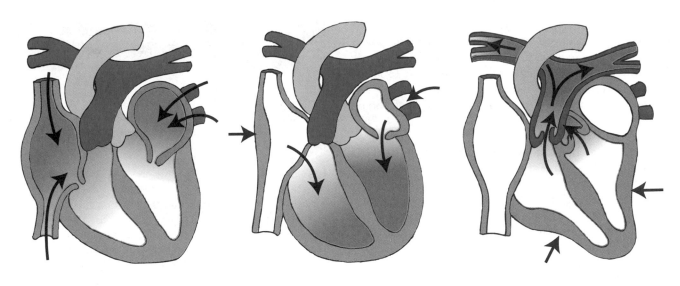

Diastole
Atria fill with blood that begins to flow into ventricles as soon as their walls relax.

Atrial systole
Contraction of atria pumps blood into the ventricles.

Ventricular systole
Contraction of ventricles pumps blood into aorta and pulmonary arteries.

FIGURE 18-2. Diastole and systole.

to measure left ventricular ejection fraction (EF). Echocardiography may show ventricular hypertrophy, decreased contractibility, and valvular disorders in the left and right ventricles. The radionuclide ventriculogram is a reliable indicator of EF. Most individuals with moderate to severe left ventricular systolic heart failure have an EF less that 35% to 40%. In general, the lower the EF, the more severe is the heart failure. Ventricular failure can occur in the left or right ventricle or in both.

Medical Treatment

Treatment involves decreasing volume overload with the use of diuretics. Diuretics decrease total blood volume and circulatory congestion. Patients with mild heart failure can usually be managed with the thiazide diuretics (eg, hydrochlorothiazide, chlorthalidone). For severe volume overload or edema that does not respond to the thiazides, a loop diuretic such as furosemide is recommended. Potassium loss (ie, hypokalemia) must be monitored closely in elderly patients receiving the thiazide diuretics or the loop diuretics. Symptoms of hypokalemia include weakness, muscle cramps, and numbness or tingling in the extremities. Other adverse reactions include postural hypotension, dizziness, headache, nausea, vomiting, diarrhea, constipation, polyuria, and impotence.

Most patients with heart failure receive one of several angiotensin-converting enzyme (ACE) inhibitors (Catopril, Enalapril). The ACE inhibitors prevent the vasoconstricting action of angiotensin II by blocking its conversion to the active form. Blockade of the vasoconstricting effect results in vasodilation. Adverse reactions of the ACE inhibitors include hypotension, hyperkalemia, renal insufficiency, cough, rash, and angioedema. ACE inhibitors minimize potassium loss, and patients receiving a diuretic and an ACE inhibitor may not exhibit hypokalemia, which is normally seen in patients taking a thiazide or loop diuretic. However, when a potassium-sparing diuretic is used in combination with an ACE inhibitor, potassium levels must be monitored for hyperkalemia (ie, high blood levels of potassium).

Digoxin (Lanoxin) is also used in the management of heart failure to strengthen myocardial contractility. While on digoxin therapy, serum digoxin levels must be monitored. Therapeutic digoxin levels range between 0.5 and 2 ng/mL. Symptoms of toxicity include anorexia, nausea, visual disturbances, abdominal pain, and bradycardia or other arrhythmias. If these symptoms are observed, the drug is withheld and the physician notified. *Older adults are at greater risk for toxicity because of the kidney's decreased ability to excrete the drug.*

Using the Nursing Process to Care for a Patient With Heart Failure

Assessment
The physical assessment provides important information about the patient's symptoms. Patients suspected of having heart failure must have pulse rate and rhythm, blood pressure, and respirations monitored.

When the patient has a diagnosis of heart failure, any abnormality observed is noted. Assessment may reveal dyspnea, especially on exertion, episodes of nighttime breathing difficulties, and difficulty breathing when lying down. The elderly patient may be confused or exhibit a change in mental or functional status.

The nurse auscultates the lungs for the presence of rales or bibasilar crackles heard best at the end of inspiration. It is important to check for abdominal discomfort or distention that may be associated with ascites (ie, collection of fluid within the peritoneal cavity). The extremities are checked for edema. The patient may complain of weight gain, fatigue, and muscle weakness.

Nursing Diagnoses

The following nursing diagnoses may be appropriate for the patient with heart failure:

> Decreased Cardiac Output related to altered myocardial contractility
>
> Fluid Volume Excess related to sodium or water retention
>
> Activity Intolerance related to dyspnea, muscle weakness, fatigue
>
> Ineffective Breathing Pattern related to dyspnea, decreased lung expansion, other (specify)
>
> Risk for Ineffective Management of Therapeutic Regimen related to lack of knowledge of disease process, treatment regimen, drug therapy, other (specify)

Other diagnoses may be appropriate to meet individual needs.

Planning and Implementation

Care of the patient with cardiovascular disease is aimed at reducing the workload of the heart, increasing myocardial contractility, and eliminating edema.

Decreased Cardiac Output. In heart failure the heart is unable to pump forcefully enough for adequate amounts of blood to reach the systemic circulation causing a decreased cardiac output. As the contractility declines, pressure builds in the pulmonary venous system, resulting in pulmonary congestion and dyspnea. The patient does not get enough oxygen to the body tissues and organs and begins to feel weak. The physician prescribes drugs to help increase the cardiac output and help the heart to work more efficiently. Display 18-2 identifies nursing interventions when caring for a patient with cardiac output.

Fluid Volume Excess. Fluid volume excess must be reduced if heart failure is to be managed. The physician usually orders a diuretic to promote diuresis and loss of excess fluid. The patient is mon-

---

DISPLAY 18-2. Nursing Interventions for Decreased Cardiac Output

- Assess heart rate and rhythm.
- Report any irregularities or a heart rate less than 60 or greater than 100 beats/minute.
- Auscultate lung sounds for rales, crackles, or rhonchi.
- Note the extent of dyspnea.
- Check lung sounds for the presence of crackles or rhonchi.
- Note any decrease in mental alertness or thought processes. The head of the bed is kept elevated and the patient in a semi- or high Fowler's position.
- Weigh the patient daily at the same time and in the same type of clothing.
- Encourage the patient to avoid straining during defecation. Straining increases venous return and increases the workload of the heart. A stool softener may be needed to prevent straining.
- Administer medications, and monitor closely for adverse drug reactions.

---

itored for adverse reactions to the medications such as hypokalemia, nausea, vomiting, tingling or numbness in the extremities, headache, diarrhea, constipation. Daily weights are used to help monitor fluid loss. The nurse reports any increase in weight of 3 pounds or more during a 48-hour period. Dietary sodium is restricted to approximately 2 to 3 g/day. Foods high in sodium are avoided, and no salt is added to foods.

Activity Intolerance. Patients with acute or worsening heart failure may become short of breath with minimal exertion. Until the heart failure is under control, these patients may be permitted only minimal activity. In general, however, activity is encouraged. Research shows that bed rest may be counterproductive and leads to complications related to immobility such as increased fatigue and muscle wasting. However, if any chest pain, dyspnea, or fatigue occurs, the activity is stopped. If the symptoms do not subside within a short period, the physician is notified.

Ineffective Breathing Pattern. Respiratory rate, depth, and pattern are monitored every 2 to 4 hours. The nurse checks the lung sounds for crackles, wheezes, or diminished breath sounds. Pulse oximetry used to monitor saturation levels may be necessary in some cases to determine hypoxemia. Oxygen by a nasal cannula may be ordered to provide supplemental oxygen. The patient dyspnea is placed with the head of the bed elevated or in the orthopneic position (ie, position in which the patient's upper trunk sits in an upright or nearly upright position in a bed or chair).

ASSESSMENT ALERT

Any evidence of worsening of breathing pattern such as increased dyspnea, orthopnea, labored or rapid respirations, or use of accessory muscles for breathing could indicate acute pulmonary edema. Bubbling sounds are heard with respirations and sputum is white or pink-tinged and frothy. Inspiratory and expiratory wheezing is present. This is a medical emergency and must be reported immediately.

Patient and Family Teaching. The nurse provides explanations in a clear, accurate, and understandable manner. Information is best retained if given over a period of time and in relatively small amounts. Written instructions are helpful to reinforce important information and to reinforce learning. Information should be given to the patient, the primary caregiver, and other family members. Information such as how to recognize signs and symptoms of fluid overload is given. For example, explain to the patient that rings or watches may feel tight or that feet may become swollen when fluid begins to collect. Daily weights are important. The physician is notified if a 3-pound weight gain occurs within 48 hours. Exercise such as walking is encouraged. Other information is included such as drug regimens, dietary restrictions, symptoms of worsening heart failure, and what to do if these symptoms occur. Display 18-3 suggests topics for the patient, family, and caregiver education and counseling.

Evaluation and Expected Outcomes

Successful care can provide the following outcomes:
   No evidence of symptoms of circulatory
      insufficiency
   Maintenance of stable weight with no evidence
      of edema
   Decreased episodes of dyspnea
   Respiratory rate, rhythm, and depth and breath
      sounds within baseline parameters
   Participation in self-care and social activities
   Expression of increased knowledge about the
      disease process, medication regimen, or other
      (specify)

CORONARY ARTERY DISEASE

Coronary artery disease is the most common disorder affecting the heart. More than 50% of deaths of individuals older than 65 years of age are caused by coro-

DISPLAY 18-3. Suggested Topics for Patient, Family, and Caregiver Education and Counseling

General counseling
   Explanation of heart failure and the reason for
      symptoms
   Cause or probable cause of heart failure
   Expected symptoms
   Symptoms of worsening heart failure
   What to do if symptoms worsen
   Self-monitoring with daily weighs
   Explanation of treatment or care plan
   Clarification of patient's responsibilities
   Importance of cessation of tobacco use
   Role of family members or other caregivers in
      the treatment or care plan
   Availability and value of qualified local support
      group
   Importance of obtaining vaccinations against
      influenza and pneumococcal disease
Prognosis
   Life expectancy
   Advance directives
   Advice for family members in the event of
      sudden death
Activity recommendations
   Recreation, leisure, and work activity
   Exercise
   Sex, sexual difficulties, and coping strategies
Dietary recommendations
   Sodium restriction
   Avoidance of excessive fluid intake
   Fluid restriction (if required)
   Alcohol restriction
Medications
   Effects of medications on quality of life and
      survival
   Dosing
   Likely side effects and what to do if they occur
   Coping mechanisms for complicated medical
      regimens
   Availability of lower cost medications or
      financial assistance
**Importance of compliance with the treatment or
care plan**

From Konstam, M., Dracup, K., Baker, D., et al. (June, 1994). *Heart failure: Evaluation and care of patients with left-ventricular systolic dysfunction. Clinical practice guideline no. 11.* AHCPR Publication No. 94-0612. Rockville, MD: Agency for Health Care Policy and Research, Public Health Service, U.S. Department of Health and Human Services.

nary artery disease. The coronary arteries supply blood and oxygen to the heart muscles. With age, the arteries, including the coronary arteries, accumulate yellowish plaques of cholesterol, lipids, and other debris on the inner surfaces of the vessels. This condition is called **atherosclerosis.** The walls of the medium-size and large arteries become thickened, causing the lumen (ie, opening) of the vessel to narrow. As the lumen accumulates debris and narrows, blood flow to areas that normally receive adequate amounts of blood decreases. Atherosclerosis is progressive, and in time, the blood supply to certain areas supplied by the arteries decreases sufficiently to cause ischemia. Ischemia results in pain as the tissues are deprived of needed oxygen and blood. When ischemia occurs in the coronary arteries, the condition is called angina pectoris. Angina pectoris refers to chest pain caused by a temporary inadequate blood supply to the heart muscle. When the heart is deprived of blood, chest pain occurs. If the ischemia becomes severe, causing damage and death of cardiac tissue, an MI occurs. When damage to the heart muscle is extensive, the heart may be unable to meet the demands of the body to maintain adequate cardiac output. When this occurs, heart failure may develop.

Angina

Angina is caused by atherosclerotic heart disease. The most prominent symptom of angina is chest pain. The chest pain with angina typically is severe and causes a feeling of tightness, pressure, or suffocation. The pain may radiate down the left side of the body to the neck, jaw, shoulders, or arms. The pain of angina may result from

- Exercise or physical exertion (eg, climbing stairs)
- Exposure to cold
- Eating a large meal (ie, pain occurs as the blood is diverted to the digestive system and away from the heart)
- Stress
- In some instances, while at rest

An older adult may not complain of "chest pain" with angina. Instead, pain may be manifested as weakness, fainting, or dyspnea. In addition to pain, the most important characteristic of angina is that the pain subsides when the cause is removed. For example, if angina is the result of exercise, it subsides with rest. If it is caused by exposure to cold, it is relieved when the individual becomes warm. Angina may remain relatively stable for a number of years. This type of angina is fairly predictable, episodic, and managed with the nitrates. However, angina that changes in frequency or severity or becomes unstable and unpredictable requires immediate medical attention.

Treatment

Treatment for angina is aimed at increasing the oxygen supply to the heart muscle and decreasing the

DISPLAY 18-4. Risk Factors for Coronary Heart Disease

- Aging
- High blood pressure
- Elevated blood pressure
- Smoking cigarettes
- Diabetes mellitus (hyperglycemia)
- Obesity
- Stress
- Lack of exercise
- Family history of a myocardial infarction

heart's oxygen demands. This is accomplished through the use of medication and patient education that focuses on modifying the lifestyle to decrease the risk of developing cardiovascular disease. Display 18-4 identifies risk factors for coronary heart disease.

Surgical treatment may be necessary if the medication regimen fails to control the angina or the angina worsens. Coronary artery bypass surgery or percutaneous transluminal coronary angioplasty (PTCA) are used along with drug therapy.

Drug Therapy

The nitrates are the most significant drugs used to manage angina pectoris. These antianginal drugs relax the smooth muscle layer of arterial blood vessels causing vasodilation (ie, increase in the size of the blood vessels). Vasodilation increases the blood flow to the affected area, resulting in complete or partial relief of pain and other symptoms associated with angina. The nitrates may be administered sublingually, transdermally, or orally.

The physician may order nitroglycerin to be left at the bedside. However, for any elderly patient who is confused or disoriented, leaving any medication at the bedside is contraindicated, because the person may forget whether the medication was taken and take more or less than the physician ordered. Side effects of nitroglycerin include headache, hypotension, dizziness, vertigo, and weakness. Flushing due to dilation of small capillaries near the surface of the skin may also be seen.

Another method of administering nitroglycerin is translingual administration. Nitroglycerin lingual aerosol (Nitrolingual spray) is a metered-spray canister that is used to terminate an acute anginal attack. The spray is directed from the canister onto or under the tongue. For some, this method of administration is more convenient than the small tablets placed under the tongue. The spray works more quickly than the tablets, giving almost immediate relief. The canister is easier to handle for many older adults, especially those with arthritic changes in the hands and those with visual impairments. The canister prolongs the potency of the drug, lasting up to 3 years. In contrast, the tablets usually stay potent for approximately 6 months.

Calcium channel blockers (eg, diltiazem, verapamil, nifedipine) are also used to treat chronic stable angina or hypertension. Side effects of calcium channel blockers include peripheral edema, dizziness, lightheadedness, nausea, skin rash, fever, and chills.

Myocardial Infarction

MI occurs when areas of the heart are deprived of blood, causing tissue death and destruction. Other words commonly used to describe an MI are heart attack and coronary occlusion. Symptoms indicating an MI include chest pain (not relieved by rest or by nitroglycerin). The pain occurs suddenly over the (lower) substernal area and is the most common symptom. The pain is often severe and unrelenting. The patient may complain of extreme pressure in the chest, shoulders, down the arms (usually the left arm), in the neck, and jaw. An important feature to help distinguish an MI from angina is that angina pain can be relieved with rest or nitroglycerin. Occasionally, the pain from an MI may be mistakenly described as a "bad case of indigestion." Pain from an MI persists, lasting for hours to days, and is not relieved by rest or any other modification of the risk factors.

✔ ASSESSMENT ALERT

The pain experienced by the elderly patient with an MI may be atypical such as fainting. Patients with dementia may be unable to express feelings of pain. In these instances, nurses must note a change in behavior or an increase in behavior symptoms (see Chapter 17).

The diagnosis after an MI is made through laboratory studies such as serum enzyme and isoenzyme determinations, electrocardiogram, and echocardiogram. Treatment is aimed at reducing the pain, stabilizing the heart rhythm, and reducing the work load of the heart. Analgesics are given to relieve the pain. Oxygen, cardiotonic drugs, antiarrhythmic drugs, and anticoagulants are usually administered in the acute stage. The patient is admitted to the cardiac care unit and placed on a cardiac monitor.

Using the Nursing Process to Care for a Patient With Coronary Artery Disease

Assessment

When assessing the patient for problems of the coronary arteries pain is the most prominent symptom. Have the patient describe the pain—its onset, location, severity, and duration. The pain may be described as pressure, tightness, squeezing, burning, or as indigestion. The pain may be substernal and radiate to the neck, shoulders, particularly the upper extremities, and more often to the left side (although the right side may be involved as well).

✔ ASSESSMENT ALERT

A distinguishing characteristic of angina is that the pain usually lasts no more than 30 minutes (averages 3 minutes to 15 minutes) and is relieved by rest or antianginal medications (nitroglycerin). The pain from an MI occurs suddenly and is unrelieved by rest or nitroglycerin.

Angina may be caused by physical exertion, emotional upset, extremes in weather, and occasionally occurs at rest. Because older adults have less subcutaneous fat to provide insulation, they may complain of chest pain quicker than younger persons. The pain of an MI is similar, but it may be more severe and radiate to the epigastric region, the elbow, jaw, abdomen, or neck. The nurse checks the vital signs (ie, blood pressure, pulse, respirations, and temperature). Vital signs are used to establish a baseline for future comparison. Dyspnea, shortness of breath, diaphoresis, or nausea and vomiting are also indicative of an MI.

✔ ASSESSMENT ALERT

The elderly experiencing an MI may not report chest pain. Older adults may have diminished pain perception or have learned to ignore symptoms, seemingly expecting a certain amount of pain with increasing age.

Nursing Diagnoses

The following nursing diagnoses may be appropriate for patients with coronary artery disease:

Pain related to ischemia of the coronary vessels

Decreased Cardiac Output related to changes in heart rate, rhythm, and conduction

Risk for Decreased Tissue Perfusion related to decreased Cardiac Output

Altered Sexuality Patterns related to pain, anxiety, other (specify)

Risk for Ineffective Management of Therapeutic Regimen related to lack of knowledge of disease process, medication regimen, other (specify)

Other nursing diagnoses may be appropriate for individual patients with coronary artery disease.

Planning and Implementation

For an older patient with an MI, immediate hospitalization in a coronary intensive care unit is necessary during the acute phase. Cardiac monitoring and administration of medications such as morphine or Demerol to control the pain along with antiarrhythmic drugs is part of the treatment plan. A cardiac rehabilitation program may be helpful for those elderly recovering from an MI. Angina may range from stable and predictable to unstable and totally unpredictable. The nitrates are used to manage angina. Older adults are taught to administer medications, monitor diet, and maintain a balance between activity and rest.

Pain. If a patient is in acute pain from an MI, a narcotic analgesic such as morphine or Demerol is administered. It is important to relieve the chest pain and reduce the heart's need for oxygen. Oxygen may be administered along with vasodilators and drugs to decrease myocardial oxygen consumption. Vital signs (ie, pulse, respirations, and blood pressure) are taken before administering of any drug to help monitor the effects of the drug and any adverse reactions. To decrease the workload of the heart, the patient is kept on bed rest. Chest pain that is not relieved is reported to the physician immediately.

For the patient with anginal pain, nitroglycerin is administered. The physician may allow the patient to keep the drug at the bedside to self-administer if pain occurs. The patient is instructed to place one tablet under the tongue when chest pain occurs. If the pain is not relieved in 5 minutes, a second tablet is taken. If the pain is not relieved after 5 more minutes, a third nitroglycerin tablet may be taken. If the pain is not relieved after taking three nitroglycerin tablets in 15 minutes, MI is suspected, and the person must notify the physician or go to the hospital emergency department for evaluation (if not already hospitalized).

If the patient is in a nursing home or a hospital and the physician has ordered nitroglycerin for angina at the bedside, the nurse must be notified when the patient takes a nitroglycerin tablet. The nurse documents when the drug was taken and the patient's response to the drug. Care must be taken to determine if an elderly patient is sufficiently alert to self-administer nitroglycerin.

ASSESSMENT ALERT

Elderly patients who are confused or disoriented may not be capable of keeping the nitroglycerin at the bedside. These patients may inadvertently take too much of the drug, causing toxic levels of the drug, or may not take enough of the drug, resulting in a lack of pain relief. Assess the patient's orientation and mental status before placing any medication at the patient's bedside.

Decreased Cardiac Output and Tissue Perfusion. A decrease in cardiac output is manifested in a change in the rate and rhythm of the heart. The nurse monitors for a weak, thready pulse; irregularities in the pulse rhythm; and hypotension. Vital signs are checked every 4 hours or more often if necessary. The nurse auscultates breath sounds for signs of the development of pulmonary congestion such as rales, rhonchi, or diminished breath sounds. Any abnormal breath sounds, dyspnea, or any abnormalities in the pulse rate or rhythm are reported immediately. A portable commode may be kept at the bedside to decrease cardiac workload. The patient is given small, frequent meals of easily digested foods. Caffeine (ie, colas, chocolate, coffee) is restricted. Supplemental oxygen is administered if ordered. Continuous cardiac monitoring is required in the acute stage. The nurse notes the effectiveness of cardiac medications and assesses frequently for adverse reactions. Intravenous medications and fluids are monitored closely. Infusion devices are necessary.

The patient is instructed to avoid activities that could cause a Valsalva maneuver (ie, increased pressure caused by forced exhalation against a closed glottis resulting in decreased pulse, decreased amount of blood returning to the heart and increased venous pressure) such as straining for a bowel movement, vomiting, forceful coughing, or isometric exercises. A stool softener may be needed to avoid straining during a bowel movement.

Risk for Altered Sexual Patterns. Most older adults have an active sex life. Any disturbance in cardiac function can cause fear and anxiety in the older adult, resulting in fear of recurrence of pain or another MI if sexual relations are resumed. The nurse checks with the physician regarding any special considerations or precautions needed during sexual activity for each patient. Most people are able to resume sexual activity within 6 weeks after an MI with minimal alterations. Precautions may be necessary, such as postponing sex for 2 or 3 hours after a heavy meal, taking a nitroglycerin tablet before sexual intercourse, or using alternate methods for expressing affection. The physician should delineate any special precautions.

Patient and Family Teaching. After a diagnosis of coronary artery disease, the patient needs a thorough explanation of the disease process, the risk factors involved, ways to modify those risk factors, the prescribed medication regimen, dietary recommendations, symptoms that should be reported, type and amount of activity allowed, and any special precautions necessary. The nurse may teach relaxation techniques to assist in managing stress. Support groups may be needed for areas where help is needed such as weight reduction or smoking cessation. It is helpful for the patient to enroll in a cardiac rehabilitation program, particularly after an MI. Other communities have wellness centers that can help to educate those with other forms of coronary artery disease, such as angina or atherosclerosis.

Cardiac Rehabilitation. Cardiac rehabilitation is comprehensive, long-term service that focuses on limiting adverse effects of cardiac disease, reducing the risk of sudden death or reinfarction, controlling cardiac symptoms, and enhancing psychosocial well-being. These programs are supervised by a physician and use a number of health care providers, such as nurses, dietitians, exercise physiologists, psychologists, physical therapists, and occupational therapists. Patients who benefit from cardiac rehabilitation include those with angina pectoris, ventricular failure, MI, cardiac transplantation, coronary artery bypass graft (CABG), and percutaneous transluminal coronary angioplasty (PTCA). Figure 18-3 illustrates a decision tree for cardiac rehabilitation services.

Functional independence is an important aspect of cardiac rehabilitation for elderly patients. Services that are provided in a cardiac rehabilitation program include
- Strength training
- Exercise training
- Smoking cessation programs
- Educational, counseling, and behavioral interventions about nutrition, hypertension, and improving psychosocial well-being

Evaluation and Expected Outcomes
Successful treatment can be gauged by the following responses of the patient:
Reports relief of chest discomfort
Appears comfortable, with the respiratory rate, heart rate, and blood pressure within normal or baseline levels
Expresses less anxiety concerning sexual activity
Complies with medication regimen and health care teachings
Expresses increased knowledge about disease process, medication regimen, risk factors, and treatment plan

Patient With a Pacemaker

Many older adults require the use of a pacemaker to maintain a normal rate and rhythm. A **pacemaker** is a device used to control the heart rate by electrical stimulation of the heart muscle. A pacemaker may be a demand pacemaker or a fixed-rate pacemaker. The demand pacemaker is set to a specific rate and it fires only when the heart does not spontaneously contract at a minimum rate. The fixed-rate pacemaker stimulates the ventricle at a constant and fixed rate without regard to the patient's own rhythm. A pacemaker may be temporarily used in an emergency situation or may be permanent. When a permanent pacemaker is needed, the pulse generator is placed underneath the skin, usually below the clavicle or in the pectoral region, with the lead wire inserted into the right ventricle.

Assessment of a Patient With a Pacemaker
In assessing a patient with a pacemaker, it is important to know the preset rate. Check the heart rate and rhythm. The patients rate may be as much as five beats more or less than the preset rate. The insertion site is inspected for evidence of infection or hematoma formation (particularly if the pacemaker is new). Normally, the site bulges slightly. Report any redness, swelling, drainage, or pain.

Nursing Care of the Patient With a Pacemaker
Initially after the pacemaker is inserted, the patient is monitored closely for signs and symptoms of infection, hematoma formation, or malfunction. After the site is healed this site is still checked but the incidence of infection decreases. The nurse reports any redness, edema, or pain to the physician. Any irregularities or any rate five beats more or less than the preset is also reported.

The functioning of the pacemaker, along with blood pressure, pulse rate, and rhythm, is monitored daily. Any pulse irregularity or significant deviation from the preset rate of five beats more or less is reported to the physician unless instructed otherwise. The nurse records type and serial numbers of pulse generator and leads, date of surgery and programmed rate of pacemaker.

Patient and Family Teaching
Patients and caregivers need to be knowledgeable about the type of pacemaker inserted and any specific manufacturer's instructions. There are more than 300 types of pacemakers with various functional abilities. The older adult may be entirely capable of monitoring the effectiveness of the pacemaker. However, it is important that family members be knowledgeable as well. Important points to

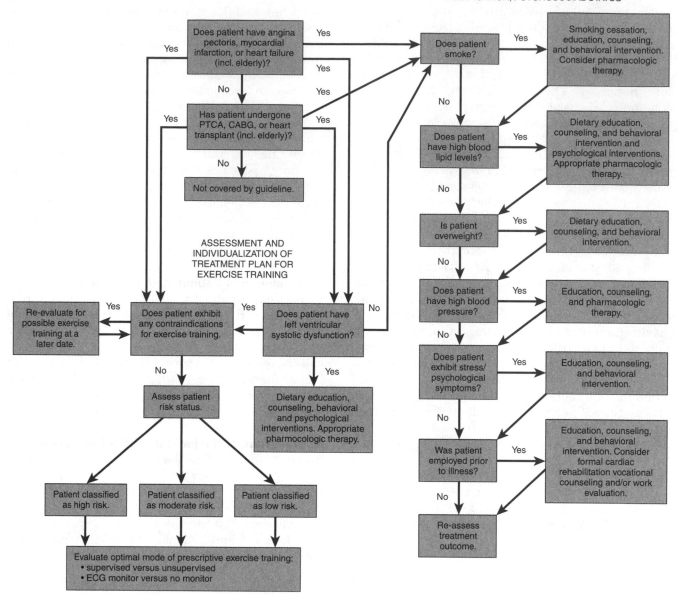

FIGURE 18-3. Decision tree for cardiac rehabilitation services. Adapted from material provided by Health Economics Research, Inc. Waltham, MA. From Wenger NK, Froelicher ES, Smith LK, et al. *Cardiac Rehabilitation as Secondary Prevention.* Clinical Practice Guideline. Quick Reference Guide for Clinicians, No. 17. Rockville, MD: U.S. Department of Health and Human Services, Public Health Service, Agency for Health Care Policy and Research and National Heart, Lung, and Blood Institute. AHCPR Pub. No. 96–0673. October 1995.

cover when giving instructions to the patient or family of the patient with a pacemaker include the importance of monitoring and maintenance of the unit.

PATIENT AND FAMILY TEACHING AID

Important points to cover when teaching the patient and the family about pacemakers:

- **Check the pulse daily. Report any increase or decrease in the pulse rate because this may indicate pacemaker malfunction or problems with the battery.**
- **Wear loose-fitting clothing over the pacemaker.**
- **Notify physician if the area becomes red or painful.**
- **Carry a pacemaker identification card with information about the pacemaker.**
- **Report any dizziness, fainting, difficulty breathing, or swelling of the hands or feet.**

- **Avoid close exposure to microwave ovens.**
- **Request hand scanning when going through security gates at the airport. Metal detectors do not harm pacemaker or alter their function. Although most walk-through metal detectors in airports do not detect a pacemaker, some are so sensitive that a pacemaker can trigger the alarm.**
- **Inform physician of the pacemaker before undergoing magnetic resonance imaging (MRI).**
- **Keep all scheduled physician appointments. The pacemaker must be checked regularly. Pacemaker batteries last 3 to 10 years, depending on the type of battery used.**

Regular monitoring of the pacemaker is done through the physician's office, pacemaker clinics, or telephone transmission of the generator's pulse rate. Special instructions are needed when monitoring is done over the telephone.

HYPERTENSION

Hypertension is a sustained elevation in blood pressure. In adults older than 60 years of age, hypertension is found in 60% of white Americans and in 61% of Hispanics. Even more alarming is the fact that 71% of African Americans older than 60 have hypertension. If on several separate occasions systolic pressure is greater than 140 mmHg or the diastolic pressure is above 90 mmHg, the patient is diagnosed with hypertension. No single blood pressure measurement is sufficient to make a diagnosis of hypertension, but it is a warning that close observation is necessary. Sustained elevated blood pressure on several different occasions is a greater indicator of hypertension than one single reading.

Research has shown that diastolic blood pressure rises until about age 55 and then declines, while systolic blood pressure increases steadily with age. A rise in systolic blood pressure becomes an important determinant for assessing the presence and severity of hypertension in the older adult. A condition called **isolated systolic hypertension (ISH)** develops when the systolic pressure is at or above 140 mmHg and the diastolic pressure is under 90 mmHg. For older Americans, ISH is the most common form of hypertension. Sixty-five percent of all hypertensive patients over age 60 have ISH.

Treatment

Treatment is aimed at maintaining a blood pressure below 140/90 mmHg, modifying risk factors, and preventing complications. In diabetic patients with hypertension, blood pressure should be kept below 130/85. Some risk factors can be modified by a more healthful lifestyle. Other risk factors such as age and sex are unable to be changed. Weight reduction, sodium restriction, limiting alcohol consumption, eliminating tobacco, learning stress reduction techniques, and exercising moderately can help in managing hypertension.

Assessment of the Patient With Hypertension

Hypertension is often called the silent killer because few or no symptoms are apparent until complications develop as the result of vascular changes. With prolonged hypertension, pathologic changes in the blood vessels occurs, particularly in the eyes, kidneys, heart, and brain. Often, the only symptom is elevated blood pressure. Occasionally, the individual may complain of headache, dizziness, or tinnitus (ie, ringing in the ears). Other symptoms include nosebleeds, visual disturbances, and nocturia. Frequent assessment of the blood pressure is important.

The nurse assesses the heart rate and rhythm because vascular changes in the arteries of the heart can affect cardiac functioning. The nurse also obtains the patient's weight, especially if a diuretic is part of the therapeutic regimen or the physician prescribes a weight loss program. Before beginning antihypertensive medication, the nurse obtains the blood pressure and pulse rate on both arms with the patient standing, sitting, and lying down.

ASSESSMENT ALERT

An elevated systolic pressure of more than 160 mmHg is particularly dangerous in the elderly. The nurse should report systolic values over 140 mmHg, even if the diastolic value is below 90 mmHg.

Caring for the Patient With Hypertension

In planning the care for a patient with hypertension, the nurse should remember that there is no one best drug or drug combination. Although there are many drugs available, not all drugs work equally well in a given patient. In some instances, the physician may prescribe a different antihypertensive drug when other less potent drugs have failed to lower the blood pressure. Two antihypertensive drugs may be given together to achieve a better response. The patient is monitored for any adverse reactions related to the medications. Common side effects of the antihypertensives include orthostatic hypotension, hypotension, dizziness, fatigue, nausea, vomiting, depression, and impotence. Obtain the blood pressure and pulse rate immediately before each dose of an antihypertensive. If the blood pressure is significantly decreased from baseline values, do not give the drug, and notify the physician if there is a significant increase in blood pressure. Diuretics are commonly prescribed for hypertension. The most common side effect with the antihypertensives include fluid and electrolyte imbalances (especially hypokalemia or hyponatremia) and dehydration. Intake and output are monitored. Some diuretics are potassium-sparing diuretics (eg, spironolactone). With the potassium-sparing diuretics, the patient is monitored for hyperkalemia (ie, muscular weakness; tingling of the hands, feet, and tongue; and slow, irregular pulse). Older adults may be more susceptible to the electrolyte disturbances of the diuretics. In older adults, medications are given at lower doses and gradually increased with longer intervals between dosage increases. Low doses of diuretics cause fewer adverse reactions and appear equally as effective as higher doses. Diuretics and beta blockers such as acebutolol, pendolol, propranolol, and timolol are the drugs used most often to treat hypertension in the elderly.

Patient and Family Teaching

The nurse explains carefully to the patient and the caregiver the importance of the drug therapy. It is important to emphasize that essential hypertension cannot be cured but can be controlled. To ensure lifetime compliance to the prescribed regimen, the nurse emphasizes the importance of drug therapy. Noncompliance is a problem in managing hypertension. Unless the patient and the caregiver have a good understanding of why the medication is needed, what adverse reactions to look for, and what adverse reactions to report compliance may be a problem. It is important to teach the caregiver and the patient important aspects of management.

 PATIENT AND FAMILY TEACHING AID

The nurse must be certain the caregiver and the patient understand the following points:
- Do not discontinue the medication except on the advise of the physician.
- Avoid the use of nonprescription drugs unless approved by the physician. Some over-the-counter drugs are capable of raising the blood pressure.
- To minimize postural hypotension and dizziness, rise slowly from a sitting or lying position.

- Contact the physician for any unusual occurrences or adverse reactions that occur.
- Follow dietary restrictions concerning sodium or fat. Do not use a salt substitute unless approved by the physician. (These substitutes sometimes contain potassium, and their use can cause an electrolyte disturbance.)
- Take the diuretics early in the morning unless directed otherwise.
- Avoid the use of alcohol.
- Lose weight if overweight.
- Weigh weekly to monitor weight loss or gain.
- Stop smoking, and reduce the intake of dietary saturated fat and cholesterol for overall cardiovascular health.
- If taking an antihypertensive that causes hypokalemia, include foods high in potassium in the diet (eg, bananas, orange juice).
- Notify the physician if any of the following symptoms occur: muscle cramps, weakness, dizziness, nausea, vomiting, diarrhea, dry mouth, general weakness, rapid pulse, or gastrointestinal disturbances.

CEREBROVASCULAR ACCIDENT

Cerebrovascular accident (CVA) or stroke is the most common cause of disability in the United States. There are approximately 3 million stroke survivors with some type of disability. Approximately one third of stroke survivors have mild impairment, one third are moderately impaired, and one third have severe impairments. The incidence of stroke increases with age (>55 years), with approximately two thirds of all strokes occurring in people 65 years of age or older. Stroke is the third leading cause of death in the United States. **CVA** is a sudden impairment of cerebral circulation caused by a partial or total blockage of one or more cerebral blood vessels. When the cells of the brain are deprived of oxygen for 7 minutes or more, cell destruction occurs. This cellular destruction leads to death of brain tissue (ie, cerebral infarction). Symptoms are highly variable and depend on the area of the brain affected, whether the blockage was total or partial, and the presence or absence of collateral circulation. Collateral circulation is a type of circulation by which smaller blood vessels are formed by branching off from the larger occluded vessels to supply the blocked or partially blocked areas with blood. Risk factors for CVA include hypertension, a history of transient ischemic attacks (TIAs), previous stroke, and atherosclerosis.

Signs and Symptoms

A CVA can occur without warning or can be preceded by one or more TIAs (Display 18-5). The TIAs can occur months to days before the stroke. Unlike a TIA, symptoms of a stroke persist. Symptoms depend on the area of the brain affected and the severity of the damage.

TIAs are a symptom of impending stroke. Other symptoms include hemiplegia (ie, paralysis on one side of the body), aphasia (ie, inability to use or understand spoken and written language), dysphagia (ie, difficulty swallowing), hemianopia (ie, seeing only one half of the normal visual field), decreased level of consciousness, and bowel and bladder dysfunction. Symptoms may subside completely, partially, or not at all, depending on the amount of brain damage that has occurred. Recovery may take days to months and require extensive rehabilitation.

Generally, if a stroke occurs in the left side of the brain, symptoms occur on the right side. If a stroke occurs in the right side of the brain, symptoms occur on the left side of the body. For example, a stroke in the left side of the brain results in hemiplegia of the right side of the body. The patient may be unconscious and comatose. The coma may last days to months. The longer the coma persists, the poorer is the prognosis. In some situations, the neurologic deficit may be minimal; in others, the deficits may be profound.

Diagnosis

Diagnosis is based on the presenting signs and symptoms and the results of a computed tomography (CT) scan or magnetic resonance imaging (MRI) showing the size and location of the infarcted area. Transcranial Doppler ultrasonography can determine the size of intracranial vessels and may locate the obstructed vessel. Other supporting tests include electroencephalogram, lumbar puncture, and angiography.

Management

Management includes rehabilitation, drug therapy, reduction of risk factors, and sometimes surgery. For example, if the stroke is caused by atherosclerosis of the carotid artery, carotid endarterectomy may be performed. Management is often supportive because there is no medical or surgical intervention to repair the damaged tissue. Drug therapy for stroke is aimed at preventing a recurrent stroke and minimizing further damage to cerebral tissue. Drugs to lower blood

---

> **DISPLAY 18-5. Understanding Transient Ischemic Attacks**
>
> Transient ischemic attacks (TIAs) are temporary episodes of cerebrovascular insufficiency. The attack typically lasts for a few minutes to 24 hours. Often called mini-strokes, these attacks may be a warning sign of an impending stroke. The incidence of TIAs depends on the area in the brain affected. The incidence of TIAs increases with age, particularly after age 50. However, older adults may ignore the symptoms of a TIA, attributing them to old age because the symptoms disappear after the attack, leaving no lingering effects. Common symptoms include visual disturbances such as blindness in one eye or double vision, speech deficiencies, headache, tinnitus, vertigo, facial weakness, ataxia, or weakness in the legs.
>
> Treatment of a TIA is often aimed at preventing a cerebrovascular accident (CVA) and consists of the administration of aspirin or anticoagulants to prevent future attacks or a CVA. Efforts are made to find the cause of the TIA and prevent a stroke. Depending on the cause of the TIA, preventative treatment may include a surgical procedure, called a carotid endarterectomy, to remove atherosclorotic plaque or thrombus from the carotid artery.

cholesterol levels, antihypertensives, anticoagulants (in selected people), and perhaps an osmotic diuretic during the acute phase to decrease cerebral edema are used. Anticoagulant therapy is not used in a hemorrhagic CVA because the drug increases bleeding.

Using the Nursing Process to Care for a Patient With a Cerebrovascular Accident

Assessment
Obtain a complete medical history from the patient or primary caregiver. Include allergies, drugs currently taken, and the occurrence of TIAs in the past 1 to 2 years. Some patients who have suffered a stroke have language and speech difficulties. Check muscular strength on both sides of the body to determine any muscular weakness. Take vital signs. The blood pressure may be elevated. Perform a complete neurologic assessment. The Glasgow coma scale (Fig. 18-4) may be used to perform the neurologic assessment. Evaluation by a speech therapist, occupational therapist, and a physical therapist may be needed, depending on the level of disability.

Nursing Diagnoses
Several diagnoses may be appropriate for a patient with a CVA, depending on the neurologic deficits

GLASGOW COMA SCALE			A.M. 7 8 9 10 11 12	P.M. 1 2 3 4 5 6 7 8 9 10 11 12	A.M. 1 2 3 4 5 6
BEST EYE OPENING RESPONSE	Spontaneously	4			
	To speech	3			
	To pain	2			
	No response	1			
BEST MOTOR RESPONSE to painful stimuli	Obeys verbal command	6			
	Localizes pain	5			
	Flexion—withdrawal	4			
	Flexion—abnormal*	3			
	Extension—abnormal**	2			
	No response	1			
BEST VERBAL RESPONSE	Oriented X 3	5			
	Conversation-confused	4			
	Speech-inappropriate	3			
	Sounds-incomprehensible	2			
	No response	1			
	* abnormal flexion—decorticate rigidity ** abnormal extension—decerebrate rigidity				

FIGURE 18-4. Glascow coma scale. Glascow coma scale for determining level of consciousness.

How to score responses:

Scoring of eye opening: **4** = If the patient opens the eyes spontaneously when the nurse approaches; **3** = If the patient opens the eyes in response to speech (spoken or shouted); **2** = If the patient opens the eyes only in response to painful stimuli such as digital squeezing around nailbeds of fingers; **1** = If the patient does not open the eyes in response to painful stimuli.

Scoring of best motor response: **6** = If the patient can obey a simple command, such as, "Lift your left hand off the bed"; **5** = If the patient moves a limb to locate the painful stimuli applied to the head or trunk and attempts to remove the source; **4** = If the patient attempts to withdraw from the source of pain; **3** = If the patient flexes only the arms at the elbows and wrist in response to painful stimuli to the nailbeds (**decorticate rigidity**): **2** = If the patient extends the arms (straightens the elbows) in response to painful stimuli (**decerebrate rigidity**): **1** = If the patient has no motor response to pain on any limb.

Scoring of best verbal response:

5 = If the patient is oriented to time, place, and person; **4** = If the patient is able to converse, although not oriented to time, place, or person (eg, "Where am I?"); **3** = If the patient speaks only in words or phrases that make little or no sense (eg. "B-H, H-K."); **2** = If the patient responds with incomprehensible sounds such as groans; **1** = If the patient does not respond verbally at all.

Adapted from Rosdahl, C.B., *Textbook of Basic Nursing,* 6th ed., (1996). Philadelphia: Lippincott-Raven.

experienced. The following nursing diagnoses are used for many patients with a CVA:

Risk for Aspiration related to impaired ability to swallow

Ineffective Airway Clearance related to a loss of consciousness

Impaired Physical Mobility related to hemiplegia, weakness

Risk for Impaired Skin Integrity related to immobility

Altered Nutrition less than body requires related to dysphagia

Constipation related to immobility

Bowel Incontinence related to decreased loss of consciousness

Urinary Incontinence related to loss of sphincter control

Self-Care Deficit related to brain damage, secondary to CVA

Impaired Verbal Communication related to aphasia, loss of muscle tone in facial muscles

Altered Thought Process related to neurologic deficit, confusion

Caregiver Role Strain related to prolonged disability

Ineffective Individual Coping related to permanent neurologic deficit

Planning and Implementation

The plan of care must be individualized for each patient depending on the neurologic deficit experienced and the severity of the deficit. The prevention of complications is an important aspect of care. The initial phase of a CVA lasts from 48 to 72 hours. During this phase, it is important to provide an ongoing assessment of neurologic status that can be compared with the initial baseline assessment. The nurse maintains a patent airway for patients who are unconscious. Bed rest is maintained until the vital signs stabilize and the patient is fully awake and alert. The less severe neurologic deficits gradually improve, leaving those that are permanent.

Action is taken to prevent future complications of immobility such as pressure ulcers and contractures. As the patient progresses, rehabilitation becomes an important part of the recovery phase. The nurse works closely with the physical therapist, occupational therapist, and speech therapist to provide the most effective treatment for each individual patient.

Aspiration and Ineffective Airway. The patient who is comatose needs careful positioning to maintain an airway and prevent aspiration. The nurse elevates the head of the bed and inserts oral airway if the patient is unable to maintain proper positioning of the tongue. Suction is applied orally and through the nasotracheal route to clear the airway. The nurse repositions the patient every 2 hours. Oxygen therapy may be needed to maintain adequate oxygenation to the body. Lungs are auscultated every 4 to 8 hours. Any abnormal sounds, difficulty breathing, or noisy respirations are reported.

Impaired Skin Integrity and Impaired Mobility

The patient is at risk for developing pressure ulcers because of the impaired mobility. Inspect bony prominences daily for evidence of breakdown (eg, redness, blanching). Turn the patient every 2 hours (ie, supine and sidelying), and position to maintain body alignment. Repositioning is necessary more often (every 1 hour) if evidence of skin breakdown is observed.

It is important to immediately begin active or passive (depending on the patient's ability) range-of-motion exercises for all extremities. The nurse may have the patient squeeze a rubber ball. The nurse uses a footboard, trochanter rolls, pillows, and splints to maintain proper alignment. A footboard or foot splint is sometimes used to maintain the foot at a 90-degree angle. Occasionally, the physician may order high-top tennis shoes to be worn to keep the patient from developing footdrop. The foot board and the tennis shoes prevent plantar flexion (ie, footdrop). The patient is not placed in a Fowler's (high or low) position for extended periods of time, because this contributes to hip flexion contracture.

The patient is positioned on the unaffected side with pillows between the legs and the affected arm resting on a pillow. A hand roll in the hand helps promote a functional position. If possible, place the patient prone (on the abdomen) for 15 to 20 minutes each day to help prevent hip deformity.

Altered Nutrition. The patient may require intravenous fluids to meet nutritional requirements, especially for the first few days after a CVA. Dysphagia (ie, difficulty swallowing) may also occur. With hemiplegia, the paralysis may extend to the face and mouth areas on the affected side, contributing to difficulty in swallowing. When feeding, keep the patient in an upright (90-degree) position for at least 30 minutes after feeding. The nurse keeps the head of the bed elevated during the feeding. Small, frequent feedings that are easy to swallow and that are a lukewarm temperature are offered. Often semisolid foods are easier to swallow than liquids. The nurse places about 5 to 10 mL of food on the unaffected side of the mouth. Swallowing may be enhanced by gently stroking the neck and side of the trachea. It may be necessary to close the patient's lips. Progress slowly with feeding to reduce the incidence of choking. Offer encouragement and praise when appropriate. A suction machine is kept at the bedside until foods and fluids are swallowed without difficulty. Nasogastric feedings or other types of feeding tubes may be necessary with severe disability.

Bowel and Bladder Function. Bowel or bladder incontinence may occur, depending on the area of the brain affected and the severity of the damage. If the patient is incontinent of urine, keep the patient dry, changing the pads and bed as needed. The nurse cleans the perineal area thoroughly and pats the area until dry. An indwelling catheter may be necessary in some situations. It is important to keep a record of the patient's fluid intake and output. The nurse observes and records the frequency and amount of urine. The bedpan or urinal is offered at frequent intervals. The nurse may palpate bladder as necessary to check for bladder distention. Begin a bladder retraining program as soon as possible (see Chapter 14).

Bowel elimination may also be affected with a CVA. The nurse observes and records frequency of bowel movement and appearance of stool (eg, color, consistency). It is important to check for impaction if the patient complains of frequent liquid stools of a small amount. The bedpan is offered at frequent intervals. The physician may order a stool softener if constipation is a problem.

Self-Care Deficit. Depending on the severity of the paralysis, the patient may or may not be able to provide self-care. If possible, the patient is encouraged to participate in self-care activities. A multidisciplinary approach with the nurse, the physical therapist, the occupational therapist, and the speech therapist working together provides the greatest potential for recovery. Assistive devices such as knife–fork combinations, long-handled brushes, extensions for picking things up from the floor, shower chairs, and raised toilets are helpful in some cases to allow greater independence in self-care.

Impaired Communication. Communication problems occur in as many as 40% of stroke patients. Occasionally, speech deficits disappear spontaneously. In other instances, speech and language deficits persist and require speech therapy. **Aphasia** is a common problem after a CVA and involves various degrees of inability to speak, write, or comprehend spoken or written language. Aphasia is manifested in a number of ways. Some individuals with aphasia understand the written and spoken word but cannot communicate verbally (ie, expressive aphasia). Others are unable to understand the written or spoken word. Global aphasia is a type of aphasia in which the patient is unable to speak, write, or understand written or spoken words. Different communication methods may be used, depending on the specific deficit, such as asking questions that require only a yes or no response. If the patient is able to write, a tablet or magic slate can be used for written communication. Pictures of activities or words that the patient can point to can also be used.

When giving instructions, the nurse should speak in a normal tone and allow ample time for the patient to respond. Talking directly to the patient using short sentences and simple phrases makes comprehension easier. The nurse should speak slowly and distinctly, giving directions one step at a time. It may be necessary to repeat instructions. It is important for the nurse to allow the patient sufficient time to process the information.

Thought Process Alterations. The patient with a CVA may have confusion and emotional lability (ie, emotional instability). Emotional outbursts such as crying, laughing, or using profanity are common after a CVA. For some, emotional lability and confusion persist indefinitely. These patients need a calm, predictable, and stable environment. Nurses and caregivers should offer support and comfort. Validation therapy or reality orientation may be used, depending on the nature and severity of the neurologic deficit (see Chapter 17). The nurse or family sets limits on behavior in a firm manner. It may be helpful to tell the patient to stop inappropriate behavior.

Ineffective Coping. Coping with the disabilities of a stroke is often difficult. Bodily changes as a result of hemiplegia, difficulty communicating, and self-care deficit can cause anxiety and depression. The nurse should encourage the expression of feelings including hostility or anger. This demonstrates acceptance by the nurse and assists the patient to deal with these feelings. The nurse gives praise and emotional support when the patient shows improvement. Encouragement at even the slightest progress may provide the impetus to continue working toward recovery. Positive feedback for accomplishments promotes independence and increases feelings of self-worth. It is important for the nurse to actively listen as the patient talks. Problems with aphasia may complicate verbal expression. The nurse allows ample time for conversation. It is important to refrain from completing the sentence or assisting the patient when talking.

Caregiver Role Strain. Prolonged disability can create stress for the caregiver. The nurse must spend time with the caregiver to establish a rapport. The caregiver is encouraged to find time for self-care activities. A support group for caregivers is helpful for some individuals. The nurse can provide information and offer referrals to organizations and agencies available to help. Display 18-6 lists available resources. The nurse takes time to talk with the caregiver and listens to expressions of feelings and concerns. Another important task is to help the caregiver to identify solutions to problems or concerns. The nurse allows the caregiver the opportunity to express anger or resentment.

Evaluation and Expected Outcomes

Successful care can provide the following outcomes for the patient:

Airway remains patent

Able to swallow without difficulty

No evidence of skin breakdown

Nutritional requirements met

Attains normal bowel functioning

Voids at regular intervals

Able to provide self-care within functional abilities

Cognitive ability improved

Demonstrates ability to cope with disease process and neurologic deficits

Caregivers express use of better coping mechanisms

Rehabilitation for Stroke Patients

A comprehensive multidisciplinary rehabilitation program can assist the patient recovering from a stroke to reach his maximum rehabilitative potential. The recommendations for stroke rehabilitation are outlined in Figure 18-5.

DISPLAY 18-6. Resources for Stroke Victims and Families

National Stroke Association
8480 East Orchard Road
Suite 1000
Englewood, CO 80111-5015
303-771-1700
800-STROKES (787-6537)

Promotes stroke prevention, treatment, rehabilitation, family support, and research and provides
Educational books, pamphlets, and audiovisual materials about stroke for stroke survivors, families, and caregivers
Information on local stroke clubs and other self-help groups
Support for stroke research
Training programs about stroke for health care professionals
Be Stroke Smart newsletter for stroke survivors, families/caregivers, and health care professionals

Rosalynn Carter Institute
Georgia Southwestern College
600 Simmons Street
Americus, GA 31709

Provides information on caregiving. Reading lists, video products, and other caregiver resources are available by writing to the address listed at left.

Stroke Clubs International
805 12th Street
Galveston, TX 77550
409-762-1022

Run by stroke survivors
Promotes hiring of people with disabilities
Provides lists of stroke clubs in each state.

The Well Spouse Foundation
P.O. Box 801
New York, NY 10023
212-724-7209
800-838-0879

Provides support for the husbands, wives, and partners of people who are chronically ill or disabled
Provides bimonthly newsletter, regional support groups, pen pal system, and an advocacy program

National Aphasia Association
P.O. Box 1887
Murray Hill Station
New York, NY 10156-0611
800-922-4622

Operates through national office and local affiliates and promotes national awareness and provides
Educational books and pamphlets about aphasia
Referral to community services

PERIPHERAL VASCULAR DISEASE

Peripheral vascular disease (PVD) includes any number of disorders that disrupts the flow of blood through the veins and arteries in the periphery of the body (away from the heart). PVD can result from venous insufficiency or arterial insufficiency. The elderly are particularly prone to PVD and the symptoms may be more pronounced than in younger adults because of chronic disease.

Venous Insufficiency

Venous insufficiency is usually the result of venous stasis, trauma to the wall of the vein, or increased coagulation of the blood. Conditions resulting from venous insufficiency include varicose veins, thrombophlebitis, and deep vein thrombosis.

Varicose Veins

Varicose veins may develop in the elderly as the veins lose elasticity and muscular support with age. The vein most often affected is the saphenous vein and its branches. **Varicose veins** are enlarged, tortuous veins usually seen in the lower extremities. Symptoms may be slight to severe. The most common symptoms include feelings of heaviness in the legs, dull aching after prolonged standing or walking, palpable nodes engorged with blood from incompetent valves, night cramps, and development of venous ulcers on the affected extremities. Treatment depends on the severity of the disorder. For mild symptoms, treatment involves rest, elevation of the extremity, and the use of elastic stockings to counteract stasis and swelling. The elastic or antiembolic stockings provide support to the vein and improve circulation. Every effort must be made to avoid any measure or activity that decreases venous return. For example, older women are instructed not to wear garters or tight girdles. Patients are instructed to avoid sitting for long periods and not to cross their legs when sitting.

For more serious varicosities, vein ligation and stripping may be necessary. Injections of a sclerosing agent (ie, agent to harden or destroy the vein) may be used for smaller varicosities. The nurse monitors for thrombophlebitis, which is a common complication. If a venous ulcer develops, the ulcer is treated with warm, moist compresses and antibiotics to prevent infection.

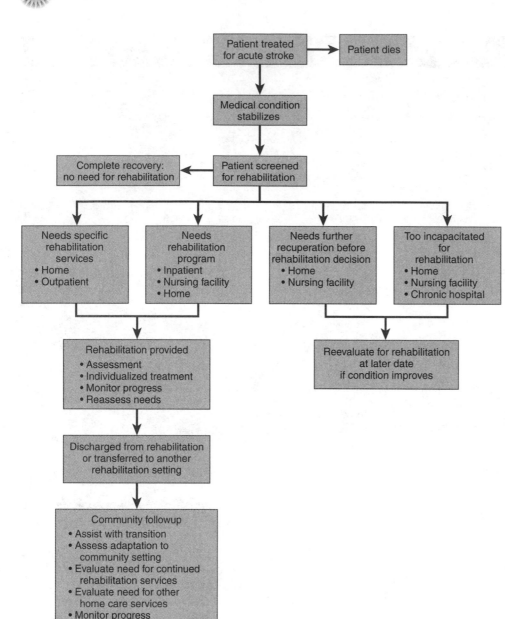

FIGURE 18-5. Clinical flow diagram for stroke rehabilitation. Gresham G.E., Dincan P.W., Stason, W.B., et al. *Post-Stroke Rehabilitation: Assessment, Referral, and Patient Management.* Clinical Practice Guideline. Quick Reference Guide for Clinicians, No. 16. Rockville, MD: U.S. Department of Health and Human Services, Public Health Serivce, Agency for Health Care Policy and Research. AHCPR Pub. No. 95-0663. May 1995.

Thrombophlebitis

Thrombophlebitis is an inflammation of superficial or deep veins with the formation of a blood clot. When the walls of the veins become inflamed resulting in venous status or when the vein is traumatized (eg, irritation from an intravenous solution), development of a thrombus (ie, clot) is a major threat. If the thrombus breaks loose from the wall of the vein, it becomes an embolus. The embolus travels until it occludes a distant vessel. For example, if a thrombus detaches from the saphenous vein in the leg and travels to the lungs, it causes a pulmonary embolism. Pulmonary embolism is a leading cause of death for elderly hospitalized patients.

Symptoms of thrombophlebitis are often vague and difficult to detect. Thrombophlebitis most often affects the lower extremities. Examine both extremities. The affected leg may feel warmer or appear red-

der than the unaffected extremity. There may be pain and tenderness in the affected leg. Measuring the circumstances of both legs at various levels with a tape measure may reveal that the affected extremity is larger. The Homans' sign (ie, calf pain with dorsiflexion of the foot) is sometimes recommended as an indicator of thrombosis in the calf. Diagnosis is made by Doppler ultrasound, phlebography, or plethysmography.

ASSESSMENT ALERT

Assess for a positive Homans sign (ie, pain in the calf when the foot is dorsiflexed). The nurse should be aware that a positive Homans sign can be detected in any painful condition of the calf and is not always accurate in detecting thrombophlebitis.

Treatment includes bed rest to prevent the clot from dislodging and analgesics for pain. Dry heat may be applied to the affected area or moist heat may be used in the form of hydrotherapy, whirlpool, or warm compresses. Elastic stockings are used to promote venous return. Usually, recovery occurs within a short time. Occasionally, surgery is performed to "tie off" the veins in which the thrombi formed. Other veins take over circulation, and collateral circulation develops.

Prevention of thrombophlebitis can be accomplished in some patients by having all patients who are immobile more than 24 hours perform active or passive range-of-motion (ROM) exercises for both extremities. Placing a pillow at the patient's feet and encouraging walking motion of the legs may be beneficial for those who cannot perform ROM exercises for the legs.

Deep Vein Thrombosis

Deep vein thrombosis (DVT) is a form of venous insufficiency. With DVT, small clots trap blood in the deep veins of the legs and pelvic region. Many patients with DVT have no symptoms. Others may complain of aching or throbbing in the affected extremity, exhibit edema of the extremity, and have a low-grade fever. Treatment involves elevation of the leg above the level of the heart. As with thrombophlebitis, observe for signs and symptoms of pulmonary embolism (eg, chest pain, dyspnea, coughing, restlessness). Anticoagulation therapy is used to prevent additional clots from forming. Urokinase or streptokinase may also be used in certain situations to dissolve the clots.

Venous Ulcers

Vascular leg ulcers are a major threat to adults 65 years of age or older. It is estimated that one in four adults older than 65 develops a vascular leg ulcer. Venous ulcers are most often treated using noninvasive measures such as elevation of the extremity, compression, and topical medications. Compression is usually accomplished using elastic stockings worn over the extremity and the ulcer (depending on the amount of drainage). Compression hose are applied before the patient gets out of bed in the morning and taken off at bedtime. Removal during the night prevents damage to the posterior popliteal fossa. Some types of compression hose have zippers that make manipulation of the hose easier for older adults with arthritic changes in the hands. These compression hose apply more compression than the elastic stockings (antiembolic) previously discussed. Other types of compression devices are available, such as the Setopress wrap, a Tubifast elastic bandage, or Unna boot. The Unna boot is a nonstretchable wrap containing gelatin, glycerin, and zinc oxide. After application, the area is covered with a spiral compression bandage and covered with successive coats of paste to produce a rigid boot. The product selected must meet the characteristics of the ulcer. The nurse consults the manufacturer's directions for specific product instructions. When an infection is suspected (eg, when the ulcer has an odor), the ulcer is not wrapped.

ASSESSMENT ALERT

Check for excessive compression by checking the capillary refill on the big toe before and after applying compression bandages. Capillary refill is normally less than 2 seconds (or almost immediate). If capillary refill is delayed, arterial circulation may be compromised by excessive pressure. Notify the physician immediately.

In older adults with thin skin and less subcutaneous tissue, skin breakdown can occur if the compression is too great. The skin is checked for evidence of breakdown, particularly over bony prominences. The patient is encouraged to elevate the feet above the level of the heart several times each day.

Arterial Insufficiency

Arterial insufficiency is caused by hypertension, increased blood cholesterol and lipid levels, obesity, smoking, diabetes, or lack of exercise. Arterial insufficiency is also called arterial occlusive disease. Arterial insufficiency is most often the result of atherosclerosis. **Intermittent claudication** or severe cramping in the extremities when walking is the most characteristic sign. This cramping is relieved with rest. The progression of the disease can be monitored by the distance a patient can walk before pain occurs. The major cause of intermittent claudication in the elderly is atherosclerosis.

With arterial insufficiency, peripheral pulses are weak or absent. The feet are cold even on warm days. The patient may complain of tingling to the extremities. If the leg is elevated, the skin color becomes pale. The affected leg may also be red with mottling (ie, discolored areas) or in some cases may be cyanotic (ie, bluish discoloration of the skin). Trophic changes in the leg produce thinning of the skin, causing a shiny appearance, loss of hair on the extremities, thickened nails, and decreased muscle mass. One or both lower extremities are affected. Sores can develop, causing arterial ulcers. The nurse notes any pain, redness, or tenderness. It is important to assess for a positive Homans sign. Both lower extremities are assessed for skin color, temperature, and size. A tape measure may be used to obtain the circumference of the legs at various intervals.

✔ ASSESSMENT ALERT

A severe arterial insufficiency occurs when the patient complains of pain in the forefoot while at rest. This pain may be worse at night. The pain may be relieved when the extremity is placed in a dependent position.

Treatment for arterial insufficiency is generally conservative with efforts made to control applicable risk factors such as quitting smoking, losing weight, and beginning a regular exercise program. If the patient has diabetes, it must be strictly managed because high glucose levels cause additional arterial damage (see Chapter 23). For intermittent claudication, pentoxifylline (Trental) is the only medication proven to be effective. If symptoms interfere with activities of daily living, surgery may be needed.

Arterial Ulcers

Most foot ulcers are arterial in origin. Venous ulcers are rarely found on the foot. Arterial ulcers most often occur on the tip of the toe, the foot, or between the toes. Goals of treatment are to prevent infection, reduce swelling, and promote healing. Most arterial ulcers require surgery to heal, but many older adults are not good candidates for surgery. Nonsurgical treatments include topical ointments, corticosteroid therapy, antibiotics and hydrogels, foams, or impregnated-gauze dressings are used to prevent or treat infection and promote healing. Necrotic tissue must be removed and infection prevented.

Arterial insufficiency is often characterized by cramping pain in the muscles when the muscle is exercised. Another type of arterial insufficiency is characterized by a burning or tingling pain accompanied by numbness of the toes that occurs at rest, usually in the night.

Nursing Care for the Patient With Peripheral Vascular Disease

Nursing care for the patient with PVD depends partly on whether the problem stems from the venous system or in the arteries. The aim of treatment is to improve circulation, relieve discomfort, and maintain skin integrity.

Venous Insufficiency

For patients with a venous occlusion such as varicose veins or thrombophlebitis, the affected extremity is elevated to promote venous return. Under no circumstances should the affected extremity be massaged. The extremity is immobilized to prevent the clot from becoming dislodged and becoming an emboli. The full length of the legs is supported when the legs are elevated. The nurse instructs the patient not to place pillows under the knees or use the knee Gatch in a hospital bed. Patient should ambulate 5 minutes every hour. Legs are elevated whenever possible (at least three times per day for 20 to 30 minutes each time). Antiembolic stockings are worn to promote venous return. To obtain maximum benefits, instruct the patient to elevate the legs approximately 15 minutes before applying the elastic stockings. If an elastic bandage is used instead of the stocking, begin wrapping the bandage at the toe and wrap upward toward the thigh, keeping the leg elevated. Stockings and bandages should be removed every 8 hours and the skin checked for indication of breakdown. The extremity's circulation is assessed every 2 to 4 hours by checking mobility, changes in temperature, and color or the extremity. The nurse measures and charts leg circumferences at specific points on the leg. Active or passive exercises while in bed, such as alternately flexing, extending, and rotating the foot, helps to promote venous return for lower extremities and reduce venous stasis.

Arterial Insufficiency

For arterial insufficiency such as arterial occlusive disease, the extremity is placed in a dependent position and maintained at rest. The extremities are kept warm because chilling can lead to vasospasm and result in increased arterial insufficiency. The patient is encouraged to avoid exposure to cold and quit smoking (if applicable).

Bed rest is maintained during the acute phase. The pain is related to the extent of circulatory deficit and inflammatory process. To enhance venous return keep the affected extremity elevated. A foot cradle may help to keep pressure off the affected leg. The extremity is kept warm to promote blood flow and decrease pain. The nurse applies moist heat to the extremity, if indicated. Any sudden or severe chest pain, especially if it is accompanied by dyspnea, tachycardia, and anxiety is reported immediately because this may indicate pulmonary edema.

Intermittent claudication can be extremely painful. However, when the patient rests, the pain subsides. Placing the extremity in a dependent position increases arterial blood supply. The drug, pentoxifylline may be prescribed to reduce the incidence of intermittent claudication. However, this drug helps relieve the signs and symptoms of claudication, allowing an increase in walking endurance, but it does not treat the underlying problem.

Patient and Family Teaching

The patient and caregiver are taught measures to promote venous return such as elevating the legs periodically during the day. Preferably, the legs should be elevated 15 to 20 minutes three times each day. Activities that compromise blood flow such as sitting or prolonged standing, crossing the legs when sitting, and wearing garters or girdles are avoided. Daily exercise such as walking is encouraged. A walking program promotes muscular contraction and provides a gentle pumping motion that increases circulation through the veins, minimizing venous pooling. If overweight, the patient is encouraged to lose weight.

For patients with arterial insufficiency experiencing intermittent claudication, walking may be prescribed to promote blood flow and encourage the development of collateral circulation. Pain is used as a guide in determining the amount of exercise. When calf pain occurs, the patient is instructed to stop walking, because this indicates an inadequate blood supply to the area. With regular walking, collateral circulation can develop, resulting in an increased walking distance before the onset of claudication. Not all patients with PVD should exercise. Be sure that the patient consults with the physician or primary caregiver before beginning an exercise program.

Teach the patient that warmth promotes arterial flow and exposure to cold temperatures causes vasoconstriction. Clothing should be warm, gloves and socks should be worn, and the patient should be encouraged to stay inside when the weather is extremely cold. The bath temperature is checked before use to decrease the possibility of burning the skin. Hot water bottles and heating pads should be avoided because the elderly patient may not be able to feel the heat, increasing the potential for being burned. Patients with arterial insufficiency should be told not to smoke because nicotine causes vasospasm and reduces circulation to the extremities.

CRITICAL THINKING EXERCISES

1. Ms. Gonzales, age 65, confides to you that her husband seems to be avoiding having sexual contact since his heart attack 6 months ago. She is concerned and asks you what she should do. How would you answer Ms. Gonzales?
2. A nursing assistant complains to you that Mr. Jones, a recent stroke patient, is difficult to care for. The nursing assistant states she is tired of his mumbling and continual gestures. What would you say to the nursing assistant? What suggestions could you make to ease the nursing assistant's frustration and to help Mr. Jones?
3. Mr. Carnes, age 75, is diagnosed with arterial insufficiency of the lower legs. What would you expect to find during an assessment? Which finding would be most significant for arterial insufficiency?

REFERENCES AND SUGGESTED READING

Easton, K. (1999). The poststroke journey: From agonizing to owning. *Geriatric Nursing, 20 (2),* 70–76.

Harris, A., Brown-Etris, M., & Troyer-Caudle, J. (1996). Managing vascular leg ulcers, part I: Assessment. *American Journal of Nursing, 96 (1),* 38–44.

Harris, A., Brown-Etris, M., & Troyer-Caudle, J. (1996). Managing vascular leg ulcers, part II: Treatment. *American Journal of Nursing, 96 (2),* 40–47.

Jaffe, M. (1996). *Medical-surgical nursing care plans* (3rd ed.). Stamford, CT: Appleton & Lange.

Konstam, M., Dracup, K., Baker, D., et al. (1994). *Heart failure: Evaluation and care of patients with left-ventricular systolic dysfunction.* Clinical practice guideline no. 11. AHCPR publication no. 95–0612. Rockville, MD: Agency for Health Care Policy and Research. Public Health Service, U.S. Department of Health and Human Services.

Leighton, C. (1998). A change of heart. *American Journal of Nursing, 98 (10),* 33–37.

Miller, C. (1999). Update on hypertension management. *Geriatric Nursing, 20 (4),* 218–219.

Miller, R., & Woo, D. (1999). Stroke: Current concepts of care. *Geriatric Nursing, 20 (2),* 66–69.

National Institutes of Health. (1997). *The sixth report of the Joint National Committee on Prevention, Detection, Evaluation and Treatment of High Blood Pressure.* Publication no. 98-4080. Bethesda, MD: National Institutes of Health.

Roach, S., & Scherer, J. (2000). *Introductory clinical pharmacology* (6th ed.). Philadelphia: Lippincott Williams & Wilkins.

Schulmeister, L. (1998). Pacemakers and environmental safety: What your patient needs to know. *Nursing, 98 28 (7),* 58–60.

Smeltzer, S., & Bare, B. (1996). *Brunner and Suddarth's textbook of medical-surgical nursing* (8th ed.). Philadelphia: Lippincott-Raven.

Stanley, M. (1999). Congestive heart failure in the elderly. *Geriatric Nursing, 20 (4),* 180–187.

CHAPTER 19

The Musculoskeletal System

CHAPTER OUTLINE

KEY TERMS
CHAPTER OBJECTIVES
NORMAL MUSCULOSKELETAL FUNCTION
AGE-RELATED CHANGES IN THE
  MUSCULOSKELETAL SYSTEM
    Changes in the Skeleton
    Changes in the Joints
    Changes in the Muscles
OSTEOPOROSIS
    Pathophysiology
    Diagnostic Tests
    Signs and Symptoms
    Treatment
    Using the Nursing Process to Manage
      Osteoporosis
    Fractures From Osteoporosis
ARTHRITIS
    Osteoarthritis
    Rheumatoid Arthritis
    Fibromyalgia
    Gout
CRITICAL THINKING EXERCISES
REFERENCES AND SUGGESTED READING

KEY TERMS

arthritis
Colles fracture
dowager's hump
fibromyalgia
gout
osteoarthritis
osteoblasts
osteoclasts
osteocyte
osteoporosis
rheumatoid arthritis
spondylosis
synovial joints
synovitis

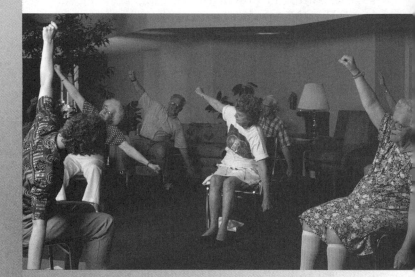

CHAPTER OBJECTIVES

At the completion of this chapter, the student will
be able to

- Discuss pathophysiology, symptoms,
  diagnostic procedures, treatment, and nursing
  care of patients with osteoarthritis

- Use the nursing process to care for patients
  with osteoporosis

- Discuss the significance and nursing
  management of fractures in patients with
  osteoporosis

- Discuss the pathophysiology, symptoms,
  diagnostic procedures, treatment and nursing
  care of patients with osteoarthritis,
  rheumatoid arthritis, and gout

- Discuss the symptoms and management of a
  patient with fibromyalgia

- Use the nursing process to care for patient
  with various forms of arthritis

- Discuss the use of joint replacement surgery in
  patients with arthritis

The bones, joints, and muscles are major components of the musculoskeletal system. Bones are attached to each other at the joints to facilitate movement of the various body parts. In the older adult, there is a generalized slowing of the growth of new bone and an increase in bone reabsorption, causing the bone to weaken. Cellular muscle loss and joint changes contribute to the musculoskeletal changes associated with aging. The changes in the bones, muscles, and joints increase the older adult's risk of developing musculoskeletal disorders such as osteoarthritis and arthritis. This chapter discusses changes that occur in the musculoskeletal system with age and the more common disorders of the musculoskeletal system facing the older adult.

NORMAL MUSCULOSKELETAL FUNCTION

Bone is composed of dense, hard, and slightly elastic connective tissue. Within the bone is an intricate network of blood vessels, lymph vessels, and nerves. **Osteoblasts** are cells located within the bone that maintain or build up the bone. The cells function in part to repair the bone after a fracture. **Osteoclasts** are the cells responsible for the breakdown and reabsorption of bone. Bone formation and bone reabsorption are ongoing processes that occur throughout life. An **osteocyte** is the main mature bone cell that regulates the concentration of calcium in body fluids by helping to release calcium from bone tissue into the blood.

The framework of the trunk is the vertebral or spinal column, which in the adult is a row of 26 separate vertebrae (ie, bones) that form a column. These vertebrae are separated by intervertebral disks that are attached to various muscles to provide strength to the spinal column. The intervertebral disks are composed of a layer of fibrocartilage that act as shock absorbers and provide a layer of padding between the vertebrae. Each vertebrae has a foramen (ie, opening) in the center. These spaces form a spinal canal that houses and protects the spinal cord.

The joints form connections between two or more bones. Joints may normally be immovable. The freely movable joints are the **synovial joints** and are the most common type of joints found in the body. Synovial joints contain a space or a joint cavity that contains synovial fluid, a thick, colorless fluid secreted by the synovial membrane that acts as a lubricant and provides nourishment to the joint space. Synovial joints include the wrist, ankle, elbow, shoulder, hip, and knee joints. The synovial joints allow freedom of movement to make changes

in position, such as flexion, extension, abduction, and adduction.

Muscle is composed of long, thin cells or fibers that contract to produce movement. In addition to movement, the muscles form a protective covering over certain areas of the body and help provide support. Muscles enable the body to perform different types of movement, such as bending, straightening, raising a body part, moving toward the midline, or away from the midline.

AGE-RELATED CHANGES IN THE MUSCULOSKELETAL SYSTEM

Age-related changes in the musculoskeletal system affect the bone, the joints, and the muscles of the older person. These changes have a significant impact on the older adult's life and can profoundly affect functional ability resulting in the loss of independence. Changes in the musculoskeletal system alter the appearance, slow movement, and affect ambulation.

Changes in the Skeleton

The skeleton is composed of 214 bones and forms the framework of the body. Bones function in support, calcium storage, and production of blood cells. Until the age of 35 to 40 years, more bone is produced than is destroyed. Around age 35 to 40, activity of the osteoblasts decreases while the activity of osteoclasts increases. Trabecular bone loss exceeds cortical bone loss. By age 80, the average man has lost approximately 27% of trabecular bone. Women lose 43% of their trabecular bone by the age of 90. Estrogen, a hormone produced by women in their childbearing years, appears to protect women against bone loss. Bone loss accelerates after menopause, when estrogen production ceases. Bone loss places the older adult at increased risk for fractures.

Height decreases with age, and posture becomes somewhat stooped. These changes in posture and height are the result of changes within the vertebral disks. The fibrocartilage of the intervertebral disks lose water and become drier and thinner. This causes the vertebrae to compress and height to diminish. Shortening of the spinal column results in a dowager's hump (ie, kyphosis of the upper thoracic spine). The extremities appear longer because of the shortening of the spinal column. Osteophytes (ie, bony outgrowths or spurs) form on the vertebral column, causing osteoarthritic changes. Height decreases by approximately 1 to 6 inches. With advancing age, the pelvis widens, and the hips and knees become slightly flexed.

Bone reabsorption causes the bone to lose calcium and have a decreased ability to produce material for the bone matrix (ie, intracellular bone), which weakens the bone. Cartilage in certain areas of the body continues to grow, particularly the cartilage in the nose and ears, resulting in widening and lengthening of the nose and lengthening of the ears.

Changes in the Joints

The freely movable synovial joints such as the joints of the knees, wrists, elbows, and hips feel the most affects of aging. The synovial membrane lines the joint cavity and secretes a lubricating fluid called synovial fluid. With age, there is a decrease in synovial fluid, and cartilage in joints become thinner. Cartilage is a special type of connective tissue that aids in joint movement. Ligaments may become shorter and less flexible. These changes result in a decreased range of motion (ROM) of the affected joints. Some joints, however, may be more mobile because ligaments are stretched.

The bursae are fluid-filled synovial sacs located at various points around the joints. The bursae make movement easier and decrease friction around the joints. With age, changes in the bursae increase the risk of inflammation causing bursitis.

Changes in the Muscles

Muscle fibers decrease with age, causing a loss of lean body mass. These muscle fibers are not replaced. Muscles become thin and flabby, particularly muscles of the arms and legs, resulting in weakness. Muscle contraction slows as the result of prolonged impulse conduction time along the motor unit in the muscle tissue. Increased muscle rigidity contributes to limited movement in areas such as the neck, hips, and knees. By the age of 80, approximately 50% of the maximum muscle mass is lost. Muscle tissue is replaced with fat. Regular physical activity can help to combat the muscle wasting (see Chapter 10).

OSTEOPOROSIS

Osteoporosis is a progressive loss of bone mass and deterioration of skeletal tissue, causing the bones to

---

DISPLAY 19-1. Risk Factors for Osteoporosis

- Being a woman
- Menopause before age 45, especially with surgical removal of both ovaries
- Low lifetime calcium intake
- Lack of exercise
- Underweight
- Being Caucasian
- Family history of osteoporosis
- Smoking

---

become porous, brittle, and weak. As the bone mass decreases, there is a increased risk for fractures. The two most common fractures that occur as the result of osteoporosis are hip fractures and vertebral fractures.

According to the National Osteoporosis Foundation, 7 to 8 million Americans have osteoporosis. Seventeen million more Americans are at risk for developing the disease. Of those affected, about 80% are women. Women are at greater risk because of their relatively smaller frame and lower peak bone mass than men. Certain risk factors place the elderly at greater risk for developing osteoporosis (Display 19-1).

Each year this disease results in approximately 1.5 million fractures. Approximately 300,000 are hip fractures and 500,000 are vertebral compression fractures. Most of these fractures occur in the elderly. Another problem associated with osteoporosis is the development of a **dowager's hump,** kyphosis of the thoracic spine, caused by collapse of the vertebrae. The dowager's hump can affect digestion because of compression of the stomach and intestine. The abdomen protrudes as the result of a relaxation of the abdominal muscles. As bone loss occurs in the spine, the vertebrae collapse, resulting in a decrease in height from 1 to 6 inches (Fig. 19-1).

Pathophysiology

For most individuals, bone mass peaks at approximately 35 years of age. After age 35, slightly more bone is lost each year than is replenished. Osteoblasts form new bone while old bone is reabsorbed by osteoclasts. Some scientists suggest that osteoporosis may occur as the result of diminishing activity of the osteoclasts and osteoblasts. Trabecular bone loss occurs more rapidly than cortical bone loss. Trabecular bone is composed of tiny spikes of bone tissue surrounded by calcified bone and found in the interior of spongy bone. The vertebral column

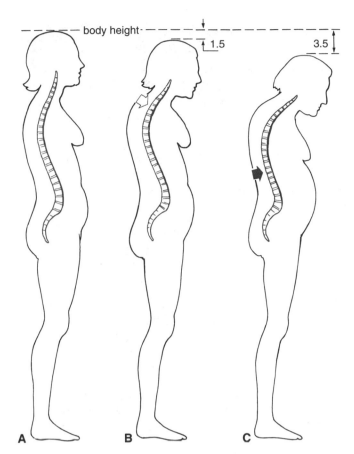

FIGURE 19-1. Typical loss of height associated with osteoporosis. (**A**) Loss at 10 years' postmenopausal. (**B**) Loss at 15 years' postmenopausal: 1.5 inches. (**C**) Loss at 25 years postmenopausal: 3.5 inches. From Rosdahl, C.B. (1995). *Textbook of Basic Nursing, 6th Edition.* Philadelphia: J.B. Lippincott Co. page 1347. Figure 85-2. Used with permission.

and the femoral neck contain trabecular bone. This accounts for the greater incidence of hip and spinal fractures.

Calcitonin, a hormone produced by the thyroid gland, acts to prevent bone reabsorption. Production of this hormone is decreased with aging, adding to the problem of bone reabsorption. Another hormone, the parathyroid hormone produced by the parathyroid gland, functions to increase bone reabsorption, and its production is increased with aging. This increased production of the parathyroid hormone is an additional factor that adds to increased bone reabsorption.

In women, estrogen inhibits bone reabsorption and helps the body absorb calcium, a mineral essential to strong bones. Older adults absorb calcium less efficiently than younger adults. This lack of absorption of calcium increases the need for dietary calcium in the elderly. In the late thirties or early forties, estrogen levels begin to decline, resulting in more bone reabsorption. The bone loss increases in

the first few years of menopause when lessening estrogen levels have the greatest impact. Although men lose bone mass at a later age than women, 1 of 3 men who are 75 years of age or older develop osteoporosis.

Diagnostic Tests

Radiographic examination for bone density, or bone densitometry, is best accomplished by the used of dual-energy x-ray absorptiometry (DEXA). DEXA is the preferred method to diagnosis osteoporosis. The DEXA measures bone density with a high degree of accuracy using only a small amount of radiation. During this test, narrow x-ray beams scan across areas of potential weakness such as the hip, the spine, or the wrist. The individual's bone density is compared with normal values for the patient's age and with normal values of healthy adults (ie, young normal values). Low readings indicate low bone density. Bone densitometry can detect low bone mass before a fracture occurs, confirm the diagnosis of osteoporosis, determine the rate of bone loss, and monitor the effects of treatment. No special preparation is required for the test.

Other methods may be used to detect osteoporosis such as the single-photon absorptiometry (SPA) or the quantitative computed tomography scan (QCT). SPA is limited to measuring the wrist. QCT is less precise than DEXA, uses more radiation, and is generally more expensive.

Signs and Symptoms

Signs and symptoms of osteoporosis include various degrees of bone pain or tenderness. Discomfort or pain in the lower back may also occur. Sometimes, no symptoms are identified, and the individual learns of osteoporosis when a fracture occurs. A dowager hump may be present if the disease has affected the spine.

Treatment

Osteoporosis is not curable but is controllable and preventable. Treatment is aimed at slowing the rate of bone reabsorption. Analgesics may decrease the pain and tenderness. Calcium supplements may be prescribed to supplement dietary calcium intake. Evidence suggests that calcium citrate is better absorbed than other forms of calcium. However, adequate calcium alone cannot stop bone loss. Estrogen replacement therapy (ERT) may be prescribed for

DISPLAY 19-2. Four Ways to Help Prevent Osteoporosis

Increase Calcium Intake. Calcium, vitamin D, and phosphorus are important nutrients to build strong bone. Milk is a good source of each of these nutrients. Before the age of 35, women can absorb calcium more easily and should build up adequate amounts of the mineral in the bone. Most adults need 1,000 to 1,500 mg of calcium each day. Older women need approximately 1,500 mg/day. Calcium carbonate supplements contain the highest amount of useful calcium. Take calcium supplements with a full glass of water and with meals. Take not more than 500 mg of calcium at a time, because small amounts are better absorbed. With age, an increased amount of calcium is needed because less calcium is absorbed in the intestine. Dairy products such as milk, cheese, and yogurt are excellent sources. Other foods high in calcium include green leafy vegetables, shellfish, sardines, oysters, tofu, and almonds. Foods such as breakfast cereals or orange juice may be fortified with calcium. A vitamin D (400 IU) supplement may be helpful for those who do not drink fortified milk, are not regularly out in the sun, or for those older than age 65.

Exercise Regularly. Weight-bearing exercises increase the force of gravity against bones and help to maintain bone mass. The performance of daily activities such as sweeping, vacuuming, and mopping may place enough stress on the bones to help with maintenance. Bone responds well when weight and moderated stress are applied. Performing activities such as ballroom or square dancing, mowing the lawn, rowing, tennis, walking, or hiking can help prevent bone loss. Weight-bearing exercising three or four times each week for 20 to 30 minutes is recommended. The older adult should check with the physician before beginning an exercise program.

Do Not Smoke. Smoking cigarettes increases the risk of fracture in people of all ages. Smoking decreases bone mass. Smoking lowers estrogen levels in women. Women who smoke enter menopause at an earlier age than nonsmokers. Another possible reason for the increased incidence of fractures in smokers is the lower overall body weight of smokers compared with nonsmokers. Cigarette smoking also increases the risk for lung cancer and cardiovascular disease.

Limit Alcohol Intake. Individuals who drink heavily have less bone mass and lose bone more rapidly than nondrinkers. Heavy drinking leads to inebriation, increasing the risk for falling and fracturing a bone. Limit alcoholic beverages to no more than two drinks per day. One alcoholic drink is equal to 12 ounces of beer, 5 ounces of wine, or 1.5 ounces of liquor.

postmenopausal women to help prevent bone loss. Osteoporosis is not an inevitable consequence of aging. Preventive measures incorporated into the lifestyle can decrease the risk of developing osteoporosis (Display 19-2).

Drug Therapy

Several drugs may be used to treat osteoporosis, including estrogen, alendronate, raloxifene, calcitonin-salmon.

Bone mass remains relatively constant until menopause. With menopause, the ovaries no longer produce estrogen, a hormone that helps maintain bone mass and retain calcium. Women lose 10% to 15% of their bone mass in the first 10 years after menopause. ERT helps to combat this bone loss and prevent osteoporosis. Estrogen may be given alone to treat osteoporosis. When estrogen is used alone, the risk of endometrial (uterine) cancer increases. Fortunately, estrogen can be combined with progestin to drastically decrease the risk of endometrial cancer. All women who have not had hysterectomies (ie, surgical removal of the uterus) should take a combination of estrogen and progestin. Estrogen only is given for women who have had hysterectomies. If progestin is given on a 10- to 14-day cycle, uterine bleeding can occur. To prevent monthly uterine bleeding, estrogen-progestin combinations are given continuously. Initially, there may be an occasional episode of bleeding, but this undesirable effect usually resolves within 6 months. ERT can reduce the risk of fracture by 50% if taken over an extended period. ERT is administered in tablet form or by a patch that is placed on the skin for intermittent release.

Nonhormonal drugs such as alendronate sodium (Fosamax) can be used to restore lost bone in many postmenopausal women. The drug increases spinal bone mass by 7% to 10% over 3 years and increases hip bone mass by 5% to 8% during the same period. This strengthens the bone and reduces the incidence of fractures. Alendronate is used for the prevention and treatment (10 mg/day) of osteoporosis. Adverse reactions with alendronate are usually mild and include abdominal pain, nausea, heartburn, irritation of the esophagus, constipation, diarrhea, or gas. The most severe adverse reaction is esophageal irritation. This reaction is greater in those patients who fail to follow dosing instructions. If pain, difficulty in swallowing, chest pain, or worsening of heartburn develops, the patient should stop the drug and contact the physician or primary health care provider. If a dose is missed, the patient should skip the dose and resume the prescribed regimen the next morning.

Because alendronate is poorly absorbed in the gastrointestinal tract, it is recommended that no

DRUG ALERT

To minimize the risk of esophageal irritation, advise the patient to use a full glass of water to swallow the drug and to stay fully upright (sitting or standing) for at least 30 minutes after the drug is taken.

food, drink, or medications be taken for 30 minutes to 1 hour after the drug is taken. The patient should take the drug first thing in the morning, 30 minutes before eating, with 6 to 8 ounces of water. Beverages such as coffee, mineral water, or orange juice decrease absorption of the drug.

Like alendronate, raloxifene (Evista) is used to treat postmenopausal women with osteoporosis. Raloxifene is a selective estrogen receptor modulator and acts by binding to estrogen receptors, producing estrogenic effects on the bone. The recommended dosage is 60 mg/day, which may be administered anytime during the day without regard to meals. The most commonly reported side effects are hot flashes and leg cramps. An infrequent but serious side effect is blood clots in the veins. The drug should be discontinued at least 72 hours before surgery and during prolonged immobilization, such as postoperative recovery or prolonged bed rest.

Another drug sometimes used to treat osteoporosis is calcitonin-salmon (Miacalcin). Once only available by injection, calcitonin-salmon is now available by nasal spray. It is used for postmenopausal women who are more than 5 years past menopause and who have low bone mass relative to healthy premenopausal women. Calcitonin-salmon allows bone formation to "catch up with" or match bone breakdown in the bone remodeling process. As an additional benefit, calcitonin-salmon has also been found to relieve lower back pain due to osteoporosis. Adverse reactions are few and mainly related to nasal irritation. The recommended dosage is 200 IU/day intranasally in conjunction with calcium and vitamin D supplementation.

Using the Nursing Process to Manage Osteoporosis

Assessment

Assessment of a patient with a diagnosis of osteoporosis requires obtaining the height and weight and determining the presence of pain, particularly in the upper and lower back or hip. Dietary assessment provides information on dietary intake of calcium-rich foods and on overall food intake. It is important to assess the coffee and carbonated beverage

intake. High-caffeine intake in coffee can increase the amount of calcium excreted in the urine, contributing to low dietary calcium levels. Carbonated beverages contain phosphorus, which can interfere with calcium absorption. The nurse questions the patient regarding cigarette smoking. Evidence suggests a greater incidence of fractures in women who smoke.

Nursing Diagnoses

One or more of the following nursing diagnoses may be used for an individual with osteoporosis:

- Pain related to compression fractures
- Altered Nutrition: Less Than Body Requirements related to lack of dietary calcium
- Anxiety related to fear of falling, disability, progression of the disease, other (specify)
- Risk for Injury related to falling
- Risk for Ineffective Management of Therapeutic Regimen due to lack of knowledge of disease process, medication regimen, preventative care, other (specify)

Planning and Implementation

Nursing interventions of the patient with osteoporosis focus on the preventive measures and treatment regimen prescribed by the physician.

Pain. Analgesics are given for pain. The nurse assesses the patient 30 minutes after medication is given to evaluate pain relief.

ASSESSMENT ALERT

The elderly patient needs careful monitoring after pain medication is administered because these drugs can cause confusion in the elderly and increase the risk of falling. Assess for changes in level of consciousness and developing or increased confusion in elderly patients receiving analgesics. Assist the patient when getting out of bed or during ambulation to prevent falling.

If the patient must stay on bed rest, the nurse gently assists the patient with position change to help maintain proper body alignment. A firm, non-sagging mattress is used. Passive ROM exercises may be performed if no fracture is present or performed on the unaffected joints even if a fracture is present. The patient is instructed to turn the body as a unit and avoid twisting. A back brace or lumbosacral corset may be prescribed for support when out of bed. The nurse instructs the patient how to put the brace or corset on correctly. Relaxation techniques may be helpful in relieving anxiety associated with pain (see Chapter 11).

Altered Nutrition. Encourage the individual to eat a well-balanced diet using the Food Guide Pyramid for planning meals (see Chapter 11). The elderly person may be prescribed 400 IU of vitamin D to promote calcium absorption and enhance its incorporation into the bones. Milk, exposure to sunlight, and dietary supplements aid in increasing vitamin D. Provide a list of foods high in calcium, including foods such as milk and milk products, canned sardines (including bones), beef, egg, peanuts, broccoli, oranges, and papaya. Optimal calcium intake for women who are older than 50 years and not on ERT is 1,500 mg/day. Recommended calcium dosage is 1,000 mg/day for women on ERT. The dosage of calcium is best absorbed if administered several times a day. Some authorities believe that only 500 mg of calcium can be absorbed at one time.

Anxiety and Risk for Injury. Anxiety develops over fear of falling and developing a fracture. The person may isolate herself, refuse to leave home, and not exercise, moving as little as possible for fear of falling. To decrease anxiety, allow the patient to express these feelings. Actively listen. Explain that inactivity worsens the problem. Physical activity strengthens muscles, prevents disuse atrophy, and slows bone loss. Encourage the implementation of an exercise program such as walking. Refer to a physical therapist to devise an exercise program to improve strength and balance. Many older adults will be forced to go to the nursing home unless they are able to remain functionally independent.

The patient is encouraged to ambulate using a normal stride. The nurse provides help with ambulation, if needed. When ambulating or exercising, fatigue is avoided. It may be necessary to modify the environment to ensure safety and promote independence. For example, the nurse may suggest that "scatter" rugs be removed, adequate lighting provided, and handles be placed in strategic areas. The nurse may instruct the older adult to avoid sudden movements such as bending or twisting and to avoid lifting heavy objects. When ambulation is poor, the nurse encourages the use of a walker, cane, or other assistive device to help reduce the incidence of falling.

Patient and Family Teaching

All patients and family members need a thorough explanation of measures to prevent further bone loss. A teaching plan for patients with osteoporosis should include information about calcium supplements and dietary considerations.

PATIENT TEACHING AID

A teaching plan for osteoporosis should include the following points:

- **Take calcium and vitamin D supplements as prescribed by the physician.**
- **Limit caffeine-containing beverages to 2 cups per day.**
- **Limit carbonated beverages to 2 cans per day.**
- **Eat a well-balanced diet.**
- **Quit smoking (if applicable).**
- **Exercise two to three times per week. Walking and weight-bearing exercise help to increase the mineral content of bone.**
- **Take analgesics as prescribed by physician.**
- **If alendronate, calcitonin-salmon, or ERT is prescribed, take as directed by the physician. Notify the physician or primary health care provider of any unusual effects or worsening of the symptoms.**

Evaluation and Expected Outcomes

Successful care can provide the following outcomes for the patient:

    No complaints of pain
    Adequate calcium and vitamin D intake
    Eating a well-balanced diet
    Decreased anxiety
    No injury as the result of a fall
    Knowledge about the disease process and
       medication regimen

Fractures From Osteoporosis

Osteoporosis results in approximately 1.5 million fractures annually. Of these, 300,000 are hip fractures, 700,000 are vertebral fractures, and 200,000 are wrist fractures. In the elderly, fractures are a major cause of death and disability. Fractures occur more frequently in the elderly with osteoporosis because the bone is so porous and weak that even the slightest stress can result in fracture. Sometimes, no fall is necessary for a fracture to occur. The patient may feel or hear the snap of a bone fracture and then fall.

Spinal or vertebral fractures occur as the vertebrae become so weakened from the disease that they collapse, causing crush fractures. Patients with vertebral crush fractures may complain of severe back pain. The most common fractures caused by osteoporosis include **Colles fracture** (ie, transverse fracture occurring just above the wrist as the result of as the result of placing the hand backward and outward), vertebral crush fractures, and hip fractures. The Colles fracture typically occurs in women as the result of a fall on an outstretched hand.

Hip Fracture

Hip fracture is the most serious of the fractures resulting from osteoporotic changes and typically occurs in the elderly after a fall. Figure 19-2 shows the common sites of hip fractures. Radiographic studies reveal the

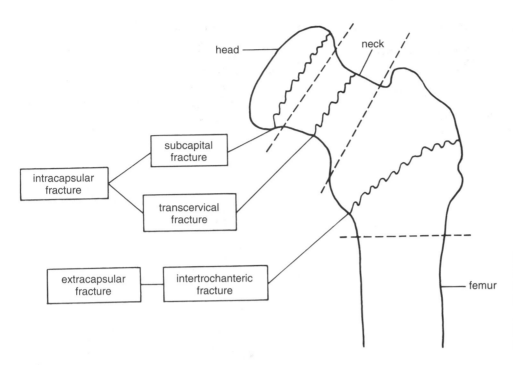

FIGURE 19-2. Common sites of hip fractures. From Scherer, J. and Timby, B. (1995). Introductory *Medical-Surgical Nursing 6th ed.* Philadelphia: Lippincott-Raven, p. 987. Used with permission.

exact location of the fracture. Typically, hip fractures are treated surgically. Traction can be used for non-ambulatory patients. Traction produces healing in 4 to 8 weeks. Treatment of hip fractures by traction increases the risk of complications from prolonged bed rest. Healing may also occur with the affected extremity out of normal alignment, resulting in shortening and external rotation of the extremity and decreased functional ability for the older adult.

Symptoms of hip fracture include pain that increases with movement. The affected extremity may appear deformed, externally rotated, and shorter than the unaffected extremity. Surgical stabilization may be accomplished with the insertion of a sliding compression hip screw that provides support and stabilization. Postoperatively, most patients can immediately begin partial to full weight-bearing ambulation with a walker. In 6 to 12 weeks, progression to a cane can usually be made.

Nursing Management of a Hip Fracture

Postoperatively, it is important to maintain good alignment of the affected leg and avoid adduction (ie, moving the leg toward the midline). When the patient is in bed, the nurse places an abduction pillow between the legs. The patient is positioned supine or on the unaffected side (depending on the physician's orders). Most often postoperative pain is moderate to severe and managed with patient-controlled analgesia (PCA), by epidural injection, or with parenteral analgesics for 1 or 2 days postoperatively. As pain intensity decreases, an oral analgesic is ordered. The nurse follows the physician's orders for ambulation and getting out of bed. Physi-

cal therapy may be prescribed by the physician. Any signs of pulmonary embolism such as respiratory distress, a change in mental status, or a sharp pain in the chest are reported immediately.

ARTHRITIS

Arthritis means inflammation of the joint and refers to more than 100 different diseases of the joints and connective tissue. The three main symptoms of arthritis are joint pain, stiffness, and joint swelling that lasts more than 2 weeks. The most common forms of arthritis are osteoarthritis, rheumatoid arthritis, fibromyalgia, and gout.

Nearly 40 million Americans have arthritis. Osteoarthritis or degenerative joint disease affects approximately 15.8 million Americans. Those older than 45 years of age are most likely to be affected. Rheumatoid arthritis is one of the most disabling forms of arthritis and affects approximately 2.1 million Americans. Fibromyalgia affects more than 2 million Americans. Although not as common as the other forms of arthritis, gout affects 1 million Americans.

Osteoarthritis

Osteoarthritis, also called degenerative joint disease, is the most common type of arthritis. The incidence of osteoarthritis rises significantly with age. Before age 45, osteoarthritis affects more men, but after age 55, it

DEGENERATIVE JOINT DISEASE (OSTEOARTHRITIS)

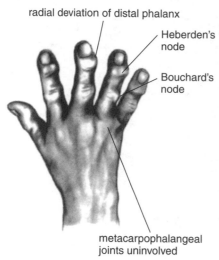

radial deviation of distal phalanx

Heberden's node

Bouchard's node

metacarpophalangeal joints uninvolved

Nodules on the dorsolateral aspects of the distal interphalangeal joints are the hallmark of degenerative joint disease, or osteoarthritis, and are called Heberden's nodes. Usually hard and painless, they affect the middle-aged or elderly and often, although not always, are associated with arthritic changes in other joints. Flexion and deviation deformities may develop. Similar nodules on the proximal interphalangeal joints, called Bouchard's nodes, are less common. The metacarpophalangeal joints are spared.

ACUTE RHEUMATOID ARTHRITIS

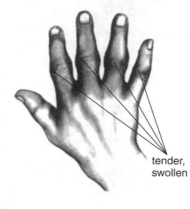

tender, swollen

Tender, painful, stiff joints characterize rheumatiod arthritis. Symmetrical involvement on both sides of the body is typical. The proximal interphalangeal, metacartophalangeal, and wrist joints are frequently affected; the distal interphalangeal joints rarely so. Patients with acute disease often present with fusiform or spindle-shaped swelling of the proximal interphalangeal joints.

CHRONIC RHEUMATIOD ARTHRITIS

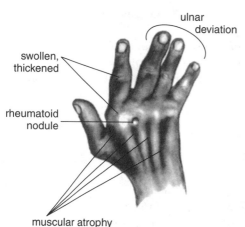

ulnar deviation

swollen, thickened

rheumatoid nodule

muscular atrophy

As the arthritic process continues and worsens, chronic swelling and thickening of the metacarpophalangeal and proximal interphalangeal joints appear. Range of motion becomes limited and the fingers may deviate toward the ulnar side. The interosseous muscles atrophy. The fingers may show "swan neck" deformities (ie, hyperextension of the proximal interphalangeal joints with fixed flexion of the distal interphalangeal joints). Less common is a boutonnière deformity, (ie, persistent flexion of the proximal interphalangeal joint with hyperextension of the distal interphalangeal joint).

Rheumatoid nodules may accompany either the acute or chronic stage.

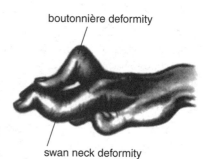

boutonnière deformity

swan neck deformity

FIGURE 19-3. Swellings and deformities of the hand.

occurs more frequently in women. Like other forms of arthritis, osteoarthritis cannot be cured but can be managed. Osteoarthritis most often affects the large weight-bearing joints, such as the hips and the knees, but joints of the hands, feet, and spine can also be affected.

Pathophysiology

The most prominent physiologic change in osteoarthritis occurs with the gradual degeneration of the articular cartilage. Cartilage covers the ends of bones, allowing smooth movement over the joint. In osteoarthritis, the cartilage degenerates with age, and in some cases, a total loss of cartilage occurs. Continued use of the joints causes inflammation, pain, and swelling. This can lead to limitation of joint mobility. New bone growth called spurs can occur around the joints as a result of the degenerative changes.

Obesity contributes to the development of osteoarthritis by adding stress to the joints and carti-

lage. Years of wear and tear from joint use and sometimes joint abuse contribute to the increased incidence of osteoarthritis in older adults. Secondary osteoarthritis is caused by another condition, such as repeated trauma, diabetes, or gout.

Symptoms

Symptoms of osteoarthritis depend on the joint affected and the severity of the disease. The most common symptom is pain in the affected joint, particularly after use. The joint pain is typically worse at the end of the day. Other symptoms include warmth, swelling, stiffness, and crepitus (ie, crackling sound heard when a joint is moved) of the affected joint. Stiffness is particularly noticeable after prolonged inactivity, such as after sitting for long periods.

Some patients may complain of few symptoms even with significant joint degeneration. Heberden nodes (ie, bony enlargements of the small joint at the end of the fingers) occur in osteoarthritis (Fig. 19-3).

Bouchard nodes also occur and are seen as bony enlargements of the middle joint of the fingers. These nodes are not painful but can be helpful identifying the disease.

When osteoarthritis affects the spine, pain typically occurs in the neck or low back. If bony spurs form in the spine, pain, numbness, and tingling can occur. Osteoarthritis of the spine is called **spondylosis.**

Osteoarthritis of the knee is associated with repeated trauma or injury. Severe osteoarthritis of the knee results in pain, limping, and joint dysfunction and may require total knee replacement.

Diagnosis

Diagnosis of osteoarthritis is made after a review of the individual's medical history and thorough physical examination, with particular attention on the painful joints. Radiographs typically reveal a loss of joint cartilage, spur formation, and narrowing of the joint space. The presence of Heberden and Bouchard nodes help establish the diagnosis.

Joint fluid analysis can be done with arthrocentesis. A joint fluid analysis can eliminate other causes of arthritis such as gout or infection. An arthrocentesis is also useful for treating the pain and inflammation by injecting a corticosteroid into the area of inflammation. Arthroscopy (ie, direct visualization of a joint with a specialized instrument called an arthroscope) is a procedure that can be used to repair damage to the cartilage and to identify the extent of damage and abnormality.

Treatment

Treatment is aimed at reducing pain and stiffness and maintaining joint mobility and function. Symptomatic treatment includes rest, exercise, weight reduction, and physical and occupational therapy. Medications include acetaminophen, the nonsteroidal anti-inflammatory drugs (NSAIDs), salicylates, and corticosteroid injections (Table 19-1). With mild pain, acetaminophen- or aspirin-based creams applied to the skin may be helpful. Acetaminophen (Tylenol) is usually the first drug prescribed for the elderly because it has fewer adverse reactions than the salicylates or NSAIDs. Although acetaminophen has no anti-inflammatory properties, it is effective in relieving the pain of osteoarthritis. The NSAIDs include celecoxib (Celebrex), rofecoxib (Vioxx), ibuprofen (Motrin), nabumtone (Relafen), and naproxen (Naprosyn). NSAIDs have analgesics and anti-inflammatory properties. The newer NSAIDs, celecoxib and rofecoxib, have fewer gastrointestinal problems than other NSAIDs. In addition, these two drugs have the advantage of once-a-day dosing.

Some physicians are also prescribing naturally occurring substances such as glucosamine and chondroitin for the treatment of osteoarthritis. Glucosamine furnishes the building blocks that the body uses to make and repair cartilage. Chondroitin is thought to make the tissue more flexible. No significant adverse reactions have been reported with the use of these two substances.

The application of heat or cold may provide short-term relief of pain and stiffness. Surgery may be needed when more conservative treatment is not effective. Arthroscopy, total knee replacement, and total hip replacement are the most common operations performed for osteoarthritis.

Rheumatoid Arthritis

Rheumatoid arthritis usually begins before age 45 and affects more women than men. Although this disease begins in young adulthood or middle age, its chronic and degenerative nature makes it one of the major causes of disability in older adults. Rheumatoid arthritis is characterized by periods of remissions (ie, periods with no symptoms) and exacerbations (ie, periods with an increase in symptoms) progressing in a downward sequence. If the disease develops in later years (after age 60), the symptoms are usually acute, and many joints are affected, but there is a greater opportunity for improvement than in the younger adult.

Symptoms

Rheumatoid arthritis affects many joints but the most common joints affected first are the small joints of the hands, wrists, and feet. Later, the knees, shoulders, hips, elbows, ankles, and cervical spine are affected. The elderly experience more muscular weakness and a greater tendency toward flexion contractures. The onset is usually abrupt, bilateral (ie, affecting both sides of the body), and symmetric (ie, occurring on corresponding sides). Affected joints are swollen, hot, and painful. Morning stiffness occurs and generally lasts more than 30 minutes after awakening.

The inflammatory process causes thickening of the tissue around the joint, destruction of the bone, deformity, and eventually disability. The course of the disease is unpredictable. Some individuals may have mild symptoms with little deformity. In others, the disease is rampant and causes crippling deformities. Any joint can be affected, but the most noticeable deformities often occur in the hands (see Fig. 19-3).

Pathophysiology

Rheumatoid arthritis begins with **synovitis,** an inflammation of the synovial membrane surrounding the joint. As synovitis persists, pathophysiologic

TABLE 19-1. Drugs Used to Treat Arthritic Conditions

Drug	Uses	Adverse Reactions	Nursing Considerations
NONSALICYLATES acetaminophen (Tylenol, Datril)	May be the initial drug for treating osteoarthritis, particularly osteorarthritis of the hip	Rash, urticaria, hepatic necrosis (if taken in excessive amounts or with alcohol)	Liver damage can occur from prolonged use or high dosages. May be taken with food or on an empty stomach. Adults may require doses up to 4,000 mg/day.
SALICYLATES aspirin, acetylsalicylic acid	Rheumatoid arthritis, osteoarthritis; pain and discomfort from musculoskeletal injuries	Tinnitus, GI upset, easy bruising, prolonged bleeding from injuries	Give with food, milk, or a full glass of water. Observe for signs and symptoms of toxicity (eg, tinnitus, dizziness, nausea, vomiting, headache). Notify physician before administering next dose. Black or dark stools or bright red blood in the stool may indicate gastrointestinal (GI) bleeding.
NONSTEROIDAL ANTI-INFLAMMATORY DRUGS (NSAIDs) etodolac (Lodine) flurbiprofen (Ansaid) ibuprofen (Advil, Motrin) indomethacin (Indocin) nabumetone (Relafen) naproxen (Naprosyn, Aleve) piroxicam (Feldene) sulindac (Clinoril) celecoxib (Celebrex) rofecoxib (Vioxx)	Rheumatoid arthritis, osteoarthritis that does not respond to acetaminophen	Nausea, vomiting, drowsiness, dizziness abdominal discomfort, epigastric pain, diarrhea, constipation, GI bleeding, gastric or duodenal ulcer	Instruct patients to take with a full glass of water 30 minutes before or 2 hours after meals. May be given with food to minimize GI upset. Black or dark stools or bright red blood in the stool may indicate GI bleeding. Avoid the use of alcohols, aspirin, acetaminophen, or other OTC drugs while taking NSAIDs. GI reactions may occur and can be serious, even fatal, especially in patients with upper GI disease. Withhold the next dose and notify physician if diarrhea, nausea, vomiting, tarry stools, or abdominal pain occurs.
MISCELLANEOUS DRUGS hydroxychloroquine	Severe rheumatoid arthritis	Irritability, nervousness, alopecia, anorexia, nausea, vomiting, ophthalmic effects, hematologic changes, dizziness, dermatoses	Administer with milk or meals to minimize GI distress. Contents of capsules may be mixed with a teaspoon of jelly or Jell-O for easier administration. Ocular damage may be minimized by wearing dark glasses in bright light. Wear protective clothing and use sunscreen to minimize dermatoses. For rheumatoid arthritis, treatment may require up to 6 months to reach full therapeutic effect.

TABLE 19-1. **Drugs Used to Treat Arthritic Conditions** *continued*

Drug	Uses	Adverse Reactions	Nursing Considerations
methotrexate (Rheumatrex)	Rheumatoid arthritis that is unresponsive to conventional therapy	Nausea, vomiting, low platelet count, leukopenia, stomatitis, diarrhea, alopecia, anemia, photosensitivity	Inform physician immediately if symptoms of infection occur. Report any unusual bleeding. Provide good oral care. Discuss possibility of hair loss. Explore coping alternatives. Instruct patient to wear sunscreens and protective clothing when exposed to sunlight.
penicillamine (Cuprimine, Neopen)	Progressive rheumatoid arthritis	Abdominal discomfort, edema, nausea, rash, indigestion, heartburn, vomiting, constipation, diarrhea, agranulocytosis	Administer on empty stomach 1 hour before or 2 hours after meals. Supplemental doses of vitamin B_6 may be needed.
DRUGS USED FOR GOUT allopurinol (Zyloprim)	Management of symptoms of gout	Rash, dermatitis, nausea, vomiting, diarrhea, abdominal pain, Stephens-Johnson syndrome	May be given with milk or meals to prevent GI upset. Avoid use of alcohol. Ensure patient maintains adequate fluid intake.
colchicine	Relief of acute attacks of gout	Nausea, vomiting, diarrhea, abdominal pain, bone marrow depression	Can be given with food or milk. Drug is administered every 1 to 2 hours, until pain is relieved or patient develops diarrhea. GI upset may continue even after drug is discontinued. Encourage fluids. Keep I & O records.
probenecid (Benemid)	Treatment of hyperuricemia of gout	Headache, anorexia, nausea, vomiting, urinary frequency, flushing, dizziness, GI upset	Administer with food or antacid to minimize GI upset. Do not take aspirin while taking this drug. May require several months of therapy for maximum effects.
GOLD COMPOUNDS aurothioglucose (Solganal)	Rheumatoid arthritis	Dermatitis, stomatitis, photosensitivity, pruritus, nausea, vomiting hematologic changes, nausea, vomiting, rash, metallic taste	Protect from exposure to ultraviolet light. Monitor older patients carefully; tolerance to gold decreases with age. Give deep IM injection. Provide good oral care to help prevent stomatitis. Observe skin for dermatitis. Patient may experience increased joint pain for 1 to 2 days after injection. Pain subsides after several injections. Provide frequent, small meals if patient has nausea.
auranofin (Ridaura)	Rheumatoid arthritis	Dermatitis, stomatitis, photosensitivity, pruritus, nausea, vomiting, glossitis hematologic changes, nausea, vomiting, rash, metallic taste	Give orally. Provide good oral care to help prevent stomatitis and glossitis. Observe skin for dermatitis. Report unusual bleeding, or bruising, fever severe diarrhea, skin rash or mouth sores. Monitor elderly patients carefully; tolerance to gold decreases with age.

changes occur, causing tissue to attach itself to the opposite joint surface, forming a band and resulting in limited movement of the joint. As the disease continues, the tissue attaching itself to the joint surface becomes calcified, resulting in osseous ankylosis (ie, immobility of a joint). In this later stage, the joint essentially no longer exists. These changes progress at different rates in different joints in those affected with arthritis. These arthritic changes influence the care of the aging adult.

Treatment

Medical Approach. Although there is no cure for rheumatoid arthritis, treatment is aimed at preventing deformity, decreasing pain and inflammation, and maintaining functional ability. Rest must be balanced with exercise; otherwise, a joint kept immobile for too long may become ankylosed (ie, immobile or fixed). Pain is managed with the salicylates or NSAIDs, which are usually prescribed at lower dosages than for younger adults. The elderly are also more prone to adverse reactions and metabolize the drugs more slowly, predisposing them to toxicity (see Table 19-1). Advanced rheumatoid arthritis may be treated with gold therapy, penicillamine, or immunosuppressive drugs such as methotrexate or azathioprine.

One of the newer drugs, Remicade, is a combination of methotrexate and infliximab. The combination drug is used in patients who have not responded to other forms of treatment, especially those who have had an inadequate response to methotrexate alone. The drug is given intravenously in 3 mg/kg doses at 0, 2, and 6 weeks and then every 8 weeks thereafter. In the first year of treatment, the patient generally receives eight infusions, and in subsequent years, the patient receives six infusions. The most common adverse reactions include upper respiratory infection, headache, nausea, sinusitis, rash, and cough. The incidence of adverse reactions is lower than in patients receiving methotrexate alone.

Joint Replacement Surgery. When medical treatment fails to control the pain of arthritis or when the joints are severely damaged so as to interfere with the performance of daily activities, joint replacement surgery may be necessary. Joint replacement can be done on any joint except the spine. Joint replacement is most commonly done on the knee or hip.

Joint replacement surgery is performed most often in those older than 65 years of age and is highly successful in older adults. The replacement device may be metallic or polyethylene (or a combination) and implanted using an acrylic cement. Another method is a coated implant that is porous enough to allow bony ingrowth. Arthroplasty is surgery for a total hip replacement. The femoral head and the acetabulum are replaced with a prosthesis (ie, artificial replacement) that is cemented into the bone.

Nursing Management of a Patient Undergoing Joint Replacement. Nursing care after a total joint replacement involves careful monitoring and meticulous care to avoid infection. The nurse takes vital signs frequently and monitors the patient for evidence of infection (eg, elevated temperature, chills, restlessness, increased respiratory rate). It is important to keep drainage devices such as the Hemovac or Jackson-Pratt patent and to measure and drain the contents at regular intervals (every 8 hours or more frequently). The nurse documents the color and amount of drainage. Purulent or malodorous drainage indicates infection and is immediately reported. Dressings are monitored for evidence of bleeding. Antibiotics are often administered prophylactically to prevent infection.

Bed rest is maintained with the affected joint in the prescribed position. A semi-Fowler position is used with caution because prolonged hip flexion may dislocate the new prosthesis. Ice may be applied to promote vasoconstriction and decrease pain. To enhance venous return, the extremity is elevated. The foot of the bed may be raised or a pillow placed the full length of the extremity, but it is important not to place pillows under the knee or allow the knee to remain bent for an extended period. The patient is turned on the operated side or as prescribed by surgeon. The operative leg is generally kept slightly abducted. Medications for pain are given before activity or procedures. Surgical pain is relieved by the use of narcotic analgesics and muscle relaxants. The surgical site is observed for evidence of healing or for signs of infection. The surgeon's directions are followed for ambulation and weight bearing. Physical therapy provides instruction and help with ambulation, weight bearing, and transfers. A walker may be used initially for support and to prevent falling.

The patient is discharged to home in approximately 10 days if able to ambulate. If assistance is required, the patient may be transferred to a nursing home until ambulatory and able to perform self-care with minimal assistance. Some individuals complain of headaches, abdominal pain, or numbness or tingling in their hands, feet, or legs.

FIBROMYALGIA

Fibromyalgia is a poorly understood chronic condition in which the patient is plagued by chronic musculoskeletal aching and pain, fatigue, morning stiffness, and sleep disturbances. Pain is the most prominent symptom and is described as burning, radiating, sore, stiff, and aching. Some individuals complain that fibromyalgia feels like a chronic case of influenza. The widespread pain affects various muscles and joints, but there is no evidence of joint swelling or degeneration. Fibromyalgia is not progressive and does not cause deformity. Many persons report severe fatigue, with lack of energy and exhaustion. Sleep problems are common.

Nursing care is particularly important because the chronic pain is difficult for the patient and there is no specific treatment. Fibromyalgia is treated with nonnarcotic analgesics, exercise programs, and relaxation techniques. The anti-inflammatory medications used to treat arthritis do not have a major effect in fibromyalgia. Aspirin, ibuprofen, or acetaminophen provide partial relief. These patients may be treated with the tricyclic antidepressants to relieve pain and to increase rapid eye movement (REM) sleep (see Chapter 10).

Each patient is treated individually, with a focus on helping the patient learn to "work through" the pain. Working through the pain involves having the patient keep going despite pain. Other forms of arthritis, such as rheumatoid arthritis and osteoarthritis, must be excluded before working through the pain is recommended. A regular exercise program, such as walking or swimming, is recommended. Although fibromyalgia is associated with chronic pain, it is not life threatening and usually does not worsen with time.

Gout

Gout is a form of arthritis that commonly affects the joints of the feet, particularly the big toe. Gout is essentially a metabolic disorder related to an excess of uric acid crystals in the body that cannot be eliminated. There is oversecretion or diminished excretion of the uric acid. Uric acid forms when the body breaks down waste products. Normally, uric acid is excreted through the kidney. In gout, this excretion

ASSESSMENT ALERT

Older adults who have had gout for 10 years or longer may have tophi, and those who have been inadequately treated often develop tophi. Tophi are deposits of uric acid crystals that collect under the skin and in the joints in cartilage, in subcutaneous tissue, and in the cartilage on the external ear. Tophi appear as hard nodules on the outer surface of the external ear (Fig. 19-4). Occasionally, tophi discharge white, chalky crystals. On the hand, tophi appear as nodules that look like knobby swellings.

CHRONIC TOPHACEOUS GOUT

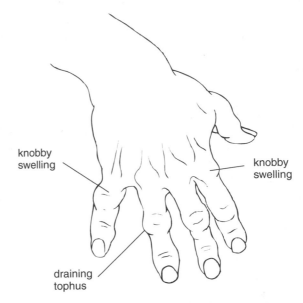

The deformities that develop in long-standing chronic tophaceous gout can sometimes mimic those of rheumatoid and osteoarthritis. Joint involvement is usually not so symmetrical as in rheumatoid arthritis. Acute inflammation may or may not be present. Knobby swelling around the joints sometimes ulcerate and discharge white chalklike urates.

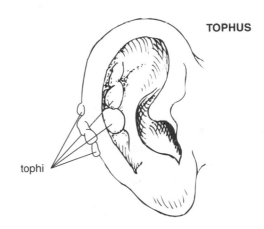

Tophi are deposits of uric acid crystals characteristic of gout. They appear as hard nodules in the helix or antihelix. They occasionally discharge white chalky crystals.

FIGURE 19-4. Tophi on the hands and around the ears.

does not readily occur, and uric acid crystals form. The uric acid crystals collect in the joints, causing pain and inflammation.

Characteristics of gout include a sudden, severe episode of pain, tenderness, redness, warmth, and swelling of usually one joint at a time. Besides the big toe, other joints affected are the knee, ankle, foot, hand, wrist, and elbow. Gout is episodic.

The individual may experience only one attack, some have several episodes, and others may have lasting joint pain and damage. Most episodes of pain and inflammation last 5 to 10 days, followed by remission of the symptoms and followed by other attacks. An attack of gout can be triggered by eating too much of the wrong food (eg, wine, beer, gravies, liver), drinking too much alcohol, an illness, or surgery. Diagnosis may be made by physical examination, medical history, and a blood test to measure the amount of uric acid in the blood.

If not treated, persistent pain and inflammation in the joint occurs. Gout cannot be cured but can be well managed with medication. Drugs used to treat gout include allopurinol, colchicine, the NSAIDs, and probenecid (see Table 19-1). The uricosuric drugs, such as probenecid, lower the uric acid level by increasing the amount of uric acid excreted by the kidney. Allopurinol (Zyloprim) reduces the amount of uric acid in the blood by slowing the manufacture of uric acid in the body.

Using the Nursing Process in Caring for Patients With Arthritis

Assessment. The nurse assesses the patient for joint pain, tenderness, redness, swelling, and stiffness. The patient is questioned concerning the increases of pain in the evening or when stress is placed on the joint. The nurse determines if there is any limitation on activity or affect on lifestyle (social or self-care activities). It is important to check for limitation of movement or decreased ROM, contractures, or deformity. The patient is weighed and questioned about recent weight loss or gain. Figure 19-5 may be used to identify and record problem areas. The nurse documents location and intensity of pain and any observations of the affected joint. Any precipitating factors of pain are noted. The joints of the extremities and external cartilage of the ears are examined for evidence of tophi. The hands are examined for deformities or nodules (see Figs. 19-3 and 19-4).

Nursing Diagnoses. One or more of the following nursing diagnoses may be used for an individual with arthritis:

Pain, acute or chronic, related to joint inflammation and swelling

Risk for Impaired Physical Mobility related to joint deformity, pain, weakness

Self-Care Deficit related to decreased strength, impaired mobility, pain on movement

Ineffective Individual Coping related to disease, loss of mobility, disability

Risk of Ineffective Management of Treatment Regimen related to lack of knowledge of disease process, treatment regimen, other (specify)

Mark on the figures below the location of pain, stiffness, or swelling.

Place "P" where you feel pain.
Place "S" where you have stiffness.
Place "X" where there is swelling

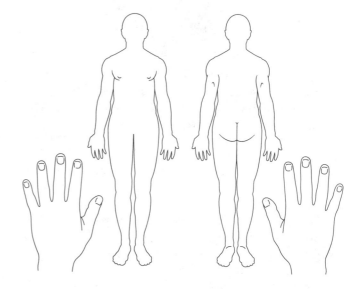

FIGURE 19-5. Assessing affected joints in arthritis.

Planning and Implementation. The care of the patient with arthritis focuses on preventing deformity, relieving pain, maintaining self-care, helping the patient to cope with a chronic disorder, and providing information about the disease and the treatment regimen.

Pain. Temporary pain relief may be accomplished by the application of heat or cold. Heat or cold applied over painful joints gives short-term relief of pain and stiffness. The choice of heat or cold may be left to the patient, or the physician may order one or the other. Some individuals prefer cold; others prefer heat. Heat relaxes the muscles and dilates superficial blood vessels, increasing circulation and decreasing edema. Cold decreases pain by numbing the area. It is important not to apply heat or cold for more than 20 minutes at a time and to make application several times each day. Heat may be applied in the form of warm compresses, warm showers, hot tubs, heated pool, or other methods approved by the physician. Cold is applied using cold compresses, an ice bag, or a bag of frozen vegetables (in the home environment).

Acetaminophen may be effective for mild pain in patients with osteoarthritis. For more severe pain, other drugs may be used (see Table 19-1). One of the newer NSAIDs, rofecoxib (Vioxx) is taken once each day and is effective for the relief of osteoarthritis pain. Rofecoxib appears to have significantly fewer gastrointestinal side effects than many other NSAIDs. Vioxx may be taken with or without food. Adverse reactions include upper and lower respiratory infection or inflammation, headache, dizziness, diarrhea, nausea, vomiting, swelling of the legs and or feet, increased blood pressure, back pain, or tiredness. Although rare, rofecoxib may cause serious stomach and intestinal bleeding.

Pennsaid Topical is a lotion used to treat osteoarthritis of the knee. Transdermal application facilitates the delivery of the drug to the site with minimal systemic absorption, decreasing adverse reactions. Pennsaid decreases stiffness and pain of the knee joint allowing for greater mobility.

With an acute attack, the patient may be placed on bed rest to decrease pain and prevent injury to the affected joints. Painful joints can be placed in splints to decrease pain and injury. However, prolonged immobility results in loss of function. As soon as pain and tenderness decrease, begin passive ROM and then active ROM.

The nurse encourages the use of relaxation techniques and imagery to decrease stress and promote relaxation (see Chapter 11). Stress can exacerbate symptoms of arthritis, and stress relief plays a role in decreasing pain.

Impaired Physical Mobility. There is always a risk for impaired physical mobility with arthritis. Schedule activities to alternate with rest periods. This helps to protect joints from the stress of repeated tasks and helps decrease fatigue. The nurse instructs the patient to change tasks frequently so the joints will not be in one position for too long of a timeframe.

If the patient is on bed rest, the nurse assists with passive or active ROM to maintain joint function. The frequency and type of ROM are determined by the individual's condition. Passive ROM is done slowly, with the extremity above and below the joint supported to prevent strain on the joint. Isometric exercise (ie, tightening and releasing large muscle groups) helps maintain muscle tone. The patient is repositioned frequently (every 1 to 2 hours), maintaining proper body alignment (Table 19-2).

A consult with a physical therapist or an occupational therapist can assist in planning an individual exercise program to maintain joint flexibility and mobility. If ambulating, the use of a cane is encouraged. The use of a cane or crutches can reduce the force of weight bearing by 50%. Mild exercise is an important component of preventing physical immobility; ROM exercise increases and maintains flexibility. These exercises should be done two or three times each day.

Walking, light weight training, and stationary cycling provide good exercise for those with arthritis. Heat can be applied before exercise and cold applied after exercise to relieve pain. Exercise is encouraged to levels that do not cause joint pain. Swimming is particularly helpful for those with arthritis because water exercise minimizes stress on the joints.

Self-Care Deficit. Self-care deficits can occur because of decreased strength or painful and inflamed joints. The inability to perform activities of daily living is a problem that can result in the elderly being placed in a nursing home. The nurse identifies the level of functioning before exacerbation or onset of the disease. Sufficient time is allowed to perform activities. The nurse assesses the need of assistive devices such as a reacher, button hook, and long-handled shoehorn. The nurse may need to arrange for help from community resources (eg, Meals on Wheels, social services, senior citizen groups, home care services). Consultation with physical therapist or occupational therapist may be necessary to help with self-care activities and to identify ways to modify tasks to maintain independence. The patient is referred to the local Arthritis Foundation to order the *Joint Savers Catalogue* (Display 19-3). This catalogue lists many helpful devices and provides tips to make daily living easier.

Ineffective Coping. The nurse encourages the expression of emotions and feelings, including anger, anxiety, fear, and guilt. Ways the person can learn to manage symptoms are explored. The problem-solving technique may be used to manage difficulties and develop solutions (see Chapter 26). The nurse encourages the individual to be open to new ideas. It is important to identify past coping skills and to reinforce positive coping mechanisms. The nurse may suggest that the patient contact the Arthritis Foundation for help in coping such as self-help classes or home study programs.

It is important to identify family members who can help with tasks or responsibilities that the patient is unable to perform. Effective methods of stress reduction are identified as well. The patient is encouraged to attend a support group for patients with arthritis or to be a volunteer for the Arthritis Foundation.

Patient and Family Teaching. When teaching patients with arthritis, the nurse focuses on ways to maintain joint function and mobility, methods to control pain, and guidelines for living with the disease. A teaching plan for a patient with arthritis should include information about the specific type of arthritis, exercise, and medication information.

TABLE 19-2. Proper Positioning

Position Characteristics	Fowler's	Lateral	Sims	Sitting
Description	Patient is supine, with head elevated 30 degrees in semi-Fowler's, 60 degrees in Fowler's, and 90 degrees in high-Fowler's	Patient is supported on right or left side. Arms are flexed toward shoulders. Hips and knees are slightly flexed.	Patient is semiprone on right or left side with opposite arm, thigh, and knee flexed and resting on bed.	Patient sits upright in chair with feet resting and knees bent at 90-degree angle.
Head support	Pillow behind head	Pillow under head to keep head, neck, and spine aligned	Pillow under head to keep head, neck, and spine aligned	Headrest
Arm support	Pillows placed under lower arm, if needed, to prevent pull on shoulders and edema in hands	Pillow under upper arm to prevent adduction and interference with respiration	Upper arm is flexed at elbow and supported with pillow	Wide armrests or pillows on overbed table to avoid pull on shoulders
Back support	Small pillow or towel roll behind lower back	Rolled pillow along back and upper buttocks to help patient maintain position	None	Small pillow or rolled towel in lumbar curve
Leg support	Pillow beneath lower legs	Hips and knees are flexed with pillow beneath upper leg to prevent adduction and internal rotation of hip	Hip and knee of upper leg are flexed and supported with pillow	Seat's edge should not press against popliteal area; legs may be elevated by footrest or footstool.
Foot support	Foot board, pillows placed against bottom of feet, high-topped sneakers, or padded, strap-on boots to prevent plantar flexion	Same as for Fowler	Same as for Fowler's	Feet may rest on floor, or legs may be elevated if ankle support (eg, high-top tennis shoes) is provided to prevent plantar flexion.
Indications	Semi-Fowler's, neurosurgical patients; Fowler's, most types of chest and abdominal surgery, heart disease, lung disease, tube feedings, obesity, high-Fowler's, severe respiratory conditions	Unilateral lung disease (with good lung down)	ARDS; left Sims for enema administration or for rectal or gynecologic examination	Mentally and physically beneficial for most patients
Contraindications	Spinal injury	Left lateral for patients with compromised oxygenation status, unless due to diseased right lung	In some cases, obesity and advanced age	Cautious use with increased intracranial pressure
Advantages	Promotes lung expansion and awareness of surroundings; facilitates coughing, deep breathing, eating, and conversation; minimizes risk of aspiration	Relieves pressure on scapulae, sacrum, and heels; can be used to improve oxygenation by increasing blood flow to dependent lung	Allows drainage of oral secretions, minimizing risk of aspiration in unconscious patients; may improve oxygenation in patients with ARDS	Promotes communication and awareness of surroundings; facilitates cardiovascular, respiratory, and gastrointestinal functions; counter many ill effects of bed rest
Disadvantages	Increases effect of gravity on coccyx; overuse may lead no flexion contracture of hips	Arms must be properly supported to avoid adduction, respiratory inhibition, and compression of brachial plexus, and medial, radial, and ulnar nerves. Left lateral position may impair oxygenation in patients with certain conditions.	Obesity and advanced age may lessen tolerance	Extended periods of sitting (>2 hours) can impede vascular return from legs. Patients may fall asleep in this position and slump into poor alignment.

Adapted from Metzler, D., & Harr, J. (1996). Positioning your patient properly: A nurse's guide to patient positioning. *American Journal of Nursing, 96 (3),* 35–36.

PATIENT TEACHING AID

The following information should be included in a teaching plan for a patient with arthritis:

- Read information about the specific type of arthritis (eg, symptoms, management, what to expect, what to report).
- Maintain normal weight. Exercise and adjusting caloric intake can prevent weight gain. Consult a dietitian if obese.
- Engage in a regular exercise program approved by the physician (eg, walking, swimming, riding a stationary bike).
- To protect joints, use the stronger joints to carry items. For example, carry bags with forearms or palms rather than fingers, or carry a purse on the shoulder rather than by the hand.
- Use canes or walkers to reduce stress on joints.
- Use assistive devices if necessary. Provide information for ordering assistive devices.
- Manage symptoms with the use of heat or cold for approximately 20 minutes several times each day.

- Use energy-saving techniques such as sitting to perform activities rather than standing.
- Use correct body positioning and posture. Avoid remaining in one position for extended periods. Keep joints extended rather than flexed. Use splints as prescribed.
- Keep all appointments with the physician, and notify the physician if an acute exacerbation occurs.
- Understand the medication regimen. This includes dosage, side effects, therapeutic effect, and signs of toxicity.
- Use enteric-coated or buffered aspirin to minimize gastric irritation. If taking unbuffered aspirin, take with an antacid.
- Take medication with meals to help prevent gastrointestinal upset.
- Understand the possible adverse drug effects, and report tinnitus, gastric intolerance, gastrointestinal bleeding, and rash.
- Take medication exactly as prescribed to obtain therapeutic effect. For example, aspirin must be taken at regular intervals to maintain therapeutic blood levels.

Evaluation and Expected Outcomes

Successful care can provide the following outcomes for the patient:

Reports pain is controlled
Uses relaxation techniques to decrease pain
Maintains functional ability in affected joint
Able to perform self-care activities
Expresses understanding of disease process and medication regimen treatments

CRITICAL THINKING EXERCISES

1. Ms. Wagoner, age 70, attends the adult day care center where you work. You observe that she has kyphosis of the thoracic spine. She smokes heavily and is very thin. What action, if any, would you take? Explain your answer.

2. Mrs. Langford, age 88, is diagnosed with osteoarthritis. She appears anxious and tells you that she is fearful of developing severe deformities. What would you tell Mrs. Langford to ease her anxiety? What suggestions could you offer Mrs. Langford to help her deal with her osteoarthritis?

3. Mr. Williams, age 65, has been retired for 2 months. Suddenly one evening, he developed severe pain in the left big toe. The doctor diagnosed Mr. Williams with gout and prescribed

probenecid (Benemid). Develop a care plan for Mr. Williams with at least three nursing diagnoses and three interventions for each diagnosis.

REFERENCES AND SUGGESTED READING

Dowd, R., & Cavalieri, R. (1999). Help your patients live with osteoporosis. *American Journal of Nursing, 99 (4),* 55–58.

Glasworthy, T.D., & Wilson, P. (1996). Osteoporosis: It steals more than bone. *American Journal of Nursing, 96 (6),* 27–34.

Kee, C., Harris, S., Booth, L., et al. (1998). Perspectives on the nursing management of osteoarthritis. *Geriatric Nursing, 19 (1),* 19–27.

Mahat, G. (1998). Clinical snapshot: Rheumatoid arthritis. *American Journal of Nursing, 98 (12),* 42–43.

Yarnold, B. (1999). Hip fracture: Caring for a fragile population. *American Journal of Nursing, 99 (2),* 36–40.

CHAPTER 20

The Respiratory System

CHAPTER OUTLINE

KEY TERMS

CHAPTER OBJECTIVES

NORMAL RESPIRATORY FUNCTION

AGE-RELATED CHANGES OF THE RESPIRATORY SYSTEM

CHRONIC OBSTRUCTIVE PULMONARY DISEASE

ASTHMA

PNEUMONIA

INFLUENZA

TUBERCULOSIS

SLEEP APNEA

CRITICAL THINKING EXERCISES

REFERENCES AND SUGGESTED READING

KEY TERMS

alveoli

asthma

bronchopneumonia

central sleep apnea

chronic bronchitis

chronic obstructive pulmonary disease (COPD)

cilia

diaphragmatic breathing

emphysema

intrinsic asthma

lobar pneumonia

Mycobacterium tuberculosis

pneumonia

pseudomembranous colitis

pursed-lip breathing

status asthmaticus

superinfection

tuberculosis

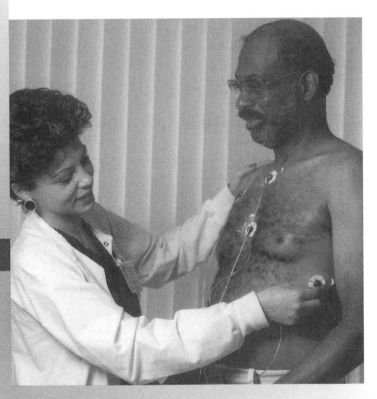

CHAPTER OBJECTIVES

At the completion of this chapter, the student will be able to

- Discuss normal respiratory function

- Identify age-related changes in the respiratory system

- Discuss signs and symptoms of a patient with chronic obstructive pulmonary disease, asthma, pneumonia, influenza, tuberculosis, and sleep apnea

- Discuss important aspects of care of the patient with chronic obstructive pulmonary disease, asthma, pneumonia, influenza, tuberculosis, and sleep apnea

- Use the nursing process to care for an older adult with chronic obstructive pulmonary disease

Many changes occur within the respiratory system of the older adult. Many of these changes can be delayed or modified by lifestyle changes such as quitting smoking or engaging in a regular exercise program. The frail elderly are particularly susceptible to respiratory disorders such as bacterial pneumonia and influenza.

This chapter describes the normal respiratory system, followed by the age-related changes that occur in the respiratory system. Common disorders discussed in the chapter include chronic obstructive pulmonary disease, asthma, pneumonia, influenza, tuberculosis, and sleep apnea.

NORMAL RESPIRATORY FUNCTION

The respiratory tract is composed of several parts that function together to provide oxygen (O_2) to all body cells and remove metabolic waste in the form of carbon dioxide (CO_2). Air normally enters the respiratory tract through the nose, where it is warmed, filtered, and moistened as it travels through the nasal cavity, down the pharynx, through the larynx, and into the trachea (Fig. 20-1). The trachea, sometimes called the windpipe, is an air tube that extends from the base of the larynx to the top of the lung. The trachea divides into two branches, or bronchi (ie, right and left bronchus). This tube is maintained by a series of C-shaped rings of cartilage that provide rigidity and support. Because they are not completely circular, the small opening allows for slight expansion when swallowing. The spaces between the rings are connected by strong fibroelastic membranes. The trachea is lined with hairlike projections called **cilia** that continuously sweep dust particles and microorganisms upward toward the pharynx, where they can be expectorated.

The trachea forms the two bronchi that enter the right and left lungs. The right bronchus is larger and straighter than the left bronchus. Each bronchus divides into smaller secondary bronchi and then into smaller and smaller tubules called bronchioles. The bronchioles branch into alveolar ducts that lead to the alveoli. The **alveoli** are grapelike clusters of air surrounded by thin membranes with networks of capillaries engulfing them. It is at these tiny capillaries at the exchange CO_2 and O_2 takes place. Each lung has more than 350 million alveoli, which provide a tremendous surface area for gas exchange. With each inhalation, lung surface area available for gas exchange is equal to that of a tennis court. Two-way gas exchange of CO_2 and O_2 takes place across the alveolar membranes.

The lungs lie in the thoracic cavity on either side of the heart and are made of spongy tissue filled with networks of tubes, air sacs, and small blood vessels. The bronchi branch out inside the lungs into bronchioles, which lead to the alveoli. The right lung has three lobes (ie, right upper lobe, right middle lobe, and right lower lobe), and the left lung has two lobes (ie, left upper lobe and left lower lobe). A two-layer membrane surrounding each lung called the pleura protects each lung. The act of breathing is a two-part process: inspiration (ie, drawing air into the lung) and expiration (ie, exhaling air from the lungs). The diaphragm is the major muscle involved in inspiration. When the diaphragm contracts, it moves downward. A pressure gradient is established and air enters the lungs. During expiration, air passively moves out of the lungs as the muscles of expiration relax, allowing the ribs and diaphragm to return to their original positions. Expiration depends on the elastic recoil of the costal cartilage and the relaxing of inspiratory muscles.

Regulation of respirations occurs primarily in the respiratory control centers of the medulla and pons in the brain. Small chemoreceptors called carotid and aortic bodies also help regulate respiration. The carotid bodies are located in the neck near the forking of the carotid arteries, whereas the aortic bodies are located in the aortic arch of the heart. These chemoreceptors monitor O_2 content in the blood. The carotid bodies increase respiratory rate when the blood O_2 levels fall below a certain level. The aortic bodies in the aorta increase the respiratory rate when sensing a lowered pH level in the blood.

AGE-RELATED CHANGES IN THE RESPIRATORY SYSTEM

The major organs of respiration, the lungs, undergo significant changes with age. The lungs are composed of spongy, elastic tissue filled with small tubules called bronchioles and air sacs called alveoli. The alveoli are engulfed in tiny capillaries through which CO_2 and O_2 are exchanged. With age, the alveoli undergo structural changes. The walls of the alveoli become thinner, the number of capillaries surrounding the alveoli decline, and the alveoli ducts become stretched, causing the alveoli enlarge or tear (Fig. 20-2). Although the number of alveoli remains relatively constant, the changes in alveolar structure decreases the amount of surface area for exchange.

The thoracic cage consists of the ribs, vertebral column, and sternum. The costal cartilages connect

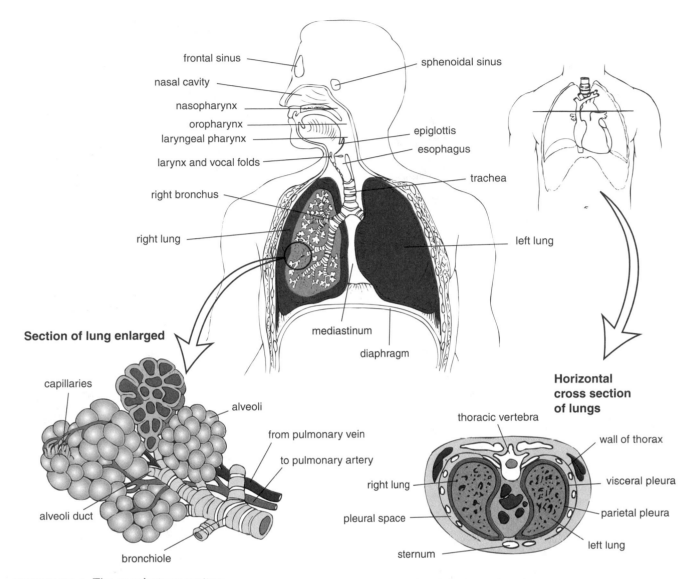

Section of lung enlarged

FIGURE 20-1. The respiratory system.

the ribs with the sternum with each other and the bodies of the thoracic vertebrae. Aging causes the costal cartilages, which connect various parts of the thoracic cage, to become more rigid and stiff resulting in decreased compliance. This change increases the need to use the accessory muscles (ie, muscles in the jaw and neck and the intercostal muscles) for breathing. The intercostal muscles that help move the chest wall atrophy and become weaker, increasing the work of breathing.

Respiratory muscle strength begins to weaken at about age 55. Changes in the musculoskeletal system also affect respiration. For example, the anteroposterior chest diameter increases, resulting in barrel-chest deformity (Fig. 20-3).

Lung volumes change with age. The bases of the lungs do not inflate well, and secretions that collect in the lungs are not easily expectorated. The older person exhales incompletely, and the residual volume (ie, amount of air that remains in the lung after a maximal expiration) increases. The increase in residual volume causes a decrease in vital capacity (ie, amount of air a person can exhale after maximal inspiration). Because parts of the lung are under ventilated, the blood coming into the lungs may be poorly oxygenated.

With age, the action of the chemoreceptors (ie, carotid bodies and aortic bodies) appear to be less responsive changes in O_2 and pH levels. Age alters these responses, making the elderly person more vulnerable to diseases affecting respiratory function such as pneumonia or emphysema. The ventilatory response to hypoxia (ie, low O_2 levels in the blood) is decreased by 51% in healthy men between the ages of 64 and 73 compared with healthy men between the ages of 22 and 30.

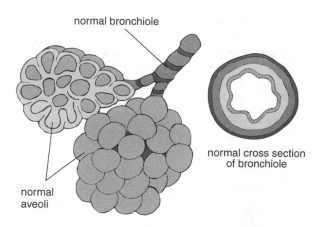

normal bronchiole

normal cross section of bronchiole

normal aveoli

Normal Breathing. In normal breathing air moves in and out of the lungs freely and easily. Any change that reduces the size of the airway can decrease the lung's ability to oxygenate the body and remove metabolic wastes.

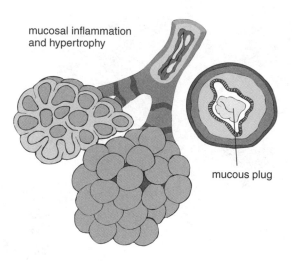

mucosal inflammation and hypertrophy

mucous plug

Chronic Bronchitis. In chronic bronchitis the air tubes narrow as a result of widespread inflammation and increased mucus production. Mucus and pus impede action of the cilia within the respiratory system. Airways narrow and mucous plugs can develop.

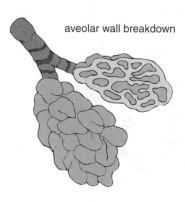

aveolar wall breakdown

Emphysema. In emphysema the walls of the individual alveoli are damaged and eventually are destroyed. Lung tissue loses elasticity and air is trapped within the lungs, resulting in a barrel-shaped chest.

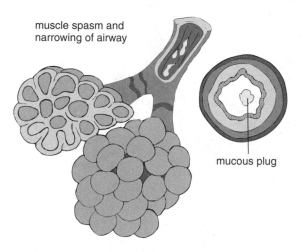

muscle spasm and narrowing of airway

mucous plug

Asthma. In asthma the mucous membranes and surrounding tissue become swollen and spasm, causing a narrowing of the airways. This mucus fills the airways and mucous plugs develop, making breathing, especially expiration, difficult. These changes are due in part to the inflammatory response.

FIGURE 20-2. Changes in the respiratory system that cause airway obstruction. Adapted from *Patient Teaching Loose-Leaf Library* (1990). Executive Director, Stanley Loeb. Respiratory Disorders, Chronic Obstructive Pulmonary Disease, page 38. Springhouse, PA: Springhouse Corp.

Even with these changes, total lung capacity is not drastically altered, but certain age-related changes place the older adult at greater risk for disorders such as pneumonia or influenza. An intact cough reflex plays an important role in clearing the respiratory tract. The elderly are not able to cough up secretions as easily as younger persons. With age, the ciliary action within the bronchial tubes is decreased, contributing to difficulty raising secre-

tions. When a patient has dysphagia or a condition that reduces consciousness, the cough reflex is impaired. The older adult is also more susceptible to influenza. Influenza destroys the epithelial cells of the respiratory tract that contain cilia to help propel the secretions upward. This destruction of the epithelial cells, combined with a decrease in the ciliary action, can lead to complications such as pneumonia or other infection.

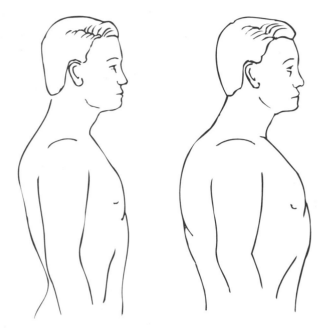

FIGURE 20-3. Barrel-chest deformity. The chest assumes a barrel shape in emphysema as the result of alveolar destruction and trapped air.

There is some controversy about whether these changes within the respiratory system are the result of a sedentary lifestyle or age. A regular exercise program can eliminate or partially eliminate some of these changes. Older adults are encouraged to participate in a regular exercise program such as walking, swimming, or cycling (see Chapter 11).

CHRONIC OBSTRUCTIVE PULMONARY DISEASE

Chronic obstructive pulmonary disease (COPD) is a term that encompasses two disorders: chronic bronchitis and emphysema. The individual diagnosed with COPD may have chronic bronchitis, emphysema, or a combination of the two. These two disorders together affect 14.8 to 15.8 million people, most of them 60 years of age or older.

The most significant risk factor in the development of COPD is smoking. Eighty-two percent of the cases of COPD are the result of smoking. Other potential causes include air pollution, exposure to irritants through job-related activities, and a genetic defect resulting in a deficiency of α_1-antitrypsin. The genetic component is linked only to the development of emphysema and is the cause of early-onset emphysema, which represents a relatively small portion of the cases.

COPD in its early stages usually manifests in a triad of symptoms: dyspnea on exertion, easy fatigability, and persistent cough. These symptoms may be attributed to the aging process. Without accurate diagnosis, treatment is delayed, and damage to the respiratory tract silently continues. COPD does not develop suddenly; it develops gradually after years of exposure to lung irritants such as cigarette smoke or asbestos.

The term COPD encompasses chronic bronchitis and pulmonary emphysema, both of which cause irreversible damage to the airway. Some textbooks consider bronchial asthma with COPD. However, asthma does not cause irreversible changes in the respiratory tract and for this reason is not considered as a component of COPD in this book.

Management of the Patient With Chronic Obstructive Pulmonary Disease

The goals of therapy in COPD is to improve quality of life and to slow progress of the disease. This is accomplished through the use of medications (Table 20-1), aerosol mist (ie, nebulization), O_2 therapy, and prevention of infection. Bronchodilators are given to relieve bronchospasm and assist in raising sputum. When bronchospasm occurs, there is a decrease in the lumen (ie, diameter) of the bronchi, which decreases the amount of air taken into the lungs. A decrease in the amount of air taken into the lungs results in respiratory distress. Use of a bronchodilating drug dilates the bronchi and allows more air to enter the lungs.

Hand-held metered-dose inhalers (MDIs) are used to deliver a specific amount of drug through an aerosol mist and provide bronchodilation and loosen bronchial secretions. This allows the medication to be administered directly to the areas of need and causes fewer systemic side effects. Lower dosages of the bronchodilators may be required for the elderly because of increased sensitivity to their effects.

Low concentrations of O_2 may be needed to improve oxygenation. Normally, O_2 should be maintained at no more than 1 to 2 L/min, because higher O_2 concentrations inhibit respiratory action in COPD patients.

Corticosteroids may be administered orally or by inhaler to control inflammation. Antibiotics are administered to prevent or treat bacterial infections that can further decrease respiratory efforts.

Emphysema

Emphysema is a condition affecting the alveoli in the lung. The alveoli are fragile, thin-walled air sacs in the lungs that are surrounded by capillary networks.

TABLE 20-1. Common Drugs Used to Manage Obstructive Conditions of the Respiratory Tract

Classification/Drug	Use and Route	Adverse Reactions	Nursing Considerations
BETA ADRENERGICS albuterol (Vevtolin, Proventil) metaproterenol (Alupent, Metaprel) terbutaline (Brethaire, Bricanyl)	Use: to relieve reversible airway obstruction in asthma or chronic obstructive pulmonary disease (COPD) Route: PO and by metered-dose inhalers (MDIs)	Nervousness, restlessness, tremor, hypertension, arrhythmias, nausea, vomiting	Usually administered on an as needed basis rather than on a regular basis. The preferred route is by MDI because the oral route increased the incidence of adverse reactions. Monitor pulmonary function tests before initiating therapy to establish baseline and during therapy to determine effectiveness of medication. Instruct on the proper use of MDI (see Table 20-2). Encourage the patient to rinse the mouth with water after each inhalation to minimize dry mouth. Encourage the patient to consult the manufacturer's instructions for use of aerosol delivery. Report any adverse reactions. If the inhaler is needed more often than every 4 hours, notify the physician. Albuterol: Instruct the patient to use albuterol before using any other inhaled medication. Allow 5 minutes before administering another inhaled medication. Terbutaline: If inhaled glucocorticoids are taken with terbutaline, the patient is instructed to take terbutaline first and allow 15 minutes to elapse before administering the glucocorticoid.
ANTICHOLINERGICS ipratropium bromide (Atrovent)	Use: to relieve asthma attack, before exercise to prevent exercise induced asthma; as a bronchodilator in maintenance therapy of airway obstruction due to asthma or COPD Route: MDI, nebulizer	Dry mouth, sore throat, dizziness, nervousness, cough, bronchospasm, palpitations, nausea	Use cautiously in patient with narrow angle glaucoma, prostatic hypertrophy, and bladder neck obstruction. Instruct on proper use of MDI (see Table 20-2). Usual dosage is 2 inhalations 4 times daily and prn up to 12 inhalations in 24 hours. Notify physician about persistent dry mouth or sore throat that lasts more than 2 weeks. Use sugarless gum or candy to relieve dry mouth. Give frequent mouth care and encourage patient to rinse mouth and gargle after using inhaler. Notify health care provider if mouth irritation occurs or dry mouth persists for more than 2 weeks. Use cautiously in older adults.
XANTHINES aminophylline (Theo-Dur)	Use: relief or prevention of bronchial asthma or bronchospasm associated with chronic bronchitis and emphysema or in severe asthma that does not respond to other medications (not used as a first-line drug) Route: PO or IV	Irritability, restlessness, dizziness, decreased appetite, palpitations, ventricular arrhythmias, tachypnea	Use of theophylline may be of no benefit in asthma when administered with a beta-adrenergic drug. Dosage based on clinical response and monitoring of the theophylline blood level (therapeutic level, 10–20 µg/mL). Report any abnormal levels. Use cautiously in the elderly with heart failure and liver disease. Do not administer time-released preparations with food (give 1 hour before or 2 hours after meals). Report any adverse reactions.

Drug	Use/Route	Side Effects/Adverse Reactions	Nursing Considerations
MAST CELL INHIBITORS cromolyn sodium (Intal, Gastrocrom)	Use: administered by inhalation for the prevention of allergic disorders such as asthmatic attacks, rhinitis, or conjunctivitis	Dizziness, headache, lacrimination, nausea, dysuria, urticaria, irritation, and dryness of the throat	Use between asthmatic attacks to prevent attacks. Do not discontinue abruptly. Taper drug when discontinuing. Store nebulizer below 30°C and protect from light. Report coughing, wheezing, or difficulty swallowing. Instruct on proper use of MDI (see Table 20-2). Does not relieve and may worsen acute attacks of asthma or bronchospasm. Report any worsening of condition or any difficulty breathing. Assess lung sounds and respiratory function before and periodically throughout therapy. Rinsing the mouth and gargling after each dose may help relieve dryness and throat irritations.
CORTICOSTERIODS Intravenous (hydrocortisone) Oral (Prednisone, Decadron) Inhalation beclomethasone (Beclovent, Beconase) dexamethasone flunisolide (AeroBid) triamcinolone (Azmacort)	Use: IV or PO for acute asthmatic attacks Inhalation: COPD, between asthma attacks to prevent an attack Route: IV, PO, or inhalation	IV, PO: depression, euphoria, personality changes, hypertension, nausea, anorexia, decreased wound healing, hirsutism, adrenal suppression, osteoporosis, increases susceptibility to infection, moon face, buffalo hump, dizziness, hypotension, muscle or joint pain occurs Inhaled: decreases side effects, throat irritation, coughing, dry mouth, hoarseness, fungal infection of mouth or throat	When changing to inhalation therapy do **not** abruptly discontinue the medication. Taper the medication slowly. Report adverse reactions. Give oral dosages with food to prevent GI upset. Inhalation: Average dosage is 2 inhalations 3 to 4 times each day; not to exceed 20 inhalations in a 24-hour period. Report redness or white patches in the mouth, sore throat or sore mouth. Assess respiratory status during therapy. Inspect oral cavity for redness, white patches, or any sign of irritation in the throat. After administration, wait 5 minutes before using other MDI. Rinse mouth after using inhaler. Follow manufacturer's instructions when using an MDI. Teach the patient the correct method of using the inhaler. Use of a spacer decreases the amount of side effects including oral fungal infections.

These capillary networks allow the exchange of CO_2 and O_2. In emphysema, there are irreversible changes in the structure of the alveoli. The walls of alveoli become damaged and break down, resulting in large air spaces where gas exchange cannot occur. The remaining alveoli enlarge, and less and less O_2 is available for the bloodstream. The lungs also lose their elasticity.

Elasticity (ie, ability to expand and contract) is lost when the elastic fibers of the lungs lose the delicate chemical balance that protect against the destruction of these elastic fibers. With the destruction of these elastic fibers, inspiration becomes difficult because of the inability of the chest to expand to allow air to enter the lungs. Expiration also becomes prolonged and difficult, often resulting in an expiratory wheeze as the air struggles to pass through the narrowed airways.

Signs and Symptoms

Many of the signs and symptoms of emphysema are related to the narrowing of the airway and the changes that occur within the respiratory system as the result of the condition:

- Exertional dyspnea
- Fatigability (breathlessness after any activity)
- Persistent productive cough of mucopurulent sputum
- Prolonged expiration with distention of the neck veins
- Use of accessory muscles (ie, muscles of the jaw and neck and the intercostal muscle) when breathing
- Increase in pulse and respiratory rates

Of those with emphysema, 64% are men, usually older men. Almost one half of those with emphysema report that the disease limits their daily activities in some way. As the disease progresses, the patient appears anxious or irritable and may speak in short, choppy sentences. Confusion, drowsiness, and irritability develop as the brain fails to obtain adequate O_2, and blood levels of CO_2 increase. The chest appears barrel shaped because of loss of lung elasticity and perpetual chest wall expansion as the result of the difficulty with exhalation.

Diagnostic Findings

Diagnosis is made after a careful history and physical examination. The patient most likely has a history of exposure to a lung irritant (eg, smoking, chemicals, asbestos). Chest radiographs, pulmonary function studies, and arterial blood gases reveal abnormalities indicative of COPD. The chest radiograph reveals hyperinflation of the lung fields and pulmonary function studies indicate difficulty with expiration of air. Arterial blood gases reveal high CO_2 levels and low O_2 levels.

Chronic Bronchitis

Chronic bronchitis is persistent inflammation of the lining of the bronchial tubes caused by exposure to an irritant, usually cigarette smoking. Other causes of chronic bronchitis include infection, allergens (eg, dust, pollen, animal dander), or airborne irritants (eg, smoke, chemicals).

In chronic bronchitis, the bronchial tubes respond to an irritant with inflammation. This inflammatory response results in an increased secretion of mucus from the goblet cells. The mucous glands enlarge as more and more mucus is produced in an effort to rid the body of the irritant. With enlargement of the mucous glands, the airways become smaller. The cilia (ie, hairlike projections that propel debris upward) cease to function, and mucus stagnates in the airway. The body coughs in an effort to remove excessive secretions. As the function of the cilia decreases, coughing becomes less effective. When the mucus remains in the respiratory tract, it becomes an excellent medium for bacteria growth and increases the incidence of bacterial infection. Secretions may also accumulate in the lungs and form mucous plugs. Unfortunately, chronic bronchitis is often not diagnosed until in the later stages, when permanent damage has occurred.

Signs and Symptoms

The most prominent early symptom is the expectoration of thick, white mucus. Coughing is most apparent in the mornings after arising and in the evening. The sputum becomes yellow, thick, and purulent when infection occurs. Typically, the individual has a cough after a cold or minor upper respiratory infection that persists for several weeks, producing large amounts of mucus. The cough may be dismissed as a "smoker's cough." The presence of a productive cough that lasts 3 months per year for 2 consecutive years is indicative of chronic bronchitis.

Diagnostic Findings

Careful interviewing often uncovers a history of smoking or exposure to another irritant. Arterial blood gas (ABG) determinations, radiographs, and pulmonary function studies reveal findings similar to those of emphysema. If infection is suspected, a culture is performed to identify the causative organism.

Using the Nursing Process to Manage a Patient With Chronic Obstructive Pulmonary Disease

Assessment

Assessment of the patient with COPD most often reveals some degree of dyspnea at rest or when performing activity. The patient may complain of fatigue, difficulty sleeping, poor appetite, and may appear anxious, confused, or irritable. The nurse obtains a history of the illness, including the amount of cigarettes smoked, how long the patient smoked, and whether the patient is still smoking. It is important to consider other irritants such as dust, fumes, cotton, asbestos, and coal dust. The patient is assessed for the presence of a cough and for the color, consistency, and amount of sputum. Pulse may be rapid, and respirations may be prolonged and shallow. The nurse observes for the use of accessory muscles during respiration. The chest may be barrel shaped (see Fig. 20-3). Skin color is usually pale with some duskiness or cyanosis of the nail beds or around the lips. In others, the skin may appear ruddy.

Nursing Diagnoses

The following nursing diagnoses may be appropriate for patients with COPD:

Impaired Gas Exchange related to changes in respiratory function, dyspnea

Ineffective Airway Clearance related to inability to expectorate secretions, persistent cough, other (specify)

Altered Nutrition, less than body requirements, related to anorexia, fatigue, other (specify)

Risk for Infection related to chronic illness, pulmonary changes, inability to expectorate sputum, other, (specify)

Risk for Ineffective Management of Therapeutic Regimen related to lack of knowledge of treatment regimen, disease process, other (specify)

Other nursing diagnoses may be applicable for individual patients.

Planning and Implementation

Planning and implementation of care requires careful monitoring of the patient and attention to maximizing remaining respiratory function. Baseline information is obtained, and continual assessment is done to detect any worsening of the patient's respiratory status.

Ineffective Breathing Pattern. Patients with COPD usually have difficulty with expiration of air. The patient is instructed in diaphragmatic and pursed-lip breathing to help prolong expiration. **Pursed-lip breathing** is accomplished by taking a slow, deep inspiration (lasting at least 3 seconds) through the nose, followed by prolonged expiration through pursed lips (lasting at least 6 seconds). A soft whistling sound is made during exhalation if pursed-lip breathing is performed correctly.

Exhalation through pursed lips is twice as long as inhalation and helps rid the body of trapped air. The nurse should explain to the patient that inhalation should be done before performing an activity and exhalation through pursed lips is done while performing an activity.

Diaphragmatic breathing also helps to decrease trapped air and makes breathing easier. This type of breathing is accomplished by having the patient consciously move the abdomen outward while taking a deep inspiration. This helps to relax the intercostal and accessory muscles used by the COPD patient when breathing. Expiration occurs as the patient slowly contracts the abdominal muscles, observing the abdomen moving inward. Explain to the patient that keeping one hand lightly on the stomach and one hand lightly on the chest helps to evaluate whether the correct procedure is being done. If performed correctly, the hand on the stomach rises during inspiration and falls during expiration. The hand on the chest remains almost still. Focused diaphragmatic breathing should be performed at least twice each day.

The patient is instructed to avoid activities that cause severe dyspnea. The nurse provides frequent rest patterns between activities. Low concentrations of O_2 (2 to 3 L/min) may be administered to promote oxygenation.

ASSESSMENT ALERT

Assess the patient on O_2 therapy for restlessness, listlessness, confusion (or if in a confused state, increased confusion), shortness of breath, and anxiety. In a normal functioning respiratory system, the stimulus for breathing is the CO_2 level in the blood. COPD CO_2 levels are continuously elevated in patients with COPD. This elevation in CO_2 disrupts normal breathing and low O_2 levels become the stimulus for breathing. If O_2 levels are given at high concentrations to the COPD patient, the hypoxic state no longer exists, and the stimulus for breathing is removed. Administration of high concentrations of O_2 (>1 to 2 L/min) can result in a decreased respiratory functioning in patients with COPD. The physician usually regulates respiratory function through ABG and pulse oximetry monitoring.

Because activity is limited, base the level of activity on the tolerance level. The patient is positioned in an upright position using two or more pillows to support head and thorax. An overbed table is placed across the bed with pillows on the table. Arms can then rest on the pillows on the overbed table.

Ineffective Airway Clearance. Patients have difficulty raising secretions from the lungs. To liquefy and loosen secretions, the nurse should increase the patient's fluid intake, if the condition permits. The patient is encouraged to drink six to eight glasses of water daily. The nurse may need to assist the patient in using an MDI or intermittent positive-pressure breathing (IPPB) treatment. Unless the MDI is used correctly, much of the medication can be deposited in the back of the throat or in the air instead of the lungs. Display 20-1 provides general information on the proper use of an MDI. It is important to read the manufacturer's directions before administering any medication administered by an MDI. Postural drainage and percussion are performed in the morning and the afternoon to help loosen and bring up secretions.

Altered Nutrition. Most patients with COPD are anorexic and lose weight. It is important to monitor the patient's weight daily. The patient may need a consultation with the dietitian for selection of foods that are well tolerated and palatable. Five or six small meals are preferable to three large meals. The nurse must allow ample time for eating with frequent rest periods. It is important to provide good oral hygiene before and after meals. Liquid nutrition supplements are provided to prevent weight loss and provide nutrient needs.

Ineffective Individual Coping. Chronic disease and limited activity may result in poor coping. The patient may become irritable, restless, and impatient with family, caregivers, and health care personnel. The patient is encouraged to do as much for themselves as possible. The nurse helps the patient to set reachable goals and assists as necessary to meet those goals. It is important to for the nurse to encourage the patient to verbalize fears and anger. The nurse actively listens and accepts the patient's feelings. Relaxation techniques (see Chapter 11) may be taught to decrease anxiety.

Risk for Infection. The risk for infection is always present in patients with COPD. Failure to raise sputum, ineffective coughing, and activity intolerance can cause secretions to pool in lower airways and become an excellent site for bacteria to grow. It is important to monitor vital signs frequently and report any elevation in temperature, pulse rate, or respiratory rate. An increase in respiratory rate of 26 to 48 is an early indicator of bacterial pneumonia in the elderly. Odorous, yellow or green sputum indicates respiratory infection. The nurse should stress the importance of good handwashing, avoiding crowds, and proper disposal of sputum to prevent infection.

Patient and Family Teaching

It is important for the older patient and the caregiver to understand the treatment plan. Understanding basic information concerning the disease process,

---

DISPLAY 20-1. General Guidelines for Using a Metered-Dose Inhaler

When a metered-dose inhaler (MDI) is prescribed, the following information should be included in a teaching plan:

- The drug is given by using an inhaler and is useful because it works quickly and goes directly into the lung, causing fewer systemic side effects than an oral or parenteral medication.
- Before use, shake the inhaler, keeping the canister above the mouthpiece.
- Tilt the head back slightly and breathe out.
- Hold the mouth open with the inhaler 1 to 2 inches away, and press down on the inhaler to release the medication as a slow inhalation is taken.
- To ensure that the medication goes into the lungs and not merely into the mouth, a spacer (ie, holding chamber) may be attached to the inhaler. Pressing on the inhaler places one puff of the medication in the holding chamber. Place the mouthpiece of the spacer in the mouth and slowly inhale. The breath is held for a short time, followed by exhalation. This procedure is repeated for each puff ordered by the physician.
- An alternate method of administrating medication with an MDI is to place the inhaler mouthpiece (without the spacer) in the mouth and have the patient breath in slowly for 5 seconds. The breath is then held for approximately 10 seconds to allow the drug to reach the lungs.
- Clean the inhaler and cap daily by rinsing it in warm water. Dry thoroughly before using again.
- Two times each week, wash the plastic mouthpiece with mild dishwashing soap and rinse well. Dry thoroughly before reuse.

  Note: These are general guidelines. The nurse should consult the manufacturer's instructions for each MDI before using it.

---

how to administer medications correctly, and important aspects of care well helps the patient remain compliant with the treatment regimen. The nurse should design a teaching plan specific to the patient's individual needs. A teaching plan for patients with COPD should include information about the disease process and medication.

PATIENT TEACHING AID

The following information should be included in a teaching plan for patients with COPD:

- **Avoid respiratory irritants (eg, cigarette smoking, dust).**
- **Humidify air in the home.**
- **Avoid crowds or persons with respiratory infections.**

- Obtain influenza and pneumococcal vaccinations.
- Teach pursed-lip and abdominal or diaphragmatic breathing techniques.
- Encourage participation in a regular exercise program to increase endurance and strength.
- Encourage the use of portable O_2 for ambulation, if ordered by the physician.
- Provide explanation concerning disease process. Answer questions and provide current information.
- Provide information about medications, adverse reactions to expect, and adverse reactions to report.
- Demonstrate technique for using metered-dose inhalant (if applicable).
- Stress the importance of stopping cigarette smoking (if applicable).

Evaluation and Expected Outcomes

Successful care can provide the following outcomes for the patient:

Less dyspnea reported

Tolerates greater activity

Progressive weight gain toward goal weight

Appetite improved

Incorporates interventions to lifestyle to decrease risk for infection

Verbalizes understanding of treatment regimen, and disease process

ASTHMA

Although considered more common in young people, asthma occurs fairly frequently in the elderly. Some elderly patients with asthma have had the disorder for many years; others experience a recurrence of childhood asthma; and others develop asthma for the first time. Asthma that occurs for the first time in older adults is most often **intrinsic asthma,** which is asthma not caused by an allergy. This type of asthma most often develops because of a bacterial or viral respiratory infection. Intrinsic asthma can also be caused by emotional factors or nonspecific irritants.

Asthma is an intermittent obstructive airway disease characterized by spasmodic constriction of the bronchi and inflammation. Attacks vary in severity from mild dyspnea and slight wheezing (ie, high-pitched musical sound) to severe dyspnea and audible wheezing. During an attack the bronchi produce large amounts of thick sputum. Asthma can complicate other disorders such as cardiovascular disease, influenza, pneumonia, or emphysema.

Signs and Symptoms

Most asthmatics report "chest tightness" or have an audible wheeze as one of the first indicators of an asthmatic attack. The patient may exhibit a classic sitting position that facilitates breathing: sitting with the body bent slightly forward and the arms at shoulder height. Signs and symptoms of asthma include

- An audible wheeze on inspiration or expiration
- An initially nonproductive cough, followed by productive cough of large amounts of thick, stingy sputum
- Pale skin
- Cyanosis in nail beds or around the lips
- Profuse diaphoresis during an attack
- Anxiety and apprehension

The attack may last several hours or several weeks. An attack that persists without response to therapy is called **status asthmaticus.** Status asthmaticus can be life threatening and must be treated aggressively.

ASSESSMENT ALERT

The elderly may not report "chest tightness" because of decreased perception of airway obstruction. In addition to a lack of sensation of tightness, the activity level of the older adult may not be sufficient to make increased demands on the respiratory system. Careful auscultation of the lungs is important to detect a wheeze. Spirometry is necessary to identify the presence and severity of airway obstruction.

Management of the Patient With Asthma

The goal of therapy is to open the airway, prevent bronchospasm, and improve breathing pattern. The use of a spirometer or a peak flow meter to measure lung volumes and capacities is a relatively simple method to measure air inhaled into and expelled from the lungs. A peak flow meter can be used for home monitoring of patients with asthma. If used on a regular basis, the peak flow meter can alert the patient or the caregiver of an impending asthma attack. Decreased air flow may precede the asthma attack by hours to a day or more. This allows the patient or the caregiver time to consult with the physician or begin a pharmacologic regimen that can avert or lessen the severity of the asthma attack.

According to the Heart, Lung, and Blood Institute, inhaled beta adrenergics are recommended for mild acute asthma; inhaled or oral beta adrenergics and an anti-inflammatory drug are for moderate asthma; and beta adrenergics and an oral corticosteroid are for severe asthma. The beta adrenergics are often used on an as needed basis instead of around the clock. Oral beta adrenergics are avoided in the elderly because of the increased incidence of adverse reactions such as nervousness, insomnia, and aggravation of cardiac arrhythmias. Table 20-1 lists the drugs used to treat obstructive respiratory disorders. The patient is monitored for improvement in respiratory function; decreased respiratory rate, decreased dyspnea, and decreased wheezing.

An inhaled corticosteroid may be used for maintenance therapy for moderate asthma. Inhaled cromolyn sodium is used prophylactically to decrease inflammation and to keep the bronchial tube dilated. Use of this drug may result in the need of less medication overall and improvement in symptoms. Inhaled corticosteroids result in fewer systemic side effects than the oral corticosteroids. When an inhaled beta-adrenergic drug and an inhaled corticosteroid are used, it is important for the elderly person to understand which inhaler is used regularly (usually the corticosteroid inhaler) and which is used on an as needed basis (usually the beta-adrenergic drug inhaler).

Many of the drugs used to manage asthma are given by an MDI. It is important that the older adult understands exactly how to use the inhaler, when to use the inhaler, and what dosage regimen to follow (see Display 20-1). The directions are contained in the package insert. The nurse should carefully go over these directions with the patient and the caregiver. A spacer is recommended for the elderly. Allowing the patient to use the inhaler in the presence of the nurse helps the nurse to correct any problems with administration. If the inhaler is not used correctly, the medication may not reach the lungs, and the full therapeutic effect is not attained.

PNEUMONIA

Pneumonia is a serious condition in the elderly. Death rates from pneumococcal infection are estimated to be almost five times higher in persons older than 65. The elderly person with pneumonia usually requires hospitalization. Chronic illness, as is common in the elderly, may complicate recovery, necessitating a longer hospital stay.

Pneumonia is an infection or inflammation of the lungs. In pneumonia, the alveoli fill with pus and exudate, causing the lungs to consolidate (ie,

become solidified). This alteration compromises gas exchange and can lead to death. If pneumonia is distributed in patchy clusters, it is called **bronchopneumonia. Lobar pneumonia** affects a segment or entire lobe of the lung. A chest radiograph confirms the diagnosis and determines the extent of the disease. Sputum cultures identify the causative organism, and drug sensitivities determine antimicrobial therapy.

The most common type of pneumonia affecting the older adult is bacterial pneumonia. Any condition in which mucus is produced increases the risk for developing bacterial pneumonia. An increased risk of developing bacterial pneumonia is also associated with those who are on bed rest, the frail elderly, those with a depressed cough reflex, and patients taking sedatives or opioids.

Signs and Symptoms

Pneumonia in the elderly manifests differently than in younger patients. The elderly may exhibit an increased respiratory rate and increased pulse rate as the first symptom of pneumonia. Respirations consistently above 26 to 28 per minute in an elderly patient with a normally lower rate may indicate pneumonia. Additional symptoms include general deterioration and changes in mental status. Typical symptoms such as cough, chest pain, production of sputum, and fever are usually not present, making pneumonia difficult to detect in the elderly.

Preventing Pneumonia

All persons older than 50 years of age should receive a yearly influenza vaccination. Pneumonia is a common complication of influenza in the elderly. A "flu" shot helps to prevent influenza and pneumonia.

A vaccine is also available against the most common type of pneumonia, pneumococcal pneumonia. All persons older than age 65, those living in nursing homes, the frail elderly, and those with cardiovascular disease should receive the pneumococcal vaccination. Most individuals have no reaction to the vaccine. A few have reported a tender, swollen, red area at the vaccination site.

Assessing the Patient for Pneumonia

Careful assessment is important for all elderly who are at increased risk, particularly those who live

TABLE 20-2. Distinguishing Lungs Sounds

Adventitious Lung Sounds*	Characteristics of the Sound	Simulation of the Sound
Crackles (previously called rales)	Best heard in the lower lung bases at the end of inspiration but can be heard during expiration Sound heard as air passes through fluid in the alveoli Heard as fluid and secretions accumulate in the bronchi Occurs with heart failure, bronchial inflammation, and pulmonary edema	Rub several pieces of hair together while holding the hairs close to the ear. Sometimes described as the fizzing sound that a carbonated beverage makes May clear with coughing
Gurgles (previously called rhonchi)	Heard throughout most lung fields during inspiration and expiration	Gurgling and bubbling May clear with coughing
Wheezes	More commonly heard in expiration but can be heard during inspiration in all lung fields Occurs as air passes through narrowed airways (ie, trachea, bronchial tubes, and bronchioles)	High-pitched musical sounds that do not clear with coughing

*Abnormal lung sounds.

alone or in a nursing facility. Home health nurses who make visits to the elderly and nurses working with the elderly in nursing homes must continually assess for bacterial pneumonia. Pneumonia bacteria are present in some healthy throats. When the body's defense are weakened, the bacteria can multiply, migrate to the lungs, and inflame the air sacs.

✔ ASSESSMENT ALERT

In assessing the older adult, the classic signs of bacterial pneumonia most likely are not present. The most important assessment measure in older adults is respiratory rate. A respiratory rate that is 24 to 48 may indicate that pneumonia is developing in an older adult. Other indicators include a change in mental status, dehydration, or increased pulse rate. The increase in respiratory rate is often the first sign in the elderly and occurs 1 to 2 days before other signs of infection.

Most older adults are hospitalized for bacterial pneumonia because the risk for complications is increased. Careful monitoring of vital signs is necessary. Report any increase in respiratory rate, increased pulse rate, or painful cough. Carefully observe sputum for amount, color, and consistency. Auscultation of the chest may reveal decreased breath sounds over the affected areas, wheezing, crackles, or gurgles. Examine nail beds, lips, and oral mucosa for cyanosis, and document findings. The patient may report fatigue decreased activity tolerance, loss of appetite, or become confused.

Caring for the Patient With Pneumonia

Planning the care of the older patient with bacterial pneumonia requires careful evaluation of assessment findings. Pharmacologic interventions are based on results of the culture and sensitivity test. Analgesics are given if pleuritic (ie, inflammation of the pleura membrane) pain is present. However, opiates are avoided in the elderly, because these patients are particularly sensitive to the respiratory depressive effects of the opiates. Temperature, pulse, respirations, and blood pressure are monitored at frequent intervals to evaluate the response to therapy.

The patient is placed in a semi-Fowler position to increase lung expansion and improve ventilation. The nurse encourages frequent position changes, or if patient is unable to change position, the nurse can reposition the patient every 2 hours. The chest is auscultated every 4 hours for lung sounds, crackles, or gurgles (Table 20-2). Oxygen therapy may be prescribed to improve oxygenation. It is important to continually monitor mental status. A change in mental status, restlessness, confusion, or drowsiness may indicate a decreased O_2 supply to the brain. Any deterioration in condition is reported immediately. Intubation and mechanical ventilation may be required for severe respiratory insufficiency. Respiratory function is monitored for rate, depth, and ease. Oxygen saturation levels (normal levels are 95%–100%) are closely monitored as well.

Maintaining the Airway

Elderly patients often have a depressed cough reflex, making expectoration of secretions more difficult. If not contraindicated, a high fluid intake (6 to 8 glasses of water per day) is encouraged to loosen secretions. Humidified air or a high-humidity mask may be necessary. The patient is encouraged to breathe deeply every 1 to 2 hours to facilitate maximum expansion of the lungs. Splinting painful areas in the chest with a pillow may decrease discomfort when coughing. Chest physiotherapy (ie, percussion and postural drainage) is also performed. Nasotracheal suctioning may be needed if the patient is unable to clear the airway by coughing.

Managing Fatigue

Older patients with bacterial pneumonia are easily fatigued and feel generalized weakness. They may have exertional dyspnea. Monitor the patient's response to activity. A quiet environment is needed to promote rest. Plan activities to alternate with frequent rest periods so as not to overtire. Assist with self-care as needed. Gradually increase activity as strength increases.

Managing Infection

The older adult is at increased risk for developing additional infections or for spread of the original infection. The patient is instructed on the importance of expectoration of mucus. Vital signs are monitored every 4 hours, and abnormalities are reported. The sputum is monitored for frequency, amount, color, and consistency. If the elderly person is unable to raise secretions, suctioning may be required. The head of the bed is kept elevated.

The physician orders an antibiotic such as penicillin, erythromycin, or clindamycin (if allergic to penicillin). The specific antibiotic is based on the results of culture and sensitivity of purulent secretions. The administration of an antibiotic places the elderly patient at increased risk to develop a superinfection. A **superinfection** is an overgrowth of bacteria or fungus not affected by the antibiotic. The antibiotic affects pathogenic (disease-causing) organisms and nonpathogenic (non–disease-causing) organisms that exist in the body. An overgrowth by an organism not affected by the antibiotic can cause a secondary infection, which can be serious and even life threatening. Diarrhea is the most prominent indication of a bacterial superinfection called **pseudomembranous colitis.** This condition is caused by an overgrowth of the microorganism *Clostridia difficile,* which produces a toxin that affects the lining of the colon. Signs and symptoms of pseudomembranous colitis include fever, abdominal cramps, and severe diarrhea that may contain blood and mucus.

ASSESSMENT ALERT

Immediately report diarrhea, abdominal cramps, and fever in older patients receiving antibiotic therapy, because they may indicate a superinfection and the need to immediately discontinue the antibiotic.

Another superinfection common to the elderly receiving antibiotics is a fungal infection called monilial (ie, candidiasis). This fungal superinfection can occur in the mouth as thrush, in the vagina (commonly called a yeast infection), and around the anal area. Signs and symptoms include anal or vaginal itching and white discharge (if in the vaginal area) and white lesions in the mouth (if thrush). Candidiasis can be treated topically with miconazole (Monostat) or clotrimazole (Lotrimin).

INFLUENZA

Influenza is a highly contagious viral infection that is particularly dangerous for the older adult. Pneumonia and influenza are the fifth leading cause of death in people older than 65 years of age. For most healthy adults, the disorder is self-limiting. For the elderly and debilitated, the condition is more severe and can be fatal. It is recommended that those 65 years of age or older have a yearly influenza vaccination to help prevent the disease.

The virus that causes influenza may be type A, B, or C. Influenza A is has the most virulent strains. Within each influenza type, there are many strains of viruses, and each year, a different strain arises. The influenza vaccination is made yearly and contains the influenza viruses most likely to be infectious that year. The recommended time for the vaccination to reach peak effectiveness is to take the vaccination sometime between October 15 and November 15 of each year.

Signs and Symptoms

Although the symptoms of influenza are respiratory in nature, the whole body is affected. Symptoms include chills, fever, weakness, loss of appetite, and generalized aching of the head, back, arms, and legs. Temperature can increase to 104°F for 2 to 3 days. However, chills, fever, and joint aching are less common in the elderly with influenza. The elderly person is at increased risk to develop pneumonia as a secondary infection.

Caring for the Patient With Influenza

No drug can cure influenza. However, antiviral drugs such as amantadine (Symmetrel), rimantadine (Flumadine), or zanamivir (Relenza) may be prescribed. The drugs must be given as soon as possible (within 48 hours) after the onset of influenza A and can shorten and reduce the severity of the illness. Zanamivir appears to be extremely effective in preventing the multiplication of the virus. An antiviral drug can also be used for prevention of influenza A if it is given daily as long as influenza cases continue to occur in a community. The physician may prescribe an antibiotic to prevent a secondary bacterial infection. The use of antiviral drugs should be considered for the elderly because influenza can be particularly severe in older adults.

Treatment consists of bed rest, increasing fluid intake, and aspirin or acetaminophen to relieve discomfort and help control temperature elevation. Preventive measures also are important. In addition to vaccination, the older adult is instructed to avoid contact with those who have influenza and crowded places such as shopping malls, grocery stores, and church.

TUBERCULOSIS

Tuberculosis (TB) is an acute or chronic infection caused by the *Mycobacterium tuberculosis* bacillus. It can be acute or chronic in nature. Although, tuberculosis primarily affects the lungs, almost any other organ can be affected. The tubercle bacillus can be dormant within the body for decades and then become reactivated years after the original infection. When the individual is first exposed to TB, the body reacts by forming granulomas, which are new tissue masses composed of live and dead bacilli surrounded by protective cells. The granulomas form a calcified scar, and the bacteria become dormant within the scar. At this point, the TB is not active. However, after many years, as the infected individual ages and becomes ill, these pockets of calcified scar tissue can open, releasing live bacilli. Reactivation of the tubercle bacilli results in recurrence of TB. Many cases of TB in the elderly occur as the result of the renewed activity of the tubercle bacillus.

Approximately 60% of the reported cases of TB occur in persons older than 45 years of age, and a significant number of these are older than 60. The elderly living in poverty, poor living conditions, in nursing homes, or in other close habitations are at increased risk for TB.

Signs and Symptoms

Older adults with TB may exhibit all of the classic symptoms of the disease:
- Low-grade fever; temperature usually rises in the afternoon
- Fatigue
- Anorexia
- Weight loss
- Persistent cough that is initially nonproductive
- cough progressing to mucopurulent discharge
- Hemoptysis
- Dyspnea
- Night sweats

✔ ASSESSMENT ALERT

The most common complaints of persons older than 60 were weight loss and anorexia. In these patients, night sweats occur less frequently than in the elderly younger than 60.

Diagnostic Findings

Traditional screening using tuberculin skin testing (PPD or Mantoux) are not reliable in the elderly. False-negative results are common. Pulmonary tuberculosis may be diagnosed by a chest radiograph and acid-fast bacilli found in the sputum.

Caring for the Patient With Tuberculosis

Treatment is aimed at relieving symptoms, preventing complications and arresting the disease. Long-term drug therapy is the mainstay of treatment. The prognosis is good if the patient continues on the drug regimen for the prescribed period, usually 6 to 12 months. A combination of two or three drugs to which the organism is susceptible prevents drug-resistant organisms from developing and cures the disease. Table 20-3 lists the first-line and second-line medications. Isoniazid (INH) may be given prophylactically to those at high risk for TB for 6 to 12 months.

Nursing care consists of monitoring adherence to drug therapy. The antituberculin drugs are capable of many adverse reactions. Any unusual occurrence or adverse reaction is reported. Monitoring the

TABLE 20-3. **Drugs Used to Treat Tuberculosis**

First-Line Drugs*	Second-Line Drugs†
Isoniazid (INH)	Capreomycin
Rifampin (RIF)	Kanamycin
Streptomycin (SM)	Ethionamide
Ethambutol (EMB)	Para-amenosalicylic acid (PAS)
Pyrazinamide (PZA)	Cycloserine

*Current recommendation—4 months with first-line drugs, follow with 2 months of INH plus RIF.
†Used for resistant strains and retreatment.

DISPLAY 20-2. **Resources for Patients With Respiratory Disorders**

American College of Chest Physicians
3300 Dundee Road
Northbrook, IL 60062-2340
(708)-498-1400

American Lung Association
1740 Broadway
New York, NY 10019-4374
1-800-LUNG-USA

Asthma and Allergy Foundation of America
1125 15th Street NW, Suite 502
Washington, DC 20005
(202)-466-7643

patient is especially important when a drug is known to be nephrotoxic or ototoxic (eg, streptomycin, capreomycin).

When administering INH, 6 to 50 mg of pyridoxine (vitamin B_6) may be administered to prevent peripheral neuropathy. When taking INH, the patient is instructed to avoid foods containing tyramine and histamine (ie, tuna, aged cheese, red wine, and yeast extract). These foods can cause lightheadedness, hypotension, headache, flushing, and headaches with INH.

Patient teaching is important for the elderly patient. The stigma associated with TB years ago persists, and the patient may fear placement away from family and friends. The patient is informed that isolation from the family is unnecessary and that compliance with the medication regimen will render them noninfectious after 2 to 3 weeks of continuous therapy. Careful teaching of the necessity of compliance to the drug regimen is critical. In some cases, the nurse may require that the patient return to an outpatient clinic to receive the medication, or the nurse may make a home visit to observe the patient taking the medication.

At the home or clinic, the medication is taken under the direct supervision of the nurse. This method is used to ensure compliance and is called direct observation therapy (DOT). The patient is instructed to cover the mouth when coughing to prevent spread of the organism. Disposable tissues are used and placed in a paper bag for disposal. The patient must provide sputum smears at periodic intervals to monitor regression of the disease.

SLEEP APNEA

Central sleep apnea is the absence for breathing of 10 seconds or longer during sleep. Central sleep apnea is a neurologic irregularity that originates in the thalamus of the brain. The body appears to "forget" to breathe. The primary symptom is omission of breathing for 10 seconds to 2 minutes (in extreme cases). After the period of apnea, the individual suddenly inhales rapidly and exhales with a snoring type of respiratory effort. These people are usually unaware of the episodes. They may complain of daytime sleepiness or drowsiness. Obesity and increasing age places the individual at increased risk. The elderly who are obese are encouraged to lose weight. Sometimes, weight loss drastically decreases symptoms.

The physician may prescribe protriptyline (Vivactil). In the geriatric population, this drug is used cautiously. Dosage is initially 5 mg, taken orally three times daily, with the dosage increased gradually until the therapeutic effect is achieved. When administered to older adults, cardiovascular status is monitored closely.

Sleep apnea may also be caused by an obstruction in the airway. In cases of mechanical obstruction, surgery may correct the problem (Display 20-2).

CRITICAL THINKING EXERCISES

1. Mr. Hernandez, age 70, has COPD. He has been rude and demanding, complaining that "no one ever listens to what I have to say." What assessments would you make to determine that cause of Mr. Hernandez's behavior? What nursing interventions could you use to help to decrease his negative behavior?
2. Mr. Hilton has smoked for 30 years. Currently, he is smoking 1 pack of cigarettes per day. He tells you that he is ready to quit but does not want to

quit "cold turkey." What suggestions could you make to Mr. Hilton?

3. Ms. Spence, age 76, is a patient in the nursing home where you work. She has been taking penicillin for pneumonia for the last 5 days. What observations would be most important for you to make when assessing Ms. Spence for adverse reactions to the antibiotic? Why are these observations important? What adverse reactions should be reported at once?

REFERENCES AND SUGGESTED READING

Berry, J., Vitalo, C., Larson, J. et al. (1999). Respiratory muscle strength in older adults. *Nursing Research, 45 (3)*, 154–160.

Borkgren, M., & Groonkiewicz, C. (1995). Update your asthma care from hospital to home. *American Journal of Nursing, 95*(1), 26–35.

Chiocca, E., & Russo, L. (1997). Action stat: Acute asthma attack. *Nursing 97, 27* (7), 43.

Frozena, C. (1998). Easing end-stage respiratory symptoms in dying patients. *Home Healthcare Nurse, 16 (4)*, 256.

Monohan, K. (1999). A joint effort to affect lives: The COPD wellness program. *Geriatric Nursing, 20 (4)*, 200–202.

O'Hanlon-Nichols, T. (1998). Basic assessment series: The adult pulmonary system. *American Journal of Nursing 98 (2)*, 39–45.

Ruppert, R. (1999). The last smoke. *American Journal of Nursing, 99 (11)*, 26–32.

Trudeau, M., & Solano-McGuire, S. (1999). Evaluating the quality of COPD care. *American Journal of Nursing, 99 (3)*, 47.

CHAPTER 21

The Gastrointestinal System

CHAPTER OUTLINE

KEY TERMS
CHAPTER OBJECTIVES
NORMAL GASTROINTESTINAL FUNCTIONING
AGE-RELATED CHANGES OF THE
    GASTROINTESTINAL TRACT
XEROSTOMIA
DYSPHAGIA
GASTRITIS
PEPTIC ULCER DISEASE
DIVERTICULOSIS AND DIVERTICULITIS
DIARRHEA
CONSTIPATION
HEMORRHOIDS
HIATAL HERNIA
GALLBLADDER DISEASE
CIRRHOSIS
HEPATITIS
CRITICAL THINKING EXERCISES
REFERENCES AND SUGGESTED READING

KEY TERMS

atrophic gastritis
biliary colic
cholecystitis
cholelithiasis
cirrhosis
constipation
diarrhea
diverticulitis
diverticulosis
dysphagia
esophageal varices
gastritis
Helicobacter pylori
hemorrhoids
hiatal hernia
portal hypertension
xerostomia

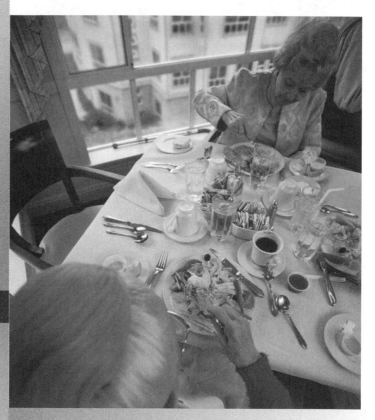

CHAPTER OBJECTIVES

At the completion of this chapter, the student will be able to

- Discuss normal gastrointestinal functioning

- Identify age-related changes that occur in the gastrointestinal tract

- Discuss signs and symptoms, treatment, and nursing care for older patients with xerostomia, dysphagia, gastritis, peptic ulcer disease, diverticulitis, diverticulosis, hemorrhoids, hiatal hernia, cirrhosis, hepatic, and gallbladder disease

- Use the nursing process to care for elderly patients with gastrointestinal disorders

FIGURE 21-1. Normal gastrointestinal tract.

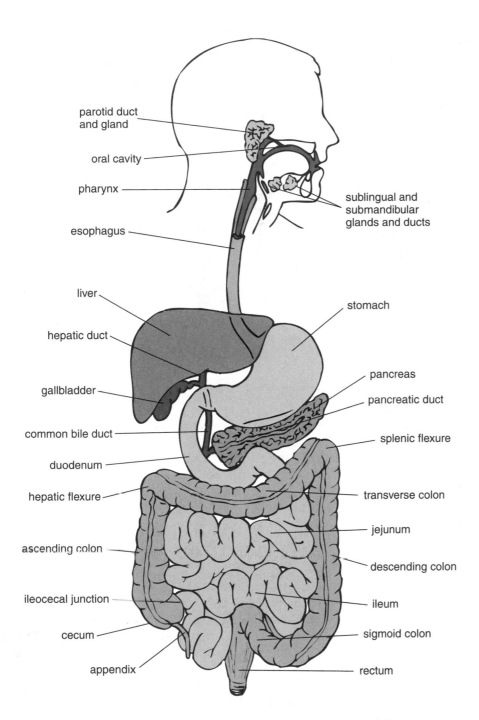

parotid duct and gland

oral cavity

pharynx

esophagus

sublingual and submandibular glands and ducts

liver

stomach

hepatic duct

gallbladder

pancreas

pancreatic duct

common bile duct

splenic flexure

duodenum

hepatic flexure

transverse colon

jejunum

ascending colon

descending colon

ileocecal junction

ileum

cecum

sigmoid colon

appendix

rectum

A normally functioning gastrointestinal tract is responsible for supplying the body with nutrients needed to maintain health. Disturbances in the function of the gastrointestinal tract can have a significant impact on the quality of an elderly person's life. Common disorders of the gastrointestinal tract affecting the older adult include xerostomia, dysphagia, gastritis, peptic ulcer disease, diverticulitis, hemorrhoids, hiatal hernia, gallbladder disease, cirrhosis, and hepatitis. This chapter discusses normal gastrointestinal functioning, the age-related changes of the gastrointestinal tract, and common disorders of the gastrointestinal tract affecting the older adult.

NORMAL GASTROINTESTINAL FUNCTIONING

The primary functions of the gastrointestinal tract are digestion of food and absorption of nutrients. Secondary functions of the accessory organs include secretion and motility. The gastrointestinal tract, also called the alimentary tract, includes the mouth, pharynx, esophagus, stomach, small intestine, and large intestine (Fig. 21-1). The gastrointestinal tract can be thought of as a tube inside the body that begins at the mouth and ends with the anus. Placed lengthwise, the tube is about 30 feet long. Accessory organs of the gastrointestinal tract include the salivary glands, liver, pancreas, and gallbladder. These accessory organs assist in the digestion of food by secreting enzymes and bile into the gastrointestinal tract through ducts.

The activity of the gastrointestinal tract begins in the mouth, where the food is prepared for digestion. Salivary amylase, secreted by the salivary glands, begins the digestion of starch. After food is lubricated by the saliva, the food bolus enters the pharynx and moves into the esophagus, where peristalsis (ie, wavelike motions that move food through the alimentary tract) propels it into the stomach.

After the stomach receives the food bolus from the esophagus, it stores, mixes, and digests the food. The mucous membrane of the stomach secretes hydrochloric acid, pepsin, mucus, and other enzymes. Most bacteria and other foreign organisms are inactivated by the acid environment in the stomach.

Absorption of most nutrients occurs in the small intestine. The small intestine is approximately 20 feet long. The first part of the small intestine is the duodenum, where the digestive process is completed and absorption begins. From the duodenum, the digested food bolus enters the jejunum and then the ilium. Most absorption occurs in the duodenum and the jejunum. Approximately 4 to 5 million finger-like projections called villi line the small intestine, greatly increasing the surface area for absorption. Each villus contains a lymph channel and a network of capillaries. Around the villi are cells with microvilli. Villi and microvilli absorb nutrients. Material that cannot be digested passes into the large intestine to be eliminated from the body. Most water used to aid in digestion is reabsorbed to prevent dehydration.

Accessory organs such as the liver, gallbladder, and pancreas play important roles in digestion. The liver is located in the upper right quadrant of the abdominal cavity. The liver secretes bile, detoxifies harmful substances, converts glucose into glycogen for later use, and helps neutralize stomach acid by secretion of the bicarbonate ion.

The main digestive function of the liver is the production of bile. Bile acts to emulsify, or break down, fats. Bile also aids in the absorption of fat in the small intestine. Bile travels by way of ducts (ie, tubes). Bile leaves the liver and enters the gallbladder by way of the common hepatic duct. The gallbladder stores bile and excretes it into the small intestine when stimulated by the presence of gastric acid and fatty food. When the gallbladder is stimulated to release bile, the bile travels through the

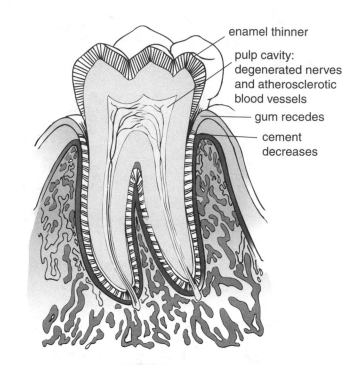

FIGURE 21-2. Age-related changes in the dental system.

common bile duct to the duodenum, the first portion of the small intestine. The pancreas produces many enzymes that assist in the digestion of fats, proteins, and carbohydrates.

AGE-RELATED CHANGES OF THE GASTROINTESTINAL TRACT

Changes occur in the gastrointestinal tract with age that can affect the nutritional status of the elderly person. For example, changes that occur within the dental system can affect the ability to chew, and other changes may affect the ability to swallow. Changes in the dental system include a generalized thinning of the enamel (ie, hard, white covering of the tooth) and discoloration of the teeth as the dentin (ie, sensitive, yellowish portion surrounding the pulp cavity of a tooth) becomes visible. Odontoblasts, the cells that produce dentin, become fewer. The gums recede, and the cement that stabilizes the tooth decreases. Within the pulp cavity, the nerves degenerate, and atherosclerosis affects the tiny vessels, causing the teeth to become brittle (Fig. 21-2). Despite these changes, becoming edentulous (ie, loss of teeth) is not inevitable.

The salivary glands produce a watery, tasteless fluid that lubricates food, moistens the walls of the mouth, and contains salivary amylase, the enzyme that initiates the digestion of carbohydrates. The

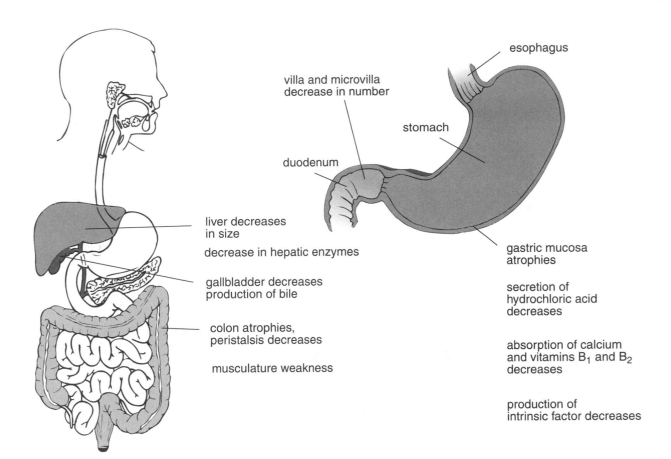

FIGURE 21-3. Age-related changes in the digestive system.

secretions of the salivary glands diminish, causing a dry mouth and sometimes making swallowing difficult. Taste buds decrease in number, contributing to decreased appetite in some older adults.

The functioning of the esophagus is essentially unchanged with age. Although many once believed that age-related changes occurred within the esophagus, it is now understood that decreased peristalsis and relaxation of the lower esophageal sphincter are more likely caused by one of several neurologic diseases commonly manifested in the aging population. There is an increased incidence of hiatal hernia with age as the result of a weakened diaphragm.

The stomach, particularly the lining of the stomach (ie, gastric mucosa), secretes hydrochloric acid, mucin, and enzymes. With age, the cells of the gastric mucosa atrophy, causing decreased production of hydrochloric acid. Absorption of calcium and vitamins B_1 and B_2 decreases, although adequate amounts appear to be absorbed. Production of intrinsic factor, necessary for the absorption of vitamin B_{12}, decreases. Decreased production, however, does not increase the risk of developing pernicious anemia. Absorption of digested food occurs through the millions of villi and microvilli.

These cells decrease with age, but because there are more than 4 million villi originally, the reduction does not significantly affect absorption of nutrients (Fig. 21-3).

The musculature of the large intestine weakens and peristalsis decreases as the person ages. Decreased peristalsis can contribute to constipation in the older adult. Constipation, although a common complaint in the aging adult, may be the result of age-related changes, inadequate diet, or a lack of exercise. Diverticulitis is common in the elderly, although it is unclear whether this condition is related to age or a result of a lack of dietary fiber.

After the age of 70, the liver decreases in size, reducing the secretion of hepatic enzymes. The decreased liver mass reduces the available space for storage within the liver. Reduced levels of hepatic enzymes makes metabolism and detoxification of drugs more difficult.

With age, the gallbladder has a more difficult time releasing bile. To add to this problem, there is a decrease in production of bile. Gallstones develop in approximately 40% of individuals by the age of 80. The formation of gallstones appears to be related to bile that is high in cholesterol.

XEROSTOMIA

Xerostomia, dryness of the mouth due to salivary gland dysfunction, is a common problem among older adults. This condition can be the result of medications (eg, anticholinergic drugs), a disease process (eg, diabetes), anxiety, mouth breathing, or a vitamin B deficiency. Saliva is needed to moisten the mouth, lubricate the food, and produce salivary amylase (ie, ptyalin). Normal salivary glands produce approximately 3 pints of saliva daily. Saliva is released into the mouth through openings in the cheeks and below the tongue.

Assessment and Intervention

Assessment reveals complaints of a dry mouth and altered taste. On examination, the oral mucosa may appear dry, inflamed, and pale. There is an increased risk for mouth ulcers and dental caries. Nursing home residents in particular must have the oral cavity assessed frequently for signs of xerostomia. Frequent mouth care before and after meals helps to decrease the discomfort from xerostomia.

Interventions are aimed at relieving the symptoms. The patient is instructed to drink frequent sips of water, suck on hard candy, or use a mouthwash frequently to help combat xerostomia. Artificial saliva, an over-the-counter agent, may be helpful. If medications are causing the xerostomia, the benefit of the drug must be weighed against the discomfort from the dry mouth. Xerostomia sometimes must be tolerated because the medication cannot be discontinued. A smaller dosage may be helpful, or changing to a different drug may alleviate the problem.

DYSPHAGIA

Dysphagia, or difficulty swallowing, is not a normal consequence of aging. It is most often the result of disease such as stroke (ie, cerebrovascular accident), traumatic brain injury, multiple sclerosis, or Parkinson disease. Patients who are confused or those with breathing problems may also be dysphasic.

Signs and Symptoms of Dysphagia

Signs and symptoms include facial weakness, weak cough, decreased gag reflex, weight loss, holding

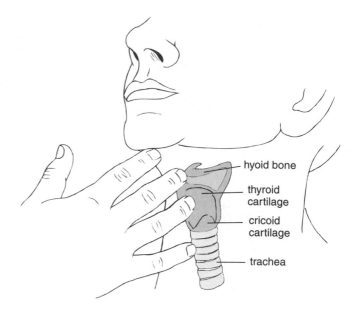

FIGURE 21-4. Assessing the swallowing reflex. When the fingers are placed as indicated in the drawing, the index finger can detect the submandibular region rising as the tongue prepares for swallowing. Simultaneously, the middle and ring finger will feel an elevation of the hyoid bone and thyroid cartilage. No movement will be felt if the swallowing reflex is absent. From Gauwitz, D. (1995). How to protect the dysphagic stroke patient. *American Journal of Nursing.* August, page 35. Used with permission.

food in the mouth, and coughing or choking during meals. Aspiration pneumonia is a serious consequence of dysphagia, particularly in the elderly. Dysphagia can be diagnosed by barium swallow or an evaluation by a speech pathologist.

Assessment and Intervention

When assessing the patient for dysphagia, examine the oral cavity for dry mucous membranes, inflamed areas in the mouth, or ulcerations. After meals, check for pockets of food remaining in the mouth. Observe the face for facial weakness or paralysis. When the person is eating, observe for gagging or choking.

✓ ASSESSMENT ALERT

To assess the swallowing reflex, place the fingers as depicted in Figure 21-4. The index finger feels the submandibular region rising as the tongue moves back for swallowing. If the swallowing reflex is intact, the middle finger and ring finger feel an elevation of the hyoid bone and the thyroid cartilage. No movement in these two areas is felt if the swallowing reflex is absent.

DISPLAY 21-1. Nursing Interventions for Patients With Dysphagia

- Allow ample time (at least 30 to 45 minutes) for feeding the patient.
- Maintain in a quiet environment away from distractions.
- Position in a high Fowler position.
- Begin with small feedings with the texture of foods the patient tolerates best. Semi-solid foods are usually tolerated best.
- Offer solid foods and liquids at different times.
- Serve foods at room temperature.
- Keep suction equipment nearby.
- Stay with the patient during a feeding, even if the patient is able to feed himself.
- If the patient has facial weakness, place the food on the unaffected side.
- Have the patient remain in an upright position for at least 45 minutes after eating.
- Inspect the oral cavity for food pockets, or have the patient do a finger sweep of the oral cavity after each bite to remove any food remaining in the mouth.
- Do not allow the patient to use a straw for liquids (unless approved by a speech pathologist). Use of straws by dysphasic patients increases the risk of aspiration because the liquid is forced too far back in the mouth.

Many patients must initially be treated with a feeding tube until the nutritional status improves. As the nutritional status improves, the patient is given oral feedings. Several types of foods may be included, depending on the patient's tolerance. For example, some patients can swallow thick liquids such as pureed foods, applesauce, or creamed soups. Other patients can tolerate soft foods such as whipped potatoes, pudding, and cooked cereals. Some patients do not tolerate pureed foods well. Chopped foods sometimes stimulate swallowing and reduce the risk of aspiration. The speech pathologist, the dietitian, and the nurse work together to determine the foods that are best tolerated. Display 21-1 identifies nursing interventions for patients with dysphagia.

GASTRITIS

Gastritis is inflammation of the stomach mucosa. Ulceration can occur and lead to hemorrhage. There are two types of gastritis: type A, or atrophic, gastritis and type B gastritis.

Type A or Atrophic Gastritis

Atrophic gastritis (ie, type A gastritis) occurs most commonly in the older adult. In **atrophic gastritis,** the mucous membrane atrophies, and hydrochloric acid secretion decreases, causing decreased absorption of iron and vitamin B_{12}. Atrophic gastritis tends to become chronic and can contribute to the development of pernicious anemia in elderly persons. Most often, there are no apparent symptoms except for the symptoms of pernicious anemia (eg, weakness, tingling in the extremities, pallor, anorexia).

Type B Gastritis

Type B gastritis is a chronic form of gastritis that is associated with *Helicobacter pylori* bacilli. Symptoms of type B gastritis include anorexia, heartburn, a bad taste in the mouth, nausea, and vomiting. Hydrochloric acid is increased in type B gastritis rather than the achlorhydria associated with type A gastritis. Type B gastritis is not associated with pernicious anemia.

Management of the Older Adult With Gastritis

Diagnosis of gastritis is made by evaluation of symptoms, endoscopy, and upper gastrointestinal radiographs. Most patients with gastritis are managed at home and must be given a thorough explanation of the disorder, the treatment regimen, and symptoms that should be reported to the physician.

Treatment of chronic gastritis is aimed at soothing the irritated gastric mucosa, providing adequate nutrition, and relieving pain. If pernicious anemia occurs, injections of vitamin B_{12} are necessary. The patient is instructed to avoid foods and beverages that are irritating. The nurse must teach the patient and family to monitor for signs of hemorrhage, such as an increased pulse rate, decreased blood pressure, or vomiting of blood. Any indication of hemorrhage is reported immediately.

Antacids or anticholinergic drugs are used to decrease acidity. However, the elderly do not respond well to anticholinergics, and use of these drugs may be limited. If hemorrhage occurs, surgery such as partial or total gastrectomy (ie, surgical removal of all or part of the stomach) or pyloroplasty (ie, surgical procedure to repair or increase the size of the pylorus) may be necessary.

PEPTIC ULCER DISEASE

Peptic ulcer is an acute or chronic ulceration of the mucosa of the stomach, duodenum, pylorus, or esophagus. Most peptic ulcers occur in the duodenum. Men suffer from peptic ulcers approximately three times more often than women. After menopause, the occurrence of peptic ulcers in women rises to become equal with men.

Ulceration occurs as the result of increased secretion of hydrochloric acid coming in contact with the mucosa wall and digesting the cells in that area. Histamine released from the injured cells stimulates the production of more hydrochloric acid. Another factor that contributes to peptic ulcer disease is damage to the gastric mucosa and decreased mucus production.

H. pylori is a contributing factor in peptic ulcer disease. *H. pylori* is a Gram-negative bacteria found in the mucosa of 80% to 90% of individuals with peptic ulcer disease. The exact relationship between the development of peptic ulcers and *H. pylori* is unclear, but it is thought that the bacteria in some way damages the gastric mucosa, rendering it more susceptible to ulceration.

Signs and Symptoms

Pain, usually occurring 2 to 3 hours after meals, is the most prominent symptom. The patient may complain of a burning, dull, or gnawing pain in the mid-epigastric region that is relieved by eating. The pain is relieved for a time, only to return. A burning sensation in the epigastric region (ie, heartburn) may lead to burping. Some individuals bleed as the first symptom of an ulcer. Bleeding may be seen as hematemesis (ie, vomiting of blood), hemorrhage, or melena (ie, blood in the stool).

Diagnosis

Diagnosis is made by visualization of gastric mucosa by an esophagogastroduodenoscopy. Hemoglobin and hematocrit levels may be low if hemorrhage is present. The presence of *H. pylori* bacteria can be confirmed by a breath test or a blood test for antibodies to *H. pylori* antigen.

Management of the Older Adult With Peptic Ulcer Disease

Nursing care involves teaching the patient about the nature of the disease and the importance of adhering to the drug regimen to eradicate the disease. A diet that is nonirritating with frequent small meals is preferred. Irritating foods and spices such as pepper, chili powder, carbonated beverages, and alcohol are omitted from the diet. The patient is instructed to report any adverse reactions to the medication and report any signs of bleeding such as spitting up blood or blood in the stool.

Treatment is aimed at relieving discomfort and preventing recurrences by controlling gastric acidity. Gastric acid is neutralized through the use of antacids (eg, Amphogel, Maalox, Mylanta, Riopan). The most frequently used drugs are the histamine receptor antagonists such as cimetidine (Tagamet), ranitidine (Zantac), and famotidine (Pepcid), which decrease the amount of acid produced. These drugs are available over the counter.

Other drugs are available by prescription and include omeprazole (Prilosec), misoprostol (Cytotec), pirenzepine (Gastrozepine), and sucralfate (Carafate). To eradicate the *H. pylori* bacteria, an anti-infective such as tetracycline or amoxicillin combined with Flagyl and bismuth salts is prescribed. Although symptoms usually disappear within a week after therapy is begun, the patient is encouraged to continue the drug regimen to allow for complete healing of the ulcer. If complete healing does not occur, the ulcer will return and again cause symptoms. If medical interventions fail to produce healing, surgery such as vagotomy or vagotomy with pyloroplasty may be performed.

Nursing Care of the Older Adult With Peptic Ulcer Disease

When assessing the older adult with peptic ulcer disease, the nurse should have the patient describe the pain. The nurse also should question the patient about the pain:

Does the pain occur after meals? If so how long after meals?

What type of pain is experienced? Burning? Gnawing?

Where is the location of the pain?

Is the pain related to eating?

An elderly, confused patient may not be able to accurately describe the pain. Assess for clues that indicate pain such as holding the chest area, increased irritability, agitation, or increased activity. The stools are observed for a black, tarry appearance, which suggests bleeding. A stool assay for occult blood may be ordered. Laboratory results such as hemoglobin and hematocrit are monitored for indications of bleeding.

The care of the patient with peptic ulcer disease is centered on managing the pain, decreasing the acid secretions of the stomach mucosa, and increasing the individual's or the caregiver's knowledge about the disease and the treatment regimen. Food sometimes relieves the pain by providing substances for the gastric secretions to act on rather than the stomach mucosa. Five or six small meals daily provide greater comfort than three larger meals. Irritating foods such as pepper, chili powder, carbonated beverages, alcohol, and coffee (caffeinated and decaffeinated) are omitted. The diet is usually individualized and its scope increased as tolerated.

Administration of histamine receptor antagonists to decrease the secretion of acid, cytoprotective agents such as misoprostol to protect the mucosal cells from acid, or the anticholinergics to decrease secretions may be helpful in controlling the pain.

Patient and Family Teaching

The nurse teaches the patient about the nature of the disease, what happens in the body, foods to avoid, and the importance of adhering to the drug regimen. Information to include in a teaching plan for the patient with an ulcer includes medication concerns, dietary suggestions, and stress-reducing techniques.

PATIENT TEACHING AID

Teaching plan for the patient with a peptic ulcer:

- **Teach the person to take medications exactly as prescribed by the primary caregiver to ensure complete healing. Symptoms may subside within a week of treatment, but caution the patient that continuation of the medication regimen is necessary until complete healing takes place. Treatment with H$_2$ antagonists may be continued for up to 1 year.**
- **Encourage the older adult to quit smoking cigarettes, because smoking increases gastric acidity. Referral to a smoking cessation support group may prove helpful (see Chapter 20).**
- **Give a written list of foods to avoid, such as spicy foods, gas-forming foods, and foods that irritate the gastric mucosa. The diet is usually individualized, and foods that cause irritation are eliminated from the diet.**
- **Instruct the patient to eat several small meals rather than three large meals.**
- **Identify and practice stress-reducing techniques (eg, relaxation techniques, walking, exercise programs, medication).**
- **Tell the person to get adequate rest.**
- **Instruct the person to report immediately any increase in symptoms (pain or discomfort) or evidence of bleeding (dark tarry stools).**

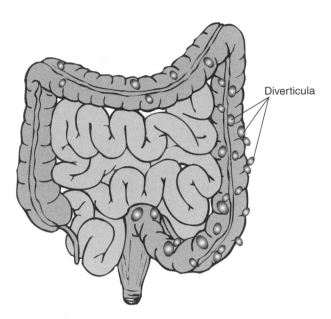

FIGURE 21-5. Diverticulosis of the colon.

DIVERTICULOSIS AND DIVERTICULITIS

Diverticulosis occurs in approximately 60% of persons older than 80 years of age. A diverticulum is a saclike pouch that forms in the mucous membrane of the intestine (Fig. 21-5). The presence of multiple diverticula is called **diverticulosis.** Diverticula usually begin to develop around the age of 50 and increase in number with age. Diverticulosis usually is asymptomatic and causes the individual no problem. However, the diverticula sometimes become pockets for the collection of fecal material. When fecal material becomes trapped, the diverticula become inflamed, causing **diverticulitis.** Inflammation spreads to the tissue around the diverticula, increasing the area of inflammation.

Signs and Symptoms

Diverticulosis may cause a change in bowel habits such as constipation or diarrhea, or it may be asymptomatic. The patient may experience pain or tenderness in the lower left abdominal quadrant that increases after eating. When inflammation occurs, diverticulosis becomes diverticulitis. Symptoms of diverticulitis include constipation alternating with diarrhea, flatulence, nausea, pain, and tenderness. Rectal bleeding can occur, resulting in a distinctive stool described as resembling current jelly. A mass may be palpated in the lower abdomen. Symptoms of diverticulosis and diverticulitis may be less severe in the older adult, making detection difficult. The older person may be asymptomatic until infection occurs. Bleeding may not be detected because of visual impairment.

Diagnosis

Diagnosis of diverticulosis is confirmed with a colonoscopy, barium enema, or a computed tomography (CT) scan. If diverticulitis is suspected, a barium enema is contraindicated because of the risk of bowel perforation.

Management of the Older Adult With Diverticulitis

No treatment is required if the patient is not experiencing any symptoms. The patient is instructed to eat a diet high in fiber (eg, whole grains, fruits, vegetables) and avoid foods that contain seeds. Constipation is prevented by use of a bulk-forming laxative such as Metamucil.

When the patient develops symptoms of diverticulitis, a low-fiber diet is recommended. Antibiotics, intravenous fluids, and resting of the bowel by withholding food and fluids are used to manage diverticulitis. Meperidine is administered to relieve pain. Oral intake is resumed as symptoms are relieved. Medical management is effective in most cases, but surgery may be performed if complications such as perforation, abscess formation, or hemorrhage occur.

DIARRHEA

Diarrhea is the frequent occurrence of loose or liquid stools. Classification by frequency is more than three loose or liquid stools per day; classification by amount is more than 200 g of stool per day. Older adults with diarrhea are at increased risk of becoming dehydrated, particularly with acute diarrhea. Acute diarrhea is characterized by the excretion of large amounts of water and electrolytes. Water enters the intestines as the result of increased osmotic pressure, causing the accumulation of large amounts of fluid in the intestine and the passage of frequent, watery stools.

Signs and Symptoms

Signs and symptoms of diarrhea include abdominal cramping, frequent watery stools, abdominal disten-

tion, increased frequency of bowel sounds, and generalized weakness. The older adult is at increased risk for hypokalemia and dehydration. Mild diarrhea may be self-limiting, lasting 2 to 3 days, but this period allows sufficient time for the older adult to become dehydrated. Any signs of dehydration such as dry mucous membranes, weakness, scanty urine output, concentrated urine, or increased pulse rate must be immediately reported. Hypokalemia is a distinct possibility in the elderly. Decreased potassium levels can cause cardiac arrhythmias and result in death.

Most cases of severe or chronic diarrhea may be the result of disorders such as Crohn's disease, lactose intolerance, or irritable bowel syndrome. Increased peristalsis causes a type of diarrhea called small-volume diarrhea. Small-volume diarrhea usually is caused by an inflammatory bowel disease such as ulcerative colitis. Diarrhea caused by an infectious organism such as *Shigella* or *Escherichia coli* is called infectious diarrhea and manifests by a watery diarrhea and increased peristalsis.

Management of the Older Adult With Diarrhea

Diarrhea is a symptom rather than a medical diagnosis and often requires numerous diagnostic examinations such as a complete blood count (CBC), stool sample for infectious or parasitic organism, and a routine stool examination to identify the underlying cause. Treatment is often symptomatic. Antidiarrheals such as diphenoxylate (Lomotil) and loperamide (Immodium) are used to control the diarrhea and prevent dehydration. Antibiotics are given if a causative organism is identified. The elderly may need intravenous therapy to rehydrate and correct a fluid imbalance.

Using the Nursing Process to Care for an Older Adult With Diarrhea

Assessment
The nurse questions the elderly person or the caregiver about the pattern of bowel movements: frequency, amount, color, and odor. A history of current drug therapy, dietary intake, and recent travel to other areas is obtained. The skin and mucous membrane of the perineal area are inspected for excoriation. The nurse takes the vital signs and weighs the patient to obtain baseline information. It is important to assess the patient for dehydration (eg, dry skin and mucous membranes; dark, scanty urine; tenting of the skin). A stool specimen is needed for laboratory examination.

Occasionally, impaction may be mistaken for diarrhea. An impaction blocks the normal passage of feces but allows seepage of liquid feces around the hardened mass. The elderly are particularly prone to fecal impaction because of decreased activity, lack of fiber, decreased amounts of fluid in the diet, or overuse of laxatives to promote bowel evacuation.

ASSESSMENT ALERT

Be alert for fecal impaction in patients that have small amounts of loose stools several times each day or seepage of liquid stools. To check for a fecal impaction, insert a gloved and lubricated index finger into the rectum in the direction of the umbilicus. A hardened fecal mass is felt if an impaction is present. The hardened stool may be broken up and removed piece by piece until all of the stool is removed. Care must be taken to prevent stimulation of the vagal nerve when the stool is removed. The elderly are particularly susceptible to vagal nerve stimulation and must be observed closely while the impaction is removed. Vagal nerve stimulation may result in changes in pulse rate and blood pressure. Check the pulse rate and rhythm and the blood pressure if the patient experiences any unusual effects and before and after removing the impaction.

Nursing Diagnoses

The following nursing diagnoses may be appropriate for patients with diarrhea:

Diarrhea related to infection, ingestion of irritating foods, medication regimen, other (specify)

Risk for Fluid Volume Deficit related to frequent watery stools

Risk for Impaired Tissue Integrity related to irritation of anal area from diarrhea

Planning and Implementation

The focus of care of the elderly person with diarrhea is to control the diarrhea, return to a normal bowel pattern, prevent dehydration and electrolyte imbalance, and maintain the mucous membranes of the anal area.

Severe Diarrhea. With severe diarrhea, the older adult is often placed on bed rest. The nurse monitors the number of diarrhea stools, as well as the color, consistency, and odor of the stools. Fluids are encouraged to replace those lost in the liquid stool. It is recommended that lukewarm (neither hot nor cold) fluids be offered to prevent additional stimulation of the gastrointestinal tract. The diet is soft and bland. Antidiarrheal drugs such as diphenoxylate or loperamide are administered.

Risk for Fluid Volume Deficit. The older adult is at great risk for dehydration with a bout of diarrhea. Confusion or irritability are common signs of dehydration in the older adult. Other symptoms of dehydration are dry mucous membranes, scanty urine, concentrated urine, confusion, or increased pulse rate. Hypokalemia (ie, low potassium level) may occur. Potassium levels should be maintained between 3.5 and 5.0 mEq/L. The nurse reports any evidence of hypokalemia such as weak pulse, hypotension, or muscle flabbiness and weakness. Serum electrolyte levels are monitored and any abnormalities reported.

ASSESSMENT ALERT

Closely monitor patients receiving the cardiac glycosides, particularly digitalis. Hypokalemia can increase the action of digitalis in the body and lead to digitalis toxicity. Normal digoxin levels should be between 0.8 and 2.0 ng/mL. Report digoxin levels above 2.0 ng/mL. Symptoms that alert to the possibility of digoxin toxicity include anorexia, nausea, vomiting, abdominal pain, visual disturbances (eg, blurred, yellow or green vision and halos; borders around dark objects), and bradycardia or other arrhythmias. If any of these symptoms develop in a patient taking digoxin (Lanoxin), withhold the next dose of the drug and notify the primary caregiver.

Impaired Tissue Integrity. The skin of an elderly person is particularly sensitive to breakdown. Check the skin around the perianal area after each bowel movement for signs of inflammation. Clean the area thoroughly with a mild soap, and rinse well. The area is then dried thoroughly. A cream may be applied to the perianal area to decrease inflammation and promote healing.

Evaluation and Expected Outcomes

Successful care can provide the following outcomes for the patient:

Normal bowel pattern restored

Adequate hydration maintained

Skin in perineal area intact and free of excoriation or irritation

CONSTIPATION

Constipation refers to the passage of abnormally hard and infrequent stools. Passage of stools is difficult and prolonged. Severe constipation can lead to fecal impaction. Constipation is not a normal occurrence with aging. Older adults have many complaints of constipation. This is seen in patients in the acute care setting, the nursing home, and in the home setting. Rather than a consequence of aging, constipation is most often related to decreased mobility, medication, (eg, tranquilizers, narcotics, antacids with aluminum), poor nutrition, inadequate fluids, or medical disorders (eg, cancer of the bowel, hypothyroidism, multiple sclerosis).

Older adults sometimes have the misconception that a daily bowel movement is necessary, and they think they are constipated if they do not have a daily bowel movement. Normal bowel movements range from three movements per day to three or fewer per week. Constipation can result from the overuse of laxatives. Chronic laxative use results in constipation by causing a loss of muscular tone in the intestine.

Management of the Older Adult With Constipation

Management is aimed at relieving the constipation and improving preventive health practices in the elderly person. Various laxatives such as bulk laxatives, fecal softeners, osmotic agents, or stimulants are available to treat constipation and help restore normal bowel function. The patient is taught preventive practices such as increasing fiber in the diet, increasing exercise, and increasing fluid intake. Instruct the patient that the overuse or routine use of laxatives to obtain a normal bowel evacuation causes a loss of muscular tone in the intestine and results in constipation.

When assessing the older adult for constipation, the nurse should question the caregiver and the elderly adult about usual bowel pattern and the use of laxatives. Some elderly persons depend on laxatives for a bowel movement. If this is the case, it is important to help them plan other methods for bowel evacuation. It is also important to obtain a description of the bowel movements (eg, consistency, frequency, hardness, color).

A diet high in fiber (eg, fresh fruits and vegetables, whole-grain breads and cereals, legumes) is provided. It is important that the older adult increases fluid intake if not contraindicated by a disease process. An individualized exercise program suitable for the patient's activity capabilities and limitations is planned. A stool softener or bulk-enhancing medication may be prescribed to promote regularity and a soft-formed stool.

HEMORRHOIDS

Hemorrhoids are dilated veins located above or below the anal sphincter. If located above the anal sphincter, the hemorrhoids are called internal hemorrhoids. If located below the anal sphincter, they are called external hemorrhoids.

Signs and Symptoms

Symptoms of hemorrhoids include itching and pain in the anal area. Internal hemorrhoids are less likely to cause pain than external hemorrhoids. Hemorrhoids bleed as dry hardened stool passes through the anal sphincter. Bleeding may be profuse or a few drops. External hemorrhoids look like small, blue-red appendages around the anus. Sometimes, internal hemorrhoids are forced out of the anus during defecation. If large, these internal hemorrhoids remain outside the anal opening. If small, internal hemorrhoids retract after defecation. Diagnosis is made by direct observation or with a proctosigmoidoscopy.

Assessment and Management of the Older Adult With Hemorrhoids

Hemorrhoids can often be managed by avoiding straining during defecation, a high-fiber diet, and the administration of a stool softener such as Colace. Sitz baths promote anorectal healing and reduce local inflammation.

✓ **ASSESSMENT ALERT**

The older adult may experience changes in blood pressure and cardiac status if exposed to water that is too hot in the anorectal area during the sitz bath. Monitor the patient carefully during and after the sitz bath. Note any changes in blood pressure and pulse rate, quality, or rhythm.

A local anesthetic agent (ie, creams, suppositories, or lotions) or astringent pads placed in the anal area may help relieve the pain and itching. Many older patients are managed with these conservative measures. For hemorrhoids that do not respond to conservative treatment, there are several procedures available such as infrared photocoagulation, bipolar diathermy, and laser therapy. Small hemorrhoids may be treated by injecting a sclerosing agent. Severe hemorrhoids may require surgical excision (ie, hemorrhoidectomy).

HIATAL HERNIA

Hiatal hernia (ie, diaphragmatic hernia) is the protrusion of the upper part of the stomach through the diaphragm. The most common type of hiatal hernia is the sliding hiatal hernia. In this type of hernia, the stomach moves into a weakened portion of the diaphragm (Fig. 21-6). When the person is lying down, the lower esophagus and the stomach move upward and slide in and out of the diaphragm. Standing causes the esophagus and stomach to slide back into normal alignment. Approximately 90% of those with hiatal hernias have sliding hernias.

Signs and Symptoms

Most older adults have small hiatal hernias. The hernia is usually asymptomatic unless reflux esophagitis is present. Symptoms, if they occur, include heartburn, regurgitation, and a feeling of epigastric discomfort after eating. Symptoms are more severe when lying down. Diagnosis is confirmed by barium contrast studies and endoscopy.

Management of the Older Adult With Hiatal Hernia

Conservative measures are used initially to manage the discomfort. The patient is instructed to remain upright for at least 1 hour after eating. Lying down causes the hernia to slide into the diaphragm. The head of the bed can be elevated on 4- to 6-inch blocks. Small, frequent meals are better tolerated than three large meals. The patient is instructed to avoid spicy foods, alcohol, caffeine, and nicotine because these foods stimulate acidity. Drug therapy includes antacids or histamine (H_2) blockers such as cimetidine (Tagamet), famotidine (Pepcid), or ranitidine (Zantac). If conservative measures are not effective, surgery may be indicated.

GALLBLADDER DISEASE

Cholelithiasis (ie, gallstone disease) is a common disorder in the elderly, and incidence is increased among

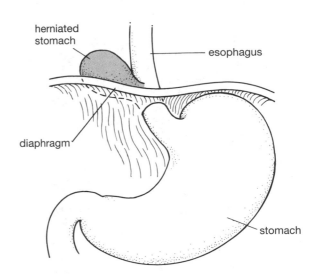

FIGURE 21-6. Sliding hiatal hernia. From Scherer, J. & Timby, B. (1996). *Introductory medical-surgical nursing.* Philadelphia: Lippincott-Raven, 675. Used with permission.

those older than age 60. Calculi (ie, stones) form in the gallbladder. It is estimated that 1 of 3 older adults has cholelithiasis by the age of 75. Gallstones are solid, crystal-like substances most commonly composed of cholesterol. Cholesterol is normally maintained in liquid form in the body by the action of bile salts. An increased amount of cholesterol in the bile prevents the bile salts from dissolving the cholesterol and causes cholesterol stones to form. Stones can also form if there is a decrease in the production of bile salts.

Gallstones may be as small as a grain of sand or as large as a lemon. Sometimes, gallstones enter the cystic ducts, the tubes through which bile travels, and become lodged in the common bile duct, obstructing the flow of bile (Fig. 21-7). When this blockage occurs, **cholecystitis** (ie, inflammation of the gallbladder) can develop. Gallstones occur more frequently in women than in men. Men and women who are overweight are also at increased risk.

Signs and Symptoms

Symptoms occur when one or more stones block the passage of bile, causing the gallbladder to distend with bile. Symptoms usually occur after a meal high in fatty foods. After a meal, the inflamed gallbladder contracts, attempting to excrete bile. When the bile cannot pass through the ducts, pain occurs. The patient complains of belching, nausea, abdominal distention, and pain in the right upper quadrant of the abdomen. The pain is called **biliary colic** and is caused by temporary obstruction of the ducts by a stone. The pain may travel to the right shoulder, back, or neck. Biliary colic sometimes mimics a heart attack.

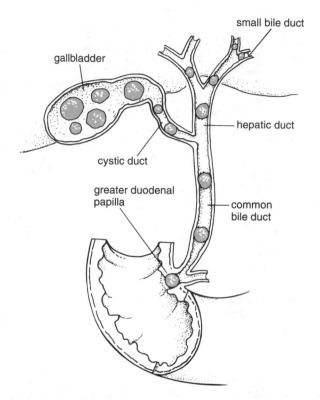

FIGURE 21-7. Potential locations of gallstones within the biliary tree. From Scherer, J. & Timby, B. (1996). *Introductory medical-surgical nursing.* Philadelphia: Lippincott-Raven, 748. Used with permission.

The gallbladder can become infected. If infection occurs, the patient develops fever. Stools may appear clay colored and the urine very dark. Symptoms of a mild inflammation may be less severe with indigestion, some pain, and tenderness in the right upper quadrant. A mass may be palpated in the upper right quadrant. Cholecystitis can become chronic and is manifested by discomfort after meals, flatulence, and nausea. Failure to obtain treatment can cause permanent damage to the gallbladder and liver. Jaundice may occur if a stone lodges in the common bile duct.

Cholelithiasis can be diagnosed by CT scan or abdominal ultrasound. Ultrasound is most often used for the elderly. It is noninvasive, is painless, has few adverse reactions, and does not require radiation.

Cholecystectomy

The most common operative procedure in the elderly is a cholecystectomy (ie, surgical removal of the gallbladder). The older person is at increased risk during surgery because of preexisting chronic diseases. However, cholecystectomy is usually well tolerated, particularly if the surgery is elective rather

than an emergency. Attacks will recur unless the gallbladder is removed.

Laparoscopic cholecystectomy is the most common procedure for removal of the gallbladder. The laparoscopic cholecystectomy does not require the abdominal muscles to be cut, but rather requires three or four small puncture sites in the abdomen. The gallbladder is drained, separated from the ducts and vessels, and removed by instrumentation through one of the puncture sites. The standard cholecystectomy requires removal through a 5- to 8-inch abdominal incision and is the recommended method for treating complicated cholecystitis.

Small cholesterol stones may be dissolved by using oral drugs such as ursodiol (Actigall) and chenodiol (Chenix). These drugs are used for those who cannot tolerate the surgical procedure and are natural bile salts that dissolve the gallstone. However, treatment may require 6 to 12 months and is only moderately successful. The rate of stone recurrence within 5 years is high.

Assessment and Management of the Older Adult With Gallbladder Disease

Assessment of the older person with cholelithiasis may be difficult because symptoms may be atypical or absent. Pain in the right upper quadrant of the abdomen is typical of gallbladder disease. The elderly or confused patient may be unable to give an accurate description of the pain. It is important that the nurse watch for signs of pain such as guarding of the abdomen, a fetal position, grimacing, restlessness, crying, or agitation. Belching, nausea, and abdominal distention may occur. An elevated temperature may indicate infection. The nurse questions the patient or caregiver about bowel movements, including frequency, color, and consistency. With gallbladder disease, stools frequently appear clay colored. The skin is examined for jaundice.

During an acute attack, the patient is maintained without oral intake (NPO), and a nasogastric tube is inserted. Analgesics and antibiotics are given until the inflammation is controlled. Surgery is delayed until the attack subsides. Approximately 80% of acute attacks subside with conservative treatment. Mild attacks respond well to a low-fat diet, avoidance of alcohol, and eating several small meals rather than three large meals. Because fat-soluble vitamins are not well absorbed from food, a supplement may be needed.

Anticholinergics, such as atropine or propantheline, may be prescribed to reduce spasms of the ducts that cause pain. Anticholinergics are used with caution in the older adult. Patients with glaucoma should not receive anticholinergic drugs because administration could initiate an acute attack of glaucoma. Analgesics such as meperidine (Demerol) may be administered to relieve pain. Note the response to pain medication, and report unrelieved pain. Morphine is not administered for biliary colic, because morphine can cause spasm in the common bile duct, resulting in increased pain. Back rubs, relaxation techniques, guided imagery, or deep breathing techniques may be used to help reduce the pain and relieve tension (see Chapter 11).

A nasogastric tube (NGT) may be inserted and connected to suction. If an NGT is required, the patient is kept NPO. The nurse measures the output from the NGT and notes color of output. If the attack is mild, the patient may be managed on a low-fat diet with frequent small meals, analgesics, and antispasmodics.

For patients with an NGT or those who are NPO, the diet may be gradually resumed after the tube is removed. A low-fat, bland diet is given to prevent stimulation of the gallbladder. Although a bland diet is sometimes described as tasteless, well-balanced, nutritious meals can be planned. Consultation with the dietitian may help the caregiver and the patient to plan meals lower in fat. Powdered protein food supplements can be added into skim milk to increase nutritive intake.

Patient and Family Teaching

The patient or caregiver may not understand the disease process, drug regimen, or the foods to be avoided. A teaching plan for the patient with gallbladder disease should include an explanation of the disease process, dietary considerations, and any drug precautions.

PATIENT TEACHING AID

Teaching plan for a patient with gallbladder disease:

- **Provide an explanation of the disease process, the treatment regimen, and the medication regimen. Answer any question that the patient or the caregiver may have.**
- **Discuss the need to loose weight if the patient is obese. Provide a consultation with the dietitian if necessary.**
- **Instruct the patient to avoid foods high in fat (eg, ice cream, whole milk, fried foods, gravies, fatty meats) and foods irritating to the gastric mucosa (eg, caffeine, carbonated beverages, cabbage, beans, spicy foods).**

- **Inform the patient using ursodiol that the drug must be taken for 6 to 12 months. Stone recurrence has been reported in up to 50% of individuals treated with ursodiol.**
- **Tell the patient to notify the primary caregiver if symptoms return or increase in severity.**
- **Surgery may be needed to relieve recurrent symptoms or to relieve acute biliary colic.**

CIRRHOSIS

Cirrhosis is a chronic disorder characterized by scarring of the liver. It is particularly common in malnourished, alcoholic men older than 50 years of age. Cirrhosis is the eighth leading cause of death of the elderly. Although there are several types of cirrhosis, the most common type is Laennec cirrhosis. Laennec cirrhosis is associated with chronic alcoholism and malnutrition. The condition develops slowly over 20 to 30 years. Over the years, the liver cells gradually die (ie, necrose) and are replaced by scar tissue. Eventually, the nonfunctioning scar tissue becomes more prevalent than normal tissue. Regardless of the type of cirrhosis, the end result in the liver and the treatment are the same.

Signs and Symptoms

Symptoms begin gradually with vague gastrointestinal problems such as anorexia, nausea, vomiting, and indigestion. The patient may complain of a dull ache in the abdominal area. The patient may experience constipation or diarrhea. Abdominal discomfort occurs because of enlargement of the liver as the cells become engorged with fat. Late in the disease process, the liver becomes a mass of scar tissue and decreases in size. Symptoms that occur late in the disease include ascites (ie, collection of fluid in the abdominal cavity causing an increase in the size of the abdomen) and esophageal varices. **Esophageal varices** are dilated and distended veins of the lower esophagus that occur as the result of portal hypertension. In cases of **portal hypertension,** blood that normally flows through the portal vein and the hepatic artery into the liver is unable to pass into the damaged liver and must find an alternate path. Varices or distended veins develop in the lower esophagus and stomach in an effort to establish an alternate pathway for the blood. These varices are unable to handle the high pressure and high volume of blood that would normally pass through the liver. Consequently, the varices have a tendency to rupture and bleed. If the varices rupture, the bleeding is massive, and the patient can die within a short period.

Patients with cirrhosis bleed easily (eg, nosebleeds, easy bruising, oozing form injection sites) and are often anemic. The skin is dry, with poor skin turgor and pruritus (ie, itching). Jaundice (ie, yellowish tinge to the skin, mucous membranes, and sclera of the eyes caused by increased levels of bilirubin in the blood) may be present. Mental function declines as hepatic encephalopathy develops because of the accumulation of ammonia in the blood.

Diagnosis

Various laboratory tests are used to diagnose cirrhosis such as determinations of serum levels of aspartate aminotransferase (AST [SGOT]) and alanine aminotransferase (ALT [SGPT]). The most definitive examination is a liver biopsy, which allows for visualization of the hepatic tissue. CT, magnetic resonance imaging (MRI), and liver scans provide additional information about the condition of the liver.

Assessment and Management of the Older Adult With Cirrhosis

A thorough nursing assessment is important because cirrhosis affects many body systems. The nurse obtains baseline vital signs and performs a thorough physical assessment. The patient is questioned about possible long-term alcohol use. Nutritional status is assessed and the patient is questioned concerning any recent weight loss or gain. Determine the patient's mental status. Note any mental confusion or mental deterioration. The nurse assesses for abdominal distention, easy bruising, pruritus, constipation, and diarrhea.

There is no cure for the disorder, and the patient is treated symptomatically. The focus of care is maintaining a normal respiratory pattern (if ascites is present), improving nutritional status, protecting the skin from injury, maintaining bed rest, and monitoring mental status. Liver transplantation may be an option for some older adults, but most are not good candidates for the procedure because of age and multiple health problems.

Patient and Family Teaching
The patient may be cared for at home, particularly after the acute phase of the disease. A teaching plan should be devised for the cirrhosis patient after the acute phase, when the patient will be cared for at home. Include information for caregivers, family members, and the patient.

 PATIENT TEACHING AID

For cirrhosis patient receiving care at home, stress the following points:
- **Eating a high-vitamin, high-carbohydrate, nutritious diet is important.**
- **Dietary sodium may be restricted.**
- **Supplemental vitamins may be needed.**
- **Eating frequent, small meals is helpful.**
- **Abstain from alcohol (refer to Alcoholics Anonymous, if indicated).**
- **Check skin for easy bruising and stools for blood (tarry or dark color).**
- **Report any worsening of symptoms or any evidence of bleeding (eg, gums, stools, vomitus), difficulty breathing, increase in abdominal girth, or mental deterioration.**

Esophageal Varices
Esophageal varices are manifested by bleeding from the dilated, tortuous veins. The bleeding is usually massive and occurs suddenly. Early symptoms may include coughing or spitting up blood or melena (ie, blood in the stool). Lifting heavy objects, coughing, vomiting, sneezing, or straining when having a stool can precipitate hemorrhage.

Treatment for esophageal varices requires immediate and aggressive care. The patient is usually admitted to the intensive care unit. Vasopressin (Pitressin) may be infused directly into the mesenteric artery to temporarily constrict the vessels and decrease bleeding. A Sengstaken-Blakemore or Minnesota tube may be inserted to control bleeding. The Sengstaken-Blakemore tube is a double-balloon tube that, after insertion, is inflated to apply pressure against the varices. An iced saline lavage can be used to help control the bleeding.

Endoscopic sclerotherapy may be used when the Sengstaken-Blakemore tube fails to control bleeding. A sclerosing agent is injected into the varices to cause thrombosis and sclerosis (ie, hardening of the tissue). Several surgical procedures have been developed for severe cases of esophageal varices, but elderly patients are at especially high risk, and complications are common.

Hepatic Encephalopathy
Hepatic encephalopathy occurs as a complication of cirrhosis, resulting in dementia and declining

mental status. Symptoms occur as ammonia accumulates in the blood. Blood ammonia levels greater than 110 µg/dL are associated with symptoms of memory loss, decreased reasoning ability, irritability, and tremor. As the condition worsens, delirium and coma can develop. Treatment consists of decreasing dietary protein, administering neomycin to decrease production of ammonia-producing bacteria, giving sorbitol to induce catharsis, or administering lactulose to decrease blood ammonia levels. Lactulose can be administered orally or as a retention enema.

HEPATITIS

Hepatitis is any inflammation of the liver. Although there are several forms of hepatitis, viral hepatitis B is the most common form found in older adults. Viral hepatitis is a systemic disease characterized by inflammation of the liver with cellular destruction and necrosis. In the early stages, the patient complains of fatigue, malaise, headache, arthralgia, anorexia, and abdominal pain. Jaundice (ie, yellowish discoloration of the skin) may or may not be present. Stools may be clay colored and the urine dark.

Diagnosis

Viral hepatitis B is most commonly spread through blood and blood products. The virus has also been found in saliva, semen, and vaginal secretions. It can be spread through the skin or mucous membranes. A diagnosis is confirmed by the presence of hepatitis B surface antigens and hepatitis B antibodies in the blood. The hepatitis B vaccine is recommended for older adults. When the hepatitis B vaccine is given, the hepatitis B antigen stimulates antibody production to provide protection from the infection. The vaccine is safe and is effective in about 90% of those vaccinated.

Assessment and Management

When assessing the patient with hepatitis, the nurse questions her about fatigue, headache, joint pain, lack of appetite, or abdominal pain. Nausea and vomiting may also be present. Fever may occur along with lymph node and liver enlargement. The nurse asks the patient to describe the color of the stools. The skin is checked for jaundice.

ASSESSMENT ALERT

Older adults may exhibit atypical symptoms, particularly acute confusion. The onset of hepatitis B in the adult may be sudden and intense. There is an increased tendency for the disease to become chronic in this patient population.

Hepatitis B is a viral infection, and no specific medication has proven to be effective. Viral hepatitis B is particularly serious in the older adult. Severe liver cell destruction leading to hepatic failure is a possibility. Older adults with hepatitis B are usually hospitalized during the acute phases. The patient is treated symptomatically, with an emphasis on maintaining bed rest until the symptoms subside and on providing adequate nutrition. Antiemetics may be prescribed to decrease nausea and prevent vomiting. In younger adults, corticosteroids may be given. However, corticosteroids are not usually given to the older adult because these drugs are more likely to cause pathogenic fractures in the elderly. Convalescence can last 12 to 16 weeks. The patient may need follow-up care for as long as 1 year to monitor for recurrence.

CRITICAL THINKING EXERCISES

1. Mr. Carpenter, age 83, is a resident in the nursing home where you work. He complains of constipation almost daily. The nurse assistant reports his complaints to you but adds, "Mr. Carpenter is just a complainer. He is preoccupied with having daily bowel movements. Just ignore him." How would you handle this situation? What would you say to the nurse assistant? How would you deal with Mr. Carpenter's complaint?
2. The nurse assistant reports that Mr. Scoggins has had loose stools for the past 10 hours. What action would you take? What assessments would be most important to make? What nursing actions would be most helpful?
3. Ms. Whitmire, age 68, is to be dismissed from the acute care facility today. She was diagnosed with diverticulosis and is currently asymptomatic. What diet instructions would be most appropriate for her? Prepare a list of 10 foods that Ms. Whitmire should include in her diet.
4. Mr. Collins has been diagnosed with internal hemorrhoids. What information is important for him to have concerning hemorrhoids? What instructions could you give Mr. Collins to help him deal with hemorrhoids on a daily basis?

REFERENCES AND SUGGESTED READING

Cohen, B.J., & Wood, D.L. (2000). *Memmler's structure and function of the human body* (7th ed.). Philadelphia: Lippincott Williams & Wilkins.

Farrell, J. (1990). *Nursing care of the older person.* Philadelphia: J.B. Lippincott.

Huston, C. (1996). Emergency! Ruptured esophageal varices. *American Journal of Nursing, 96 (4),* 43.

Matteson, M.A., McConnell, E.S., & Linton, A.D. (1997). *Gerontological nursing concepts and practice* (2nd ed.). Philadelphia: W.B. Saunders.

Ruth-Sahd, L. (1995). Emergency! Renal calculi. *American Journal of Nursing, 95 (11),* 50.

Smeltzer, S., & Bare, B. (1996). *Brunner and Suddarth's textbook of medical-surgical nursing.* Philadelphia: Lippincott-Raven Publishing.

Timby, B., Scherer, J. & Smith, N. (1999). *Introductory medical-surgical nursing* (7th ed.). Philadelphia: Lippincott Williams & Wilkins.

CHAPTER 22

The Genitourinary System

CHAPTER OUTLINE

KEY TERMS
CHAPTER OBJECTIVES
NORMAL GENITOURINARY FUNCTIONING
AGE-RELATED CHANGES OF THE GENITOURINARY TRACT
URINARY TRACT INFECTIONS
URINARY INCONTINENCE
NOSOCOMIAL URINARY TRACT INFECTIONS
BENIGN PROSTATIC HYPERPLASIA
PROSTATITIS
CANCER OF THE PROSTATE
RENAL FAILURE
CYSTOCELE
CRITICAL THINKING EXERCISES
REFERENCES AND SUGGESTED READING

KEY TERMS

acute renal failure
benign prostatic hyperplasia
chronic renal failure
cystitis
cystocele
glomerular filtration rate
glomerulus
nephrons
pessary
prostate gland
prostate-specific antigen
prostatitis
pyelonephritis
renal failure
urinary incontinence

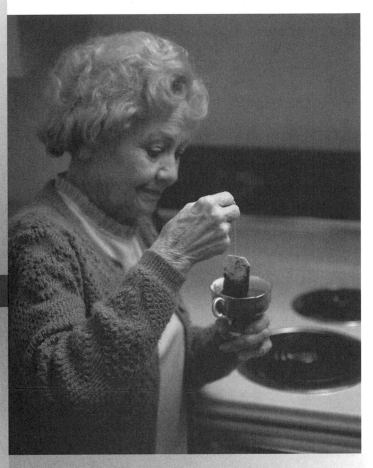

CHAPTER OBJECTIVES

At the completion of this chapter, the student will be able to

- Discuss normal genitourinary functioning

- Describe age-related changes that occur in the genitourinary system

- Discuss the signs and symptoms, diagnosis, and treatment of older adults with urinary tract infections, urinary incontinence, benign prostatic hyperplasia, prostatitis, cancer of the prostate, acute and chronic renal failure, and cystocele

- Use the nursing process to care for elderly patients with common disorders of the urinary tract

Genitourinary dysfunction presents many obstacles for the aging adult. The older adult suffering from urinary incontinence may be embarrassed and reluctant to discuss the issue. These adults may become socially isolated and virtually withdrawn from life. Other older adults may have decreased libido or sexual dysfunction as the result of medication or prostatectomy. These older adults present a challenge to gerontological nurses. Nurses must be sensitive, caring, and willing to devote the time needed to assist the older adult in dealing with these and other problems of the genitourinary tract. This chapter discusses normal genitourinary functioning, age-related changes, and genitourinary diseases common in the older adult.

NORMAL GENITOURINARY FUNCTIONING

The genitourinary system consists of the kidneys, the ureters, urinary bladder, and the urethra (Fig. 22-1). In the male, the prostate gland lies under the urinary bladder and encircles the first part of the urethra.

The kidneys remove waste products and unneeded substances from the blood to form urine. The two kidneys are located in the posterior portion of the abdomen, with one kidney on each side of the spine. The kidneys are highly vascular. Approximately 1.3 liters of blood pass through the kidneys each minute. Urine is formed within the nephrons of the kidney. The **nephron** is the functional unit of the kidney, and it filters blood, selectively reabsorbs substances needed by the body, and secretes unnecessary substances from the blood into the filtrate. Through selective reabsorption of water and electrolytes, the nephron helps to maintain fluid and electrolyte balance in the body.

The nephron is composed of the renal corpuscle, the proximal convoluted tubule, the descending and ascending loop of Henle, the distal convoluted tubule, and the collecting tubule. These tubes form a tiny coil with a bulb at one end called Bowman's capsule. The fluid travels through the pathway established by these tubules, where water and various substances needed by the body are reabsorbed into the blood. The water and waste products remaining in the tubules become urine.

The **glomerulus** is a mass of capillaries located in Bowman's capsule that function to bring blood to the nephron where urine formation begins. Glomerular filtration occurs as pressure forces water and substances through the thin membranes of the glomerulus into the nephron tubules. The resulting fluid is called the glomerular filtrate.

The **glomerular filtration rate** (GFR) is the amount of filtrate formed in the capsule each minute. The filtrate then travels through the nephron tubules. Approximately 160 liters of filtrate are formed daily by the kidneys. From this filtrate approximately 1 to 1.5 liters of urine are formed. Most of the fluid that passes into the filtrate is reabsorbed into the blood stream. Urea and nitrogenous wastes are retained in the tubules as urine. The urine goes to the renal pelvis for storage until it passes down the ureters (ie, tubes from the kidneys) into the urinary bladder (ie, the storage reservoir). A single tubule called the urethra allows the passage of urine from the bladder to the outside of the body.

In the male, the **prostate gland** surrounds the neck of the bladder and the urethra. It is a firm, chestnut-size structure that contains ducts through which secretions of the gland pass into the urethra. These alkaline secretions enhance the motility of the spermatozoa. The prostate gland contracts to aid in the ejaculation of seminal fluid (ie, mixture of sperm and other secretions from various glands of the male reproductive tract) from the body.

AGE-RELATED CHANGES OF THE GENITOURINARY TRACT

Each kidney contains approximately 1 million nephrons at birth. Beginning around the age of 40, there is a gradual decrease in size and number of nephrons. By the age of 80, up to 50% of the nephrons are lost. Although large numbers of nephrons are lost, each kidney requires only approximately 25% of its nephrons to maintain normal function. The membranes of the nephron thicken, and the vascular system degenerates with age. Rates of filtration, excretion, and reabsorption decline. A decline in the GFR predisposes the elderly person to problems excreting medications eliminated by the kidney.

The older adult is likely to have a higher renal threshold for glucose. An older adult may be able to "hold more sugar" in the blood before it spills over into the urine, causing glycosuria.

With age, the kidney has a decreased ability to concentrate urine because of the decreased number of nephrons. This diminished ability to concentrate urine can affect water balance. The elderly person is at increased risk for dehydration, particularly if the person is allowed nothing by mouth before a diagnostic examination or also has fever, diarrhea, or vomiting.

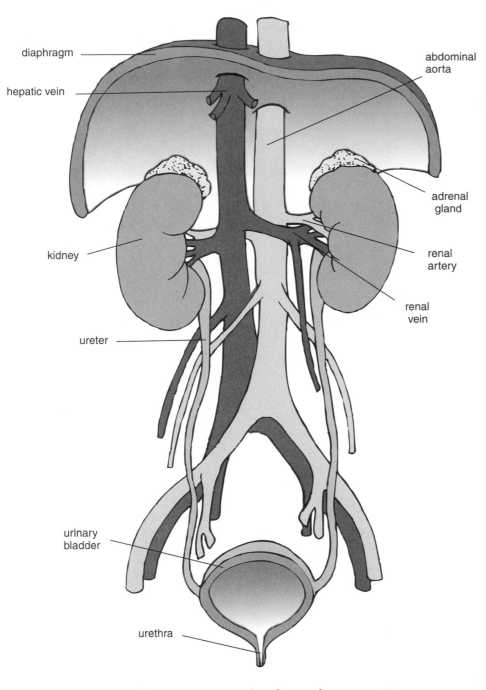

FIGURE 22-1. The urinary system, with blood vessels.

diaphragm

hepatic vein

kidney

ureter

urinary bladder

urethra

abdominal aorta

adrenal gland

renal artery

renal vein

The potential for dehydration is increased as the result of a decreased thirst sensation in the elderly.

Electrolyte imbalances may occur more rapidly in the elderly. Hyperkalemia (ie, high levels of potassium in the blood) or hyponatremia (ie, low sodium levels) can occur in part because of the decreased GFR. These changes in kidney function alter the renal excretion of drugs. Drugs that are excreted unchanged by the kidney are excreted more slowly, increasing the risk of the development of toxic drug levels. Drugs that are excreted more slowly, such as digitalis or the aminoglycosides, are prescribed at a reduced dose, or the dosing intervals are increased.

ASSESSMENT ALERT

When administrating medications eliminated by the kidney, creatinine clearance is used rather than serum creatinine levels. Serum creatinine levels may give a false indication of renal function and are not recommended for use to monitor renal function in the older adult. Creatinine clearance is a 24-hour urine collection that measures GFR (milliliters of filtrate made by the kidneys per minute). The GFR decreases with age and in certain disease conditions such as glomerulonephritis. The decreased GFR can affect the excretion of some drugs, causing toxic levels to build up in the blood.

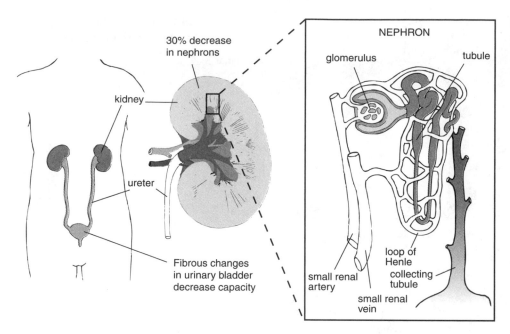

30% decrease in nephrons

kidney

ureter

Fibrous changes in urinary bladder decrease capacity

NEPHRON

glomerulus

tubule

small renal artery

loop of Henle

collecting tubule

small renal vein

FIGURE 22-2. Age-related changes in the urinary system.

The bladder is a muscular storage bag for urine. With age, the smooth muscle and elastic tissue of the bladder are replaced with fibrous tissue. Small sacs, or diverticula, can develop within the bladder as well. Capacity for holding urine is decreased, and there is incomplete emptying of the urine. The incomplete emptying of the bladder increases the risk for urinary tract infection. Figure 22-2 depicts changes in the genitourinary system that occur with age.

Men and women may have difficulty passing urine through the urethra because of problems opening the external sphincter because of a delay in the reflux that relaxes the sphincter. Childbearing may cause the pelvic floor muscles in the female to relax, resulting in leakage of urine with increased pressure from coughing, sneezing, or laughing. In the male, hyperplasia (ie, enlargement) of the prostate gland may cause obstruction of the flow of urine and increased pressure within the kidney. Permanent kidney damage can occur if this condition goes untreated.

URINARY TRACT INFECTIONS

Urinary tract infections (UTIs) are common in the older adult. Factors that increase the risk of an UTI with age include urinary stasis, institutionalization, sexual activity, and catheterization. Normal urine is sterile (ie, free of bacteria). Infection occurs when microorganisms begin to grow in the urethra, the bladder, or the kidneys. Most UTIs are caused by a common organism living in the colon, *Escherichia coli*. When *E. coli* leaves the colon and enters the urinary tract, a serious infection is likely to occur. Other organisms that can cause urinary infection include *Proteus, Enterobacter, Klebsiella, Pseudomonas,* and *Staphylococcus aureus.* An infection usually begins growing in the urethra, resulting in urethritis. The bacteria can travel up the urethra and enter the bladder, causing **cystitis** (ie, bladder infection). If cystitis is not treated, the infectious organism "crawls" up the narrow pathways of the ureters and invades the kidney, causing **pyelonephritis** (ie, infection of the kidney). Bacteria can also be pushed up the female urethra during sexual activity. If untreated, permanent damage to the urinary tract can occur. In general, the prognosis for a simple UTI is good. However, recurrence may occur especially in those elderly who are frail, debilitated, or have an indwelling urinary catheter.

Risk Factors

Some individuals are at greater risk for developing UTIs than others. Men with an enlarged prostate gland are at increased risk for infection from urinary retention and slowed urine flow. The elderly who have an indwelling Foley catheter or a suprapubic catheter are prone to UTIs. Bacteria on the catheter can travel to the bladder causing infection.

Individuals with diabetes have a higher risk of a UTI. In women, the incidence of UTI increases with age. The cause of this increase is unclear. In general, a woman's urethra is short, and the bacteria have only a short distance to travel to reach the ureter. The urethra's proximity to the anus and the vagina may also contribute to the increased incidence of

UTIs in women. For many women, sexual intercourse triggers a urinary infection.

Signs and Symptoms

Some individuals with a UTI may be asymptomatic. Other, more common symptoms may occur that are usually related to urination. These symptoms are identified in Display 22-1.

Even though the urge to void occurs frequently, only small amounts of urine may be excreted. The urine may appear milky, cloudy, or reddish (if blood is present). Nausea and vomiting may be experienced.

Diagnosis

Diagnosis is made by a laboratory analysis of a urine sample. Accurate diagnosis depends on a properly obtained urine specimen and culture. The urine is examined microscopically for bacteria identification and growth. Antibiotic sensitivity is identified 24 to 48 hours after the specimen is collected. If the individual shows signs of a UTI and has pyuria but the culture fails to identify offending bacteria, the physician may suspect *Chlamydia* or *Mycoplasma.* The two organisms can only be identified with a special culture. In some situations, additional diagnostic measures may be needed such as an ultrasound, intravenous pyelogram (IVP), or a cystoscopy.

Management

UTIs are treated with an antibiotic. The choice of drug depends on the culture and sensitivity tests that identify the offending bacteria and the drugs to which the organism is sensitive. The most commonly used drugs to treat UTIs are trimethoprim-sulfamethoxazole (TMP-SMZ, Bactrim, Septra), trimethoprim (Trimpex), amoxicillin (Amoxil, Trimox), nitrofurantoin (Furadantin), and ampicillin. Table 22-1 provides more information about drugs used to treat UTIs.

After taking the antibiotics for 1 to 2 days, the symptoms may subside. However, infection may recur if the antibiotics are discontinued before the full course of treatment (usually 10 days to 22 weeks) is completed. Longer treatment with tetracycline, TMP-SMZ, or doxycycline is required for a UTI caused by *Mycoplasma* or *Chlamydia.* After the full treatment regimen recommended by the health care provider is completed, a follow-up urinalysis may be done to confirm that the urinary tract is infection free. Recurrent UTIs may be treated with

---

DISPLAY 22-1. Symptoms of Urinary Tract Infections

- Pain and discomfort when urinating (burning, itching)
- Frequent urination (especially at night)
- Urethral discharge (usually clear but may contain a small amount of pus)
- Generalized feelings of malaise
- Women may feel discomfort or pressure above the pubic bone
- Men may experience a feeling of fullness in the rectum
- Generalized abdominal pain
- Fever
- Blood in the urine
- Back pain (low back pain is associated with prostatitis; high back pain is associated with kidney infection)

TMP-SMZ or nitrofurantoin for at least 6 months or a 1- to 2-day antibiotic treatment regimen when symptoms of UTI appear.

Using the Nursing Process to Care for the Older Adult With a Urinary Tract Infection

Assessment

When assessing a person for a UTI, careful questioning is necessary to obtain accurate information. If the elderly person is confused, the nurse verifies the answers obtained in the interview with the caregiver or a family member. It is important to question the patient concerning the type of pain, the location of the pain, frequency of urination, amount of urine excreted, and the color and odor of the urine. The nurse obtains a clean catch urine specimen to be sent to the laboratory for a culture and sensitivity analysis. The nurse takes the vital signs for baseline comparisons. The presence and location of any back pain, nausea, or malaise are documented. Assessment is more complicated if the patient is confused and unable to recognize or communicate the pain, discomfort, or problems with urination.

ASSESSMENT ALERT

Patients in the nursing home must be monitored closely for UTI. Sometimes, no specific symptoms are experienced except generalized weakness and fatigue. At other times, the classic symptoms are present. The nurse must be alert for signs and symptoms of UTI in all patients, particularly those who are frail, chronically ill, or have an indwelling catheter.

TABLE 22-1. Drugs Used to Treat Urinary Tract Infections

Drug	Nursing Considerations
trimethoprim (Proloprim, Trimpex)	For geriatric patients or those with renal impairment, do not administer if creatinine clearance is less than 15 mL/min.
	Monitor for adverse reactions: epigastric pain, rash, fever, distress, nausea, vomiting, pruritus, thrombocytopenia, leukopenia, and neutropenia.
	Take the full-dosage regimen prescribed.
	The 200-mg tablets must be protected from light.
	Monitor blood counts periodically during therapy.
	Administer 1 hour before or 2 hours after meals.
sulfamethoxazole (Gantanol)	Administer the drug on an empty stomach 1 hour before or 2 hours after meal with a full glass of water.
	Monitor for the following adverse reactions: nausea, vomiting, rash, fever, dizziness, ataxia, depression, confusion, crystalluria, photosensitivity, superinfection, hypersensitivity reactions, aplastic anemia, and agranulocytosis.
	Instruct the patient to use sunscreen and protective clothing to prevent photosensitivity reactions.
	Report unusual bleeding or bruising, sore throat, chills, fever, or rash.
	If the elder has difficulty swallowing, tablets may be crushed and taken with any fluid.
	Fluid intake should be approximately 1,500 to 2,000 mL/day to prevent crystalluria.
amoxicillin (Amoxil)	Give 1 hour before or 2 hours after meals. Absorption is delayed if administered with food. The drug is available only as an oral preparation.
	Monitor for the following adverse reactions: glossitis, stomatitis, gastritis, sore mouth, furry tongue, nausea, vomiting, diarrhea, abdominal pain, pseudomembranous colitis, anemia, blood dyscrasias, rash, and fever.
	Obtain a urine culture before beginning therapy.
	Report unusual bleeding or bruising, sore throat, fever, rash, severe diarrhea, or difficulty swallowing.
ampicillin (Principen)	Available for administering IV, IM, or PO.
nitrofurantoin (Furadantin, Macrobid)	Use cautiously in diabetic patients. May worsen peripheral neuropathy.
	Monitor for the following adverse reactions: nausea, vomiting, anorexia, dizziness, headache, drowsiness, nystagmus, chest pain, diarrhea, abdominal pain, rust-brown discoloration of urine, photosensitivity, and blood dyscrasias.
	Administer with food or milk to minimize gastrointestinal irritation.
	Do not crush tablets. Oral preparations may be mixed with water, milk, or fruit juice.
	Rinse mouth with water after administering oral preparation.
	Inform the patient that urine may turn rust-yellow to brown.
	Instruct the patient to use a sunscreen and wear protective clothing when exposed to the sun.
trimethoprim-sulfamethoxazole (Bactrim, Septra, Sulfatrim)	Obtain urine for culture and sensitivity before beginning therapy.
	Report the following adverse reactions: nausea, vomiting, rash, phlebitis at the IV site, allergic reactions, photosensitivity, diarrhea, insomnia, fatigue, depression, and hallucinations.
	Inspect the IV site frequently for signs of inflammation, redness, or pain.
	Administer 1 hour before or 2 hours after meals.
	Instruct the patient to use a sunscreen and wear protective clothing when exposed to the sun.

Nursing Diagnoses

The following nursing diagnoses are used for a patient with a urinary tract infection:

Pain related to localized inflammation, discomfort, infection

Alteration in Urinary Elimination Patterns related to inflammation, pain, need to urinate frequently

Risk for Ineffective Management of Therapeutic Regimen related to lack of knowledge regarding disease process, therapeutic regimen, prevention of recurrent UTIs

Other nursing diagnoses may be appropriate for individual patients.

Planning and Implementation

In planning the care for a patient with a UTI, the nurse must carefully monitor the patient, voiding patterns, and amount and clarity of the urine. Vital signs are taken every 4 hours, and any abnormality is reported. The older adult may not report the typical symptoms of a UTI, making careful monitoring essential. For example, the elderly patient may not exhibit an elevated temperature. Even a slight temperature elevation may be significant. Behavior changes may indicate the beginning of an infection or an exacerbation of an existing infection. Any change in the patient's condition is reported.

Pain. The nurse informs the patient that the discomfort will diminish after the infection is under control (1 to 2 days). Warm sitz baths are used to relieve discomfort. The nurse observes the patient for reduction of pain, decreased urinary cloudiness, and the presence of an odor. Any recurrence of symptoms is reported. It is important to monitor for adverse reactions to antibiotic therapy (see Table 22-1). The nurse encourages the patient to drink fluids (3,000 mL/day) if the patient's condition permits. Phenazopyridine (Pyridium) acts as a local analgesic and may be given to provide symptomatic relief of pain, itching, or burning. If phenazopyridine is administered, the nurse informs the patient that the urine may be an orange-red color and can stain clothing. A sanitary napkin can be used to protect clothing.

Altered Urinary Elimination Pattern. With a UTI, the patient may experience a disturbance in elimination. The urge to void may be persistent, yet only small amounts of urine is excreted. The nurse explains to the patient the importance of emptying the bladder completely when urinating. The previous pattern of elimination is determined and compared with the current pattern. The bladder may be palpated to assess retention. Fluids up to 3,000 mL/day (if the patient can tolerate this) are encouraged to provide a natural bladder irrigation. It is important to develop toileting routines or offer the bedpan at regular intervals. Some physicians recommend cranberry juice to acidify the urine. In these cases, offer cranberry juice at frequent intervals (eg, every 1 to 2 hours).

For patients with an indwelling catheter, the nurse keeps a record of fluid intake and output. The color and odor of urinary output is monitored. The catheter is removed as soon as possible to reestablish a normal voiding pattern. The nurse is careful to keep the catheter drainage tubing positioned in a way that facilitates drainage. The system is not broken when obtaining a specimen for laboratory analysis; urine is removed from the collection port on the tubing.

Patient and Family Teaching

The nurse instructs the patient and family members on the disease process, ways to prevent recurrent infection, and the treatment regimen. It is important to emphasize that a few simple life changes can help prevent future UTIs. A patient and family teaching plan about UTIs should include an explanation of the treatment plan, as well as advice about medication.

PATIENT AND FAMILY TEACHING AID

Information to be included when teaching the patient or family about UTIs:

- **Explain the disease and treatment regimen.**
- **Take medication exactly as prescribed by the primary care giver. Do not stop the medication when the symptoms subside or the infection may recur.**
- **Empty the bladder whenever the urge to urinate is present. Females should void after sexual activity.**
- **Drink 6 to 8 glasses of water daily.**
- **Avoid spicy foods, caffeine, and alcohol, which aggravate a UTI.**
- **Drink cranberry juice at frequent intervals (every 1 to 2 hours) during the day.**
- **Always clean after urinating or defecating by wiping from front to back.**
- **Keep follow-up appointments with the primary care giver.**
- **Report any return of symptoms or any adverse drug effects immediately.**
- **If possible, take showers instead of tub baths.**
- **Avoid using feminine hygiene sprays, bubble baths, or scented douches, which may irritate the urethra.**

Evaluation and Expected Outcomes

Successful treatment can be gauged by the following responses:

Pain is decreased or eliminated.

Normal elimination patterns are restored.

Patient expresses knowledge of disease process, treatment regimen, and ways to prevent recurrent UTIs.

DISPLAY 22-2. Types of Incontinence

Type of Incontinence	Description
Stress incontinence	Involuntary loss of urine as the result of a sudden increase in intra-abdominal pressure; caused by damage to the pelvic muscles; occurs with exercise, coughing, sneezing, or laughing
Urge incontinence	Occurs when the patient is able to sense the need to void but is unable to hold urine long enough to reach the toilet. The urge to void cannot be consciously stopped.
Overflow incontinence	Frequent loss of urine from the bladder that occurs because the amount of urine exceeds the bladder's capacity
Functional incontinence	Patient is unable to identify the need to void as the result of cognitive or physical impairment.
Surgical incontinence	Occurs after surgical procedures such as hysterectomy, prostatectomy, lower intestinal surgery, or rectal surgery
Mixed incontinence	Incontinence as the result of a combination of several physical or functional problems

---

URINARY INCONTINENCE

Causes and Diagnosis

Urinary incontinence, or loss of bladder control, is a symptom not a disease. Normally, the bladder holds urine until the volume of urine in the bladder is approximately 250 to 400 mL (less in the older adult). When the volume of urine is sufficient the micturition reflex is activated causing the bladder to contract. Approximately 50% of older adults living at home or in nursing homes are incontinent. Of those affected by incontinence, approximately 80% can be helped. Diagnostic examinations include radiographs, cystoscopy, blood tests, urinalysis, and tests to determine bladder capacity, sphincter control, and residual urine. The method of treatment depends on the cause of the incontinence. In the elderly, the most common cause of urinary incontinence is detrusor muscle (ie, muscular layer in the bladder) instability, causing abnormal bladder contractions. Display 22-2 lists the various types of incontinence. Incontinence can be transitory or established. Until proven otherwise, incontinence is considered treatable. Causes of incontinence include weakness of the pelvic floor, benign prostatic hyperplasia, impaired mobility, certain drugs (Display 22-3), and pathologic conditions such as infection, fecal impaction, hyperglycemia, and delirium. Treatment of the cause can eliminate the incontinence. For example, treating an urinary tract infection can eliminate incontinence caused by the infection.

Older adults should be encouraged to see the physician or primary health care provider for specific treatment. At times, the older adult may feel embarrassed to discuss the problem of incontinence or feel that nothing can be done. Actively listen and

DISPLAY 22-3. Drugs That Can Cause Urinary Incontinence

chlordiazepoxide (Librium)
clonidine (Catapres)
diazepam (Valium)
digitalis (Lanoxin)
furosemide (Lasix)
isoproterenol (Isuprel)
levodopa (L-dopa, Larodopa)
lithium (Lithotabs, Lithane)
methadone (Methadose, Dolophine)
metronidazole (Flagyl)
neostigmine (Prostigmin)
phenytoin (Dilantin)
terbutaline (Brethine)
valproic acid (Depakene)
vasopressin (Pitressin)

provide a sympathetic response to the patient's fears and concerns. The problem of incontinence can cause the older adult to be reluctant to socialize with others because of embarrassment or anxiety.

If the patient is alert, the nurse asks the patient keep a voiding record for 4 or 5 days. It the patient is unable to do so, the nurse records the time and amount the person voids. A log is kept of the solid and liquid foods consumed. The nurse notes the medications taken and the times of administration. Simple dietary changes or discontinuing or reducing the dosages of certain medications sometimes can help relieve the incontinence.

Treatment

Treatment includes behavioral strategies, medications, or surgery. Behavior strategies includes scheduled toileting (ie, placing the person on a regular voiding schedule every 2 to 4 hours), bladder retraining, and Kegel exercises (see Chapter 14). Medications such as oxybutynin (Ditropan) may be used to treat incontinence. Oxybutynin is a urinary antispasmodic and can be used to treat neurogenic bladder. Side effects include drowsiness, dizziness, blurred vision, dry mouth, nausea, urinary hesitancy, and retention. Surgical treatment can be performed if nonsurgical methods fail to achieve the desired results. Another drug, tolterodine tartrate (Detrol), may be administered to patients with an overactive bladder with symptoms of urinary frequency, urgency, or urge incontinence. The drug is given orally with or without food. The usual dosage is 2 mg twice each day. Patients with significantly reduced hepatic function should not take more than 1 mg twice daily. Adverse reactions of tolterodine include dry mouth, constipation, visual difficulties, and urinary retention. Procedures that are used to treat urinary incontinence include bladder neck suspension, collagen injections around the urethra, and surgical creation of an artificial urinary sphincter.

Urinary retention or failure to empty the bladder increases the possibility of infection. Increasing fluids helps to keep urine diluted and decreases possibility of infection. The nurse must note the color and clarity of urine. Cloudiness or reddish urine is reported to the physician. Vital signs are monitored for increase in temperature. It is important for the nurse to palpate bladder and report any bladder distention. Antibiotics are administered to treat infection. Incontinence is not an inevitable change of aging; it most often is a reversible condition common in older adults. Chapter 14 provides additional information concerning incontinence and the nursing interventions used to manage this common disorder.

NOSOCOMIAL URINARY TRACT INFECTIONS

UTIs are the most common type of nosocomial (ie, hospital-acquired) infection. Nosocomial UTIs occur most often in patients with indwelling Foley catheters. The catheter irritates the cells of the urethra and bladder making them more vulnerable to bacterial invasion. The catheter may allow a residual pool of urine in the bladder that fosters bacterial colonization. Improper hand washing, breaking, or disconnecting the catheter tubing to obtain a specimen or irrigating the catheter can increase the risk of

---

DISPLAY 22-4. Ways to Help Prevent Institutionally Acquired Urinary Tract Infections

- Always wash hands between patients and when hands become contaminated.
- Monitor the patient for chills, fever, dysuria, frequent or painful urination, back pain, and tenderness over the bladder.
- Catheterize only if absolutely necessary, not for the convenience of the nursing staff.
- Begin a bladder training program as soon as feasible.
- If catheterization is necessary, use aseptic technique.
- Maintain a closed, sterile drainage system.
- Only obtain urine specimens using the sample port.
- Keep catheter bag below the level of the bladder.
- Provide good meatal care at least twice each day with soap and water.
- Use gloves when emptying the drainage bag.
- Monitor intake and output.
- Document color, amount, and odor of urine.

---

infection. Diagnosis, as for all of UTIs, is based on culture and sensitivity study results to determine the causative organism and the antibiotic that can destroy the organism.

Institutionally acquired UTIs are a significant problem in nursing homes and acute care facilities, especially in patients with Foley catheters. Display 22-4 identifies ways to help prevent institutional acquired UTIs.

BENIGN PROSTATIC HYPERPLASIA

Benign prostatic hyperplasia (BPH) is a common disorder in the aging man. BPH is a nonmalignant enlargement of the prostate gland that constricts the urethra and causes various degrees of urinary flow restriction. By age 60, more than 50% of men have some degree of prostatic hyperplasia. Approximately one of four men experiences symptoms of BPH that require treatment by the age of 80.

Signs and Symptoms

Symptoms of BPH develop slowly. At first, the patient may notice a narrowing of the urinary stream or difficulty initiating a stream. Other symptoms include urinary frequency, nocturia, urgency, straining to urinate, hesitancy, weak or intermittent urinary stream, and a sensation of incomplete emptying. Untreated BPH can result in renal insufficiency, urinary tract infections, gross hematuria, or bladder stones.

Diagnostic Evaluation

After obtaining a medical history focusing on the urinary tract, the physician performs a digital rectal examination (Fig. 22-3). Other diagnostic procedures are a urinalysis, serum creatinine, creatinine clearance, uroflowmetry, postvoid residual urine, pressure-flow studies, and prostate ultrasound.

Management

Watchful Waiting and Surgery
If the patient is asymptomatic, no treatment is generally required. "Watchful waiting" is the treatment of choice for most patients exhibiting no or few symptoms. Careful medical follow-up on a yearly basis is appropriate. If symptoms develop the primary care giver is notified. BPH usually progresses slowly, allowing the option to watch and wait.

Surgery can alleviate the symptoms of BPH. Two operations are commonly used: transurethral resection of the prostate (TURP) and transurethral incision of the prostate (TUIP). Although TURP is the most common procedure, TUIP is just as effective in most cases. TURP is the removal of the hypertrophied prostate tissue by means of an endoscope passed through the urethra. With TURP, only the hypertrophied tissue is chipped off and washed out by an irrigating solution leaving only normal prostatic tissue and the outer capsule intact. TURP requires no incision and a short hospital stay.

TUIP is the most effective when removing prostate tissue weighing 30 g or less. In TUIP, the endoscope is passed through the urethra to the prostate gland, where one or two incisions are made on the prostate and the prostate capsule to reduce pressure on the urethra and relieve the constriction. An advantage of TUIP is that it can be done on an outpatient basis. Fewer complications are experienced with TUIP. TURP and TUIP may need to be repeated if the prostate gland again enlarges and constricts the urethra. Prostatectomy is performed when the prostate tissue is greatly hypertrophied. Display 22-5 discusses different types of prostatectomies.

Drug Therapy
The alpha$_1$-adrenergic blocking drugs are used to relieve the symptoms of BPH. One such drug is tera-

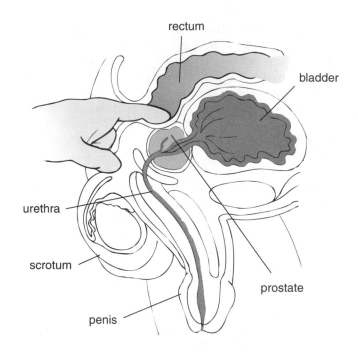

One important way doctors check for prostate abnormalities is by inserting a rubber-gloved finger into the rectum, where the prostate can be explored by touch. The exam is performed with the patient in a bent-over position.

FIGURE 22-3. Digital rectal exam. From *Prostate Cancer: New Tests Create Treatment Dilemmas.* (1995). Department of Health and Human Services, Food and Drug Administration, HFI-40, Rockville, MD, 20857. Pub. No. 95-1220 (FDA).

zosin (Hytrin), which decreases contractions in smooth muscle of the prostate capsules, decreasing the symptoms of prostatic hypertrophy. Side effects include dizziness, weakness, headache, palpations, nasal congestion, blurred vision, nausea, and vomiting. The first dose should be administered just before bedtime to lessen likelihood of fainting, postural hypotension, and dizziness.

Tamsulosin HCl (Flomax) is another alpha-adrenergic blocking drug used to treat men with an enlarged prostate. This drug helps to relieve the signs and symptoms of BPH. Because an enlarged prostate and cancer of the prostate cause many of the same symptoms, it is important to exclude cancer of the prostate before administering any drug for BPH. Tamsulosin (0.4 mg) is given once daily, approximately one-half hour after the same meal each day. The physician may increase the dosage to 0.8 mg daily if it is needed for a therapeutic response. Common adverse reactions include orthostatic hypotension,

DISPLAY 22-5. Surgeries Commonly Performed for Prostate Cancer

Types	Characteristics
Perineal prostatectomy	Removal of the gland through an incision in the perineum between the scrotum and the rectum. Used for large tumors located low in the pelvic area. May result in impotence or incontinence. Location of incision near the rectum may complicate healing because of contamination.
Retropubic prostatectomy	Prostate gland is removed through a low abdominal incision. Suitable for large glands located high in the pelvis. Hemorrhage and infection of incisional site may occur.
Suprapubic prostatectomy	Removal of the prostate gland through an abdominal incision made in the bladder. This technique provides a wide area of exploration during procedure. Hemorrhage may occur. Indicated for tumors weighing more than 60 g.
Transurethral resection of the prostate (TURP)	Prostate tissue is removed by means of an endoscope inserted through the urethra. The gland is removed in small pieces with an electrical cutting device. No incision is required. Rarely causes erectile dysfunction. May cause retrograde ejaculation, causing seminal fluid to flow out through the bladder and giving urine a cloudy appearance.

dizziness, fainting, decrease in amount of semen, rhinitis (ie, stuffy nose), and headache.

Finasteride (Proscar) is also used for long-term symptomatic relief of BPH. The drug is taken orally once daily to reduce the size of the prostate gland. At least 6 to 12 months of therapy may be needed before a therapeutic response is observed. Side effects include decreased libido, impotence, abdominal upset, and decreased volume of ejaculation.

Using the Nursing Process to Care for an Older Adult With Benign Prostatic Hyperplasia

Assessment

When assessing for BPH, the nurse questions the patient about urinary patterns including frequency of urination, hesitancy, inability to empty bladder, dysuria, or nocturia. The patient may report a decrease in the force of ejaculation and concerns about the effects of the disorder on sexuality. It is important to identify any medications that may contribute to problems with urination, such as antihypertensives, antidepressants, or over-the-counter cold or allergy medications. The nurse determines color and clarity of urine. Urine may be cloudy, concentrated, or may be dark or a reddish color. Urine should be analyzed microscopically in the laboratory.

Nursing Diagnoses

The following nursing diagnoses are used for patients with BPH:

Altered Urinary Elimination related to enlarged prostate

Pain related to bladder distention

Anxiety related to inability to void, sexual dysfunction, change in health status other (specify)

Risk of Ineffective Management of Therapeutic Regimen related to lack of knowledge about the disease process, prognosis, or treatment regimen

Other nursing diagnoses may be appropriate for individual patients.

Planning and Implementation

In planning the care for the patient with BPH, the nurse strives to maintain normal urinary elimination, relieve pain, reduce anxiety, and provide patient teaching concerning the disease process and treatment regimen.

Altered Urinary Elimination and Pain. To prevent urinary distention, the patient is encouraged to void every 2 hours. The nurse documents the force and size of urinary stream at each voiding. The patient is assessed for pain in the abdominal area and when voiding. The nurse monitors the intake and output. Fluids (up to 2 L/day) are encouraged if medical condition permits. Fluids may be restricted in the evening if nocturia is a problem. Vital signs are monitored closely. The nurse reports any abnormalities of the vital signs.

Warm sitz baths may relieve pain and promote muscle relaxation. The bladder may be palpated to check for distention. Catheterization is prescribed if the patient is unable to void or to determine amount of residual urine. It is important to provide privacy and easy access to the toilet. Some elderly may need assistance in ambulating to the bathroom.

Antispasmodics (eg, oxybutynin) may be administered to relieve bladder spasms. Alpha$_1$-adrenergic blocking drugs (eg, terazocin) may be administered to provide symptomatic relief. The nurse monitors and reports any side effects of terazocin (eg, dizziness, hypotension, weakness, headache, edema, nausea, nasal congestion). The initial dose is administered before bedtime to minimize effects of dizziness and orthostatic hypotension. Subsequent doses may be administered at bedtime if dizziness or orthostatic hypotension persists. The blood pressure is monitored before administering drugs. The physician or primary care giver is notified of a significant change.

Anxiety. Men with BPH may be anxious because of the change in health status, the inability to void, or a fear of sexual dysfunction. The nurse should be available to answer questions, provide accurate information, and listen to the patient's anxieties and fears. It is important to encourage verbalization of these fears and actively listen as the patient speaks. The nurse needs to maintain a trusting and open relationship.

Any decrease in sexual desire or impotence should be reported to the primary care giver. The patient may need assistance to identify alternative ways of sexual expression. The patient is informed that certain medications (eg, finasteride) may affect sexual functioning. Medication may need to be changed or the patient referred to a nurse practitioner, clinical nurse specialist, or a professional counselor.

Patient and Family Teaching

A lack of knowledge of the disease process and treatment regimen can contribute to anxiety and noncompliance. A teaching plan for BPH should include the following: information concerning the disease process, a discussion of sexual concerns, and the importance of following the treatment regimen.

PATIENT TEACHING AID

Information to include in a teaching program for BPH:

- **Provide specific information concerning the disease process and the medication or treatment regimen.**
- **Discuss sexual concerns. Sexual activity may increase pain during an acute episode of urinary retention. However, frequent ejaculation may help to decrease discomfort in chronic disease.**
- **Discuss concerns and fears to correct any misconceptions and give accurate information.**
- **Emphasize contacting the primary health care provider if unable to void or symptoms worsen.**
- **Emphasize the importance of following the treatment regimen and keeping follow-up appointments with the health care provider.**
- **Drugs must be taken as directed at the same time each day. If a dose is missed, the patient should take it immediately but not double the dose.**

DRUG ALERT

Inform patients of the possible side effects of the following drugs commonly used to treat BPH:

Terazocin (Hytrin)

- **This drug may cause orthostatic hypotension or dizziness. The initial dose should be taken at bedtime to minimize the dizziness and orthostatic hypotension that may occur with this drug. Subsequent doses may also be taken at bedtime if these symptoms persist. Instruct the patient to weigh twice each week and check feet, ankles, and fingers for fluid retention. The patient should avoid the use of over-the-counter drugs unless approved by health care provider. The physician is notified if fainting or dizziness persists or if edema is noted.**

Tamsulosin (Flomax)

- **Inform the patient of the possibility of orthostatic hypotension. The patient should rise slowly from a sitting to a standing position. The physician is notified if fainting or dizziness persists. Caution should be exerted when driving.**

Finasteride (Proscar)

- **This drug must be taken for 6 to 12 months before symptoms improve.**
- **Alert the male that libido may decrease. The volume of ejaculate may also decrease.**

Evaluation and Expected Outcomes

Successful treatment can be gauged by the following responses:

Normal urination pattern is maintained.
Pain is relieved.
No evidence of infection is seen.
Anxiety is decreased.
Patient expresses knowledge of the disease process and treatment regimen.

PROSTATITIS

Prostatitis is inflammation of the prostate gland. It can be acute or chronic. Acute prostatitis is most often caused by a bacterial infection from one of several organisms, but most commonly *E. coli*. Organisms on the urethra meatus can quickly ascend to the prostate gland and cause infection. Chronic prostatitis can lead to recurrent UTIs and is found in approximately 35% of men older than age 50.

Symptoms and Diagnosis

Symptoms of acute prostatitis include sudden fever, chills, and perineal, rectal, or low back pain and urinary symptoms such as burning frequency, urgency, and nocturia. The prostate gland may be tender, firm, and warm to the touch. Chronic prostatitis is more difficult to recognize. Some patients may be asymptomatic, but most exhibit symptoms similar to acute prostatitis except to a lesser degree. Diagnosis is made by rectal examination, reported symptoms of prostatitis, and bacterial urine culture identifying the offending organism. After the organism is identified, appropriate antibiotic therapy can be started.

Management

Antibiotic therapy is administered for 10 to 14 days. If chronic infection of the prostate gland is a problem, continuous low-dose antibiotic therapy may be indicated. Nursing care is mainly supportive. Warm sitz baths, stool softeners, and administration of analgesics can provide some relief of the discomfort.

Patient and Family Teaching

Many patients with prostatitis are treated in the outpatient setting, making patient education an important part of care. Instructions to the patient with prostatitis should stress the importance of strict adherence to prescribed medication regimens.

PATIENT TEACHING AID

Information to include when teaching patients with prostatitis:

- **Follow medication regimen exactly as prescribed by primary caregiver.**
- **Keep all follow-up appointments and immediately report any increase or recurrence of symptoms.**
- **Take warm sitz baths two or three times each day for 20 minutes.**
- **During acute attacks, avoid sexual intercourse. In cases of chronic prostatitis, sexual intercourse may help relieve discomfort from prostatic fluids.**

CANCER OF THE PROSTATE

More than 75% of the cases of prostate cancer are men age 65 or older. Cancer of the prostate is the sec-ond most common cancer in men. Fewer than 10% of the cases occur before the age of 50. This cancer rarely results from BPH that commonly affects the older male.

Typically, cancer of the prostate is slow growing, with few signs and symptoms until it is in advanced stages. As the malignancy spreads, symptoms of back or hip pain may occur, indicating that the cancer has metastasized to the bone. In advanced disease, edema of the scrotum or the leg may occur.

Early Detection

Prostate-specific antigen (PSA) is a laboratory blood test that measures a protein made only by the prostate gland. Normally, a small amount of PSA is found in the blood. Higher blood levels of PSA may be found in prostatic hypertrophy, infection of the prostate, or prostatic cancer.

✓ ASSESSMENT ALERT

An elevated PSA level alerts the caregiver that there is a problem occurring with the prostate gland. Normal PSA findings are values less than 4 ng/mL. In general, levels are greatly increased in men with prostate cancer.

PSA may also be used to monitor the patients response to therapy and recurrence of the cancer after treatment. Some men undergoing treatment for BPH may have low or normal PSA levels.

Because a PSA may indicate problems other than malignancy, a digital rectal examination (DRE) is also done. The physician palpates the prostate gland by inserting a gloved, well-lubricated finger into the rectum, where the prostate can be palpated (see Fig. 22-3). When a suspicious area is identified by DRE, a biopsy is performed. The DRE is the most commonly used and cost-effective assessment of the prostatic gland. Other diagnostic examinations include transrectal ultrasonography, magnetic resonance imaging (MRI), and computed tomography (CT).

Medical Management

After the diagnosis of malignancy is established a choice is made to treat the disorder with surgery, radiation therapy, or hormonal therapy or to watch and monitor the patient. Surgical removal of the

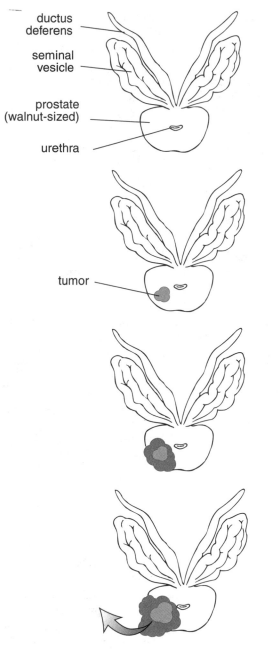

Stage A

Tumor is microscopic and confined to the prostate. Doctor cannot feel it and it causes no symptoms.

Stage B

Tumor is confined to only one side of the prostate and is smaller than 3/5 inch. (Stage B2: Cancer is found on both sides of the prostate and exceeds 4/5 inch.)

Stage C

Cancer has penetrated the prostate covering (capsule) or spread more extensively beyond the prostate wall to surrounding tissue. The glands that produce semen (seminal vesicles) may be involved.

Stage D

Cancer has spread to pelvic lymph nodes or to organs distant from the prostate. At this stage, cancer is rarely curable.

FIGURE 22-4. Prostate cancer stages. From *Prostate Cancer: New Tests Create Treatment Dilemmas.* (1995). Department of Health and Human Services, Food and Drug Administration, HFI-40, Rockville, MD, 20857. Pub. No. 95-1220 (FDA).

prostate (ie, prostatectomy) can result in complications related to bladder or sexual functioning such as incontinence or impotency. For men in their late sixties with small tumors, some physicians are advocating a philosophy of watchful waiting. Proponents of the watchful waiting philosophy point out that the trauma and adverse effects of surgery or irradiation could outweigh the benefits, especially because the older men are more likely to have cardiac and respiratory problems.

Some cases of prostatic cancer are treated by orchiectomy (ie, surgical removal of the testes) and the administration of oral estrogens. Tumors of the prostate gland are stimulated by androgens (ie, male hormones). Removal of the testes decreases andro-gen levels and inhibits tumor growth. Administration of oral estrogens such as diethylstilbestrol (DES) also decreases androgen levels, inhibits tumor growth, and decreases pain.

Staging

Staging is the method of categorizing tremors according to the extent of the disease and the organs involved (Fig. 22-4). Stages range from stage A, in which the tumor is microscopic and confined to the prostate, to stage D, in which the cancer has metastasized to other areas of the body. In general, the lower the stage the better the prognosis.

Nursing Management

Nursing management depends on the type of treatment prescribed. It is important to provide clear accurate explanations of the disease process and the treatment regimen. The patient is encouraged to express feelings and concerns. Concerns about sexual functioning and are often of utmost importance to the man. The American Cancer Society has a publication entitled *Sexuality & Cancer* for the man with cancer and his partner that provides good information, particularly concerning sexual issues and offers practical suggestions to help alleviate certain associated problems. Display 22-6 provides information on how to obtain this booklet and other resources. The patient must be made aware of the possibility of impotence, dribbling of urine, or incontinence with surgery. In general, impotence occurs when perineal nerves are cut during radical procedures (see Display 22-5).

In surgeries that do not involve the prostate capsule, impotence and sterility do not usually occur. Sexual activity may be resumed in 6 to 8 weeks after less radical procedures. A penile prosthesis may be used to correct problems with obtaining an erection after prostatectomy.

If metastasis has occurred, pain may be a concern. The nurse evaluates pain and effectiveness of analgesics. The patient is questioned for signs of urinary dysfunction. The nurse monitors urinary intake and output. PSA levels may be used to monitor the patient's response to therapy and detect early recurrence.

If radiation therapy is used, the patient is monitored for adverse effects such as prostatitis, diarrhea, urinary frequency, bladder spasms, and rectal irritation. The patient is encouraged to increase fluids (up to 2 to 3 L/day) unless the patient's condition prohibits. Analgesics are administered for pain, and antispasmodics are given to relieve the discomfort of bladder spasms.

If cancer of the prostate is treated with hormonal therapy, the patient is monitored for adverse reactions such as fluid retention, nausea, vomiting, gynecomastia (ie, breast enlargement), and decreased libido. Hormonal therapy with DES increases the risk of thromboembolism, myocardial infarction, and stroke.

RENAL FAILURE

Renal failure is a condition in which the kidneys fail to excrete waste, concentrate urine, and main-

---

DISPLAY 22-6. Resources for Patients With Urinary Disorders

American Cancer Society
1-800-ACS-2345
Request the following brochures: *Facts on Prostate Cancer* and *Sexuality & Cancer For the Man Who Has Cancer, and His Partner.*
Other pamphlets and brochures are available.

American Foundation for Urologic Disease
Request booklet *Prostate Cancer: What Every Man Over 40 Should Know.*
1-800-242-2383
Other pamphlets and brochures are available.

Mathews Foundation for Prostate Cancer Research
1-800-234-6284
Request information on prostate cancer. Trained personnel are available to answer questions.

Us Too
Subscribe to a monthly newsletter for prostate cancer survivors.
1-800-828-7866

National Association for Continence (NAFC)
1-800-BLADDER

National Kidney and Urologic Disease Information Clearinghouse
301-468-6345
Box NKUDIC, 9000
Rockville Pike
Bethesda, MD 20892

---

tain electrolyte and water balance. The two types of renal failure are acute renal failure and chronic renal failure. Chronic renal failure is an irreversible condition that results in the continued need for hemodialysis or peritoneal dialysis.

Acute Renal Failure

Acute renal failure (ARF) is the sudden loss of kidney function. It may be reversible or irreversible. ARF is caused by tubular destruction and necrosis as the result of trauma, obstruction of the renal artery, toxic injury to the kidney from medications, or exposure to metals or radiographic contrast. Any condition causing extreme hypotension (eg, burns, hemorrhage, shock) can result in a decreased blood flow to the kidney and result in ARF. The older adult is at increased risk because the elderly are more prone to disorders that precipitate ARF such as dehydration, diabetes mellitus, heart failure, surgery, and athero-sclerosis. Certain drugs are especially toxic to the kidney and can result in ARF. ARF can progress to chronic renal failure in some instances.

Symptoms and Diagnosis

Signs and symptoms of ARF occur suddenly and include

> Decreased or no urinary output (oliguria, anuria)
>
> Generalized edema, particularly noticeable in the ankles, feet, and legs
>
> Changes in mental status (agitation, drowsiness, lethargy, confusion, delirium, moodiness, attention deficit)
>
> Nausea, vomiting
>
> Prolonged bleeding, easy bruising
>
> Hypertension or hypotension

Diagnostic studies include renal function tests (eg, urinalysis, serum creatinine, creatinine clearance, blood urea nitrogen [BUN]). Serum potassium may be increased. Kidney or abdominal ultrasound, renal arteriography, and abdominal CT scan or MRI may aid in the diagnosis of ARF.

Management

The goal of treatment of ARF is to identify and promptly treat reversible causes. Reversible causes of renal failure include conditions such as obstruction or the administration of nephrotoxic medications. ARF is most often treated with hemodialysis or peritoneal dialysis.

For patients with ARF, fluid intake may be restricted. Dietary modifications include a diet that is high in carbohydrates, low in protein, and low in sodium and potassium.

Hyperkalemia (ie, high blood levels of potassium) is a potentially serious problem and potassium levels are monitored closely. Symptoms of hyperkalemia include irritability, diarrhea, nausea, vomiting, and changes in the electrocardiogram. The normal potassium blood level range is 3.5 to 5.0 mEq/L. Critical values are levels below 2.5 mEq/L or greater than 6.5 mEq/L. Any abnormalities in potassium levels should be reported because even small changes in the concentration can have significant consequences, particularly on cardiac functioning.

Although the aging kidney can recover from an episode of ARF, more than 50% of older adults do not survive. A few individuals progress from ARF to chronic renal failure. Death occurs more frequently for those who also suffer from heart disease, respiratory disorders, or recent cerebrovascular vascular accident (ie, stroke).

Chronic Renal Failure

Chronic renal failure (CRF) is a slow, progressive and permanent loss of kidney function. Disorders such as glomerulonephritis, polycystic kidney disease, hypertension, obstructive kidney disease, kidney stones, and diabetes mellitus may result in CRF. With CRF, there is irreversible damage to the kidney nephrons, causing gradual destruction of the kidney. Progression may continue to end-stage renal disease.

Signs and Symptoms

The destruction of the kidney nephrons in CRF usually occurs slowly over several years. Initially, there may be no symptoms. Nonspecific symptoms such as anorexia, headache, nausea, and vomiting may be present. Sometimes, the individual experiences frequent hiccups or generalized pruritus (ie, itching). Later symptoms include increased or decreased urinary output, easy bruising or bleeding, drowsiness, lethargy, mental confusion, delirium, diarrhea or constipation, edema, anemia, and muscle cramps. Urination may be excessive at night. The individual may awaken several times during the night to void. Skin may have increased pigmentation, causing the skin to appear yellow or brown. Halitosis (ie, breath odor) and body odor characteristic of urine may occur (compare with symptoms of ARF).

Hypertension usually occurs with CRF. Blood pressure may be mild to severe. Edema occurs as the result of the inability of the kidneys to excrete water and sodium. Uremic frost (ie, deposits of white crystals) appears on the skin. CRF usually ends with uremia (ie, the bodily condition resulting from renal failure) and azotemia (ie, accumulation of nitrogenous substances in the blood). Many body systems are affected by CRF.

Diagnosis

Diagnostic examinations include IVP, percutaneous kidney biopsy, and abdominal MRI or CT. An abnormal urinalysis result may occur up to 10 years before symptoms occur. Laboratory examination reveals a gradually increasing creatinine and BUN, decreasing creatinine clearance, and hyperkalemia.

Management

Hemodialysis or peritoneal dialysis is the most effective treatment. The number of older adults on dialysis is increasing. Older adults can be managed successfully on hemodialysis if vascular access is not compromised by vascular changes such as atherosclerosis.

Peritoneal dialysis may be more practical for some elderly, particularly those with cardiovascular disease, respiratory problems, or diabetes. Kidney transplantation is successful in some older adults, providing a donor can be found. Complications after a transplantation are more common in the older adult.

Using the Nursing Process to Care for an Older Adult With Renal Failure

Assessment

It is important to identify, if possible, the underlying cause of the renal failure and determine whether the condition is acute or chronic. Age or altered thought processes from the uremia may prohibit the patient from giving accurate health information. Having the caregiver and family present aid in obtaining a history of the illness. The nurse observes the patient's general appearance. Skin may be pale, or there may be increased pigmentation, making the skin appear yellow or brown. It is important to check for uremic frost and pruritus. The skin may also be dry and scaly.

The nurse assesses mental status. The patient may be confused, disoriented, or delirious. If other disease processes are present, it may be difficult to distinguish if the altered mental status is the result of CRF or another disorder. The nurse keeps a record of the urinary intake and output. Urinary output sometimes is normal but is decreased or increased at other times. Nocturia may occur. Blood urea nitrogen and serum creatinine levels are obtained to establish a baseline.

✔ ASSESSMENT ALERT

Serum creatinine levels greater than 10 mg/dL and BUN levels greater than 120 mg/dL generally indicate the need for dialysis. When levels reach this point, hemodialysis or peritoneal dialysis is begun to remove excess fluids and waste products from the blood.

Anorexia, nausea, and vomiting may be present. The patient may have halitosis or a characteristic odor of urine. It is important to obtain and record a baseline weight. The patient may complain of a metallic taste.

The nurse takes and records the vital signs. Hypertension is a common problem in CRF, and establishing a baseline reading is helpful for later comparisons. It is important to check extremities for edema. Generalized edema may also occur. The skin is assessed for bruises. Mucous membranes of the mouth and the stools are examined for bleeding.

Nursing Diagnoses

The following nursing diagnoses are used for patients with renal failure:

Altered Urinary Elimination related to oliguria anuria

Impaired Skin Integrity related to uremic frost, dry skin, edema, reduced activity

Altered Oral Mucous Membrane related to dehydration, dry mouth

Altered Nutrition: Less Than Body Requirements related to nausea, vomiting, anorexia

Altered Thought Process related to disorientation, increased nitrogenous waste in the blood, behavioral changes

Risk for Injury related to anemia, bleeding tendencies

Risk for Decreased Cardiac Output related to electrolyte imbalances, alterations in heart rate, rhythm

Risk of Ineffective Management of Therapeutic Regimen related to cognitive loss, lack of understanding of the disease process, other (specify)

Additional nursing diagnoses may be appropriate for specific patients.

Planning and Implementation

Treatment focuses on lifelong symptom control and minimizing complications. Controlling hypertension, anemia, and acidosis are important aspects of treatment. Normal serum potassium, sodium, calcium, and phosphate levels are priorities in preserving electrolyte balance within the body. Medication dosages are adjusted to account for the decreased kidney function. Peritoneal or hemodialysis are used to rid the body of unwanted waste products.

Altered Urinary Elimination. Urinary output may be less than 400 mL/day. An indwelling catheter may be inserted to prevent urinary stasis. The nurse keeps a record of oral intake and urinary output. Hemodialysis or peritoneal dialysis are required to remove the nitrogenous waste that accumulates because of the nonfunctional kidneys. The patient is monitored for edema or elevated blood pressure and the primary health care giver notified of any edema or if an elevation in blood pressure occurs. A diuretic or antihypertensive may be needed to prevent complications such as heart failure or pulmonary edema.

Impaired Skin Integrity. The skin is rinsed with warm water or a solution of weak baking soda and water to decrease itching and rinse off uremic frost. Uremic frost is usually controlled if the patient is on dialysis. The nurse applies lotion to areas of dry skin. The patient's nails are trimmed short. The patient is instructed to wear loose-fitting cotton clothing. The patient's position is changed every 2 hours. A foam or low-pressure mattress is used to prevent skin breakdown. The skin and bony prominence are inspected for areas of redness, breakdown, bruising, or dryness. Daily perineal care is given using soap and water.

Altered Oral Mucous Membrane. The nurse examines the oral cavity daily for evidence of dryness, ulcerations, or inflammation. Oral care is best given with soft toothbrush or sponge tip after each meal. It is important to offer fluids at regular intervals within the prescribed fluid limitations. Hard candy, gum, or mints are provided between meals to help alleviate dry mouth and metallic taste. Artificial saliva is provided if needed.

Altered Nutrition. The nurse monitors the weight and daily food intake. It is important to offer four or five small meals rather than three larger meals. A dietary consultation may be necessary if the patient is having problems eating. High-potassium and high-sodium foods may be restricted. In some instances, protein and fluids may also be restricted. Adherence to dietary restrictions is encouraged. To prevent constipation the diet should contain sufficient fiber.

Altered Thought Process. The nurse assesses the extent of confusion and altered mental status. It is important to provide a quiet atmosphere. It may be necessary to orient the patient to the surroundings. A family member is encouraged to stay with the patient. The use of restraints is avoided. The nurse presents reality calmly but does not challenge illogical thought patterns. Short, simple sentences are used. A regular, predictable routine is maintained.

Risk for Injury. It is important to answer the call light immediately. The nurse assists the patient as necessary to the bathroom or with ambulation. The ability to ambulate and risk for falling are evaluated. The patient may need some orientation to the surroundings. A night light may be used at night. Injury may occur because of capillary fragility and bleeding tendencies. Side rails are padded to keep the patient from slight trauma when hitting extremities against the rails. It is important to apply pressure to venipuncture sites until oozing has stopped. The mucous membranes are observed for bleeding. A soft-bristle toothbrush is used to prevent irritation of gums. The stools are observed for bright red blood or a tarry color.

Risk for Decreased Cardiac Output. The nurse auscultates the lungs for crackles, rhonchi, and decreased lung sounds (see Chapter 20). A record of the patient's intake and urinary output is kept. The patient is weighed daily. Weight gain may indicate generalized edema. The nurse must assess for signs

of hyperkalemia, such as leg cramping, muscular weakness, weak pulse, and changes in the electrocardiogram. The heart rate and rhythm is monitored. Increased blood pressure, increase or decrease in heart rate, and any irregular rhythm of the heart is reported. Dialysis may correct electrolyte imbalances, decrease edema, and control hypertension.

Patient and Family Teaching

The patient and family, especially the primary caregiver, need to understand the disease process and treatment regimen. A teaching plan for an older adult with CRF should include dietary guidelines and information about integumentary concerns.

 PATIENT TEACHING AID

Information to include when teaching the patient with CRF:

- Dietary guidelines and restrictions must be followed. Provide the patient with a list of foods to include in the diet and foods to avoid. A dietitian may be helpful in assisting the caregiver and patient in meal planning.
- Unless prescribed by the physician, do not use salt substitutes because many are high in potassium and contribute to hyperkalemia.
- Explain hemodialysis or peritoneal dialysis. Give specific instructions on the care of the dialysis site.
- Maintain fluid limitation as prescribed.
- Avoid exposure to infection (eg, colds, flu, sore throats).
- Keep the skin clean and dry. Shower or bathe daily. Use lotion or cream to help control itching and dryness.
- Weigh daily. Report rapid weight gain or loss.
- Observe for and report signs of bleeding in the stool, urine, or vomitus.
- Monitor blood pressure and pulse at home and report any significant change.
- Contact the physician if any of the following occurs: chills, fever, sore throat, cough, easy bleeding or bruising, extreme fatigue, inability to urinate, or any marked change in urinary pattern.
- Suggest that the patient wear a medical identification bracelet.

Evaluation and Expected Outcomes

Successful treatment can be gauged by the following responses:

Elimination of waste products occurs by peritoneal or hemodialysis.

Skin remains intact, moist, free of infection, edema, and uremic frost.

Mucous membranes are free of irritation and inflammation.

Nutritional intake is within dietary guidelines.

Patient regains and maintains normal mental abilities.

Patient expresses understanding of the disease process.

CYSTOCELE

A **cystocele** is displacement of the bladder into the vagina. This causes the bladder to protrude into the vaginal cavity. The cystocele becomes apparent during the aging process with generalized relaxation of the pelvic muscles and genital atrophy. Having given birth to several children predisposes women to this condition.

Symptoms

Symptoms may not be apparent in the early stages. However, with aging, symptoms appear and include

Feelings of pressure or heaviness in the pelvic region

Urinary symptoms (eg, frequency, urgency, incontinence, or leakage of urine)

Nervousness and fatigue

Backache

This condition is made worse by activities that increase intra-abdominal pressure such as coughing, sneezing, or straining to defecate. Obesity also aggravates the symptoms.

Diagnosis and Treatment

The diagnosis is made by visual examination of the pelvic region. A urine specimen may be ordered to determine if the infection is present. Treatment is often symptomatic initially. For example, symptoms of heaviness and pressure may be relieved by having the patient lie down. An antibiotic is ordered if infection is present. If the cystocele is large and interferes with voiding, surgery may be performed.

Using the Nursing Process to Care for an Older Adult With a Cystocele

Assessment
When assessing a patient suspected of having a cystocele, obtain a thorough history of pregnancies, voiding patterns, feelings of heaviness or pressure in the pelvic area, backache, and for any urinary symptoms (ie, frequency, urgency, incontinent episodes,

or leakage of urine). To obtain a visual assessment, have the patient lie down with the legs apart. Spread the walls of the labia and ask the patient to bear down as if having a bowel movement. A cystocele appears as a downward protrusion of tissue into the anterior vaginal wall. (*Note:* Rectocele, a protrusion of the rectum into the posterior vaginal wall, is also possible.) Document all findings carefully.

Nursing Diagnoses
The following nursing diagnoses may be suitable for a patient with cystocele:

Pain related to pressure of bladder in peritoneal region

Urinary Incontinence related to weakened perineal muscles

Other nursing diagnoses may be appropriate for individual patients.

Planning and Implementation
Careful nursing care can help alleviate the discomfort of a cystocele. The nurse provides the patient with information concerning the condition to help decrease any anxiety associated with the condition. Carefully document voiding patterns and the presence of discomfort, as well as the presence and size of the cystocele.

Pain and Incontinence. A thorough record of voiding patterns is necessary. The nurse establishes a schedule for voiding based on the patient's usual voiding pattern. The bladder may be palpated for overdistention. Incontinence pads may be necessary if cognitive ability is not sufficient to determine the need to void. Kegel exercises can help alleviate incontinence if performed regularly (see Chapter 14).

If surgery is not an option because of advanced age or ill health, a **pessary** may be used to assist in keeping the bladder in proper alignment and alleviating discomfort. Pessaries are devices designed to keep the bladder in place and prevent further prolapse. They are made of rubber or plastic material and usually shaped like a ring. The physician or nurse practitioner determines the size and the type of pessary most suitable for each individual patient. If the patient is alert and has no condition that limits hand mobility, she is taught to insert, remove, and clean the device. If the patient is unable to manage insertion or removal of a pessary, family members or the primary care giver may be taught to perform the procedure. Some pessaries are removed at night and reinserted in the morning. Others remain in place for a longer period. Instruct the patient to report any discomfort, discharge, or irritation in the perineal area, which would indicate possible problems such as infection. In general, a pessary should not cause any discomfort, irritation, or discharge.

Evaluation and Expected Outcomes

Successful treatment can be gauged by the following responses:

No pain or discomfort from cystocele is reported.

Episodes of incontinence decrease or are eliminated.

CRITICAL THINKING EXERCISES

1. Mr. Caso, age 78, is diagnosed with cancer of the prostate. The physician suggests that Mr. Caso use the strategy of "watchful waiting" to manage his prostate cancer. Mr. Caso reveals to you that he is afraid his cancer is going to spread and does not understand why his physician does not want to do anything to help him. What would you say to Mr. Caso to ease his fears? What would be the best action for you to take?

2. Ms. Henderson, an elderly resident of the nursing home, has been incontinent for the past 5 days. Normally, she is able to go to the bathroom with minimal or no assistance. She seems a little withdrawn and is staying in her room more than she usual. How would you assess this situation? What questions would be most important for you to ask Ms. Henderson?

3. Mrs. Baker, age 88, lives at home with her daughter and son-in-law. She comes to the senior citizens' center every day to play dominos, visit with her friends, and eat lunch. For the past 2 days, you notice that Mrs. Baker is making frequent trips to the bathroom and has a slight urine odor. She tells you that she is not feeling well. How would you approach Mrs. Baker about this problem? What questions would help you collect the most pertinent data? What four suggestions could you give Mrs. Baker? What is the most important suggestion for Mrs. Baker to have a through understanding?

REFERENCES AND SUGGESTED READING

Johnson, S. (2000). From incontinence to confidence. *American Journal of Nursing, 100 (2)*, 69–76.

Kelly, M. (1996). Nursing rounds: Chronic renal failure. *American Journal of Nursing, 96 (1)*, 36–37.

King, B. (1997). Preserving Renal function. *RN, 60 (8)*, 34–39.

Roach, S., & Scherer, J. (2000). *Introductory clinical pharmacology* (6th ed.). Philadelphia: Lippincott Williams & Wilkins.

Timby, B., Scherer, J., & Smith, N. (1999). *Introductory medical-surgical nursing* (7th ed.). Philadelphia: Lippincott Williams & Wilkins.

CHAPTER 23

The Endocrine System

CHAPTER OUTLINE

KEY TERMS
CHAPTER OBJECTIVES
NORMAL ENDOCRINE FUNCTION
THYROID DYSFUNCTION IN THE OLDER ADULT
DIABETES MELLITUS IN THE OLDER ADULT
CRITICAL THINKING EXERCISES
REFERENCES AND SUGGESTED READING

KEY TERMS

diabetes mellitus

diabetic ketoacidosis

endocrine system

euthyroid

glycosylated hemoglobin

Graves disease

Hashimoto thyroiditis

hyperglycemia

hyperglycemic hyperosmolar nonketotic syndrome

hyperthyroidism

hypoglycemia

hypothyroidism

intensive insulin therapy

ketone

negative feedback mechanism

neuropathy

nonproliferative retinopathy

peripheral neuropathy

proliferative retinopathy

retinopathy

sulfonylureas

thyroid crisis

type I diabetes mellitus

type II diabetes mellitus

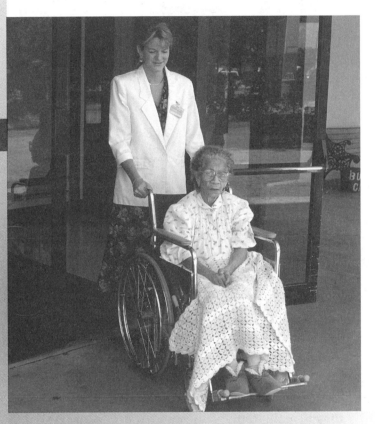

CHAPTER OBJECTIVES

At the completion of this chapter, the student will be able to

- Describe basic endocrine functioning

- Discuss age-related changes in the endocrine system

- Identify signs and symptoms, diagnosis, and treatment of diabetes mellitus, hypothyroidism, and hyperthyroidism

- Discuss general recommendations for older adults with diabetes mellitus

The endocrine system is composed of glands that secrete hormones necessary for the normal functioning of the body. Endocrine glands include the thyroid gland, parathyroid gland, adrenal gland, pituitary gland, pancreas, testes, and ovaries (Fig. 23-1).

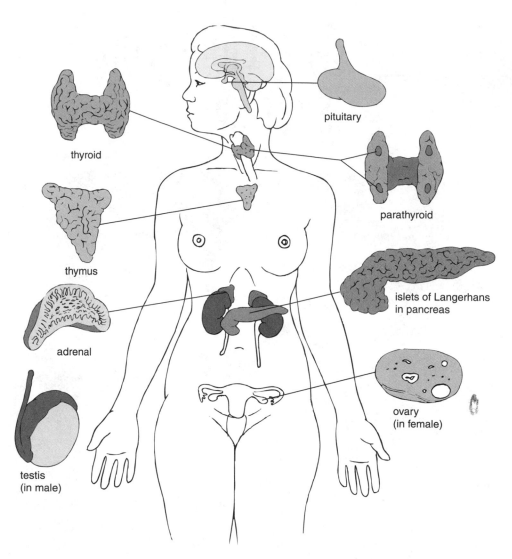

FIGURE 23-1. Endocrine glands. Adapted from Rosdahl, C.B. (1995). *Textbook of basic nursing,* Ch. 19, 198. Philadelphia: Lippincott-Raven. Used with permission.

In the older adult, the most common disorders of the endocrine system occur with dysfunction of the pancreas and thyroid gland.

NORMAL ENDOCRINE FUNCTION

The **endocrine system** is a complex system that helps to regulate body processes. Endocrine glands and the hormones they secrete are the basic components of the endocrine system. The endocrine glands secrete their respective hormones directly into the capillaries, where they immediately become a part of the circulatory system. Each hormone has a target organ or tissue on which the effects of the hormone are felt. Table 23-1 lists the endocrine glands, the hormones secreted, and functions.

Hormones are released by the gland as the result of changes that occur in the body indicating a need for a specific hormone. These changes provide the stimulus that cause the gland to increase or decrease production of the hormone specific for that endocrine gland. As the hormone is released, the stimulus is removed, and the gland decreases production of the hormone. When the changes again occur creating a stimulus, the gland increases production of the hormone. This type of feedback is called negative feedback mechanism. In the **negative feedback mechanism,** a sensory stimuli causes a change in the internal environment of the body that produces an opposing or different response from the initial stimulus within the body. This mechanism helps to maintain homeostasis or balance within the body.

An example of the negative feedback mechanism is the secretion of insulin by the beta cells of the islets of Langerhans in the pancreas in response to hyperglycemia (high blood glucose levels). When hyperglycemia occurs, the pancreas secretes insulin that enables glucose to leave the blood and enter the cell. As insulin leaves the blood and enters the cell, blood glucose levels decrease. Insulin secretion

TABLE 23-1. Endocrine Glands: Hormone Secreted and Function

Endocrine Gland	Hormone(s)	Function
Thyroid gland	Thyroxine (T_4) Triodothyronine (T_3)	Regulates body metabolism
Parathyroid glands	Parathormone	Stimulates bones to release calcium and enter bone
Pancreas		
Alpha cells	Glucagon	Increases blood glucose by stimulating the conversion of glycogen to glucose
Beta cells	Insulin	Enables glucose to enter cells; lowers blood sugar
Gonads		
Testes (males)	Testosterone	Development of male sex characteristics
Ovaries (females)	Estrogen	Regulates female sex characteristics (eg, menstruation)
Pituitary gland		
Anterior	Adrenocorticotropic hormone (ACTH)	Stimulates adrenal cortex to produce cortisol
	Thyroid-stimulating hormone (TSH)	Regulates thyroid hormone
	Follicle-stimulating hormone (FSH)	Stimulates growth and secretion of eggs in ovaries
	Luteinizing hormone (LH)	Helps to control ovulation and menstruation; important in sustaining pregnancy
	Growth hormone (GH)	Controls bone and tissue growth
	Oxytocin	Causes contractions of the uterus; stimulates milk production
Posterior	Vasopressin (ADH)	Raises blood pressure; promotes reabsorption of water in kidney

decreases until blood glucose levels again increase, creating the stimulus for the secretion of insulin.

Thyroid Gland

The thyroid gland is the largest endocrine gland and is located in the front and sides of the neck. Hormones produced by the thyroid gland include thyroxine (T_4), triiodothyronine (T_3), and calcitonin. T_4 and T_3 increase the rate of energy metabolism and protein metabolism. Iodine is necessary for the production of the thyroid hormones. Calcitonin functions to lower the amount of calcium in the blood.

Parathyroid Gland

The parathyroid glands lie behind and are somewhat embedded within the thyroid gland. The parathyroid hormone (PTH) helps to regulate calcium and metabolism. PTH increases the amount of calcium in the blood, and calcitonin lowers the amount of calcium in the blood.

Pancreas

The pancreas is a large, elongated gland located behind the stomach. Scattered throughout the pan-

creas are small groups of specialized cells called the islets of Langerhans. These islets are the endocrine areas of pancreatic function. The islets of Langerhans secrete insulin, which lowers blood glucose levels. Alpha cells in the islets produce glucagon, which raises blood glucose levels. A major disorder of the pancreas is diabetes.

Adrenal Gland

The adrenal glands located above each kidney are divided into the adrenal medulla (ie, inner portion of the gland) and the adrenal cortex (ie, outer portion). Each part of the gland releases specific hormones. The adrenal medulla secretes the two neurotransmitters of the sympathetic nervous system, epinephrine and norepinephrine. These hormones prepare the body for action by increasing the heart rate and metabolic rate, by dilation of the bronchioles, and by increasing blood pressure.

The adrenal cortex secretes the glucocorticoids, mineralocorticoids, and sex hormones. The glucocorticoids have many functions, particularly in metabolism and in aiding the body to fight inflammation by suppressing the inflammatory response within the body. The mineralocorticoids function in regulation of sodium and potassium balance. Sex hormones secreted by the adrenal cortex have minimal effects within the body.

Pituitary Gland

The pituitary gland is located deep within the skull directly below the hypothalamus. The pituitary gland is divided into the anterior and posterior pituitary. Each part has separate and distinct functions. The anterior pituitary produces thyroid-stimulating hormone (TSH), follicle stimulating hormone (FSH), luteinizing hormone (LH), growth hormone (somatotropin), prolactin, and adrenocorticotropin (ACTH). Except for growth hormone, these hormones control the activities of their target gland (eg, the thyroid, ovaries, testes, mammary glands, adrenal cortex). Somatotropin affects every part of the body that is associated with growth. The posterior pituitary gland secretes the antidiuretic hormone (ADH) and oxytocin. The pituitary gland is sometimes called the master gland because of its wide range of effects within the body on growth, metabolism, the reproductive cycle, electrolyte balance, and water retention or loss.

Gonads

The sex organs, or gonads, are the testes in the male and ovaries in the female. The gonads secrete hormones that help to regulate reproduction. The testes produce testosterone, which stimulates the production of sperm and helps to promote male sexual development and activity. The major ovarian hormones are the estrogens and progesterone, which help to regulate female reproductive functioning.

Age-Related Changes of the Endocrine System

During middle age, the pituitary gland reaches its peak size at about 1 g. As age increases, the gland gradually diminishes in size. The vascular bed of the pituitary gland decreases, and there is a loss of cell mass. No change appears to occur in the secretion of the hormones, with the exception of FSH, which increases in women after menopause. Secretion of FSH is unchanged in men.

With age, the thyroid gland undergoes some gradual structural changes. Fibrosis (ie, degeneration of fibrous tissue) of the gland occurs. Small nodular goiters may form on the gland. Even with these structural changes, no change in function is noted. T_4 levels remain relatively unchanged throughout the aging process. T_3 levels, however, decrease by as much as 40%. The basal metabolic rate decreases with age. This metabolic decline is gradual but can be significant. This decline, along with a lack of exercise, contributes to a gradual weight gain in the older adult.

Some structural changes occur in the parathyroid gland. However, degeneration and loss of function appear to be minimal.

Secretion of hormones or glucocorticoids from the adrenal cortex decreases with age. For example, cortisol (the principal glucocorticoid or hormone secreted by the adrenal cortex) secretion rate drops approximately 25%. Even with a decrease in the secretion of the glucocorticoids, no adverse effects are observed.

With age, glucose tolerance declines, and there appears to be a decrease in insulin sensitivity. Receptor sites on the cells become less sensitive to insulin with age. Fasting plasma glucose levels generally increase 1 mg/dL per decade with advancing age. This age-related change increases the risk of the older adult developing diabetes with age.

The gonads are the ovaries in the female and testes in the male. In women, a gradual decrease in the secretion of estrogen by the aging ovaries begins around age 40 and continues for several years. This decline in the secretion of estrogen occurs more as surges and remissions of the hormone rather than by a gradual reduction. Menopause, or the cessation of menstruation, occurs in approximately 95% of women by age 55. Estrogen production decreases approximately 80%. After menopause, progesterone secretion by the ovaries also decreases. As the estrogen level decreases, changes occur in the reproductive organs, including a decrease in size of the ovaries, uterus, cervix, and fallopian tubes. There is also a decrease in the number of mammary ducts. The vaginal canal shortens and becomes drier, increasing the risk for infection and inflammation.

In the male, sperm production declines but does not prevent reproduction. Testosterone secretion decreases in the male. However, the ovaries continue to secrete testosterone after menopause. The ability to have a penile erection is slowed and is somewhat less intense than in the younger male. An erection can be sustained for a longer period, but the volume of semen expelled when ejaculation occurs is less. These changes in sexual function appear to be related to changes occurring in the structure of the reproductive organs in the male rather than from a decline in hormonal production.

The most common disorders of the endocrine system in the older adult include hypothyroidism, hyperthyroidism, and diabetes mellitus (type II).

THYROID DYSFUNCTION IN THE OLDER ADULT

Thyroid disease is not uncommon in the aging population. The risk of thyroid disease increases with age. Two types of thyroid dysfunction occur in the elderly: hypothyroidism and hyperthyroidism. Of the two, hypothyroidism is more common and occurs more often in women than men. Thyroid disease may go undetected because symptoms are often mistaken for changes associated with aging, such as cognitive changes, slowing of functional ability, lower body temperature, or intolerance to cold.

Hypothyroidism

Hypothyroidism is a condition in which the thyroid gland secretes inadequate amounts of the thyroid hormones. The most common cause of hypothyroidism is chronic lymphocytic thyroiditis or Hashimoto thyroiditis. **Hashimoto thyroiditis** is an autoimmune condition in which the body views the thyroid tissue as foreign and "attacks" the tissue. Thyroiditis occurs up to 10 times more often in women than in men.

Hypothyroidism can occur after a thyroidectomy (ie, surgical removal of the thyroid gland) is performed to treat cancer of the thyroid gland. When the thyroid gland is removed, no source of the thyroid hormones remains, and hypothyroidism develops. The use of radioactive iodine to treat hyperthyroidism can also cause hypothyroidism. Drugs such as propylthiouracil (PTU) or methimazole (Tapazole) sometimes are used to treat an overactive thyroid gland. Adverse effects of these drugs can result in hypothyroidism.

Signs and Symptoms

Mild hypothyroidism usually causes no symptoms. As the condition worsens, symptoms become more apparent. Display 23-1 identifies the common signs and symptoms of hypothyroidism.

Symptoms may be overlooked in the elderly or attributed to the normal aging process. Sometimes, symptoms are so vague that hypothyroidism is detected only by laboratory findings.

Diagnosis

Diagnosis is based on the presence of signs and symptoms, increased TSH blood levels, and decreased T_4 levels. An elevated blood TSH level is the most significant laboratory finding.

DISPLAY 23-1. Signs and Symptoms of Hypothyroidism

- Intolerance to cold
- Anorexia
- Fatigue, weakness
- Constipation
- Weight gain
- Muscle cramps
- Dry skin
- Increased blood cholesterol level
- Dry coarse hair or hair loss
- Slow speech, thought, and movement

Assessment and Management

Because the symptoms of hypothyroidism are nonspecific in the elderly, assessment is sometimes difficult. To obtain an accurate assessment, the nurse questions the patient about the extent of fatigue, anorexia, weakness, and intolerance to cold. The patient is weighed. It is important for the nurse to inquire about recent weight gain or loss. The nurse also determines whether constipation is a problem. The skin is inspected for dryness, redness, or lesions. Hair may be dry, course, and thin. Speech may be slow and mental ability dull.

ASSESSMENT ALERT

Hypothyroidism causes dementia in the elderly. Carefully evaluate all elderly patients for confusion and decrease in mental status.

The pulse rate may be slow and temperatures subnormal. The patient may complain of feeling cold regardless of how warm the environmental temperature is. Serum blood cholesterol levels may be elevated.

When diagnosed, hypothyroidism is easily treated with thyroid hormone replacement therapy such as a synthetic form of T_4 called levothyroxine (Synthroid) or T_3 triiodothyronine (Triostat). In the elderly, these drugs are generally started at the lowest possible dosage and increased gradually over several weeks. Adverse effects include irritability, nervousness, insomnia, tachycardia, arrhythmias, weight loss, and heat intolerance. The medication is given orally before breakfast to prevent sleep disturbances. Dosage is withheld and the physician notified if the pulse rate is greater than 100 beats per minute. There are many drug-drug reactions that must be taken into consideration when administering the thyroid hormone.

The average dose is less than dosages prescribed for younger adults, particularly if there is a history of cardiovascular disease. The elderly are more prone to adverse reactions with replacement therapy than younger adults. Cardiac complications may occur if thyroid replacement therapy is excessive or if coexisting cardiovascular problems exist.

Hyperthyroidism

Hyperthyroidism occurs when excessive amounts of thyroid hormones (T_3 and T_4) are secreted by the thyroid gland. The prevalence of hyperthyroidism is at least seven times greater in individuals older than 60 years of age than in younger adults. Hyperthyroidism has several causes, including Graves disease, toxic nodules (ie, goiter), high dosages of thyroid medication, iodine excess, and thyroiditis.

Graves disease is a condition of overactivity of the thyroid gland resulting in hypertrophy of the thyroid gland. The most common manifestations of Graves disease includes hypertrophy of the thyroid gland, exophthalmos (ie, protruding of the eyes), and skin changes. Exophthalmos gives the person a startled expression, causes increased sensitivity to light, and may cause visual disturbances. The characteristic skin lesions are painless, red, lumpy areas occurring on the front of the legs. Older adults may report dry skin and pruritus.

Nodules can develop on the thyroid gland. These toxic nodules produce excessive amounts of T_3 and T_4, leading to symptoms of hyperthyroidism. Certain medications contribute to the development of hyperthyroidism. For example, amiodarone (Cordarone), an adrenergic drug used to treat cardiac arrhythmias, contains large amounts of iodine and may contribute to hyperthyroidism. Overdosage of the thyroid hormone when treating hypothyroidism can also result in hyperthyroidism.

Signs and Symptoms

Symptoms that are found in younger adults but generally not found in older adults with hyperthyroidism include hyperactivity, nervousness, and exophthalmus, and warm, moist skin. Symptoms of hyperthyroidism found in the elderly are found in Display 23-2.

Diagnosis

Diagnosis is difficult in the elderly because of the other illnesses that are present, atypical symptoms, and symptoms that mimic the aging process. When hyperthyroidism is suspected, laboratory examination reveals elevated levels of T_4, resin T_3 uptake, and serum free T_4. TSH levels are decreased.

DISPLAY 23-2. Symptoms of Hyperthyroidism in the Elderly

- Weight loss
- Heat intolerance
- Anorexia
- Depression
- Palpitations
- Tremor
- Dry skin, pruritus
- Fatigue
- New or worsening CHF
- Insomnia
- Hair loss
- Decreased ability to concentrate

Assessment and Management

The nurse assesses the patient for weight loss and lack of appetite. It is important to determine mental status. The nurse notes depression, decreased mental ability, or decreased ability to concentrate. The skin temperature is checked for hydration. Hair loss may be seen. If hyperthyroidism is present, a rapid pulse (>90 beats/min) or an irregularity in the pulse may be noted. The patient may report palpitations, hand tremors, or pruritus.

The nurse monitors the elderly patient frequently for a rare but serious complication of hyperthyroidism, **thyroid crisis** (ie, sudden increase of the symptoms of hyperthyroidism in which all body functions increase to dangerously high levels).

ASSESSMENT ALERT

Symptoms of thyroid crisis that should be reported immediately include elevated temperature, diarrhea, arrhythmias, tachycardia (up to 200 beats/min), dehydration, and extreme irritation.

Thyroid crisis can result in death if not adequately treated. Treatment includes drugs to depress hormone secretion in the overactive gland.

The most effective treatment of hyperthyroidism is the administration of radioactive iodine. The drug is given orally and migrates to the overactive gland to destroy it. Between 8 to 12 weeks is needed for full therapeutic effect (ie, for the gland to become normal).

Before the administration of radioactive iodine, antithyroid medications such as PTU or methimazole are used to normalize thyroid function. When the thyroid gland becomes **euthyroid,** or normal, usually after 3 to 6 months of treatment, the patient is ready for the permanent treatment with radioactive iodine. Beta-adrenergic blocking drugs or sedatives may be used as adjuncts to treatment to manage symptoms such as tremor, nervousness, and rapid heart rate.

DIABETES MELLITUS IN THE OLDER ADULT

Diabetes mellitus is a metabolic disorder of the pancreas resulting in various degrees of insulin insufficiency. Without sufficient insulin, glucose cannot enter the cell to produce energy. A deficiency of insulin allows glucose to remain in the blood, resulting in hyperglycemia. The two major types of diabetes mellitus are type I or insulin-dependent diabetes mellitus (IDDM) and type II or non–insulin-dependent diabetes mellitus (NIDDM).

Type I Diabetes Mellitus

In **type I diabetes mellitus,** the pancreas does not produce any insulin, and the body is unable to regulate carbohydrate or glucose metabolism. This inability to metabolize carbohydrates causes blood glucose levels to increase, sometimes to dangerously high levels. A lack of insulin affects the metabolism of fats, proteins, and carbohydrates. Type I diabetes is also called IDDM because the patient must receive daily insulin injections to survive. Of the 14 million Americans with diabetes mellitus, about 5% to 10% have type I. Type I diabetes is most often diagnosed in people younger than 30 years of age. Most older adults with type I diabetes have had the disease for many years. Older adults more commonly have type II diabetes that was diagnosed later in life.

Signs and Symptoms

The classic signs and symptoms of type I diabetes mellitus are polyphagia (ie, excessive hunger), polydipsia (ie, excessive thirst), polyuria (ie, excessive urination), and **hyperglycemia** (ie, high blood glucose levels). Along with the classic symptoms, the patient may exhibit weight loss, nausea, vomiting, and extreme fatigue. **Diabetic ketoacidosis** (DKA), or a severe insulin deficiency, can develop. Symptoms of DKA include severe abdominal pain, fruity odor to the breath, Kussmaul respirations (ie, deep and rapid respirations), and coma.

Diagnosis

Diagnosis is made on the basis of signs and symptoms. However, in the elderly, the symptoms may be vague or attributed to other causes. For example, symptoms of polyuria may be mistakenly diagnosed as urinary incontinence. Other symptoms such as weight loss or fatigue may be attributed to the aging process. Polydipsia may not be experienced because of the decreased sensation of thirst in the elderly.

Diagnosis can be made when a random blood glucose level exceeds 200 mg/dL or more and the patient has the classic signs of diabetes or two fasting blood glucose levels above 126 mg/dL. Signs and symptoms of DKA helps to confirm the diagnosis.

Treatment

The goal of treatment in type I diabetes mellitus is to maintain blood glucose levels within normal limits as much as possible. For an elderly patient, blood glucose levels below 140 mg/dL is a reasonable goal. For a young to middle-aged adult, the goal is a fasting blood glucose level of 120 mg/dL or less. However, an older person is at a greater risk for hypoglycemia (ie, low blood glucose levels), and a higher fasting blood glucose helps to minimize that risk. The 2-hour postprandial level is also increased somewhat from a normal of 140 mg/dL or less in a young to middle-aged adult to 200 mg/dL or less in the elderly.

In type I diabetes, insulin must be administered on a daily basis. The type and amount of insulin varies with the patients condition. Regular blood glucose monitoring with a glucometer is essential to determine insulin requirements. In addition to insulin, diet and exercise play important roles in managing diabetes mellitus.

Regular medical care is essential to help prevent complications such as poor wound healing, increased incidence of infection, atherosclerosis, blindness, or kidney disease.

Insulin. Maintaining "tight control" over blood glucose levels by maintaining levels as close to normal as possible can prevent or slow the progress of complications. For tight control, **intensive insulin therapy** or multiple daily insulin injections may be given. For example, the individual usually takes an injection of short-acting insulin (ie, regular insulin) before each meal and intermediate- or long-acting insulin at bedtime. Another method to gain tight control is to wear an insulin pump that releases insulin into the body continually, with extra insulin released when needed (eg, before a meal). Blood glucose levels are monitored several times each day. Intensive insulin therapy is not for everyone with diabetes. Older adults are generally not placed on intensive insulin therapy.

Because insulin is given on a constant basis, hypoglycemic reactions occur more frequently. Hypoglycemia is a particularly dangerous condition in the older adult because low blood glucose levels can cause stroke or myocardial infarction, seizures, or angina.

In many instances, the older adult is managed on a regimen of subcutaneous insulin administration once or twice daily. The physician prescribes the insulin regimen that provides the best control for each individual patient. Sometimes, the diabetic may be managed well on one injection of intermediate-acting insulin in the morning, whereas others require an additional injection of insulin in the evening. Some patients may need the morning dosage of intermediate-acting insulin combined with a shorter-acting insulin to best manage the disease. The insulin regimen is highly individualized, and the physician's recommendations must be followed.

The first new insulin since the early 1980s, lispro insulin (Humalog), is absorbed more rapidly, reaches higher peak concentrations, and has a shorter duration of action than regular insulin. Because lispro insulin more closely mimics the action of natural human insulin, more stable glucose levels are possible. Lispro insulin should be injected 15 minutes before meals rather than the traditional 30 minutes before meals because of its more rapid onset of action than regular insulin.

Type II Diabetes Mellitus

Type II diabetes mellitus (NIDDM), can occur at any age, but approximately 50% of the 13 million type II diabetics are older than 65. In type II diabetes, the body is usually able to produce some insulin. However, the beta cells often function inadequately and are unable to produce sufficient insulin. Insulin resistance often develops, resulting in the inability of the cells to use the insulin that is available. The number of insulin receptor sites on the cells appear to decrease, causing a problem with receptor binding.

Signs and Symptoms

The signs and symptoms of type II diabetes are vague, and the onset is gradual. Symptoms usually develop during middle age or later. If symptoms occur, they are usually mild and include fatigue, irritability, polyuria, polydipsia, poor wound healing, and blurred vision. Usually, the individual is overweight or obese. In the older adult, these symptoms may be less prominent or absent. For example, because the renal threshold for glucose increases with age, typical polydipsia and polyuria may not be seen even when blood glucose levels are greater than 200 mg/dL. Older diabetics are likely to present severely dehydrated and comatose. Common symptoms may be attributed to the aging process rather than diabetes. For example, complaints such as blurred vision may be attributed to cataracts rather than as a result of hyperglycemia. Sluggishness or fatigue may also be attributed to aging.

Diagnosis

Diagnosis may be detected with routine laboratory examinations not performed specifically as a result of symptomatology. Random blood glucose levels greater than 200 mg/dL and fasting plasma glucose greater than 126 mg/dL on more than one occasion help establish a diagnosis. An oral glucose tolerance test (OGTT) with levels greater than 200 mg/dL is also used to diagnose diabetes.

Although the reasons are unclear, blood glucose levels rise with age. Some researchers believe that certain physiologic changes that occur with age causes glucose intolerance leading to diabetes. Heredity, obesity, and decreased activity are also associated with type II diabetes.

Treatment

Treatment consists of diet therapy to maintain a healthy weight and overall good nutrition and regular exercise to help improve the insulin activity. Good nutrition and regular exercise may be all that is necessary to maintain normal or near normal blood glucose levels. Oral hypoglycemic agents may be added to the treatment regimen if blood glucose cannot be managed with diet and exercise alone. A practical goal for the older adult is a fasting blood glucose level between 100 and 140 mg/dL and a 2-hour postprandial level up to 200 mg/dL.

Type II diabetics may become resistant to the oral drugs commonly used and require insulin to manage the diabetes. This need for insulin, however, does not "convert" the disease state from type II to type I diabetes mellitus.

Control of diabetes in the older adult is complicated by many factors. Terpstra and Terpstra (1998) identified several factors that affect diabetes control in the older adult (Display 23-3).

General Recommendations for Diabetics

Exercise. Some older adults with physical limitations as a result of arthritis or other musculoskeletal disorders may be unable to exercise adequately. Problems can occur if the elderly exercise too strenuously.

If the patient experiences exercise-induced hypoglycemia, the physician carefully monitors the blood glucose level before, during, and after exercise. Recommendations may be to eat more food or adjust the amount of medication on the days designated for exercise. In some cases, the exercise regimen may require modification.

ASSESSMENT ALERT

One potential problem with the older diabetic is exercise-induced hypoglycemia that can occur up to 24 hours after exercise. Symptoms include extreme fatigue, tremors, sweating, and headache. These symptoms are treated with immediate administration of orange juice, Lifesaver candies, or a commercially prepared drink or candy designed to be used for hypoglycemic reactions.extreme fatigue, tremors, sweating, and headache. These symptoms are treated with immediate administration of orange juice, Lifesaver candies, or a commercially prepared drink or candy designed to be used for hypoglycemic reactions.

DISPLAY 23-3. Factors That Affect Diabetes Control

- Decline in visual acuity affects the patient's ability to read medication labels, insulin syringes, and dietary instructions.
- Hearing impairments can hamper the patient's ability to hear and understand instructions concerning the diet and medication regimen.
- Altered taste can affect food choices and nutritional status
- Poor dentition or changes in the gastrointestinal system can cause problems with digestion.
- Changes in hepatic or renal function can alter the effects of medication.
- Arthritis or other disorders can affect the ability to self-administer medications.
- Practice of polypharmacy can cause dangerous interactions with diabetic medications.
- Depression affects motivation for self-care.
- Cognitive impairments affect the ability to manage the therapeutic regimen.

Exercise need not be strenuous to be effective. Aerobic conditioning is preferable. Recommended types of exercise for older adults is walking, swimming, or riding a stationary bicycle (see Chapter 14). Exercise should be carefully planned with the diabetic educator, geriatric nurse practitioner, or other health care provider. Some elders walk in groups at the mall or on specially designed walking tracks.

Diet Therapy. Although nutrition is a key component of diabetes management, the trend is a less restrictive diet than in the past. The older adult may be asked to restrict concentrated sugars, fatty foods, salt, and alcohol while adhering to a required meal schedule. Although older adults may be overweight, a severe weight loss program is usually not recommended unless they are significantly overweight (ie, approximately 1.5 times their normal weight). Older adults are more likely to be nutritionally deficient as the result of poor dentition, decreased appetite, decreased taste sensation, or chronic illness. Self-care deficient may cause difficulties in food preparation. A well-balanced diet, eating at regular intervals, and avoidance of concentrated sweets help to prevent episodes of hypoglycemia that occur more frequently in the elderly. Fruits, vegetables, and whole-grain breads and cereals provide the bulk of the diet. If obesity is a problem and weight loss is required, a gradual weight loss is recommended.

Medication Therapy

Oral hypoglycemic agents are used when diet and exercise do not control type II diabetes. In older adults, the lowest effective dose of the drug is given to decrease the incidence of adverse reactions. If necessary the dosage can be increased gradually until the desired effect is reached. Occasionally, oral drugs used to treat type II diabetes may become ineffective after several months or even years. The patient may respond to a different drug, or insulin may be required

to control the diabetes. The nurse should keep in mind that the more complicated the treatment regimen, the less likely the older adult is to remain compliant.

Sulfonylureas. A group of oral hypoglycemic agents, called the **sulfonylureas,** are commonly prescribed for the older adult. Sulfonylureas stimulate insulin secretion of the pancreas and improve the action of insulin. Sulfonylureas used for the older adult with the type II diabetes mellitus include glyburide (DiaBeta, Micronase), glipizide (Glucotrol), or tolbutamide (Orinase). Chlorpropramide (Diabinese) is not safe for use in the elderly because the prolonged action increases the risk of a severe hypoglycemic reaction in older adults. If fasting blood glucose levels are more than 250 mg/dL, the physician may use insulin instead of the oral drugs.

Combination therapy, such as an oral drug in combination with insulin, may also be used. When the older adult is under stress or during an illness, insulin needs increase and the patient may require insulin to maintain control of the diabetes.

Metformin. Metformin (Glucophage) may be administered alone or in conjunction with the sulfonylureas for type II diabetes mellitus. Metformin is a biguanide that acts to lower blood glucose levels by decreasing hepatic glucose production, decreasing intestinal absorption of glucose, and improving insulin sensitivity. An advantage of metformin is that it does not cause hypoglycemia.

Metformin is used in conjunction with diet to treat type II diabetes mellitus or in combination with a sulfonylurea when diet and metformin do not result in

ASSESSMENT ALERT

Before initiating therapy with metformin and during treatment with metformin, renal function must be assessed and monitored closely. Because metformin is excreted by the kidneys, it can pose a threat to older adults with decreased renal function. In older adults, decreasing kidney function can cause an accumulation of the drug in the body that results in lactic acidosis. Lactic acidosis is a rare but serious condition. The onset of lactic acidosis is insidious, with complaints of malaise, respiratory distress, abdominal distress, and muscular aches and pains. Blood metformin levels greater than 5 μg/mL are usually found with metformin-induced lactic acidosis. Dialysis is recommended to remove the metformin from the bloodstream.

blood glucose control. Common adverse reaction of metformin include diarrhea, nausea, vomiting, abdominal bloating, gas, and loss of appetite. Diarrhea in the elderly can cause dehydration. A potential benefit in the older adult who has a history of constipation is a normalization of stool patterns.

Acarbose. Acarbose (Precose) is also used in the management of type II diabetes. Acarbose delays the digestion of carbohydrates causing a smaller increase in blood glucose levels after eating. This drug may be used in combination with diet to treat type II diabetes mellitus or in combination with a sulfonylureas and diet. Acarbose when used alone does not cause hypoglycemia, but when combined with a sulfonylureas, it may result in hypoglycemia. Common adverse reactions when using acarbose are related to the gastrointestinal tract and include abdominal pain, diarrhea, and flatulence. These side effects tend to decrease with time.

Thiazolidinediones. The thiazolidinediones include pioglitazone (Actos) and rosiglitazone (Avandia). These drugs are used for type II diabetes with a sulfonylurea or insulin (pioglitazone) or with metformin (rosiglitazone, pioglitazone) to improve control of diabetes. Pioglitazone may be given alone to manage type II diabetes. The risk of a hypoglycemic reaction is increased when administered with insulin. Rosiglitazone is given as a single dose or in divided doses twice daily. Pioglitazone is given once daily without regard to meals. When taking these drugs it is important that patients follow dietary instructions and have blood glucose and glycosylated hemoglobin levels tested regularly.

Self-Monitoring of Blood Glucose

Regular blood glucose monitoring is necessary if diabetes is to be controlled. Glucose meters or glucometers are used to monitor blood glucose levels. Today's meters are easy to use, accurate, and come in various price ranges. Manufacturer's directions must be followed.

Even though blood glucose levels are more stable in type II diabetes, monitoring is still important. Self-monitoring using a glucometer of blood glucose levels is the best method of maintaining control.

Problems in using a glucose monitor may be experienced by the elderly who have musculoskeletal disorders, such as arthritis or whose vision is not adequate to reach the glucometer. Patients with a decrease in mental status or those who are confused may also be unable to use a self-monitoring device. If self-monitoring is not possible, a family member or a caregiver can be taught to monitor daily glucose levels. In the hospital or nursing home the nursing staff monitors blood glucose levels.

With type II diabetes, testing blood glucose levels 2 hours after a meal enables the diabetic or caregiver to identify how various foods affect blood glucose levels. Self-monitoring is also helpful for patients not taking insulin to monitor the effectiveness of exercise, diet, or oral agents. Blood glucose levels taken before meals and at bedtime is a means to determine insulin requirements and to monitor the effectiveness of the insulin regimen for patients requiring daily insulin.

Glycosylated Hemoglobin. The most common laboratory examination used to monitor diabetes control over a 2- to 3-month period is the **glycosylated hemoglobin** determination. In hyperglycemia, glucose attaches to hemoglobin in a red blood cell. The longer hyperglycemia is present, the more glucose attaches itself to the blood cells. When glucose attaches to hemoglobin, the result is glycosylated hemoglobin. This attachment lasts for the 4-month lifespan of the hemoglobin. The higher the glycosylated hemoglobin, the higher the glucose levels have been over the past several months. This indicates poor control. Normal values vary slightly from laboratory to laboratory and range from 4% to 8%. When the glycosylated hemoglobin levels are normal or near normal, blood glucose levels for the past 2 to 3 months have been within a normal range.

Urine Testing. Ketones are acids that appear in the urine when fat is burned to obtain the needed energy because the body does not have enough insulin. Urine testing is not accurate for monitoring blood glucose levels, but urine testing for ketones is recommended when blood glucose levels are more than 240 mg/dL. Testing for the presence of ketones every 4 to 6 hours is also recommended during an illness such as the flu.

The physician or health care provider is notified when urine testing shows large ketone levels, large

TABLE 23-2. Characteristics of Hypoglycemia and Ketoacidosis

Reaction	Onset	Urine Glucose/ Acetones	CNS Symptoms	Respiration Symptoms	Gastrointestinal Symptoms	Skin
Hypoglycemic (insulin reaction)	Sudden	Neg/neg	Fatigue weakness, nervousness, confusion, headache, diplopia, convulsions, psychoses, dizziness, unconsciousness	Normal to rapid	Hunger, nausea	Pale, moist, cool
Ketoacidosis (diabetic coma)	Gradual (hours or days)	Pos/small, medium, or large	Drowsiness, dim vision	Deep, rapid	Thirst, acetone breath, nausea, vomiting, abdominal pain, loss of appetite	Dry, flushed

ketone and high blood sugar levels, or moderate amounts of ketones in two tests. High ketone content in the urine and hyperglycemia may indicate that the diabetes is out of control and that immediate treatment is needed.

ASSESSMENT ALERT

Because the renal glucose threshold is higher in older adults, this method of testing is not reliable in older adults and therefore is not routinely recommended.

Acute Complications

Acute complications for diabetes mellitus include hypoglycemia, hyperglycemia, DKA, and hyperglycemic hyperosmolar nonketotic syndrome.

Hypoglycemia. Hypoglycemia occurs whenever the blood sugar level falls below 60 mg/dL. This occurs from eating little food, exercising excessively, taking too much insulin, or as an adverse reaction to the oral hypoglycemic agents (Table 23-2).

ASSESSMENT ALERT

A hypoglycemic reaction can occur at any time but commonly occurs before meals, particularly if meals are delayed or snacks omitted. The older adult is especially prone to hypoglycemia. Common symptoms of hypoglycemia include diaphoresis (ie, sweating), palpitations, tachycardia, hunger, headache, nervousness, confusion, emotional changes, visual disturbances, and drowsiness. When the hypoglycemia becomes severe,

ASSESSMENT ALERT

seizures and loss of consciousness can occur. Careful monitoring of the older adult is necessary because the symptoms of hypoglycemia can mimic other conditions such as stroke.

Confusion may be dismissed as a normal occurrence in older age. Confusion, particularly sudden confusion, is a symptom of an underlying problem, and its causes must be investigated (see Chapter 14). The older adult is particularly susceptible to confusion when hypoglycemia is present.

Immediate treatment must be given when hypoglycemia occurs. If the patient is conscious and able to swallow the nurse would administer one of the following:

- 4 to 6 ounces of fruit juice (usually orange juice)
- 4 to 6 ounces of a carbonated beverage (not diet)
- 6 to 8 hard candies such as Lifesavers
- 2 to 3 teaspoons of honey or sugar

After administration, monitor the patient carefully for 10 to 15 minutes. The symptoms should subside within a few minutes. If symptoms persist after 15 minutes, the treatment is repeated. A blood glucose level is taken and the physician notified of the patient's condition. After the hypoglycemia is corrected, a snack is given containing a protein and a starch to provide sustained elevation of the blood glucose level. The snack may consist of milk and graham crackers or 1 oz. of turkey or chicken and crackers. If a meal is to be eaten within the next 30 minutes, no snack is necessary. Diabetic patients are encouraged to keep some form of simple sugar with them at all times to use when symptoms of hypoglycemia occur.

Diabetic Ketoacidosis. DKA is a potentially life-threatening deficiency of insulin resulting in severe hyperglycemia. DKA is caused by

Severe stress such as an illness or infection

Receiving too little insulin or missing a dose of insulin

Initial undiagnosed diabetes

DKA requires immediate administration of insulin. Because insulin is unavailable to allow glucose to enter the cell, dangerously high levels of glucose build up in the blood, causing hyperglycemia. The body requires energy and begins to break down fat to obtain this energy. As fats are broken down, ketone bodies are produced. The liver is unable to metabolize these bodies and releases them into the bloodstream. As more and more fats are broken down, higher levels of ketones accumulate in the blood. This increase in ketones disrupts the acid–base balance in the body, causing an acidotic condition called DKA.

Elevated blood glucose levels (>200 mg/dL) are indicative of DKA. The severity of DKA, however, is not proportionately related to blood glucose levels. Some patients may have blood glucose levels of 500 or more but show no signs of DKA, whereas others with blood glucose levels of 200 mg/dL may have severe acidosis. If DKA is suspected or if the patient shows any symptoms of hyperglycemia, the urine is checked, usually using a dipstick method, as described in the section on urine testing. Symptoms of DKA must be reported immediately (Display 23-4).

This is a serious condition that requires immediate administration of insulin, treatment restoring electrolyte balance, and reversing the acidosis. Insulin is given intravenously along with 0.9% normal saline to correct the dehydration. Electrolyte balance is restored by adding potassium to the intravenous solution. Patients with DKA are treated in the acute care setting where they can be closely monitored. Life-threatening arrhythmias can occur if the condition is not treated promptly.

Fortunately, older diabetics are less prone to DKA than younger or middle-aged adults. Patients with type I diabetes are the most likely to suffer this complication. The most important aspect in managing DKA is prevention. Taking insulin as prescribed, regular monitoring of blood glucose levels, and urine testing for ketones help prevent DKA from developing. Table 23-2 compares DKA with hypoglycemia.

Hyperglycemic Hyperosmolar Nonketotic Syndrome. **Hyperglycemic hyperosmolar nonketotic syndrome** (HHNS) is a syndrome that occurs as a result of undiagnosed type II diabetes mellitus or as the result of a stressor such as acute illness. HHNS is characterized by blood glucose levels above

---

DISPLAY 23-4. Symptoms of Diabetic Ketoacidosis

- Hyperglycemia
- Headache
- Increased thirst
- Epigastric pain
- Nausea, vomiting
- Hot, dry, flushed skin
- Restlessness
- Fruity odor to the breath
- Deep, rapid respirations (Kussmaul respiration)

---

600 mg/dL, severe mental impairment, and hyperosmolarity resulting in dehydration. The hyperglycemia and hyperosmolarity results in cellular dehydration and excessive urination. Symptoms of HHNS resemble symptoms of DKA (Display 23-5).

A serious consequence is an electrolyte imbalance caused by a loss of sodium (ie, hyponatremia) and potassium (ie, hypokalemia) during diuresis. Ketoacidosis does not occur in HHNS. Treatment consists of administration of intravenous insulin and correction of fluid and electrolyte imbalance. The elderly patient must be continually monitored for signs and symptoms of fluid overload (eg, increased confusion, orthopnea, shortness of breath, pulmonary congestion, weight gain).

Long-Term Complications

Long-term complications are a serious threat to a diabetic. Long-term complications affect the small arterioles and vessels as well as the large vessels in various parts of the body such as the kidneys, the eyes, and the extremities. Long-term complications include retinopathy, circulatory problems of the feet and legs, neuropathy, and kidney disease.

Retinopathy. **Retinopathy** (ie, disease of the retina) results from changes in the small blood vessels in the retina of the eye. These changes are thought to occur when hyperglycemia is left unchecked and becomes chronic. Background or **nonproliferative retinopathy** usually develops within 5 to 15 years of the diagnosis of diabetes. In this type of retinopathy, there are no symptoms and vision is not affected. Some people with background retinopathy develop macular edema. When macular edema develops, the diabetic has visual distortion and loss of central vision.

Proliferative retinopathy presents the most significant threat to vision. In proliferative retinopathy, thin fragile vessels of the retina rupture, allowing blood to enter the chamber behind the eye and mix with the vitreous humor. This hemorrhage clouds the vitreous and causes visual disturbances that

DISPLAY 23-5. Symptoms of Hyperglycemic Hyperosmolar Nonketotic Syndrome (HHNS)

- Blood glucose levels greater than 600 mg/dL
- Increased urinary output
- Warm, flushed, dry skin
- Poor skin turgor
- Dry mucous membranes
- Weight loss and fatigue
- Confusion
- Lethargy
- Coma, if left untreated

leads to blindness. A significant degree of proliferative retinopathy can occur before symptoms occur.

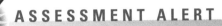

ASSESSMENT ALERT

When the diabetic reports visual disturbances of any type, such as floaters, spots, specks, or cobwebs, a referral to the ophthalmologist (ie, physician who specializes in treatment of the eye and disorders of the eye) is needed.

Laser surgery by photocoagulation is used to seal the blood vessels and prevent the leakage of fluids into the vitreous humor. This complication occurs in type I and type II diabetics.

Circulatory Complications of the Feet and Legs. Up to 75% of the amputations performed on the lower extremities are on individuals with diabetes. Many amputations can be prevented if the diabetic gives proper attention and care to the feet. Decreased sensation in the lower extremities prevents the diabetic from feeling injuries of the feet and legs. As the result of diabetes, healing is prolonged. The damaged vessels in the feet are not able to provide the necessary oxygen and nutrients to the injury for healing to occur. Infection and necrosis spread, leading to the need for amputation.

Neuropathy. Neuropathy (ie, pathologic changes of the nervous system) results from damage to nerves of the gastrointestinal system, genitourinary system, and the cardiovascular system. Gastrointestinal neuropathy manifestations include delayed gastric emptying, bloating, nausea, vomiting, constipation, or diarrhea. Neurogenic bladder and impotence are the result of genitourinary neuropathy. Cardiovascular manifestations include postural hypotension, resting tachycardia, and a painless myocardial infarction. The occurrence of neuropathies increase with age.

Of particular concern in the older diabetic is **peripheral neuropathy.** Peripheral neuropathy affects the nerves of the lower extremities. Symptoms include tingling, prickling, or burning sensations in the lower extremities. Symptoms may be more prominent at night. Pain, which can be extremely uncomfortable, may subside within 6 to 8 months or can continue for years. Eventually, the feet become numb. This numbness contributes to the foot problems commonly seen in diabetes. The diabetic does not feel the injury to the foot and therefore does not provide the necessary care to promote healing. For this reason, preventive care of the feet becomes an important issue with the diabetic.

Kidney Disease. Kidney disease is a serious and common complication in type I and type II diabetes mellitus. Approximately 60% of all type II diabetes develop kidney disease within 10 years of diagnosis. Although kidney disease is less common in type I diabetes, approximately 30% of these individuals develop kidney disease within 20 years of diagnosis. Patients who develop kidney failure need dialysis.

Using the Nursing Process to Care for an Older Adult With Type II Diabetes Mellitus

Assessment

Assessing the older adult with diabetes requires skillful questioning by the nurse because the symptoms of type II diabetes mellitus may appear slowly over a number of years. Symptoms are often mild and can go undetected or be attributed to another cause. The nurse assesses the patient's emotional status, level of consciousness, and memory impairment. The patient is questioned concerning

- Signs and symptoms of diabetes (eg, fatigue, irritability, increased thirst, increased hunger)
- Poor wound healing
- Visual disturbances
- Vaginal itching
- Nausea, vomiting, or abdominal pain
- Headaches
- Family history of diabetes, heart disease, hypertension, or stroke

A careful medication history is important, because many drugs may interfere with blood glucose control. Some drugs can potentiate hypoglycemic effects, and others can potentiate hyperglycemia (Table 23-3).

The nurse must assess the feet and legs of the diabetic. The nurse carefully examines legs and feet for signs of cuts, lesions, or abrasions. The patient may report numbness, tingling, or burning in the lower extremities. The diabetic often does not feel any discomfort when injuries occur, and observation is the only method to detect these injuries. The nurse checks the lower extremities for signs of vascular

TABLE 23-3. Drugs That Commonly Interfere With Blood Glucose Control

Potentiates Hypoglycemia	Potentiates Hyperglycemia
alcohol	corticosteroids, such as prednisone (Deltasone)
allopurinol (Lopurin)	diuretics, such as furosemide (Lasix) and all thiazide diuretics
anticholinergics, such as dicyclomine (Bentyl)	epinephrine (Primatene Mist)
beta-adrenergic antagonists, such as atenolol (Tenormin) and metaprolol (Lopressor)	estrogens
clofibrate (Novofibrate)	niacin (Vitamin B_3)
haloperidol (Haldol)	phenothiazines, such as chlorpromazine (Thorazine)
H_2-receptor antagonists, such as cimetidine (Tagamet) and ranitidine (Zantac)	phenytoin (Dilantin)
monoamine oxidase inhibitors, such as phenelzine sulfate (Nardil)	rifampin (Rifadin)
phenylbutazone (Azolid)	sympathomimetics, such as theophylline (Duraphyl)
salicylates, such as aspirin	
sulfonamides, such as trimethoprim-sulfamethoxazole (TMP-SMX; Bactrim)	

From Deakins, D. (1994). Teaching elderly patients about diabetes. *American Journal of Nursing, 94*(5), 41.

insufficiency: coldness, loss of hair, shiny skin, pallor on elevation, rubor (ie, redness) on dependency, and hypertrophic (ie, increase in volume of cells) changes of the toe nails. Pulses (ie, pedal, posterior tibial, and popliteal) may be weak or absent. Capillary refill may be insufficient, occurring in up to 20 seconds. If lesions or abrasions are present, the nurse documents the exact location or draws the lesion location on a special flowsheet designed to show the extremities. Determine if the patient smokes cigarettes and if so how many.

It is of utmost importance to assess coordination, self-care ability, and educational potential of the older adult. Coordination and visual ability are needed to use the glucometer and administer insulin (if this is required). Coordination and self-care ability are assessed while observing the patient perform tasks such as reading the newspaper, dressing, eating, or using a pencil to write. The nurse must determine whether the patient can follow simple commands and recall current medication regimen (if applicable). The nurse also assesses the extent of knowledge of diabetes, complications of diabetes, and the treatment regimen. The nurse determines the level of the patient's anxiety.

It is important to assess nutritional status. The nurse obtains the patient's weight and asks if there has been a recent weight gain or weight loss. Type II diabetes mellitus is associated with obesity. The nurse also obtains a history of eating patterns and food preferences.

Nursing Diagnoses
The following nursing diagnoses may be used for an older adult with type II diabetes mellitus:

Altered Nutrition, related to insulin deficiency, lack of proper diet, other (specify)

Anxiety related to inability to manage disease, complications other (specify)

Risk for Impaired Skin Integrity related to circulatory changes, delayed healing

Risk for Ineffective Management of Therapeutic Regimen related to lack of knowledge of dietary requirements, medication regimen, disease process

Other nursing diagnoses may be appropriate for individual patients.

Planning and Implementation
After stabilizing the blood sugar, planning the care of a type II diabetic usually centers on teaching the patient and the caregiver the information necessary to maintain blood glucose levels within a normal range. Diet, exercise, and medication are the major treatment modalities.

Altered Nutrition. Diet is a mainstay in the treatment of diabetes. The correct diet helps to maintain blood glucose levels within a normal range, decreased weight to a more normal level, and prevent complications. During the past several years, dietary guidelines have been modified to allow more flexibility. The dietitian plans the dietary regimen based on the patient's eating habits, blood glucose levels, serum lipid levels, and desired weight. Consult with the dietitian, if needed (see the section on dietary teaching). Promote pleasant relaxing atmosphere when eating. Encourage the patient to select foods that are appealing. Review the drug regimen and potential problems when the dietary regimen is not followed. Help the patient in identifying resources such as The American Dietetic Association and other community resources that can provide assistance.

Anxiety. The new diabetic may have difficulty accepting the diagnosis, and the complexity of the therapeutic regimen can seem overwhelming. Before patients can be responsible for managing their diabetes, they must deal with their feelings about having the disorder. The nurse must acknowledge the patient's anxiety and actively listen as the patient expresses feelings. A therapeutic relationship with the nurse is essential in helping these patients gradually accept the diagnoses and understand their feelings. Referral to a diabetic support group may be appropriate. The nurse encourages the use of stress reducing techniques such as a calm environment, soft music, or back rubs.

Anxiety may be manifested in a number of ways, such as avoiding a discussion of the diabetes, expressing fears or concerns, or acting withdrawn or anxious. The nurse provides opportunities for the patient to discuss anxiety or fears. It is important to actively listen as the patient talks. The nurse must provide accurate information about diabetes and correct any misconceptions. Referral to a dietitian or diabetic nurse educator is necessary if more information is needed.

Impaired Skin Integrity. Numbness, tingling, or burning in extremities indicates peripheral neuropathy. The patient is encouraged to change positions at least every 2 hours while in bed. The nurse instructs the patient to avoid prolonged standing. The patient is taught how to inspect the skin daily for evidence of skin breakdown. Warm (not hot) water and mild soap is used to clean the skin. The skin must be patted dry rather than rubbed vigorously. The areas between the toes and the soles of the feet are inspected for irritation. It is important for the patient to use a moisturizer or powder on the feet. Lamb's skin may be placed between the toes for protection. Foot care on a daily basis is imperative if the diabetic is to avoid complications. Referral to a podiatrist may be necessary for nail trimming and care. The nurse reviews importance of skin care and measures to maintain skin integrity. Emphasis is placed on the importance of wearing properly fitting shoes, avoiding the use of heating pads, and not going without shoes.

Patient and Family Teaching

Failure to comply with the prescribed medication regimen may be a problem for patients taking the oral antidiabetic drugs because of the erroneous belief that not having to take insulin means that the disease is not serious and does not require strict adherence to the prescribed regimen. Dietary guidelines may not be followed for the same reason. The nurse must inform these patients that control of type II diabetes mellitus is just as significant as controlling insulin-dependent diabetes. It is important to emphasize that control is achieved only with adherence to the prescribed treatment regimen. Family members can be taught to premeasure insulin for the older patient's use. If vision is poor, the older adult may use a magnifier to read insulin dosages. The use of an insulin pen may be more convenient that a vial and syringe for the older adult. Display 23-6 gives some general information to include when teaching the older adult about diabetes and the treatment regimen.

Dietary Teaching

The American Diabetes Association currently allows sugar in moderation if the patient is not overweight and does not exceed the daily carbohydrate limit. Patients are instructed that sugar substitutes such as aspartame or saccharin can be used to sweeten foods and beverages.

The diabetic diet usually consists of 50% to 60% carbohydrates, 15% to 20% protein, and 30% fat, individualized to meet specific food preferences and patient needs. Any illness, vomiting, or decreased appetite should be reported.

The patient is encouraged to follow the diet prescribed by the physician. The following are general dietary instructions for the diabetic:

- Eat at approximately the same times each day. Do not skip meals.
- Avoid alcohol, dieting, commercial weight loss products, and strenuous exercise programs unless approved by the physician.
- Reduce fat intake by eating poultry rather than the higher-fat meats such as beef or pork.
- Bake, broil, or roast foods rather than fry.
- Use polyunsaturated safflower or corn oil for cooking. If cholesterol levels are high, monounsaturated fats such as olive and canola oils may be included.
- Use whole-grain breads and cereals.
- Eat fresh fruits, vegetables, and beans daily.
- Avoid adding extra salt to foods.
- Eat several small meals rather than two or three large meals. Do not skip meals.

Evaluation and Expected Outcomes

Successful treatment can be gauged by the following responses:

Patient follows dietary regimen.

Blood glucose levels are within normal range.

Patient expresses less anxiety.

Patient can manage the disease and complies with therapeutic regimen.

DISPLAY 23-6. Information to Include in the Diabetic Teaching Plan

- Take the drug exactly as prescribed (eg, tolbutamide is taken with food to prevent gastric upset; glipizide is given 30 minutes before a meal in the morning or in divided doses; glyburide is given with breakfast or with the first main meal of the day).
- Never stop taking the prescribed drug or increase or decrease the dosage unless told to do so by the physician.
- Take the drug at the same time or times of the day.
- Test blood for glucose and urine for ketones as instructed by the physician. Keep a record of test results and bring this record to the physician or the clinic for each visit. Urine may be tested periodically for ketones.
- Carry some form of concentrated sugar such as hard candy (eg, Lifesavers) to take if signs of hypoglycemia occur.
- Notify the physician if episodes of hypoglycemia occur, blood glucose levels rise above 160 mg/dL, urine is positive for ketones, cuts or scratches do not quickly heal, or any illness occurs such as gastrointestinal upset, fever, sore throat, diarrhea, rash, or unusual bleeding or bruising of the skin.
- Give printed information with symptoms of hypoglycemia and diabetic ketoacidosis. Explain the method recommended by the physician for terminating a hypoglycemic reaction.
- Exercise should be balanced with diet. Recommended exercises for the older adult include walking, swimming, and riding a stationary bike.
- Maintain good foot and skin care.
- Have routine eye and dental examinations for early detection of complications that occur in some diabetics.

- Wear identification such as a Medic-Alert to inform medical personnel and others of diabetes and the drug or drugs used to treat the disease.
- Occasionally, type II diabetes cannot be managed with diet, exercise, and the oral antidiabetic drugs alone. Insulin may be added to the treatment regimen. In this instance, information on types of insulin, dosage of insulin, how to administer insulin injections, and special precautions when administering insulin are given.
- Provide follow-up appointments with the Nurse Diabetic Educator, if necessary.
- Refer to an organization dealing with diabetes:

American Diabetes Association
Diabetes Information Service Center
1660 Duke Street
Alexandria, VA 22314
1-800-ADA-DISC
American Dietetic Association
216 West Jackson Boulevard
Chicago, IL 60666
1-800-877-1600
American Association of Diabetes Educators
444 North Michigan Ave
Suite 1240
Chicago, IL 60611
1-312-644-AADE
National Diabetes Information Clearing House
Box NDIC
1801 Rockville Pike
Bethesda, MD 20892
Juvenile Diabetes Foundation
423 Park Ave South
New York, NY 10011
1-800-JDF-CURE

Skin remains intact and free of lesions.
Patient follows the medication regimen.
Patient participates in daily foot care.

CRITICAL THINKING EXERCISES

1. Mr. Carter, age 69, was recently diagnosed with type II diabetes mellitus. The physician ordered a diabetic diet and placed him on chlorpropamide (Diabinese). Until approximately 3 months ago, he was very active and played tennis two or three times each week. He tells you that he is eager to play tennis again and asks you how soon he can resume this activity. What would you tell Mr. Carter? What is the most important consideration in his care? What, if any, action should you take?

2. Ms. Little, age 79, is an insulin-dependent diabetic (type II). She is a resident at the nursing home where you work. For the past several days, Ms. Little has had an upper respiratory infection and is taking antibiotics. What interventions would be most important for you to take in monitoring Ms. Little? What complications would she most likely experience? What assessments would you make when monitoring for these complications?

3. Mr. Landry, age 84, is diagnosed with hypothyroidism. The physician prescribes levothyroxine (Synthroid). What information would you give Mr. Landry about this drug? What precautions should Mr. Landry observe when taking levothyroxine?

4. Mr. Haley, age 68, recently had a thyroidectomy. He comes daily to the adult day care center where you work. Mr. Haley initially recovered well after his surgery, but lately you notice that his hair is coarse and dry, he appears weak, and he is not eating his meals. What action would you take first? What assessments would you make? What information would you give Mr. Haley?

REFERENCES AND SUGGESTED READING

Cirone, N., & Schwartz, N. (1996). Diabetes in the elderly, part II: Finding the balance for drug therapy. *Nursing, 96,* 40–45.

Depree, P. (1998). Lispro insulin: A short course on a quick performer. *Nursing 98,* 28 (11), 54–55.

Fleming, D. (1999). Challenging traditional insulin injection practices. *American Journal of Nursing, 99 (2),* 72–74.

Haplan-Landry, J., & Goldsmith, S. (1999). Feet first: Diabetes care. *American Journal of Nursing, 99 (2),* 26–33.

Hernandez, D. (1998). Assessing microvascular complications of diabetes. *American Journal of Nursing, 98 (6),* 26–32.

Jankowski, C. (1996). Irradiating the thyroid: How to protect yourself and others. *American Journal of Nursing, 96 (10),* 50–54.

Miller, C. (1998). Keeping up with new drugs for diabetes. *Geriatric Nursing, 19 (1),* 55–56.

O'Hanlon-Nichols, T. (1996). Hyperglycemic hyperosmolar nonketotic syndrome. *American Journal of Nursing, 96 (3),* 38.

Reed, R., & Mooradian, A. (1998). Management of diabetes in the nursing home. *The Annals of Long-Term Care, 6 (3),* 100–106.

Robertson, C. (1995). Diabetes 2000: Chronic complications. *Registered Nurse, 58(9),* 34–39.

Terpstra, T., & Terpstra, T. (1998). The elderly type II diabetic: A treatment challenge. *Geriatric Nursing, 19 (5),* 253–260.

Tomky, D. (1995). Diabetes 2000: Advances in monitoring. *Registered Nurse, 58(3),* 38–45.

CHAPTER **24**

CHAPTER OUTLINE

KEY TERMS
CHAPTER OBJECTIVES
NORMAL VISION
AGE-RELATED CHANGES IN THE EYE
THE EAR
AGE-RELATED CHANGES IN THE EAR
OTHER SENSORY ORGANS
CRITICAL THINKING EXERCISES
REFERENCES AND SUGGESTED READING

The Sensory Organs

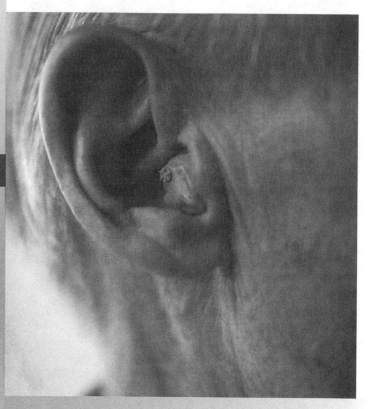

KEY TERMS

accommodation

age-related macular degeneration

aphakia

cataract

cerumen

closed-angle glaucoma

conductive hearing loss

ectropion

entropion

extracapsular cataract extraction

open-angle glaucoma

phacoemulsification

presbycusis

recruitment

sensorineural hearing loss

tinnitus

tonometer

trabeculectomy

trabeculoplasty

tympanic membrane

vertigo

CHAPTER OBJECTIVES

At the completion of this chapter, the student will be able to

- **Describe important aspects of normal vision and hearing**

- **Discuss age-related changes that occur within the eye and ear**

- **Discuss symptoms and treatment for common disorders affecting vision in the older adult**

- **Use the nursing process to care for an elderly adult with a visual or hearing impairment**

- **Distinguish between conductive hearing loss and sensorineural hearing loss**

- **Identify important aspects of managing older adults with a hearing loss**

- **Discuss the importance of the other senses: taste, smell, and touch**

The eye and the ear play vital roles in maintaining an active and independent lifestyle. Sometimes, changes occur with vision and hearing as the result of the aging process that affects self-care ability. Older adults who develop vision or hearing problems may experience social isolation and diminished self-care ability, increasing their risk for entering a nursing home. Minor adjustments often can enhance the older adults lifestyle and enable them to remain independent in the home environment. This chapter discusses visual and hearing impairments, as well as the senses of taste, smell, and touch.

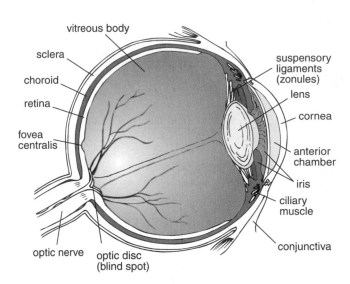

FIGURE 24-1. The normal eye.

NORMAL VISION

The eye is the organ of vision. The eye is a spherical organ set within the orbital cavity. Three supportive layers form a protective covering for the eye: sclera, choroid, and retina (Fig. 24-1). The outermost layer is the white covering of the eyeball called the sclera. The sclera is made of tough connective tissue to protect the delicate layer underneath. The cornea is a continuation of the sclera and forms a transparent layer on the front of the eyeball. Light enters through the cornea. The middle layer of the eyeball, the choroid, is filled with a tiny meshwork of blood vessels. The third and innermost layer is the retina. The retina contains the receptors for vision, the rods and the cones.

The light rays bend as they pass through the eye to focus on the retina. This bending of the light rays is called refraction and is accomplished with the help of three structures: aqueous humor, lens, and vitreous humor. The aqueous humor is a watery fluid that fills the anterior cavity of the eye. The lens is an elastic transparent body of cells that functions in **accommodation** (ie, focusing light rays on the retina). The lens adjusts its shape to focus on objects nearby or faraway. The ciliary body is a thickened area that connects the choroid (ie, the middle layer) with the iris. The ciliary body contains muscles that contract to help control the thickness of the lens and to function in accommodation.

The last of the structures that affects refraction is the vitreous body, a soft, jelly-like substance that fills the cavity behind the lens. The aqueous humor and the vitreous body maintain a relatively constant amount of solution within their respective cavities that helps maintain the shape of the eyeball as well as functioning in refraction. From the retina, the nerve impulses travel to the optic nerve, which transmits the impulses to the brain.

The iris is the colored or pigmented part of the eye. The muscular action of the iris causes the circular opening of the eye, the pupil, to contract or dilate. In this way, the size of the pupil is regulated, and light entering the eye is controlled. Lacrimal ducts near the nasal area of the eye drain tears and small particles into the nose. The tears are produced by the lacrimal glands located on the upper outer corner of each eye.

AGE-RELATED CHANGES IN THE EYE

Multiple structural changes occur within the aging eye. The cornea, lens, ciliary body, iris, vitreous body, and aqueous humor all undergo changes with age. The cornea has a generalized decrease in sensitivity, causing the older adult to be less aware of injury to the eye. Epithelial cells within the cornea decrease in number. The production of aqueous humor is decreased with age, but it does not greatly affect the balance of intraocular pressure. The thick fluid of the vitreous body becomes thinner, and floaters may appear within the visual field. In addition to becoming larger and more rigid, the lens becomes discolored and opaque, affecting visual acuity and leading to age-related cataracts.

As the eye ages, there is an accumulation of what is thought to be lipids that collect on the outer edge of the cornea. This lipid ring appears as a grayish ring surrounding the iris called the arcus senilis (Fig. 24-2). There is no pathology associated with arcus senilis. The iris itself losses pigment with age, leaving most older adults with a light blue or grayish iris. With increasing age, the pupil becomes smaller. By the age of 60, the pupil is only two

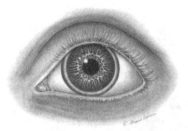

FIGURE 24-2. Arcus senilis. Seen as a thin grayish-white circle not quite at the edge of the cornea.

thirds of the size of the pupil of a young adult. The decrease in pupil size contributes to the loss of visual acuity.

The process of accommodation is the ability of the eye to focus on objects close by and objects far away. Accommodation is accomplished through coordination of the ciliary body and the muscle fibers of the iris. As the ciliary body contracts, the lens thickens, and the muscle fibers of the iris contract, resulting in a smaller pupil. In this manner, the ciliary muscle changes the curvature of the lens. Age, however, causes the ciliary muscle to decrease in length and become less elastic. The muscle is replaced with connective tissue, resulting in a decreased ability to change the shape of the lens and focus clearly on nearby objects. The lens becomes less elastic and larger as cellular debris collects within the lens capsule contributing to a loss of accommodation. This change in accommodation results in a condition called presbyopia, or "old sightedness."

Loss of Visual Acuity

Visual acuity (ie, ability to see clearly) decreases with age. Several factors contribute to the loss of acuity. The progressively smaller pupil, the clouding and yellowing of the lens, the thinning of the vitreous solution, and the presence of floaters in the vitreous body all contribute to a loss of visual acuity. Peripheral vision decreases, night vision diminishes, and there is an increased sensitivity to glare.

The changes can result in the older adult having problems driving (especially at night), engaging in social activities, and in the performance of activities of daily living. Most older adults older than the age of 60 lose visual acuity to a point that glasses must be worn. However, loss of vision is not inevitable and some older adults do not lose the ability to see well as age increases.

The most common visual disorders of the older adult are age-related macular degeneration, cataracts, glaucoma, and diabetic retinopathy (see Chapter 24).

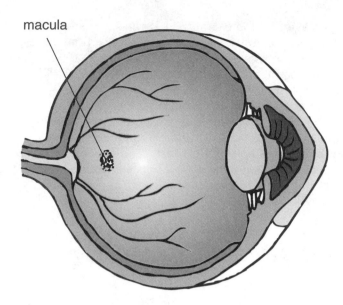

macula

FIGURE 24-3. Macula position. The macula is located in the center of the retina and provides sight in the center of the visual field. The macula is responsible for sharp, straight-ahead vision necessary for driving or doing close work, such as sewing, reading, or recognition of faces.

Age-Related Macular Degeneration

Age-related macular degeneration (ARMD) occurs most often in individuals older than age 50 and is the leading cause of visual loss for those older than 65. As the population ages, the incidence of this disorder is expected to increase. The macula is located on the retina directly behind the lens (Fig. 24-3). The cones are located within the macula, providing sharp central vision and color vision. The cells within the macula diminish in functional ability with age, and replacement of the damaged cells is decreased, causing irreversible damage to the macula. This loss of functional ability results in a loss of central vision.

Signs and Symptoms
Initial signs and symptoms are vague, and patients may simply sense that something is wrong with their vision. Images are fuzzy or distorted. Objects may appear to be the wrong size or shape, and straight lines appear wavy or crooked. There is a progressive loss of central vision, increased sensitivity to glare, blurring of vision, and diminishing color vision. Peripheral vision is not affected. Eventually there is a total loss of central vision. Diagnosis is made by an ophthalmologist who measures visual acuity. A specialized diagnostic test called intravenous fluorescein angiography is used to confirm a diagnosis of ARMD.

Management
Some cases of ARMD can be treated with a laser if the problem is discovered in the early stages. Laser

treatment can prevent or delay extension of the degeneration process in only a limited number of cases. Unfortunately, no treatment is available for most cases of ARMD.

Nursing management involves assisting the patient in dealing with the loss of vision, retaining self-care abilities, and providing patient and family teaching to increase understanding of the disease and treatment options. In most cases, the retention of peripheral vision allows the patient to remain relatively independent, although modifications must be made.

Glaucoma

Although glaucoma can occur at any age, those most at risk are older adults older than age 60. Vision lost as the result of glaucoma cannot be restored, but with medication and surgery, further damage and visual loss can be controlled. Glaucoma occurs as the result of increased intraocular pressure (IOP).

The front portion of the eye is filled with aqueous humor. This fluid is constantly produced by the ciliary body and nourishes the eye. The fluid flows out of the inner part of the eye through a meshwork of small drainage tubules located around the outer edge of the iris. The amount of fluid within the eye determines the IOP. Normally the IOP stays with a range that allows the eye to function well. With glaucoma, the drainage tubules become clogged, preventing the outflow of fluid. The ciliary body continues to produce aqueous humor, but with no means for drainage, the fluid builds and increases the IOP. If the IOP becomes too high for too long, the excessive pressure can damage the optic nerve leading to visual problems or blindness.

Types of Glaucoma

There are two main types of glaucoma: open-angle glaucoma or chronic glaucoma and closed-angle or acute glaucoma (Fig. 24-4). **Open-angle glaucoma** is the most common form of glaucoma. Approximately 90% of those diagnosed with glaucoma have open-angle glaucoma. The course of the disease is slow, with symptoms appearing gradually as the drainage tubules become clogged. IOP increases because aqueous fluid cannot drain in adequate amounts. As the name open-angle implies, the angle where the iris meets the cornea is wide and open.

In **closed-angle glaucoma,** the angle between the iris and the cornea is too narrow, hampering the drainage of fluid. Pressure builds up very quickly because the drainage tubules are blocked. Symptoms occur suddenly, and immediate medical attention is needed to prevent permanent visual damage. Acute glaucoma is rare.

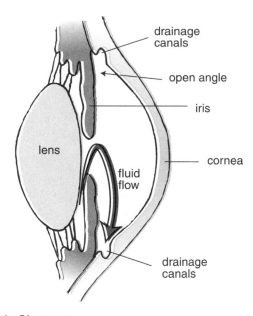

Open-Angle Glaucoma
The most common type of glaucoma. It progresses very slowly as the eye's drainage system gradually becomes blocked, causing an increase in IOP. Notice that the angle where the iris meets the cornea is "open."

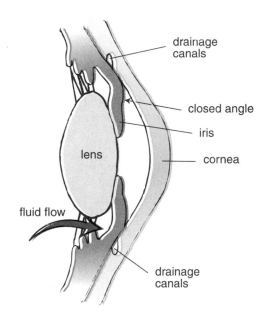

Closed-Angle Glaucoma
A less common type of glaucoma in which the IOP increases very rapidly due to a blockage in the trabecular networks. Notice that the angle where the iris meets the cornea is "closed."

FIGURE 24-4. Types of glaucoma.

Signs and Symptoms
Open-angle or chronic glaucoma is often difficult to detect. The onset is insidious, and the disease progresses slowly. Symptoms occur bilaterally and include mild aching of the eyes, loss of peripheral

vision, halos around lights, and decreased visual acuity. The loss of peripheral vision leads to a tunnel vision effect.

Acute closed-angle glaucoma is unilateral, and symptoms occur suddenly. Symptoms include severe eye pain, seeing halos around lights, redness, and blurred vision. Nausea, vomiting, or bradycardia may accompany the severe pain.

Treatment

When signs and symptoms are present, further diagnostic tests are necessary. The **tonometer** is an instrument used to measure pressure in the eye. Applanation tonometry requires the eye to be anesthetized with drops. Using a slit lamp, a plastic prism is pushed lightly against the eye, measuring the IOP. If air tonometry is used, a puff of air is administered on the cornea to obtain a measurement. The ophthalmologist (ie, physician who specializes in diagnosis and treatment of disorders of the eye) can view the color and appearance of the optic nerve to determine the extent of the glaucoma and identify any damage. Visual field testing may be done manually or using a computer to determine the individual's field of vision.

When glaucoma is diagnosed early and treatment instituted, blindness is almost always preventable. Problems arise because extensive damage can occur before any symptoms appear. To detect glaucoma early, it is recommended that older adults have an eye examination by an ophthalmologist yearly. There is no cure for glaucoma, but it may be controlled with medication to reduce aqueous humor or surgery to provide a drainage pathway for the aqueous humor.

For acute glaucoma, treatment involves a type of laser surgery to unblock the drainage tubules. When laser surgery is used for open-angle glaucoma, the procedure is called laser **trabeculoplasty.** During laser trabeculoplasty, the laser is focused on the trabecular meshwork, causing a shrinkage of some of the trabecular meshwork and allowing the fluid to escape and IOP to decrease. Many patients may be able to discontinue some of their antiglaucoma medication after a trabeculoplasty.

A more traditional surgical procedure is the **trabeculectomy** (ie, surgical removal of a small section of trabecular mesh). After a trabeculectomy, IOP decreases because the aqueous humor is able to drain out of the anterior portion of the eye. Most patient are able to discontinue all of their antiglaucoma medication after this procedure. Regular follow-up examinations are required, even after successful treatment, because chronic glaucoma can develop years later.

Medication such as pilocarpine or timolol maleate can also be used to manage glaucoma. Timolol (Timoptic) is commonly prescribed, and it decreases the rate at which fluid flows into the eye. Timolol, however, can worsen pulmonary symptoms, causing respiratory distress and decreased pulse rate. Betaxolol (Betoptic) is recommended for patients who have asthma or emphysema. Pilocarpine causes miosis (ie, constriction) of the pupil, opening the blocked channels and allowing normal passage of fluid. Other drugs, such as brimonidine (Alphagan), decrease the formation of aqueous humor.

Oral carbonic anhydrase inhibitors such as acetazolamide (Diamox) reduces fluid flow into the eye. Traditionally these drugs are used as a last resort because of poorly tolerated side effects such as frequent urination, tingling sensation in the fingers and toes, kidney stones and aplastic anemia. Other disturbing side effects are depression, fatigue and lethargy. Dorzolamide (Trusopt) is the first topical carbonic anhydrase inhibitor and is reasonably well tolerated with significantly less side effects than the more traditional oral medication.

Latanoprost (Xalatan) increases the rate at which aqueous humor flows out of the eye. This drugs has the advantage of once-daily dosing. Latanoprost may cause the iris suntan syndrome, which is an increased amount of brown pigment in the eyes of patients with hazel, green-brown, or blue-brown eyes. This change occurs slowly and may not be immediately evident.

When taking eyedrops, it is important for the patient or the caregiver to understand the importance of taking the medication exactly as prescribed by the ophthalmologist. Some medications have a duration of 6 hours and must be taken at regular intervals to assure that the drug's effectiveness is maintained for the full 24-hour day.

Older patients taking these drugs must be carefully monitored. Instruction on the correct method of administration of an ophthalmic drug is necessary. It is important to assess the older adult's ability to instill drops. Arthritis or other musculoskeletal disorders may make instillation difficult. The patient's mental status is important. Forgetting to instill the drops may result in an attack of acute glaucoma. In most instances, the drug must be continued for life. The individual is instructed to keep the eyes closed for 1 to 2 minutes after administration and press lightly against the nasal corner of the eyelids. This closes the duct that drains into the nose and minimizes absorption into the systemic circulation. The physician is notified if eye discomfort or inflammation occurs. Vision may be blurred immediately after instillation of medication but should clear within 15 to 20 minutes. Notify the health care provider if blurred vision persists. If more than one ophthalmic medication is prescribed, wait 15 minutes between each instillation. Periodic eye examinations are necessary to monitor progress.

Cataracts

A **cataract** is clouding of the eye's lens that prevents light from focusing properly on the retina. The lens focuses light rays on the retina (ie, innermost layer of the eyeball that transmits visual stimuli to the optic nerve) and produces an image. The lens functions in accommodation, allowing the eye to focus on close and distant objects.

Although cataracts can occur at any age, the highest incidence is found in individuals older than age 55. Cataracts usually develop slowly over a number of years and develop bilaterally, although often at different times. For example, an older adult may develop visual problems as the result of a cataract and may have surgery to correct the problem. In several months to several years, a cataract may develop in the other eye and require surgery.

Signs and Symptoms

The lens contains, among other things, protein molecules and water. With age, changes within the lens cause the protein to bind together and cloud the lens. Over time, the entire lens may become opaque (ie, cloudy), making clear vision almost impossible. The physician may use the phrase "ripening" when referring to the cataract. The cataract is considered ripe when swelling occurs within the lens as a result of water being drawn into the lens. Although a cataract begins small with little visual disturbance, in time, vision is blurred as in looking through a water fall or cloudy glass. In addition to blurred or hazy vision, other symptoms include

- Increased problems with glare
- Need for more light to perform tasks such as reading that require good visual acuity
- Increased nearsightedness
- Poor vision at night
- Need for frequent eyeglass prescription changes
- Double vision

Treatment

Initially, glasses or contacts may be used to improve vision. The only effective treatment for a cataract is surgical removal of the lens. Cataract surgery is one of the most common surgeries performed in the United States each year. Surgery is unnecessary when a cataract is present but is indicated when the cataract interferes with daily activity.

DISPLAY 24-1. Patient Teaching After Cataract Surgery

- Perform usual activities in moderation. For example, watching television or reading is permitted, but only for short periods.
- Do not bend over the sink or tub or place the head down below the waist. When washing hair, tilt the head slightly backward.
- Sleep on the back or side, not the abdomen.
- Wear sunglasses for protection.
- Do not rub eyes, squeeze eyelids, or cough.
- Take a stool softener to avoid straining during a bowel movement.
- Follow the physician's recommendations concerning resuming sexual activity.
- Do not lift anything heavier that 15 pounds.
- Take medications as prescribed by the physician.
- Use sterile cotton or gauze moistened with sterile water or normal saline to clean the eye.
- When instilling eye drops, tilt the head back, gently pull down the lower conjunctival sac, and instill the correct number of drops.
- Wear a protective shield at night if prescribed by the physician.
- Immediately report any of the following symptoms: eye pain, redness, swelling, inflammation, discharge from the eye, changes in visual acuity, light flashes, spots in the visual field, or halos around lights.

The most effective surgical procedures to treat cataracts are phacoemulsification and extracapsular extraction. During the surgery, the lens is removed and replaced with a clear plastic lens (ie, lens implant).

During **extracapsular cataract extraction,** the surgeon makes an incision at the point where the cornea and sclera meet. The surgeon enters the eye through the incision and opens the front of the capsule and removes the nucleus of the lens. The surgeon then gently suctions the remainder of the lens, leaving the capsule in place. In **phacoemulsification,** the surgeon breaks up the lens with ultrasound and then suctions these fragments from the eye through a small incision.

Aphakia is the term used to describe an eye with no lens. An intraocular lens implant is usually performed during cataract surgery. A clear plastic lens is implanted into the eye in place of the natural lens. This implant functions like the natural functioning eye and is more convenient for the elderly than wearing cataract eye glasses or contact lenses. Display 24-1 provides information to include when teaching the patient or caregiver after cataract surgery.

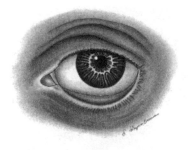

Ectropion
Note that the margin of the lid is turned outward, exposing the inner conjuctiva.

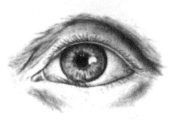

Entropion
Note the inward turning of the lid margin, making the lower lashes invisible because they are turned inward.

FIGURE 24-5. Ectropion and entropion.

Entropion and Ectropion

Entropion and ectropion are disorders that commonly occur in older adults. These conditions do not cause vision loss but are uncomfortable. **Entropion** is an inward turning of the lid margin (Fig. 24-5). The lower lashes may not be visible and can irritate the conjunctiva, causing watering and redness of the eye. The inversion of the lower lid is caused by a generalized wasting of muscle and tissue surrounding the eye.

Ectropion is an outward turning of the margin of the lid, exposing the conjunctiva. Ectropion interferes with draining of the tears, and increased tearing may occur. Like entropion, in the elderly, it is most often caused by a generalized weakening and atrophy of the tissues and muscles surrounding the eye. Surgery is indicated to correct ectropion and entropion.

Using the Nursing Process to Care for an Elderly Adult With a Visual Impairment

Assessment

Because the aging process leads to a gradual decline in visual acuity, all older adults are assessed for visual impairment. A Snellen eye chart may be used to assess visual acuity. The individual stands at a distance of 20 feet, covers one eye, and reads each line of the chart until the print can no longer be distinguished. For a patient who cannot read, the Snellen E chart can be used. In this chart, the E appears in four different positions. The indi-

vidual's visual acuity is tested by having the person indicate the direction of the E orally or by placing the fingers in the direction the E is pointing. With age, there is decreased ability to focus on close objects or see small print (ie, presbyopia), reduced capacity to adjust to changes in light and dark (ie, accommodation), and decreased ability to distinguish color.

It is important to assess nursing home residents and those living alone because the impact of visual impairment is far-reaching. Visual defects can affect social interactions, self-care ability, self-esteem, and rehabilitation potential. A visual problem may affect the resident's ability to eat, walk, recognize staff, or navigate within the environment.

Obtain a family history of eye disorders (eg, glaucoma, diabetes, vascular disorders). Display 24-2 identifies ways to assess visual impairment.

ASSESSMENT ALERT

Eye pain, blurred or fuzzy vision, double vision, or sudden loss of vision are usually associated with acute eye disorders and should be immediately reported to the physician or health care provider.

The nurse also obtains a history of past and current illnesses or diseases. Disorders such as cerebrovascular accident, dementia, or myasthenia gravis (ie, neuromuscular disorder characterized by severe muscular weakness) produce visual disturbances not related to disease of the eye.

Assessing for visual impairment in older adults with dementia, those with a decreased mental status, or those with a communication deficit may be difficult, because they may be unable to understand questions or follow directions necessary to test visual acuity. In these situations, the nurse must be alert for nonverbal clues that indicate possible visual disturbances, such as eating difficulties, difficulty navigating in the environment, bumping into things, or squinting the eyes when trying to see.

Many older adults wear eye glasses or contact lenses. The nurse assesses manual dexterity to determine whether the individual is able to place the contact lens in the eye. Eyeglasses are checked for scratches and cleanliness. The patient's ability to function within the environment is assessed. Does a visual problem decrease the ability to eat food, walk safely within the environment, or interact with others? Can the individual see to read or watch television? The nurse refers to an ophthalmologist for further assessment if indicated. The older adult should have an eye examination at

---

DISPLAY 24-2 **Assessment of Visual Impairment**

- Visual disturbances (eg, blurred, cloudy, or hazy vision, loss of peripheral vision, halos, tunnel vision, and loss of central vision)
- Glare or increased sensation to light
- Frequent need to change eyeglasses or eyeglass change does not result in improved vision
- Increased tearing
- Pain or pressure in the eye (severe pain in the eye is an emergency and requires immediate treatment)
- Headache
- Self-care ability
- Poor night vision
- Problems distinguishing color
- During eye examination, note any gray or milky white appearance of pupil. The size of pupil and pupillary response is documented.

---

least yearly or more often if any visual impairment occurs or any worsening of a previous visual impairment occurs.

Nursing Diagnoses

The following nursing diagnoses may be used for an older adult with a visual impairment:

> Impaired Home Maintenance Management related to lack of assistance
>
> Self-Care Deficit (specify type) related to visual disturbances
>
> Situational Low Self-Esteem related to adjusting to vision loss
>
> Social Isolation related to inability to see clearly, move freely in environment, other (specify)
>
> Risk for Injury related to impaired vision, unfamiliar surroundings, other (specify)
>
> Knowledge Deficit of assistive agencies
>
> Diversional Activity Deficit related to difficulty performing usual activities (reading) because of diminished vision

Other nursing diagnoses may be appropriate for individual patients.

Planning and Implementation

Planning the care of an older adult with a visual impairment requires careful attention to providing the individual with a safe home environment, promoting self-esteem, preventing social isolation, creating the means to continue pleasurable diversionary activities, and correcting any knowledge deficit.

Impaired Home Maintenance. Older adults living at home who have poor vision must learn to manage the home environment. Environmental changes such as low-glare floors, large-print signs marking specific rooms, color-coded tape on the dresser drawers, or large numbers on the telephone may allow the older adult more independence in the home or nursing home environment. If glare is a problem, the individual may wear a yellow-tinted visor and a pair of sunglasses. Fluorescent lighting increases the glare and should be avoided.

Sometimes, assistance may be needed because of loss of vision. Planning care with a multidisciplinary team helps to maintain a high quality of care that meets the individual's needs. The patient may require assistance such as a home health nurse to make periodic visits, homemaker services, Meals-on-Wheels, or social services. The nurse assists with obtaining any specialized equipment, such as a cane to recognize objects in the path and makes arrangements for needed services. The family and friends are involved in the care. Shopping, cleaning, banking, and transporting the patient are all ways for the family to assist the older adult with home maintenance. Identify community resources and support systems and involve them in the care.

Self-Care Deficit. Problems with self-care can arise in older adults with visual problems. The patient's room or house is kept the same. Objects and furniture are left in the same place. Smaller items such as toilet articles, grooming aids, clothing, shoes, or the urinal are kept in specific places where the patient is aware of them and where the items are easily accessible. The doors are left wide open or totally closed. A thorough orientation is needed to any new environment.

For eating, have the patient use the face of a clock to identify the image of the location of specific foods on the plate. Twelve o'clock is the top of the plate, and 6 o'clock is the bottom of the plate. The nurse or staff member describes the various foods on the plate in relation to the clock face. Food is "pushed" toward the center of the plate with a roll or a piece of bread.

Another method to help with self-care for those with partial site is to use bright colors that provide a sharp contrast to other colors. This makes vision easier. For example, towels that contrast with bathroom walls are easier to locate than towels the same or similar color. Hand rails may be painted a color that contrasts with the walls.

The patient may need simple reminders to put glasses on daily. Sometimes, eye glasses can provide enough vision to promote self-care. If manual dexterity is a problem, the nurse or caregiver can provide the needed assistance. Glasses are cleaned with dish soap and wiped with a soft cloth.

Situational Low Self-Esteem. Self-esteem may be affected when the patient is no longer able to participate in activities requiring sight. Encourage expression of feelings and anxieties. The nurse must actively listen and convey confidence in the patient's coping abilities. Positive feedback is given. It is important to help the patient to develop goals that can be attained to build confidence. The patient is allowed to make decisions about care and have control over the environment. The family and caregivers are involved as much as possible. The patient is encouraged to attend a support group. The nurse promotes self-care, socialization, and the use of diversionary activities to combat low self-esteem.

Social Isolation. When faced with visual impairment, some older adults may withdraw from social activities and isolate themselves from interaction with others. For example, a nursing home resident may refuse to participate in group activities or come to the dining hall to eat and remain alone in the room.

Sighted guides may be assigned to lead a visually impaired person from place to place. The sighted guide may be a nurse assistant, a fellow patient, a family member, a friend, or another member of the health care team. These guides walk from place to place with the visually impaired person to assist her around the home, outside, in the acute care facility, or in the nursing home. If the patient agrees to have a guide, the guide offers his elbow or arm. The visually impaired person takes the arm slightly above the elbow. During ambulation, the guide remains slightly ahead. While walking, the guide describes the surroundings.

The nurse must actively listen as the patient expresses feelings and emotions. Time spent with the individual shows a genuine interest in the patient's welfare. It is also important to encourage socialization. In some cases, the nurse must mobilize the individual's support system. Senior citizen centers, church groups, day care centers, and foster grandparent programs may also be used to increase opportunities for socialization.

Risk for Injury. Older adults are at an increased risk for injury, especially from falls. A visual disturbance places the older adult at an even greater risk for injury. When caring for a person with a visual impairment, it is important to orient them to the physical environment. The nurse describes where furnishings are located and the location of the closet or the bathroom. Objects are kept in the same place in the environment. The area is kept clean and uncluttered. Environmental hazards, such as throw rugs or spills, must be taken care of as soon as possible. It is important to provide names, addresses, and phone numbers of organizations that offer help to the visually impaired. Family members or caregivers are taught ways to keep the home environment safe.

When assisting with ambulation, walk slowly and stand to the side slightly ahead of the visually impaired person. The patient grasps the nurse's or caregiver's elbow when walking. The nurse should not grasp the patient's elbow and pull the person along or push the individual. By allowing the visually impaired person to hold the elbow or arm, tension and anxiety are reduced, and there is less risk for injury.

The home or physical surroundings must be well lighted. Visually impaired individuals need three or four times more light than a normally sighted person. The nurse makes sure environment does not produce glares. For example, nonfluorescent lighting produces less glare than other forms of lighting. For those with partial sight, it is important to keep large printed signs to mark rooms and large numbers on phones. The patient is taught how to use a cane for ambulating.

Diversional Activity Deficit. The patient is encouraged to acknowledge his or her feelings and reality of the current situation. Activity options are explored taking into consideration the loss of vision. Modifications or adjustments are made so activities the individual previously enjoyed can still be a source of pleasure. For example, if the patient enjoyed reading, suggest that large print books or magazines be used or that the individual listen to audiotapes of books. Large-print books or magazines and taped books may be found in the public library or modestly priced at most book stores. If partial vision remains, keep areas well lighted. It may be necessary to use a 300-watt bulb when reading.

The patient may want to have a magnifying glass available. Magnifiers are one of the most basic and valuable tools for the patient with low vision. Magnifiers come in various forms: hand held, stand, and lighted. Radios, compact discs, and tapes offer the opportunity for diversion and relaxation without the need for a magnifier.

The patient is referred to support groups or self-help agencies. For those interested in learning Braille refer to the appropriate agency (Display 24-3). Names of individuals who agree to be "telephone buddies" are provided. These individuals can talk to the patient, provide encouragement, and offer an enjoyable alternative during long days.

Assistive Agencies. Numerous agencies are available to assist those with visual disturbances. The patient and family may not be aware of these resources. The nurse can provide a listing of these resources (Display 24-4).

Evaluation and Expected Outcomes
Successful treatment can be gauged by the following responses:

Assistance is obtained for home care.

Family becomes involved in home care.

DISPLAY 24-3. Ready Resources for Those With Visual Impairment

American Foundation for the Blind
11 Penn Plaza, Suite 300
New York, NY 10001
800-232-5463
The Center for the Partially Sighted
12301 Wilshire Blvd, Suite 600
Los Angeles, CA 90025
800-481-3937
National Association for Visually Handicapped
22 West 21st Street
New York, NY 10010
212-889-3141
Association for Macular Diseases, Inc.
210 East 64th Street
New York, NY 10021
The Glaucoma Foundation
33 Maiden Lane
New York, NY 10038
800-GLAUCOMA
(http://www.glaucoma-foundation.org/info)
American Academy of Ophthalmology
P.O. Box 7472
San Francisco, CA 94120-7424
(http://www.eyenet.org)
For information on eye care for low-income older
   people, call 800-222-3937
**National Eye Institute/National Institutes
   of Health**
2020 Vision Place
Bethesda, MD 20892-3655
National Braille Association
1290 University Ave
Rochester, NY 14607
Taping for the Blind
3935 Essex Lane
New York, NY 10022

DISPLAY 24-4. Nursing Interventions for the Hearing Impaired

- When speaking, increase volume of the voice, but do not increase the pitch.
- Do not shout.
- Speak into the "good" ear, being careful to stay at a distance of 2 to 3 feet.
- Articulate words carefully, speak slowly, and rephrase if necessary.
- Face the individual you are speaking with.
- Use gestures if necessary, but keep the hands away from the face.
- Reduce or eliminate background noise by turning off the radio or television.
- Avoid appearing frustrated.
- Test for accuracy of hearing by having the older adult repeat the information.
- Write messages if necessary for easier communication.
- Use a light to indicate the doorbell is ringing.
- Place an amplifier on the telephone.
- Use earphones with an amplifier for listening to the television.

Patient provides self-care within limitations.

Patient relates feelings of improved self-esteem.

Patient participates in social activities.

Patient relates use of safety measures to prevent injury.

Patient relates ability to enjoy diversionary activities.

Patient expresses increased awareness of assistive agencies.

THE EAR

The ear functions in hearing and in maintaining equilibrium. The ear is composed of three main parts; the external ear, middle ear, and the internal ear. The outermost part of the external ear is the auricle, followed by the external auditory canal that provides a route for sound waves to travel to the middle ear. The beginning external auditory canal is lined with glands known as ceruminous glands that excrete **cerumen,** or ear wax. Sometimes, the cerumen can be so thick and dry that it becomes hard and impacted in the canal. Impacted cerumen can interfere with hearing and must be removed.

The **tympanic membrane** receives the sound waves from the auditory canal and serves as a protective barrier for the innermost parts of the ear. Sound waves cause the tympanic membrane to vibrate, resulting in the transmission of sound to the middle ear. The tiny bones of the middle ear, the malleus, incus, and stapes amplify the sound waves received from the tympanic membrane and transmit the sounds through the oval window to the internal ear (Fig. 24-6).

The cochlea and the semicircular canals of the internal ear contain a fluid through which sound waves travel. The organ of Corti, located at the base of the cochlear duct, is essentially the organ of hearing. The organ of Corti has hairlike cilia that are extremely sensitive to the vibrations of the sound waves. These hairlike cilia propagate the nerve impulses that travel to the cochlear nerve.

Equilibrium or balance, is also controlled by the structures of the inner ear. Receptors for the sense of balance are also located on the cilia of the organ of

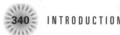

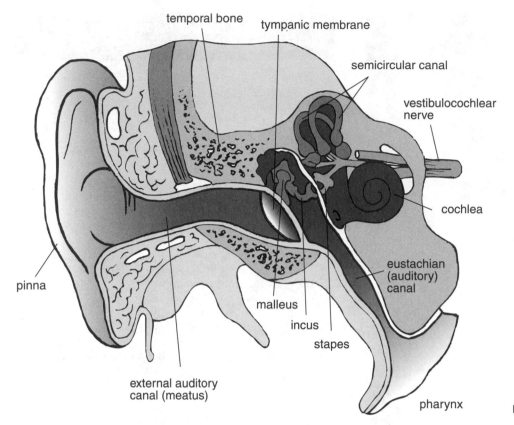

temporal bone

tympanic membrane

semicircular canal

vestibulocochlear nerve

cochlea

eustachian (auditory) canal

pinna

malleus

incus

stapes

external auditory canal (meatus)

pharynx

FIGURE 24-6. The normal ear.

Corti. The cilia innervate fibers of the vestibular nerve. The vestibular nerve and cochlear nerve then join to form the eight cranial nerve or the vestibulocochlear nerve.

AGE-RELATED CHANGES IN THE EAR

Hearing deficits have been reported in approximately 55% of those older than age 65 and in 66% of individuals older than age 80. Although some degree of hearing loss occurs in about two thirds of the elderly, the loss is not always caused by age-related changes. Many individuals suffer hearing loss from non–age-relate disorders such as exposure to loud noise or as an adverse effect of medication. In general, hearing loss occurs in three forms: conductive hearing loss, sensorineural hearing loss, and mixed (ie, sensorineural and conductive).

Conductive hearing loss occurs as the result of problems involving the external and middle ear. A conductive loss typically involves interference with the passage of sound waves through the middle and external ear. **Sensorineural hearing loss** involves damage to the structures of the inner ear, particularly the cochlear nerve. In the elderly, the most common cause of diminished hearing is mixed hear-

ing loss, which is a combination of conductive hearing loss and sensorineural hearing loss.

Conductive Hearing Loss

Conductive hearing loss can occur in the elderly because of previous injury to the tympanic membrane resulting in scaring or inflammation or from a disease such as otosclerosis (ie, disease of the middle ear, resulting in the tiny ossicles being unable to pass vibrations on to the inner ear) or because of impacted cerumen. Cerumen excreted by ceruminous glands is drier and more solid in the older adult. This dry, hardened cerumen easily becomes impacted within the ear, causing a conductive hearing loss. This type of hearing loss is more common in elderly men.

Sensorineural Hearing Loss

Sensorineural hearing loss in the elderly is usually bilateral and becomes slowly but progressively worse with age. Total deafness usually does not occur. **Presbycusis** is the term used to describe progressive sensorineural hearing loss occurring as the result of changes in the innermost parts of the ear. Some degree of presbycusis affects approximately 60% of adults older than age 65. As with conductive loss, men are more often affected than women. Structured changes in the inner ear include loss of hair cells and atrophy in the organ of Corti, as well as atrophy of vestibular structures, causing problems with equilibrium.

Decreased speech discrimination often accompanies sensorineural loss. A decreased ability to hear high-frequency sounds results in the decreased ability to discriminate between sounds. Vowels are more easily heard because they are lower pitched, but consonants pose a problem for many older adults. Distinguishing between the sounds *sh* and *ch* or *p* and *d* is often difficult. Rapid speech and background noise make hearing more difficult for the older adult. **Recruitment** (ie, loud sounds heard abnormally loud) also occurs in the older adult, making speech difficult to understand.

Tinnitus

Another age-related problem that interferes with hearing is the presence of **tinnitus,** or ringing in the ears. Tinnitus may occur in sensorineural and in conductive hearing loss. The sound is described as a ringing, buzzing, or hissing noise. Tinnitus may occur as the result of a disease process such as otosclerosis or Ménière disease or as an adverse reaction to certain ototoxic drugs such as gentamicin or aspirin. Typically, tinnitus occurring as the result of a conductive hearing loss is low pitched; whereas, with sensorineural hearing loss, the tinnitus is high pitched.

Management of Hearing Loss in the Elderly Adult

Management of a hearing loss in the elderly adult depends on the type of hearing loss. For example, a hearing aid may be quite helpful for a conductive hearing loss but of no value in sensorineural hearing loss. Simple interventions (see Display 24-4) may prove beneficial in increasing the ability to hear in conductive and in sensorineural hearing loss.

Correcting hearing problems in the elderly is complicated when the older adult accepts hearing loss as a normal consequence of aging and decides that nothing can be done. Withdrawal, social isolation, and loneliness can needlessly occur when this type of attitude is taken. When hearing problems are not corrected, communication is virtually impossible, causing frustration and resentment for the older adult as well as family and friends.

Clearing the auditory canal of impacted cerumen may greatly improve conductive hearing loss. Removal of the cerumen can be accomplished by gentle irrigation of the ear canal. If the tympanic membrane is unbroken, irrigation with normal saline at body temperature can clear the cerumen. The intact tympanic membrane can be viewed with an otoscope after removing some of the cerumen. Irrigation is never attempted unless the tympanic membrane is intact. A normal tympanic membrane appears pearly gray when viewed through a otoscope. When talking with the older adult, it is important to emphasize that objects such as bobbie pins or cotton swabs should not be used to remove cerumen.

Ear wax can also be removed using one of several over-the-counter eardrops such as Cerumenex. When used as directed on the package insert, these medications can be effective in ridding the ear of cerumen. Some physicians, however, advise against using over-the-counter drugs because infection and irritation can occur.

Although there is no cure for sensorineural deafness, various interventions can enhance the ability to hear. Display 24-3 gives guidelines to assist the older adult to hear.

An evaluation by an otologist (ie, physician who specializes in disorders of the ear) or an audiologist (ie, specialist who evaluates hearing function) is necessary to determine the exact cause of a hearing deficit. The older adult may have a disease of the ear that causes the hearing loss. For this reason, it is important not to indiscriminately attribute hearing loss to old age without a thorough evaluation by a physician to rule out other causes.

Tinnitus is a symptom, not a disease. However, it is common and can be extremely troublesome. Tinnitus should never be casually dismissed. Sometimes, the tinnitus is not noticeable until its severity varies. For some, tinnitus is masked by environmental noises and is not noticeable unless in an unusually quiet environment. For others, the tinnitus is severe and causes great anxiety. Treatment is often ineffective. Sometimes, soft music or other environment noise can be used as competing sound to diminish or relieve the tinnitus. For others, time diminishes or alleviates the problem.

Hearing Aids

Hearing aids may be useful for some types of hearing loss. An examination by an audiologist may reveal the need for a hearing aid and provide suggestions as to the type of device needed. However, for most people, a hearing aid does not correct a hearing problem as efficiently as glasses correct a visual impairment. Improvement in hearing using a hearing aid may be minimal or moderate. One particularly bothersome effect is the amplification of background noise.

For the older adult, the manual dexterity required to insert a hearing aid or replace a battery may present a problem. Even turning the volume up or down

DISPLAY 24-5. Guidelines for Hearing Aid Use

- Determine if the hearing aid is for the left or the right ear.
- Before removing any hearing aid, the volume should be turned down and the aid off, if possible. If there is an on-off switch, make sure the aid is off when not in use. Some hearing aids are regulated by opening or closing the battery door.
- When inserting the hearing aid, the volume is turned low and gradually turned up until able to hear and understand comfortably.
- Treat the hearing aid with care. Although hearing aids can take considerable amount of everyday wear, they are still delicate instruments that should be protected.
- Never leave the hearing aid unprotected on a table or exposed to direct sunlight.
- Do not use hair spray while the hearing aid is in the ear.
- Clean the ear mold very carefully with a special tool available form the hearing aid manufacturer. Ear mold for behind-the-ear, eyeglass, and body-worn aids are washed with mild soap and water. Do not immerse in water, but wipe the hearing aid with a cloth.
- If the hearing aid suddenly quits working, the battery is probably no longer functioning. When replacing a hearing aid battery, be sure that the new battery is exactly the same type as the old one. Check the number on the old battery to determine the exact type. Before changing the battery, check to see if the volume is turned down.
- If feedback or a whistling sound is not heard when the volume is on, change the battery. If still no feedback is heard, there is a problem with the instrument.
- Replace any cracked, broken, or twisted sound tubing.
- Feedback may be caused by an improper fit of the ear mold. Contact a hearing aid specialist if feedback continues.
- In confused patients a change in behavior such as isolating self, developing behavior problems, or general disinterest in surroundings may indicate a problem with the hearing aid.
- Remove the hearing aid before going to bed, bathing, or showering.

Adapted from Farrell, J. (1990). *Nursing care of the older person.* pp 241–246, Philadelphia: J. B. Lippincott.

DISPLAY 24-6. Assessment for Hearing Impairment

- Indifference when conversing
- Social withdrawal
- Suspicion that others are talking about them
- Excessively loud or soft speech
- Constantly asking the speaker to repeat what was said
- Cupping the hand behind the ear
- Tendency to dominate conversation in an effort to control the topic of conversation
- Words slurred or flat-sounding speech
- Expression of frustration or anger

Using the Nursing Process to Care for an Elderly Adult With a Hearing Impairment

Assessment

Hearing impairment may be mild, moderate, profound, or severe. In assessing for hearing loss the patient is observed for signs that indicate a hearing impairment (Display 24-6).

ASSESSMENT ALERT

Hearing loss should not be considered a normal consequence of aging. If a problem with hearing is suspected, referral to an otologist is necessary.

The external ear is examined. The nurse observes the external ear for tophi (ie, chalky uric acid deposit that often appears on the external ear), lesions, or cysts. Pain that occurs when the auricle is moved is reported. Pain caused by movement of the auricle is indicative of acute otitis media (ie, inflammation of the middle ear). An otoscope (ie, instrument used to visualize the external canal and tympanic membrane) may be used to visualize the tympanic membrane. Normally, the tympanic membrane appears pearly gray, is intact, and transmits light. Any deviation from normal is reported. If the tympanic membrane cannot be visualized with an otoscope, impacted cerumen may have blocked the canal. Report any inflammation, discharge, or pain in or around the ear.

The whisper test may be used to detect hearing impairment. The patient's ability to hear the nurse's whisper from 1 to 2 feet away is assessed. One ear is tested at a time. Numbers may be whispered and the patient asked to repeat the numbers. When testing, one ear is covered with the palm of the hand.

The Weber and the Rinne test may be used to distinguish conductive loss from sensorineural loss. The physician may use audiometric testing to diagnose

or using the on/off switch (if there is one) may prove difficult. Some areas provide programs that teach hearing aid use and speech reading and provide counseling for those needing additional help. Display 24-5 gives some guidelines for hearing aid use.

the extent of hearing loss. These tests are used if a more detailed assessment is needed.

The nurse questions the patient about the presence of tinnitus. Tinnitus may be described as ringing, buzzing, or humming. The nurse must also assess for dizziness or loss of balance.

✔ ASSESSMENT ALERT

It is important to obtain information concerning all medications the patient is taking. Many drugs are ototoxic and can damage the eighth cranial nerve or the organs of hearing and balance. Ototoxicity is often irreversible, making it imperative to obtain an accurate medication history. Regular assessment of hearing is important if the older adult is prescribed ototoxic drugs. Table 24-1 provides examples of ototoxic drugs commonly prescribed.

Nursing Diagnoses

The following nursing diagnoses may be used for an older adult with a hearing deficit:

Impaired Verbal Communication related to hearing impairment

Diversional Activity Deficit related to inability to engage in desired activities because of hearing loss

Impaired Home Maintenance Management related to hearing loss

Impaired Social Interaction related to sensory losses

Other nursing diagnoses may be appropriate for specific individuals with other needs.

Planning and Implementation

When caring for a patient with a hearing impairment, the focus of care revolves around improving communication, preventing social isolation, identifying diversionary activities, and improving home care.

Impaired Communication. Communication is always a problem with a hearing loss. Depending on the degree of hearing loss, various interventions may be used to assist the older adult in communication. Sign language or speech reading (ie, lip reading) may be used by some with impaired hearing. Educational facilities are available especially for those with hearing impairment to teach speech reading. Display 24-3 provides some guidelines for communicating with the hearing impaired. The caregiver and family members are taught techniques for communication. If a hearing aid is used, be sure it is in good working order (see Display 24-5). It is important to have a new battery available in case a replacement is needed.

Impaired Social Interaction. Impaired hearing is frustrating for the person who has a hearing problem

TABLE 24-1. Examples of Ototoxic Drugs

Classification	Examples of Drugs
Aminoglycoside antibiotics	Amikacin
	Gentamicin
	Kanamycin
	Neomycin
	Streptomycin
	Tobramycin
Anti-inflammatory agents	Aspirin
	Indomethacin
Chemotherapeutic agents	Cisplatin
	Nitrogen Mustard
Chemicals	Alcohol
	Arsenic
Diuretics	Ethacrynic acid
	Furosemide
	Acetazolamide
Metals	Gold
	Mercury
	Lead
Other antibiotics	Erythromycin
	Minocycline
	Polymyxin
	Vancomycin

Adapted from Smeltzer, S., & Bare, B. (1996). *Brunner and Suddarth's textbook of medical-surgical nursing (8th ed).* Philadelphia: Lippincott-Raven Publishing, 1667.

and for the individual trying to communicate with the affected person. Rather than face the frustration of trying to communicate, the older adult often withdraws from engaging in any social interaction. It is important to encourage the older adult to remain socially active with friends and loved ones. Telephones may be adapted with an amplifier to increase the sound from callers making communication via the telephone possible. A telecommunication device for the deaf (TDD) can be obtained for those with a severe hearing impairment. The TDD is a combination typewriter and telephone.

Diversional Activity Deficit. The individual with a hearing loss may be able to continue with certain diversionary activities such as reading, knitting, or crocheting. However, other pleasant diversionary activities are limited. Listening to music or television may be activities that were once enjoyed, but with a hearing loss become almost impossible. However, some television programs are transmitted using closed-caption inserts in which the dialogue is printed on the bottom of the screen. Amplifiers in headsets are sometimes available in theaters or churches for those with a hearing impairment. The older adult is encouraged to use assistive devices that help to improve hearing such as hearing aids or amplifiers.

Impaired Home Maintenance. The home environment must be modified in order for the older adult to function with normality. The home can be equipped with various devices to assist the older adult to live more comfortably and safely in the home environment. For example, light-activated alarms used in smoke detectors, alarm clocks, door bells, or telephones are useful for those with a hearing impairment. These alarms flash a light to gain the attention of the hearing-impaired individual. Assistance from various agencies (Display 24-7) or support groups may be helpful in providing an avenue of support and in identifying available assistive devices for the hearing impaired. The family and friends should be involved in the care.

Evaluation and Expected Outcomes

Successful treatment can be gauged by the following responses:

Communication improves.

Patient can communicate effectively within personal limitations.

Patient interacts with others socially.

Patient increases use of diversionary activities.

Patient participates in enjoyable diversionary activities.

Home maintenance is improved through use of assistive devices.

Vertigo

More than 100,000 hip fractures in the older adult are thought to be associated with disorders of balance. **Vertigo** is a feeling of motion and often results in problems with balance. With vertigo, the individual feels that the surrounding environment is moving or spinning. Vertigo is often caused by a dysfunction of the inner ear (ie, labyrinth). Dizziness is a vague term that generally includes the sensation of vertigo and ataxia (ie, unsteadiness and disequilibrium).

Nursing Interventions for an Older Adult Experiencing Vertigo

Careful assessment is needed for an older adult. Many conditions contribute to vertigo such as inner ear dysfunction, cardiovascular problems, fluid and electrolyte disturbances, alcohol, and certain medications. The patient is asked to give a description of the sensations. The nurse evaluates the older adult's ability to ambulate and get up and down from the bed or chairs. Assistance is provided as necessary. The person is advised to change positions slowly. A chair, walker, or cane is kept close by to use to steady oneself if necessary. It may be necessary to have the patient stand a few minutes before going on to each step. Some loss of balance and dizziness is normal with increasing age, but it often diminishes

---

DISPLAY 24-7. Resources for those with a Hearing Impairment

American Academy of Audiology
1735 North Lynn Street
Arlington, VA 22209
American Speech-Language-Hearing Association
10801 Rockville Pike, Dept. AP
Rockville, MD 20852
American Tinnitus Association
P.O. Box 5
Portland, OR 97207
National Hearing Aid Society
20361 Middlebelt
Livonia, MI 48152
National Institute on Deafness and Other Communication Disorders
National Institutes of Health
Building 31, Room 3C35
9000 Rockville Pike
Bethesda, MD 20892
Self Help for Hard of Hearing People
4848 Battery Lane, Dept. E
Bethesda, MD 20814
The Deafness Research Foundation
55 East 34th Street
New York, NY 10016

---

with slower movement. A cane or walker is kept available for ambulation. The nurse must be ready to provide assistance if necessary. Meclizine (Antivert) may be used to manage the vertigo. Adverse reactions to meclizine include drowsiness, blurred vision, and dry mouth. Elderly patients are assessed frequently for the effectiveness of the treatment (ie, decreased dizziness).

OTHER SENSORY ORGANS

Taste and Smell

The organs of taste are the tastebuds located toward the back and on the sides of the tongue. The center of the tongue contains few taste buds. There are four basic tastes: sweet, sour, salt, and bitter. Sweet and salty taste buds are located on the front of the tongue, sour taste buds along the edges, and bitter taste buds at the back of the tongue. With age, taste buds gradually diminish in number, resulting in some loss of taste, especially the taste of sweetness, but recent data indicate that changes in taste are relatively small.

The sensation of bad taste is a common complaint of old age. This bad taste is not related to the presence or absence of taste buds, but rather to a dry mouth (ie, xerostomia) that alters the taste of food, producing an unpleasant taste. Contributing to a dry mouth and consequently to a bad taste in the mouth are drugs such as diuretics or anticholinergics.

Other problems that adversely affect taste is years of cigarette smoking, poor dental status, or poor oral hygiene. The loss of taste contributes to a decreased food intake and interest in food. In an effort to regain taste sensations, excessive salt or sugar may be added to food to enhance the taste.

The enjoyment of food is enhanced by the ability to smell. The sense of smell (ie, olfactory sense) enables detection of odors and depends on the stimulation of the sense organs in the nose. Small patches of olfactory cells in the nasal mucosa are connected to the brain by the olfactory nerve. The nerve endings detect odors inhaled on the air currents and pass these sensations to the olfactory nerve and then to the brain.

With age, there is a generalized decline in olfactory function and moderate loss of neurons. Although many older adults complain of a decrease in taste and smell, others do not. More research is needed to determine the exact changes in the sensations of taste and smell.

Nursing Interventions to Enhance Taste and Smell

The nurse can teach the older adult or caregiver ways to maximize taste and smell. A pleasant mealtime environment makes eating more pleasurable. Using seasonings such as herbs, spices (if the patient can tolerate them), and lemon instead of salt or sugar is encouraged. The nurse may need to explain age-related changes. The older adult is encouraged to have regular dental examinations, brush the teeth several times each day, and use a gentle mouthwash. If the sense of smell has severely declined, it is important to encourage the use of a smoke detector to alert the patient of a fire.

Touch

The sense of touch is extremely important. Perhaps more than any other sense, touch expresses a message. Touching can convey caring and reduce feelings of isolation and loneliness. Nurses play an important role in conveying caring to the older adult through touch. The older adult often is isolated from social contacts and other family members. The simple act of touching by the nurse provides an increased sense of well-being. The nurse can use touch through back rubs, foot massage, a bed bath, a hug, or a simple pat on the shoulder. Animals such as cats or dogs can be used to encourage touching.

CRITICAL THINKING EXERCISES

1. Mr. Olivera, age 78, lives at home alone. He was recently diagnosed with ARMD. Mr. Olivera is concerned about his loss of vision and states that he is afraid he will be unable to care for himself. What questions would you ask Mr. Olivera initially? What information can you give him about his loss of vision? How could you help him remain independent?

2. Hattie Stone, age 58, was recently diagnosed with chronic glaucoma in the right eye. She is prescribed timolol (Timoptic). What information would you include in a teaching plan for Hattie. Be sure to include information on the medication and the disease process. Before developing the teaching plan, what information concerning Hattie would be most helpful for the nurse to know?

3. Mr. Guthrie, age 77, has Alzheimer's disease and shows symptoms of confusion and irritability. Explain how you would assess for a visual impairment in Mr. Guthrie?

4. Charlie Riley, age 92, lives in a nursing home. He wears a hearing aid but often forgets to put it on. What three interventions could be included in Mr. Riley's care plan to assist him in hearing? What actions could the staff at the nursing home take to maximize communication with Charlie?

5. Prepare a teaching outline for the nursing home staff to teach the nursing assistants how to care for and use a hearing aid. What information would be most important for the staff to know?

REFERENCES AND SUGGESTED READING

Kavanaugh, K.M., & Tate, B. (1996). Recognizing and helping older persons with vision impairments. *Geriatric Nursing, 17 (2),* 68–71.

Matteson, M.A., McConnell, E.S., & Linton, A.D. (1997). *Gerontological nursing: Concepts and practice* (2nd ed.). Philadelphia: W.B. Saunders.

McConnell, E. (1998). Clinical do's and don'ts communicating with a hearing impaired patient. *Nursing 98 (1),* 32.

Miller, C. (1998). Keeping an eye on the hidden effects of eye drops. *Geriatric Nursing, 19 (5),* 293–294.

CHAPTER **25**

Developing Leadership and Management Skills

CHAPTER OUTLINE

KEY TERMS
CHAPTER OBJECTIVES
MANAGEMENT VERSUS LEADERSHIP
PROBLEM SOLVING
PASSIVE, AGGRESSIVE, AND ASSERTIVE
   BEHAVIORS
RESPONSIBILITIES OF A MANAGER
CRITICAL THINKING EXERCISES
REFERENCES AND SUGGESTED READING

KEY TERMS

aggressive behavior
assertive behavior
authoritarian leadership
autocratic leadership
change agent
compromise
conflict
democratic leadership
halo effect
laissez-faire leadership
leadership
management
participative leadership
passive behavior
situational leadership theory

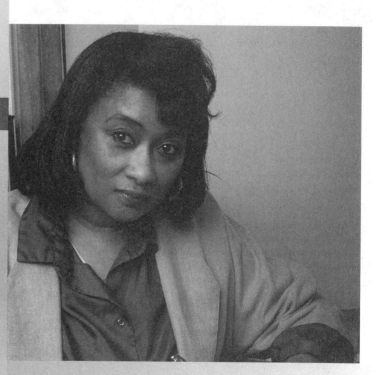

CHAPTER OBJECTIVES

At the completion of this chapter, the student will be able to

- Identify characteristics of effective leaders

- Describe autocratic, laissez-faire, democratic, and participative leadership styles

- Discuss situational leadership theory

- Identify guidelines for leaders

- Use problem solving techniques to develop solutions to problems

- Distinguish between assertive, aggressive, and passive behaviors

- Describe the steps of conflict resolution

- Discuss the responsibilities of a manager

- Describe the basic concepts involving change

Practical nurses function in many situations requiring leadership skills. The practical nurse may be a team leader in a nursing home or long-term care facility with the responsibility of coordinating the care of the patients on a specific unit. Supervising the work of several nurses, medical assistants, or other unlicensed assistive personnel (UAP) requires the ability to function in a leadership role. Supervisors direct and manage the work performance of another individual or group to see that specific tasks are accomplished. Although each state has different guidelines, the role of the practical nurse in caring for the gerontological patient is one of increasing responsibility.

MANAGEMENT VERSUS LEADERSHIP

Although management and leadership are closely related, they are not the same. **Leadership** can be defined as the ability to guide or direct the actions of another to accomplish a specific goal or task. Individuals who desire a leadership role can become leaders by developing the personal characteristics of leaders. Many leaders have a certain charisma that inspires others to follow.

Management is the establishment of an effective environment that focuses on reaching organizational goals. Managers coordinate and direct people, supplies, and activities to accomplish goals. Because an effective manager should have the qualities of a good leader, leadership and management are discussed together in this chapter.

Characteristics of Effective Leadership

Tappan (1989) identifies and describes 6 characteristics (Fig. 25-1) of good leaders. According to Tappan good leaders are
- Goal oriented
- Skillful and knowledgeable
- Self-aware
- Able to communicate
- Energetic
- Decisive

Goal-Oriented Leaders
Good leaders set clear, achievable goals. With effective leadership, the group tends to take the goals of the leader and make them their own. In general, a leader has more influence on the group than the group has on the leader.

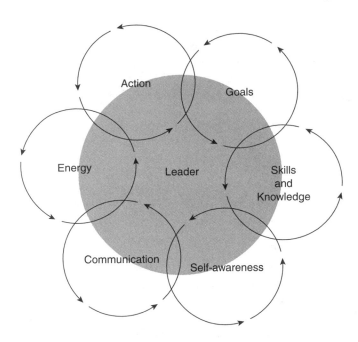

FIGURE 25-1. Components of effective leadership. From Tappen, R.M. (1989). *Nursing leadership and management: Concepts and practice,* 2nd ed, p 58. Philadelphia: F.A. Davis. Used with permission.

Skillful and Knowledgeable Leaders
A good leader has the skills and knowledge that result in respect from members of the group. To be an effective nurse leader, it is important to be a skillful nurse and to have a basic knowledge of principles of leadership. The nurse can improve knowledge of leadership through attending leadership seminars and incorporating leadership skills into nursing practice. A basic knowledge of the job is essential for effective leadership. In general, the more skilled the nurse, the greater the respect from others in the group. When an individual is viewed with respect and admiration, her ability to lead is greatly enhanced.

Self-Aware Leaders
Self-awareness is an increased insight into one's own self. Self-knowledge involves being in tune with your inner self. Understanding personal motives, reactions, and inner feelings provides the nurse with personal insight that leads to self-awareness and self-acceptance. Without self-awareness, the nurse tends to be defensive and dependent on others for approval, traits not desirable in a leader. Self-awareness can be increased by obtaining feedback from others. Questioning and analyzing one's behavior to understand the reasons for certain actions helps the nurse gain insight. The leader should listen to feedback from others, whether it is in the form of criticism or encouragement. When

a deeper understanding of self is achieved, the nurse is better able to understand and guide others in a constructive manner.

Communication by Leaders

The ability to communicate is perhaps the single most important characteristic of leadership. Without the ability to communicate, the nurse leader has no method to give instructions, initiate action, or evaluate the effectiveness of activities. Chapter 5 provides information on basic communication skills. The ability to communicate assertively is essential for a good leader. Information on assertive communication is given later in this chapter.

The leader must be able to communicate feedback on the performance of those being supervised. Positive and negative feedback mechanisms are used. Positive feedback provides encouragement and an impetus to accomplish goals. Negative feedback is given without demeaning or belittling the individual. The focus of negative feedback is on the unacceptable behavior not on the person as unacceptable. All communication must be in a respectful and compassionate manner whether it be with a patient or with a coworker. A good leader is careful not to embarrass others.

Energetic Leaders

An effective leader is energetic and imparts that energy to others. One who accepts a role with a high energy level is not only able to accomplish much, but inspire others to greater performance.

Decisive Leaders

A leader is decisive and is not afraid to act. Without action, nothing could be accomplished. Many worthwhile projects and plans never come to be because no one has the initiative to put a plan into action.

Leadership Styles

To become an effective leader, a basic understanding of the various leadership styles is important. Leadership styles (ie, approaches a leader uses to accomplish goals) may be autocratic or authoritarian, laissez-faire, democratic, or participative.

Autocratic or Authoritarian Leadership

Using **authoritarian or autocratic leadership** style, the leader leads by giving very specific directions (orders) while allowing only minimal input from the workers. All decisions are made by the leader. This style is restrictive and controlling. The leader remains aloof from the group and views the workers as incapable of making decisions for themselves and unable to accomplish a task without specific instructions. Autocratic leaders are described as firm and dominating. They make all the rules and tell the workers exactly how to accomplish the job at hand.

When this style is used exclusively, the leader is generally not well liked, and the workers feel pressured, used, or forced to do the job. Organizational goals are not supported and the workers must have almost constant supervision to accomplish the desired task. The autocratic leader values the accomplishment of tasks or goals and places little importance on the worker who provides the means to meet the goal. Workers are discouraged from offering personal opinions and suggestions for improvement.

Although this style seems harsh and of little value, it can be effective in certain situations, particularly in health care settings. Autocratic leadership is effective in emergency situations requiring immediate, nonquestioning action, such as when a patient suddenly stops breathing and a code is called. Individuals who are lacking in knowledge or skills may also benefit from this type of leadership. When knowledge or skills are inadequate, an authoritarian leader may be the type of leader who is able to "get the job done" in the quickest and most efficient manner.

Laissez-Faire Leadership

When **laissez-faire leadership** style is used, the leader allows the group to make all decisions with little or no direction or input from the leader. This style is sometimes referred to as permissive leadership style. The individual becomes the focus of the group rather than the accomplishment of the task or the goal. The laissez-faire leadership style is based on the assumption that all workers are responsible and willing to work toward the goal of the organization. The relationship between the group and the leader is open and friendly, but it lacks focus and guidance. This type of leadership style promotes frustration and tension because of lack of accomplishment. Laissez-faire leadership may provide some highly motivated and self-directed individuals with an avenue to accomplish a given task, such as a group of researchers doing research in an area of interest. Most health care settings are not suitable for this style of leadership.

Democratic Leadership

In **democratic leadership,** the leader includes all members of the group in the decision-making process. The leader encourages and guides the group in making decisions, establishing priorities, and determining the best methods to meet goals. Democratic leaders value the workers more than the task to be accomplished. The leader develops a trusting, collaborative working environment. Ideally, all members of the group participate, and each member is considered responsible for contributing to the welfare of the group. For this type of leadership to be effective, group members must be motivated, mature, able to work independently, and have good communication skills. The leader maintains some control over final decision making and participates in the group process. Groups with democratic leadership are highly supportive and have a high level of job satisfaction.

Participative Leadership

Participative leadership combines the best traits of autocratic and democratic leaders. Participative leadership is sometimes referred to as multicratic leadership. In this type of leadership, the leader analyzes the situation and makes suggestions or proposals to the group and then elicits feedback from the group. After hearing the comments and criticism from the group, the participative leader makes the final decision, taking into account the feedback received.

This type of leadership has proven quite successful. The workers feel empowered through their participation within the decision-making process. Ideas are shared freely, and the workers feel a greater sense of self-esteem than with the autocratic or democratic leadership styles. The participative leader is usually one that workers look up to, admire, and desire to follow.

Situational Leadership Theory

Paul Hersey and Kenneth Blanchard (2000) developed the **situational leadership theory.** The situational leadership theory states that the situation dictates the type of leadership used. According to Hersey and Blanchard, the behavior of leaders can be divided into two categories:

- Behavior that focuses on the accomplishment of activities or tasks
- Behavior that focuses on the relationship with workers or group members

The accomplishment of tasks requires behaviors that communicate to the worker the information concerning the tasks to be accomplished (eg, how, when, and where tasks are to be accomplished). A leader that is task oriented focuses on the accomplishment of the task with little consideration about the workers being supervised.

Relationship behaviors are behaviors with which the leader communicates, provides emotional support, and interacts with the workers. Leaders that place more importance on the relationship with the workers are considered to be people oriented or rela-

tionship oriented rather than task oriented. Relationship behaviors are particularly important when individuals are not highly motivated to perform the task. Words of praise or encouragement can provide an incentive to become a more active and productive worker.

Rather than a leader becoming purely task oriented or relationship oriented, the ideal is to balance task and relationship behaviors to manage different situations. Four combinations of leadership behaviors are identified in situational leadership:

1. High relationship–low task leadership behavior
2. High task–high relationship leadership behavior
3. Low relationship–low task leadership behavior
4. High task–low relationship leadership behavior

The decision to use a specific combination depends on the situation (ie, situational leadership). Maturity of the group or individual to be supervised is a major consideration in selecting the leadership style. Maturity refers to the ability to accurately and responsibly perform the task. In general, an individual with low task maturity needs a leader who is highly task oriented. As the level of maturity increases (eg, the ability to perform the task increases), the leader can become more relationship oriented.

Traditionally, nursing has focused on the needs of the patient. The accomplishment of tasks has traditionally been the goal with little consideration to the needs of the nurse. High task–low relationship style is used when nursing is viewed as a series of tasks to be accomplished (eg, administering medication, following physician orders, performing treatments).

The most effective style appears to be one in which the leader assesses the maturity of the group to be supervised and selects the leadership style that would be most effective. No single leadership style is appropriate in every situation. When a specific task must be accomplished for the patient, the nurse as a leader must be in complete control to assure that the task is performed correctly. For example, medications must be administered accurately and in a timely manner observing the Six Rights (see Chapter 13). The leader's responsibility to see that those performing nursing tasks for the patient are competent to complete the assignment promptly, accurately, and with consideration for the patient. In areas that are not critical, such as making daily assignments, scheduling breaks, and assigning routine tasks, a more democratic, people-oriented approach is appropriate. Table 25-1 identifies the various situational leadership behavior combinations, characteristics, and provides examples of effective use in nursing situations.

TABLE 25-1. Situational Leadership Combinations: Characteristics and Uses

Leadership Behaviors	Characteristics	Use
High task/low relationship	Leader identifies the jobs and gives specific direction on how, when, and where to do the job. One-way communications occurs. As workers understand the job and gain expertise, the leader can be more relationship oriented. Requires close supervision.	Used when the worker cannot perform the job well, but wants to learn *Example:* To give directions for a procedure; when orienting new employees
High task/high relationship	Leader must give specific and clear directions for the job. Leader seeks to develop a relationship with the worker by providing praise, support, and direction. Leader seeks to motivate the worker to desire to perform the task.	Used when the worker is not able to perform the job well and is not motivated to do the job *Example:* Joe Garza is a new nurse assistant. He is unsure of his nursing skills and seems disinterested in learning or improving his job performance.
Low relationship/low task	Leader can delegate task to the worker. Unit will run well, even if the leader is not present. Leader can allow considerable freedom. Minimal supervision does not decrease job performance.	Used when the worker is motivated to do the job and is skilled in job performance *Example:* J. Doner, LPN, has worked on a particular unit for 5 years. She loves her work and has consistently received superior work performance evaluations. She manages the nurse assistants under her supervision well.
Low task/high relationship	Leader and worker share in decision making. Two-way communication is necessary. Leader's role is to offer support and praise.	Used when the worker is able to perform the task well, but is not motivated to perform the job *Example:* S. Martin transferred to the nursing unit where you are the charge nurse. She has worked for the nursing home for more than 1 year and knows her job well. The director of nursing transferred her to your unit because, although her task performance is good, she does not seem interested in her work and shows little interest in her job.

The practical nurse must use sound judgment in making leadership decisions. Understanding the various leadership styles allows greater ease in choosing an appropriate leadership style. Time and patience are necessary to develop the ability to become skillful in selecting the most suitable leadership style. Display 25-1 provides some general guidelines for leaders.

PROBLEM SOLVING

The problem-solving process is much like the nursing process. Like the nursing process, there are five steps in the problem-solving process:

1. Identify the problem.
2. Diagnose the problem.
3. Develop strategies for solving the problem.
4. Implement the selected strategies.
5. Evaluate the outcome for success.

Nurses use the problem-solving process to solve problems that arise as a result of leadership responsibilities and when planning and implementing patient care.

Identify the Problem

The first step in the problem-solving process is to identify or define the problem. The more accurate and clear the problem is defined, the easier the remainder of the problem-solving process is to complete. Vague problems do not produce good solutions, and a problem may continue because it was not adequately defined. In identifying the problem, accurate information is essential. If a problem is

DISPLAY 25-1. General Guidelines for Leaders

- Become knowledgeable about the different leadership styles and the appropriate use for each style.
- Try to balance task-oriented leadership with people-oriented leadership. In the health care setting, there are times when the tasks to be accomplished take precedence over the people accomplishing those tasks. However, a good leader is quick to identify situations when support and concern for the needs of the nurse assistant or other health care provider is possible. A word of encouragement, asking for the opinion of another in a situation, or a quick coffee break with a troubled staff member can be effective in letting the staff know you are concerned about them and value their thoughts and feelings.
- Develop people skills. Become an active listener. Try to understand what your staff member is attempting to say. Keep lines of communication open.
- Give positive reinforcement whenever possible.
- Be an expert caregiver. Value doing the task correctly. Be able to perform the task correctly yourself. Put the patient first and set excellent care as your priority.
- Set the example. If you expect your staff to be at work on time, you should be on time. If you expect your staff to follow the facility's dress code, follow the dress code yourself.
- Be interested in those who are supervised. A simple voice of concern will let others know that you care. Do not, however, become the counselor or one who continually listens to and solves problems. Communicate with your supervisor and find sources of referral for those with problems or concerns.
- Be decisive and follow through. When a decision is made, stay with that decision unless it becomes obvious that it is wrong and then admit your mistake. Use the problem solving process to develop strategies.
- Continually aim for self-improvement. Identify your weak areas and work on them. Attend workshops or continuing education programs to keep yourself knowledgeable with the most current information.
- Observe leaders you admire. Observe your supervisor. Identify strengths and weaknesses. Seek to improve your own leadership ability.
- Don't be afraid to ask for help, if necessary. If a situation arises that you are unsure of, talk with your supervisor. Brainstorm and discuss various solutions.

identified, decide whether the problem is important enough to continue with the process or is not particularly significant and can be ignored.

Analyze the Problem

The second step is to analyze the problem to determine the extent and cause of the problem. Gather as much information (data) about the problem as possible. Do not show bias toward any individual or fact or group of individuals or facts. Findings may indicate an inability to communicate, personality conflicts, or inadequate knowledge on the part of an individual or a group of individuals. Try to view the situation from every viewpoint.

Develop Strategies

Third, list all possible strategies to solve the problem. Brainstorm and list all solutions, even ones that at first may not seem the most appropriate. Then analyze all possible identified strategies. For example, if a lack of knowledge is identified as the cause of the problem, identify the method of education that would be most appropriate to increase the individual's knowledge level. If there is a problem with communication within the unit, develop strategies

that facilitate communication. Identify all barriers to each strategy. Explore all possible consequences.

Implementation and Evaluation

Fourth, select and implement the strategy or strategies that seem best. If possible remove any barriers that were identified. Evaluate the results. If the strategies did not result in the desired outcome, new strategies must be identified. The problem goes back to the beginning stages of the problem-solving sequence, identification and analysis. Sometimes further clarification is needed to identify more effective strategies to solve the problem.

Problem solving is not a long, complicated process, but a systematic active process that can be accomplished in a relatively short time frame. Use of problem-solving techniques is helpful when used by the practical nurse in a leadership role.

PASSIVE, AGGRESSIVE, AND ASSERTIVE BEHAVIORS

Three basic types of behavioral styles are used to communicate: passive, aggressive, and assertive.

TABLE 25-2. Passive, Aggressive, and Assertive Responses

Situation	Passive Response	Aggressive Response	Assertive Response
The head nurse criticizes you for the manner in which you are working with the nurse assistants.	"Oh, I'm really sorry. I will try to change my behavior." (No attempt is made to clarify criticism and an apology was made too quickly.)	"That's ridiculous! I can do my job without any assistance from someone who sits in an office all day. I am the one who knows these people best!" (This response is demeaning and is rude.)	"Please explain more fully. I want to be sure that I understand what you are saying. Can you give me some examples." (The nurse is clarifying the criticism without trying to justify actions.)
Your supervisor asks you to work an extra shift tomorrow because one of the other nurses wants to attend a special activity with her husband.	"Well, I had plans but I guess I could stay." (Even though the nurse had plans no resistance was offered.)	"You can't expect me to do anything for you or any one else if you ask me this late. What kind of manager are you anyway? I have plans tomorrow." (This response is vicious and insulting to the manager.)	"I know this is important, but I cannot work an extra shift tomorrow. I have already made plans. Ask me again another time." (This response acknowledges the importance of the request, refuses with no guilt, and leaves the door open to help if a similar incident occurs in the future.)
Your patient, Mr. Hubbard, is 70 years old. He had surgery several days ago and returned to the nursing home yesterday. The physician ordered that he ambulate at least two times each day. He refused this morning. Now it is 4:30 PM, and he is still refusing to ambulate.	Mr. Hubbard, do you want to try to ambulate this afternoon? I know you are really hurting and if you don't want to, it's okay." (This response is powerless and gives the patient an easy out from an activity that is uncomfortable. By allowing Mr. Hubbard to remain in bed and not ambulate, the nurse is placing him at risk for complications.)	"Mr. Hubbard, you are going to get out of bed and walk down the hall. I will not leave this room until you do. You will get pneumonia and can die if you don't do as I say." (This statement is intimidating and not an appropriate way to communicate with a patient.)	Mr. Hubbard, I need you to ambulate. I will help you walk down the hall and back. Walking is an important part of your recovery. It will help prevent complications from the surgery and promote healing of your wound." (This response is straightforward and clear. It provides Mr. Hubbard with an explanation of the importance of ambulation.)

Passive behavior allows individuals to avoid direct confrontation. By avoiding direct contact, communication is blocked and interpersonal relations are strained. Those who practice aggressive behavior use anger to gain results. Aggressive behavior humiliates others and often embarrasses the aggressor. Assertive behavior is particularly useful for those in leadership roles. Individuals who practice assertiveness express thoughts directly but in a manner that values the opinions and feelings of others. Table 25-2 provides examples of passive, aggressive, and assertive responses.

Passive Behavior

Passive behavior is behavior that allows others to make decisions and take control while offering little feedback. These individuals are inhibited, timid, and apologetic. Individuals who act passively generally do not question, ask for clarification, or respond directly to others. Passive people are the ones who cry "I'm sorry; I tried," "I guess I just didn't understand," or "That's unfair." These statements may not be made directly to the offending party. Individuals who behave passively feel inadequate and insecure. Display 25-2 gives examples of passive behavior.

Aggressive Behavior

Aggressive behavior is behavior that is aimed at hurting or intimidating others. Aggressive individuals are overbearing and often use sarcasm or offensive language. These individuals exercise their rights without regard to others. With aggressive

DISPLAY 25-2. Examples of Passive Behavior

- A new nurse overwhelmed by the patient care assignment says nothing. Rather than ask for help, the nurse decides to request a transfer to another unit.
- A nurse in an outpatient clinic is reprimanded unjustly by the physician. The nurse is angry but says nothing to the physician.
- The director of nursing asks the practical nurse to take on additional responsibilities because "we are so short-handed." The nurse does not feel these responsibilities are within her scope of practice but agrees to assume the responsibilities. Later she complains to her coworkers about the additional work she is required to do.
- A nurse avoids contact with a patient because the patient is demanding.

DISPLAY 25-3 Examples of Aggressive Behaviors

- When having a disagreement with a nurse assistant the practical nurse says, "I don't care what you think, I am the boss around here."
- A patient is frequently using the call light to make insignificant requests of the nurse. After answering the call light numerous times, the nurse states, "Mr. Cauley, don't put that call light on again unless it is an emergency. You are annoying me. I have other patients that require care, and I won't be answering yours again until I have helped the other patients."
- The medication aide reports a medication error on an elderly patient to the vocational/practical nurse in charge of a group of elderly patients. The nurse is rude and tells the medication aide that she is "stupid and does not know how to pass medications safely."

behavior, communication is one way. Leaders who behave in an aggressive manner are not viewed as sensitive, understanding, or approachable. They are easily angered and prone to emotional outbursts. Staff members become stressed and feel anxious when managers behave aggressively. Display 25-3 identifies examples of aggressive behaviors.

Assertive Behavior

Assertive behavior is behavior that allows an individual to act in his own best interest and to defend his rights without denying the rights or others. Assertive behavior is honest, straightforward, and clear. It is not blunt or hurtful but instead shows consideration for the feelings of others. Assertive behavior does not mean that the outcome will always be exactly as desired; it allows the individual to maintain a sense of control and not feel manipulated. Nurses in a leadership role who acknowledge the rights of others and communicate in an assertive manner are well respected because they communicate clearly, value the rights of the people they manage, and are open to feedback. This type of behavior reduces misunderstandings and negativism in the work environment.

Nurses can use declarative statements to communicate assertively. Declarative statements clearly and concisely state the wants or needs of the nurse. The following are examples of declarative statements:

I need you to bathe Mr. Struthers in Room 142.
I want you to take the vital signs for all patients that come in the clinic today.
Take these reports to the radiology department now.
Mr. Jones, I need you to ambulate now.

These declarative statements provide specific instruction without belittling or demeaning others. The use of "I" statements is an effective way to communicate assertively, because they let others know your needs without assigning blame or belittling another. Messages beginning with "you" place the other person on the defensive and block communication. For example, "I feel concerned (alarmed) when you do not report abnormal vital signs because this could endanger the patient" is an assertive communication. Making a "you" statement, such as "You placed the patient in danger when you did not report those vital signs," is belittling and blocks communication. The individual feels the need to defend his action of lack or action. The "I" statement presents the same message as the "you" statement but in a less threatening format.

A simple format to use when practicing assertive statements is "I feel when because." For example, I feel upset when the patients are not turned every 2 hours because this could result in the formation of pressure ulcers." This statement could be followed with "I expect you to turn the patients every two hours and document this on the flow sheet."

Guidelines for Becoming More Assertive

The following guidelines can help the nurse to become more assertive:

Learn the characteristics of assertive, passive, and aggressive behavior. Identify these behaviors in yourself and others.
Modify personal behavior to become more assertive.

Use "I" statements rather than "you" statements to discuss issues.

Respect the feelings and rights of patients, coworkers, and supervisors.

Keep communication clear by stating the situations specifically and in a positive manner. Use declarative statements. Ask for what is needed.

Conflict Resolution

Whenever groups of people work together, conflict occurs. The nurse who is knowledgeable about conflict resolution can better deal with conflict when it occurs. Webster's defines **conflict** as a sharp disagreement, as of interests or ideas. In a conflict, two or more views or feelings about an idea, situation, or person exist.

Conflict resolution results in one of three outcomes:
• Win–lose outcome
• Lose–lose outcome
• Win–win outcome

In a win–lose outcome, one person or group wins by dominating the other group or individual. This results in one group feeling satisfaction and the other group feeling resentful, hurt, and dissatisfied. The conflict is usually only temporarily resolved and may resurface at a later time.

In a lose–lose solution, neither party feels satisfied. There is no willingness to understand the other's viewpoint. Resolution occurs by coercion, intimidation, or withdrawal. Both sides feel dissatisfied and let down.

The goal of conflict resolution is to resolve the conflict by finding an outcome that leaves both parties feeling satisfied. This results in a win–win situation, and the conflict has a good chance for complete resolution. For a win–win outcome to occur, all people involved must communicate openly and honestly. Each side must be willing to accept responsibility and commit themselves to resolving the conflict.

Win–win outcomes occur most often when a form of problem solving is used. Figure 25-2 identifies the steps involved in conflict resolution. Confrontation is necessary to resolve a conflict. The purpose of confrontation is to define the problem and begin a discussion that will lead to a win–win solution that is satisfactory to everyone involved.

Another means of conflict resolution is to use compromise. **Compromise** occurs when both parties make concessions. However, when a compromise is reached, both parties may feel that they "gave" too much, and the solution to the conflict is viewed as having a lose–lose outcome. If only one party feels too much was given, a win–lose outcome occurs.

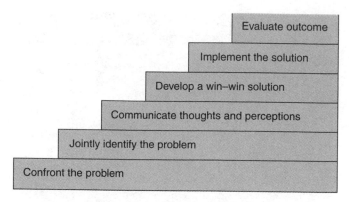

FIGURE 25-2. Steps in conflict resolution.

The role of the practical nurse in conflict resolution among staff members is to facilitate communication between all parties, to provide an atmosphere of mutual respect, and to seek and win–win outcome. If a solution is reached collaboratively, it has a greater opportunity to succeed. The following guidelines can be used to promote a win–win resolution to conflict:

Openly and honestly discuss feelings about the conflict. Use nonthreatening speech and behavior. Use "I" statements rather that "you" statements.

Direct any anger in the conflict toward the issue rather than toward an individual.

Try to see the conflict form the viewpoint of everyone involved. Encourage all parties to fully express feeling and perceptions.

Do not insult, belittle, or act rudely to anyone.

Define the conflict as specifically as possible. A vague problem is more difficult to solve.

All individuals involved in the conflict need to be satisfied with the result. Each party should view the solution as a win–win solution.

Several weeks after implementing the solution, evaluate the effectiveness of the solution. If the conflict still exists, try again by reworking the steps of conflict resolution.

RESPONSIBILITIES OF A MANAGER

A manager coordinates the activities of individuals to meet organizational goals. Nurse managers must be able to motivate others, direct the activities of UAP, and evaluate the performance of others.

Motivating Staff Members

Motivating others to perform their jobs well is an important responsibility of the manager. People are motivated in a job in various ways. Salary, employee benefits, and working conditions are motivators that are most likely set by the organization. The manager has minimal control over motivators set by the organization. Mangers must use other motivators such as job satisfaction, recognition, and positive reinforcement to enhance job performance.

Providing positive reinforcement for a job well done motivates most people to perform better. Mangers must be careful not to focus on mistakes and inadequacies. Continual criticism decreases an individual's desire to try to improve. Positive reinforcement in the form of praise shows that the manager cares and motivates staff to improve job performance. For praise to be effective, it must be meaningful and sincere. If praise is given too freely or is overdone, it becomes phony.

Job satisfaction is a powerful motivator. Increasing job satisfaction may be difficult. Caring for the elderly requires a genuine concern for the elderly, eliminating attitudes of ageism, and a sincere desire to help others. Individuals who do not truly care for the elderly may not be satisfied working with older adults. Sometimes job satisfaction can be increased in simple ways, such as providing a change in scheduling to allow a nurse assistant to go to a special family event, varying the patient care assignment with a particularly difficult patient, or decreasing or increasing the opportunity for working overtime.

Recognition can also be a motivator. For example, some organizations select an "Employee of the Month." A special parking place or a special meal may be given to the honoree. Other organizations have yearly recognition parties or receptions with some special type of recognition given to designated employees. A note written to commend an individual for a job well done is a strong motivator for some individuals. Actions by the manager have a significant impact on an individual's motivation to perform well. Display 25-4 offers suggestions for managers about how to motivate others to improve job performance.

Managing Unlicensed Assistive Personnel

In the nursing home and outpatient settings practical nurses are often asked to manage UAP, including nursing assistants, medical assistants, attendants, and others who are involved in patient care. Most states have regulatory agencies that monitor the training of nurse assistants.

The nurse in charge of UAP has the responsibility to know each individual's strengths and weaknesses. If weaknesses are identified in the perfor-

---

DISPLAY 25-4. Tips to Motivate Others to Improve Job Performance

- Provide clear instructions regarding patient care assignments.
- Make assignments based on the individual's ability.
- Provide positive reinforcement.
- Be available to help answer questions.
- Show no favoritism; treat everyone equally.
- Make each person feel valued and an important part of the team.
- Keep employee issues confidential.

---

mance of patient care activities, the person is taught the correct method of performing the task or providing care. Nurse assistants must be competent in tasks such as personal care skills and basic restorative care and have an understanding of resident or patient rights and communication skills. The vocational or practical nurse may be the health care provider that ensures that UAP are competent caregivers. Continuous monitoring of the UAP in the performance of the assigned tasks provides the nurse the opportunity to correct any identified problems immediately, thereby protecting the patient's safety. Using the strategies to enhance job performance in Display 25-4 can help in motivating the UAP to achieve peak performance.

Knowing the capabilities of the UAP, their strengths and weaknesses, assists in making assignments that match the skill level of each UAP with the needs of a particular patient. When delegating tasks, it is imperative that UAP are able to perform the task correctly and safely. While patients are cared for by UAP, the practical or vocational nurse must continually monitor the patient's condition closely for any change.

Evaluating the Performance of Others

When evaluating the performance of others, it is important that the individuals being evaluated have a clear understanding of what behaviors are expected. Besides modeling the desired behaviors, managers must provide clear job descriptions and instruction on what is expected. Give praise for jobs well done. Praise provides positive feedback, and it lets the person know you are aware of his strengths.

When individuals are not meeting the job expectations, a counseling session may be necessary. Follow organizational guidelines concerning counseling UAP. For example, some organizations require written counseling forms on each incident. Others may want an oral counseling session, followed by a more formal written summary if the problem continues.

Even when individuals are not meeting the job expectations, try to begin the counseling session with a review of his or her successful areas. Be specific about problem areas. Take care not to attack the person, only the performance. Ask for their suggestions about how the situation can be handled. Allow the individual being counseled to express feelings and concerns. Offer your suggestions, and be clear about expected behavior. Set a time for reevaluation. When preparing a yearly performance evaluation, avoid the **halo effect.** The halo effect is the tendency of some mangers to rate all traits positive because one trait is positive. Consider the entire performance, not just one aspect of the performance. Consider the entire year, rather than the past few months. Notes or documentation of positive and negative behaviors during the past year can be helpful. Although the practical nurse may not be responsible for the yearly performance evaluation, input of the UAP's performance is expected.

Adjusting to Change

Change is inevitable. Contrary to popular belief, some individuals adapt well to change and even relish the idea of change. Others find change threatening or at the very least the source of great anxiety. Nurses are faced with changes on a daily basis. Changes in physician orders, new equipment that must be mastered, changing job demands, and even a promotion can present steady challenges for the nurse. Many of these changes become a part of the daily nursing routine. Certain changes occurring within the health care community such as downsizing, more complex technology, and managed care can cause even the seasoned nurse to be overwhelmed. Major changes can cause emotional turmoil, depression, and exhaustion. To minimize the impact of change, nurses must be aware of some basic concepts of change.

Unplanned Change

Unplanned changes are dealt with in the health care environment on a daily basis. Learning to effectively manage unplanned change is an important goal for the nurse manager. Use of the problem-solving process can assist the nurse manager in managing unplanned change. The first rule is to remain calm and keep a clear head. Think the situation through, analyze the situation, and plan potential solutions. Determine priorities. Make the decision, and implement the solution. If time is available, discuss the situation with your supervisor or other nurses.

Unplanned change can cause anxiety in managers and other personnel. A manager who adapts to unplanned changes in a calm and efficient manner sets the example for staff members to follow.

Planned Change

Planned change occurs when an organization, individual or group of individuals determine to make changes in the system to improved the organization's effectiveness. Ideally, these changes occur slowly, with individuals within the system receiving preparation to meet the challenges created by the change. If done in an organized manner, planned change is effective and meets with minimal resistance.

The Change Theory

The change theory was introduced by Kurt Lewin in 1951. According to Lewin the change process consists of three phases: unfreezing, changing, and refreezing. The initial step in Lewin's change theory is unfreezing. Unfreezing occurs as the staff members see the need for change. This stage prepares the staff for the change. Change occurs as the staff members internalize the new ideas, behaviors, and concepts of the change. Freezing occurs when the change is fully internalized and the new behaviors are accepted by those individuals within the organization. Practicing and becoming comfortable with the change is necessary before refreezing is complete.

A **change agent** is one who is responsible for implementing the change. A manager, a consultant, or an individual appointed by the organization can serve as the change agent. Change agents educate the staff concerning the change, model the behaviors indicated by the change, and solve problems that arise as the result of the change. Display 25-5 offers an example of how the change process works.

CRITICAL THINKING EXERCISES

1. Identify a nurse leader you admire, and analyze this leader's leadership style (ie, democratic, autocratic, laissez-faire, or participative). State the rationale for your choice. What personal qualities do you see that make this person a good leader?
2. Analyze your personal qualities as a leader using Tappen's six characteristics of a good leader. Choose one or two traits that you would like to develop more fully. Devise a plan to help you develop these characteristics.

DISPLAY 25-5. An Example of How the Change Process Evolves

The Desired Change: The nursing home decided to change from a manual charting system to a computerized charting system. Many of the nurses in the facility were unfamiliar with computers and were extremely anxious and resistant to the change.

The Change Agent: One of the nurses at the nursing home was selected to oversee implementation of the change and to serve as change agent. This nurse received special training to become familiar with the new system and in working with the computer.

Unfreezing: Unfreezing was accomplished gradually as the staff was educated on the uses of the computer and the need for the change. Staff members were assigned times to work on the computer. They attended classes pertaining to the use of the computer. A few simple computer games were devised to help the staff become comfortable working on the computer. In time, all but a few of the most resistant were ready for the change.

Change: The new system was implemented with the change agent nurse using the computer system to chart on the patient record. The change agent modeled the desired behavior and then helped the staff members to practice the new behavior.

Re-freezing: In time, all individuals internalized this behavior and felt comfortable using the computer when charting. Many of the nurses involved expressed a feeling that the new computerized system was superior to the old manual method of charting. Freezing was complete.

3. Write a passive, aggressive, and assertive response to each of the following situations. Share your responses with your classmates.

   Situation 1: A family member of a resident in the nursing home where you work complains to you that someone in the facility is stealing her mother's personal items. She is in the lobby, talking loudly and making derogatory statements about the nursing home.

   Situation 2: One of the nurse assistants is talking with a family member. The information she is giving about the resident is incorrect.

   Situation 3: Your instructor embarrasses you by pointing out your mistakes in front of the patient. This makes you so nervous that you are unable to perform well.

4. You have been appointed to oversee a number of changes at the community center for older adults where you work. The new owner plans to change the daily schedule of activities to one that is less flexible and more structured. The older adults at the center are complaining about the new system. How would you assist these older adults to adjust to the change? Explain how you could use your knowledge of the change theory in managing this problem.

REFERENCES AND SUGGESTED READING

Anderson, M.A. (1997). *Nursing leadership, management, and professional practice for the LPN/LVN.* Philadelphia: F.A. Davis.

Deering, C. (1996). Learning to say no. *American Journal of Nursing, 96 (4),* 62.

Herschfelt, D., & Brill, S. (2000). *Effective communication for health professionals.* Philadelphia: W.B. Saunders.

Hersey, P., Blanchard, K., & Johnson, D. (1996). *Management of organizational behavior: Utilizing human resources* (7th ed.). Englewood Cliffs, NJ: Prentice-Hall.

Ireson, C., & McGillis, G. (1998.) A multidisciplinary shared governance model. *Nursing Management, 29 (2),* 37–39.

Lewin, S. (1951). *Field theory in social science.* New York: Harper & Row.

Longenecke, P. (1998). Managing nurse managers—What is the secret? *Nursing Management, 29 (3),* 35–37.

Parsons, L. (1997). Delegation decision making. *Journal of Nursing Administration, 27 (2),* 47.

Shindul-Rothschild, J., et al. (1997). 10 Keys to quality care. *American Journal of Nursing, 97 (11),* 35.

Tappan, R.M. (1995). *Nursing leadership and management: Concepts and practice* (3rd ed.). Philadelphia: F.A. Davis.

Weiss, L. (1998). How to work with a difficult manager. *Nursing 98, 28 (2),* 64.

A Patient's Bill of Rights

INTRODUCTION

Effective health care requires collaboration between patients, physicians, and other health care professionals. Open and honest communication, respect for personal and professional values, and sensitivity *to differences* are integral to optimal patient care. As the setting for the provision of health services, hospitals must provide a foundation for understanding and respecting the rights and responsibilities of patients, their families, physicians, and other caregivers. They must also ensure a health care ethic that respects the role of patients in decision making about treatment choices and other aspects of their care. Finally, hospitals must be sensitive to cultural, racial, linguistic, religious, age, gender, and other differences as well as the needs of persons with disabilities.

The American Hospital Association presents this *Patient's Bill of Rights* with the expectation that it will contribute to more effective patient care and be supported by the hospital on behalf of the institution, its medical staff, employees, and patients. The American Hospital Association encourages health care institutions to tailor this bill of rights to their patient community by translating and/or simplifying its language as may be necessary to ensure that patients and their families understand their rights and responsibilities.

BILL OF RIGHTS*

1. The patient has the right to considerate and respectful care.
2. The patient has the right to and is encouraged to obtain from physicians and other direct caregivers relevant, current, and understandable information concerning diagnosis, treatment, and prognosis.

Except in emergencies when the patient lacks decision-making capacity and the need for treatment is urgent, the patient is entitled to the opportunity to discuss and request information related to the specific procedures and/or treatments, the risks involved, the possible length of recuperation, and the medically reasonable alternatives and their accompanying risks and benefits.

Patients have the right to know the identity of physicians, nurses, and others involved in their care, including those who are students, residents, or other trainees. The patient also has the right to know the immediate and long-term financial implications of treatment choices, insofar as they are known.

3. The patient has the right to make decisions about the plan of care prior to and during the course of treatment, to refuse a recommended treatment or plan of care to the extent permitted by law and hospital policy, and to be informed of the medical consequences of this action. In case of such refusal, the patient is entitled to receive other appropriate care and services that the hospital provides or to transfer to another hospital. The hospital should notify patients of any policy that might affect patient choice within the institution.
4. The patient has the right to have an advance directive (such as a living will, health care proxy, or durable power of attorney for health care) concerning treatment or designating a surrogate decision maker with the expectation that the hospital will honor the intent of that directive to the extent permitted by law and hospital policy.

Health care institutions must advise patients of their right under state law and hospital policy to make informed medical choices, ask if the patient has an advance directive, and include that information in patient records. The patient has the right to timely information about any hospital policy that might limit its ability to implement fully a legally valid advance directive.

*These rights can be exercised on the patient's behalf by a legally designated surrogate or proxy decision maker if the patient lacks decision-making capacity, is legally incompetent, or is a minor. Reprinted with permission of the American Hospital Association. © 1992.

5. The patient has the right to every consideration of privacy. Case discussion, consultation, examination, and treatment should be conducted so as to protect each patient's privacy.

6. The patient has the right to expect that all communications and records pertaining to his/her care will be treated as confidential by the hospital, except in cases such as suspected abuse and public health hazards when reporting is permitted or required by law. The patient has the right to expect that the hospital will emphasize the confidentiality of this information when it releases his/her records to any other parties entitled to review them.

7. The patient has the right to review the records pertaining to his/her medical care and to have the information explained or interpreted as necessary, except when restricted by law.

8. The patient has the right to expect that, within its capacity and policies, a hospital will make reasonable response to the request of a patient for appropriate and medically indicated care and services. The hospital must provide evaluation, service, and/or referral as indicated by the urgency of the case. When medically appropriate and legally permissible, or when he/she has so requested, a patient may be transferred to another facility. The institution to which the patient is to be transferred must first have accepted him/her for transfer. The patient must also have the benefit of complete information and explanation concerning the need for, risks, benefits, and alternatives to such a transfer.

9. The patient has the right to ask about and be informed of the existence of business relationships *among* the hospital, educational institutions, other health care providers, and payers that may influence the patient's treatment and care.

10. The patient has the right to consent to or decline to participate in proposed research studies or human experimentation affecting care and treatment or requiring direct patient involvement, and to have those studies fully explained prior to consent. A patient who declines to participate in research or experimentation is entitled to the most effective care that the hospital can otherwise provide.

11. The patient has the right to expect reasonable continuity of care when appropriate and to be informed by physicians and other caregivers of available and realistic patient care options when hospital care is no longer appropriate.

12. The patient has the right to be informed of hospital policies and practices that relate to patient care, treatment, and responsibilities. The patient has the right to be informed of available resources for resolving disputes, grievances, and conflicts, such as ethics committees, patient representatives, or other mechanisms available in the institution. The patient has the right to be informed of the hospital's charges for services and available payment methods.

The collaborative nature of health care requires that patients, or their families/surrogates, participate in their care. The effectiveness of care and patient satisfaction with the course of treatment depend in part on the patient fulfilling certain responsibilities. Patients are responsible for providing information about past illnesses, hospitalizations, medications, and other matters related to health status. To participate effectively in decision making, patients must be encouraged to take responsibility for requesting additional information or clarification about their health status or treatment when they do not fully understand information and instructions. Patients are also responsible for ensuring that the health care institution has a copy of their written advance directive if they have one. Patients are responsible for informing their physicians and other caregivers if they anticipate problems in following the prescribed treatment.

Patients should also be aware of the hospital's obligation to be reasonably efficient and equitable in providing care to other patients and the community. The hospital's rules and regulations are designed to help the hospital meet this obligation. Patients and their families are responsible for making reasonable accommodations to the needs of the hospital, other patients, medical staff, and hospital employees. Patients are responsible for providing necessary information for insurance claims and for working with the hospital to make payment arrangements, when necessary.

A person's health depends on much more than health care services. Patients are responsible for recognizing the impact of their lifestyle on their personal health.

CONCLUSION

Hospitals have many functions to perform, including the enhancement of health status, health promotion, and the prevention and treatment of injury and disease; the immediate and ongoing care and rehabilitation of patients; the education of health professionals, patients, and the community; and research. All these activities must be conducted with an overriding concern for the value and dignity of each patient.

APPENDIX B

Directive to Physicians and Family or Surrogates

Instructions For Completing This Document

This is an important legal document known as an "advance directive." It is designed to help you communicate your wishes about medical treatment at some time in the future when you are unable to make your wishes known because of illness or injury. These wishes usually are based on personal values. In particular, you may want to consider what burdens or hardships of treatment you would be willing to accept for a particular amount of benefit obtained if you were seriously ill.

You are encouraged to discuss your values and wishes with your family or chosen spokesperson, as well as your physician. Your physician, other health care provider, or medical institution may provide you with various resources to assist you in completing your advance directive. Brief definitions are listed below and may aid you in your discussions and planning. Initial the treatment choices that best reflect your personal preferences. Provide a copy of your directive to your physician, usual hospital, and family or spokesperson. Consider a periodic review of this document to best assure that it reflects your preferences.

In addition to this advance directive, Texas law provides for two other types of directives that can be important during a serious illness. These are the Medical Power of Attorney and the Out-of-Hospital Do-Not-Resuscitate Order. You may wish to discuss these with your physician, family, hospital representative or other advisers. You also may wish to complete a directive related to the donation of organs and tissues.

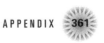

Directive

I, _____(insert your name), recognize that the best health care is based upon a partnership of trust and communication with my physician. My physician and I will make health care decisions together as long as I am of sound mind and able to make my wishes known. If there comes a time that I am unable to make medical decisions about myself because of illness or injury, I direct that the following treatment preferences be honored:

If, in the judgment of my physician, I am suffering with a terminal condition from which I am expected to die within six months, even with available life-sustaining treatment provided in accordance with prevailing standards of medical care:

_____ I request that all treatments other than those needed to keep me comfortable be discontinued or withheld, and my physician allow me to die as gently as possible; OR

_____ I request that I be kept alive in this terminal condition using available life-sustaining treatment. (THIS SELECTION DOES NOT APPLY TO HOSPICE CARE.)

If, in the judgment of my physician, I am suffering with an irreversible condition so that I cannot care for myself or make decisions for myself and am expected to die without life-sustaining treatment provided in accordance with prevailing standards of care:

_____ I request that all treatments other than those needed to keep me comfortable be discontinued or withheld, and my physician allow me to die as gently as possible; OR

_____ I request that I be kept alive in this irreversible condition using available life-sustaining treatment. (THIS SELECTION DOES NOT APPLY TO HOSPICE CARE.)

Additional requests: (After discussion with your physician, you may wish to consider listing particular treatments in this space that you do or do *not* want in specific circumstances, such as artificial nutrition and fluids, intravenous antibiotics, etc. Be sure to state whether you *do* or *do not* want the particular treatment.)

_____

_____

_____

After signing this directive, if my representative or I elect hospice care, I understand and agree that only those treatments needed to keep me comfortable would be provided and I would not be given available life-sustaining treatments.

(If a Medical Power of Attorney has been executed, then an agent already has been named and you should not list additional names in this document.)

If I do not have a Medical Power of Attorney, and I am unable to make my wishes known, I designate the following person(s) to make treatment decisions with my physician compatible with my personal values:

1. _____

2. _____

If the above persons are not available, or if I have not designated a spokesperson, I understand that a spokesperson will be chosen for me following standards specified in the laws of Texas. If, in the judgment of my physician, my death is imminent within minutes or hours, even with the use of all available medical treatment provided within the prevailing standard of care, I acknowledge that all treatments may be withheld or removed except those needed to maintain my comfort. I understand that under Texas law this directive has no effect if I have been diagnosed as pregnant. This directive will remain in effect until I revoke it. No other person may do so.

Signed _____ Date_____
City, County, State of Residence _____

Two competent adult witnesses must sign below, acknowledging the signature of the declarant. The witness designated as Witness 1 may not be a person designated to make a treatment decision for the patient and may not be related to the patient by blood or marriage. This witness may not be entitled to any part of the estate and may not have a claim against the estate of the patient. This witness may not be the attending physician or an employee of the attending physician. If this witness is an employee of a health care facility in which the patient is being cared for, this witness may not be involved in providing direct patient care to the patient. This witness may not be an officer, director, partner or business office employee of a health care facility in which the patient is being cared for or of any parent organization of the health care facility.

Witness 1 _____Witness 2 _____

DEFINITIONS:

- **"Artificial nutrition and hydration"** means the provision of nutrients or fluids by a tube inserted in a vein, under the skin in the subcutaneous tissues, or in the stomach (gastrointestinal tract).
- **"Irreversible condition"** means a condition, injury or illness:
  (1) that may be treated, but can never be cured or eliminated;
  (2) that leaves a person unable to care for or make decisions for himself/herself; and
  (3) that, without life-sustaining treatment provided in accordance with the prevailing standard of medical care, is fatal.

Explanation: Many serious illnesses such as cancer, failure of major organs (kidney, heart, liver, or lung), and serious brain disease such as Alzheimer's dementia, may be considered irreversible early on. There is no cure, but the patient may be kept alive for prolonged periods of time if the patient receives life-sustaining treatments. Late in the course of the same illness, the disease may be considered terminal when, even with treatment, the patient is expected to die. You may wish to consider which burdens of treatment you would be willing to accept in an effort to achieve a particular outcome. This is a very personal decision that you may wish to discuss with your physician, family, or other important people in your life.

- **"Life-sustaining treatment"** means treatment that, based on reasonable medical judgment, sustains the life of a patient and without which the patient will die. The term includes both life-sustaining medications and artificial life support, such as mechanical breathing machines, kidney dialysis treatment, and artificial hydration and nutrition. The term does not include the administration of pain management medication, the performance of a medical procedure necessary to provide comfort care, or any other medical care provided to alleviate a patient's pain.

- **"Terminal condition"** means an incurable condition caused by injury, disease or illness that according to reasonable medical judgment will produce death within six months, even with available life-sustaining treatment provided in accordance with the prevailing standard of medical care.

Explanation: Many serious illnesses may be considered irreversible early in the course of the illness, but they may not be considered terminal until the disease is fairly advanced. In thinking about terminal illness and its treatment, you again may wish to consider the relative benefits and burdens of treatment and discuss your wishes with your physician, family or other important people in your life.

Medical Power of Attorney

DESIGNATION OF HEALTH CARE AGENT

I, _____ (insert your name) appoint:

Name: _____

Address: _____

_____ Phone: _____

as my agent to make any and all health care decisions for me, except to the extent that I state otherwise in this document. This Medical Power of Attorney takes effect if I become unable to make my own health care decisions and this fact is certified in writing by my physician.

LIMITATIONS ON THE DECISION-MAKING AUTHORITY OF MY AGENT ARE AS FOLLOWS:

_____

_____

DESIGNATION OF ALTERNATE AGENT

(You are not required to designate an alternate agent, but you may do so. An alternate agent may make the same health care decisions as the designated agent if the designated agent is unable or unwilling to act as your agent. If the agent designated is your spouse, the designation automatically is revoked by law if your marriage is dissolved.)

If the person designated as my agent is unable or unwilling to make health care decisions for me, I designate the following persons to serve as my agent to make health care decisions for me as authorized by this document, who serve in the following order:

A. First Alternate Agent

Name: _____

Address: _____

_____ Phone: _____

B. Second Alternate Agent

Name: _____

Address: _____

_____ Phone: _____

The original of this document is kept at:

_____

_____

The following individuals or institutions have signed copies:

Name: _____

Address: _____

Name: _____

Address: _____

DURATION

I understand that this power of attorney exists indefinitely from the date I execute this document unless I establish a shorter time or revoke the power of attorney. If I am unable to make health care decisions for myself when this power of attorney expires, the authority I have granted my agent continues to exist until the time I become able to make health care decisions for myself.

(If applicable) This power of attorney ends on the following date:_____

PRIOR DESIGNATIONS REVOKED

I revoke any prior Medical Power of Attorney.

ACKNOWLEDGMENT OF DISCLOSURE STATEMENT

I have been provided with a disclosure statement explaining the effect of this document. I have read and understand that information contained in the disclosure statement.

(YOU MUST DATE AND SIGN THIS POWER OF ATTORNEY.)

I sign my name to this Medical Power of Attorney on _____ day of

_____ (month) _____ (year) at

_____
(City and State)

_____
(Signature)

_____
(Print Name)

STATEMENT OF FIRST WITNESS

I am not the person appointed as agent by this document. I am not related to the principal by blood or marriage. I would not be entitled to any portion of the principal's estate in the event of the principal's death. I am not the attending physician of the principal or an employee of the attending physician. I have no claim against any portion of the principal's estate in the event of the principal's death. Furthermore, if I am an employee of a health care facility in which the principal is a patient, I am not involved in providing direct patient care to the principal and am not an officer, director, partner or business office employee of the health care facility or of any parent organization of the health care facility.

Signature: _____

Print Name: _____ Date: _____

Address: _____

SIGNATURE OF SECOND WITNESS

Signature: _____

Print Name: _____ Date: _____

Address: _____

Artificial Nutrition and Hydration: Comfort Care or Medical Treatment?

In theory, decisions about using life support are reasoned and logical: the benefits and burdens of the treatment are weighed in light of the patient's wishes. But in real life, those decisions can be messy and emotionally wrenching. For many families, the toughest decision of all is whether to use artificial nutrition and hydration (ANH) when their loved one is dying.

"It is very common that people near the end of life quit eating, or at least quit eating much, and quit drinking," explains Joanne Lynn, MD, a geriatrician and Senior Associate Professor at Dartmouth Medical School. "The question becomes whether we should use artificial means to circumvent their stopping eating, and that turns on whether it does them any good." How could being fed *not* do good? Most of us assume that it must be painful to go without food, to die from malnutrition or dehydration. The medical evidence, however, contradicts this assumption.

THE DYING PROCESS

Most people (including many medical professionals) do not realize that dying people often feel little or no hunger or thirst, and that those patients will not suffer without nourishment. As well, people often do not understand how tube feeding can do harm rather than good. Yet clinicians who work with dying patients attest to this phenomenon, as does the med-

ical literature. In a 1993 article in the *Journal of General Internal Medicine,* Robert Sullivan, MD and MPh, of Duke University reviews the medical literature on the physiological changes that accompany the withholding of nutrition and hydration. Not only does he find that a person who has stopped all food and fluid intake is unlikely to experience pain, he also warns that administration of small amounts of food or even the small amount of dextrose found in many IV solutions can rekindle a sense of hunger. He concludes: "It is likely that prolonged dehydration and starvation induce no pain and only limited discomfort from a dry mouth, which can be controlled. For individuals carrying an intolerable burden of illness and disability, or those who have no hope of ever again enjoying meaningful human interaction, the withdrawal of food and fluid may be considered without concern that it will add to the misery."

A Fundamental Sign of Caring

The notion that dying patients must be provided with nutrition and fluids nonetheless continues to be a powerful one. Dr. Lynn suggests some reasons for this when she notes: "Our instinct is to provide food. Feeding another person is the way of showing that you care about them, and failure to feed is ordinarily a way of showing that you *don't* care."

Normally, feeding a helpless person—a baby, an invalid—is a lifesaving and deeply caring act. When someone is dying and there is "nothing more to be done," that urge may become even stronger. The desire to do *something* to show our caring often reflects a sense of powerlessness in the face of death.

The Power of Symbols

It is one thing when a competent dying person refuses tube feeding and can explain her choice, while reassuring her loved ones that she is not in pain. It is another to make that decision for someone who is unconscious or incompetent.

The symbolism of feeding can be so powerful that families who know that their loved one would not want to be kept alive may still feel that stopping artificial feeding is taboo. In such cases, according to Dr. Lynn and other geriatricians, a compromise can often be reached. "Usually you can honor the symbol without hurting the patient," Dr. Lynn explains. "You can run an IV with the family's awareness that it's at a very low rate," thereby reassuring the family without causing edema or other side effects. The moment when family members are watching a loved one die is not the time to debate their assumptions or educate them about the physiology of the dying process.

Decision Making

"Some families and patients find tube feeding to be just like Grandma's chicken soup—others find it to be just like respirators," Dr. Lynn points out. If you are in the latter group, however, it is important to recognize that your loved ones or future caregivers may not see tube feeding the way you do.

The emotional issues surrounding the use of tube feeding are complex. Even state law may handle these treatments differently from other medical treatments. Because so much controversy surrounds the use of artificial nutrition and hydration, it is important that you state specifically whether or not you would want these treatments when preparing your advance directive.

Decisions about withholding or withdrawing artificial nutrition and hydration are greatly influenced by the attitudes of the health care facility and physician who may be unfamiliar or misinformed about state law. Therefore, it is important that you become familiar with your rights before completing your advance directive.

Your Right to Refuse Tube Feeding

You have both a federal constitutional and a state law right to refuse tube feeding. In 1990, the U.S. Supreme Court decided in the case of Nancy Cruzan that a competent patient has "a constitutionally protected right to refuse lifesaving hydration and nutrition." In addition, state laws allow you to refuse artificial nutrition and hydration in case of future incapacity, by means of advance directives. However, state laws do vary with what you must do to preserve your right to refuse tube feeding through advance directives.

Most states have one advance directive law for living wills and a second for durable (medical) powers of attorney for health care, which let you appoint a health care agent to direct your care if you are unable to make decisions for yourself. Historically, living wills were developed first and apply to a limited set of medical conditions, such as end-stage terminal illness or persistent vegetative state. Durable (medical) powers of attorney for health care were designed later to be more flexible and generally apply anytime you lose the ability to make medical decisions for yourself.

Adapted and reprinted with permission from Choice in Dying, 1036 30th Street, Washington, DC.

Numeric Identifier _____

MINIMUM DATA SET (MDS) - *VERSION 2.0*
FOR NURSING HOME RESIDENT ASSESSMENT AND CARE SCREENING

BASIC ASSESSMENT TRACKING FORM

SECTION AA. IDENTIFICATION INFORMATION

1.	**RESIDENT NAME***	a.(First) b.(Middle Initial) c.(Last) d.(Jr/Sr)

> **GENERAL INSTRUCTIONS**
> *Complete this information for submission with all full and quarterly assessments (Admission, Annual, Significant Change, State or Medicare required assessments, or Quarterly Reviews, etc.)*

2.	**GENDER***	1. Male 2. Female
3.	**BIRTHDATE***	☐☐ - ☐☐ - ☐☐☐☐ Month Day Year
4.	**RACE/* ETHNICITY**	1. American Indian/Alaskan Native 4. Hispanic 2. Asian/Pacific Islander 5. White, not of 3. Black, not of Hispanic origin Hispanic origin
5.	**SOCIAL SECURITY* AND MEDICARE NUMBERS* [C in 1st box if non med. no.]**	a. Social Security Number ☐☐☐ - ☐☐ - ☐☐☐☐ b. Medicare number (or comparable railroad insurance number)
6.	**FACILITY PROVIDER NO.***	a.State No. b.Federal No.
7.	**MEDICAID NO. [" + " if pending, "N" if not a Medicaid recipient] ***	
8.	**REASONS FOR ASSESS-MENT**	[Note - Other codes do not apply to this form] a. Primary reason for assessment 01.Admission assessment (required by day 14) 02.Annual assessment 03.Significant change in status assessment 04.Significant correction of prior full assessment 05.Quarterly review assessment 10.Significant correction of prior quarterly assessment 00.*NONE OF ABOVE* b. *Codes for assessments required for Medicare PPS or the State* *1. Medicare 5 day assessment* *2. Medicare 30 day assessment* *3. Medicare 60 day assessment* *4. Medicare 90 day assessment* *5. Medicare readmission/return assessment* *6. Other state required assessment* *7. Medicare 14 day assessment* *8. Other Medicare required assessment*
9.	**SIGNATURES OF PERSONS COMPLETING THESE ITEMS:**	

a. Signatures   Title   Date

b.   Date

* = Key items for computerized resident tracking

☐ = When box blank, must enter number or letter   [a.] = When letter in box, check if condition applies

MDS 2.0 01/30/98

Resident _____   Numeric Identifier _____

MINIMUM DATA SET (MDS) - *VERSION 2.0*
FOR NURSING HOME RESIDENT ASSESSMENT AND CARE SCREENING

BACKGROUND (FACE SHEET) INFORMATION AT ADMISSION

SECTION AB. DEMOGRAPHIC INFORMATION

1.	DATE OF ENTRY	*Date the stay began. Note - Does not include readmission if record was closed at time of temporary discharge to hospital, etc. In such cases, use prior admission date* ☐☐ - ☐☐ - ☐☐☐☐ Month　　　Day　　　Year
2.	ADMITTED FROM (AT ENTRY)	1. Private home/apt. with no home health services 2. Private home/apt. with home health services 3. Board and care/assisted living/group home 4. Nursing home 5. Acute care hospital 6. Psychiatric hospital, MR/DD facility 7. Rehabilitation hospital 8. Other
3.	LIVED ALONE (PRIOR TO ENTRY)	0. No 1. Yes 2. In other facility
4.	ZIP CODE OF PRIOR PRIMARY RESIDENCE	☐☐☐☐☐
5.	RESIDENTIAL HISTORY 5 YEARS PRIOR TO ENTRY	*(Check all settings resident lived in during 5 years prior to date of entry given in item AB1 above)* a. Prior stay at this nursing home ... a. b. Stay in other nursing home ... b. c. Other residential facility-board and care home, assisted living, group home ... c. d. MH/psychiatric setting ... d. e. MR/DD setting ... e. f. *NONE OF ABOVE* ... f.
6.	LIFETIME OCCUPA-TION(S) [Put "/" between two occupations]	☐
7.	EDUCATION *(Highest Level Completed)*	1. No schooling　　5. Technical or trade school 2. 8th grade/less　　6. Some college 3. 9-11 grades　　　7. Bachelor's degree 4. High school　　　8. Graduate degree
8.	LANGUAGE	*(Code for correct response)* a. Primary Language 0.English　　1.Spanish　　2.French　　3.Other b. If other, specify ☐☐☐☐☐☐☐
9.	MENTAL HEALTH HISTORY	Does resident's RECORD indicate any history of mental retardation, mental illness, or developmental disability problem? 0. No　　　　1. Yes
10.	CONDITIONS RELATED TO MR/DD STATUS	*(Check all conditions that are related to MR/DD status that were manifested before age 22, and are likely to continue indefinitely)* a. Not applicable - no MR/DD (Skip to AB11) ... a. 　MR/DD with organic condition b. Down's syndrome ... b. c. Autism ... c. d. Epilepsy ... d. e. Other organic condition related to MR/DD ... e. f. MR/DD with no organic condition ... f.
11.	DATE BACK-GROUND INFORMA-TION COMPLETED	☐☐ - ☐☐ - ☐☐☐☐ Month　　　Day　　　Year

SECTION AC. CUSTOMARY ROUTINE

1.	CUSTOMARY ROUTINE *(In year prior to DATE OF ENTRY to this nursing home, or year last in community if now being admitted from another nursing home)*	*(Check all that apply. If all information UNKNOWN, check last box only.)* **CYCLE OF DAILY EVENTS** a.Stays up late at night (e.g., after 9 pm) ... a. b.Naps regularly during day (at least 1 hour) ... b. c.Goes out 1+ days a week ... c. d.Stays busy with hobbies, reading, or fixed daily routine ... d. e.Spends most time alone or watching TV ... e. f.Moves independently indoors (with appliances, if used) ... f. g. Use of tobacco products at least daily ... g. h.*NONE OF ABOVE* ... h. **EATING PATTERNS** i. Distinct food preferences ... i. j. Eats between meals all or most days ... j. k.Use of alcoholic beverage(s) at least weekly ... k. l. *NONE OF ABOVE* ... l. **ADL PATTERNS** m.In bedclothes much of day ... m. n. Wakens to toilet all or most nights ... n. o. Has irregular bowel movement pattern ... o. p. Showers for bathing ... p. q. Bathing in PM ... q. r. *NONE OF ABOVE* ... r. **INVOLVEMENT PATTERNS** s. Daily contact with relatives/close friends ... s. t. Usually attends church, temple, synagogue (etc.) ... t. u. Finds strength in faith ... u. v. Daily animal companion/presence ... v. w. Involved in group activities ... w. x. *NONE OF ABOVE* ... x. y. UNKNOWN - Resident/family unable to provide information ... y.

[END]

SECTION AD. FACE SHEET SIGNATURES

SIGNATURES OF PERSONS COMPLETING FACE SHEET:

a. Signature of RN Assessment Coordinator			Date
b. Signatures	Title	Sections	Date
c.			Date
d.			Date
e.			Date
f.			Date
g.			Date

☐ = When box blank, must enter number or letter　　a. = When letter in box, check if condition applies

MDS 2.0　01/30/98

- 2 -

Resident _____ Numeric Identifier _____

MINIMUM DATA SET (MDS) - *VERSION 2.0*
FOR NURSING HOME RESIDENT ASSESSMENT AND CARE SCREENING
FULL ASSESSMENT FORM
(Status in last 7 days, unless other time frame indicated)

SECTION A. IDENTIFICATION AND BACKGROUND INFORMATION

1.	RESIDENT NAME	a.(First)　　　b.(Middle Initial)　　　c.(Last)　　　d.(Jr/Sr)

2.	ROOM NUMBER	

3.	ASSESS-MENT REFERENCE DATE	a. *Last day of MDS observation period* ☐☐ - ☐☐ - ☐☐☐☐ Month　　Day　　Year b. Original (0) or corrected copy of form (enter number of correction)

4a.	DATE OF REENTRY	Date of reentry from most recent temporary discharge to a hospital in last 90 days (or since last assessment or admission if less than 90 days) ☐☐ - ☐☐ - ☐☐☐☐ Month　　Day　　Year

5.	MARITAL STATUS	1. Never married　　3. Widowed　　5. Divorced 2. Married　　4. Separated

6.	MEDICAL RECORD NO.	

7.	CURRENT PAYMENT SOURCES FOR N.H. STAY	*(Billing Office to indicate; check all that apply in last 30 days)* a. Medicaid per diem ☐　　f. VA per diem ☐ b. Medicare per diem ☐　　g. Self or family pays for full per diem ☐ c. Medicare ancillary part A ☐　　h. Medicaid resident liability or Medicare co-payment ☐ d. Medicare ancillary part B ☐　　i. Private insurance per diem (including co-payment) ☐ e. CHAMPUS per diem ☐　　j. Other per diem ☐

8.	REASONS FOR ASSESS-MENT [Note - If this is a discharge or reentry assessment, only a limited subset of MDS items need be completed]	a. Primary reason for assessment 01. Admission assessment (required by day 14) 02. Annual assessment 03. Significant change in status assessment 04. Significant correction of prior full assessment 05. Quarterly review assessment 06. Discharged - return not anticipated 07. Discharged - return anticipated 08. Discharged prior to completing initial assessment 09. Reentry 10. Significant correction of prior quarterly assessment 00. *NONE OF ABOVE* b. **Codes for assessments required for Medicare PPS or the State** 1. Medicare 5 day assessment 2. Medicare 30 day assessment 3. Medicare 60 day assessment 4. Medicare 90 day assessment 5. Medicare readmission/return assessment 6. Other state required assessment 7. Medicare 14 day assessment 8. Other Medicare required assessment

9.	RESPONSI-BILITY/LEGAL GUARDIAN	*(Check all that apply)* a. Legal guardian ☐　　d. Durable power attorney/financial ☐ b. Other legal oversight ☐　　e. Family member responsible ☐ c. Durable power of attorney/health care ☐　　f. Patient responsible for self ☐ g. *NONE OF ABOVE* ☐

10.	ADVANCED DIRECTIVES	*(For those items with supporting documentation in the medical record, check all that apply)* a. Living will ☐　　f. Feeding restrictions ☐ b. Do not resuscitate ☐　　g. Medication restrictions ☐ c. Do not hospitalize ☐　　h. Other treatment restrictions ☐ d. Organ donation ☐　　i. *NONE OF ABOVE* ☐ e. Autopsy request ☐

SECTION B. COGNITIVE PATTERNS

1.	COMATOSE	*(Persistent vegetative state/no discernible consciousness)* 0. No　　1. Yes　　**(If yes, skip to Section G)**

2.	MEMORY	*(Recall of what was learned or known)* a. Short-term memory OK-seems/appears to recall after 5 minutes 0. Memory OK　　1. Memory problem b. Long-term memory OK-seems/appears to recall long past 0. Memory OK　　1. Memory problem

3.	MEMORY/ RECALL ABILITY	*(Check all that resident was normally able to recall during last 7 days)* a. Current season ☐　　d. That he/she is in a nursing home ☐ b. Location of own room ☐　　e. *NONE OF ABOVE* are recalled ☐ c. Staff names/faces ☐

4.	COGNITIVE SKILLS FOR DAILY DECISION-MAKING	*(Made decisions regarding tasks of daily life)* 0. INDEPENDENT - decisions consistent/reasonable 1. *MODIFIED INDEPENDENCE* - some difficulty in new situations only 2. *MODERATELY IMPAIRED* - decisions poor; cues/ supervision required 3. *SEVERELY IMPAIRED* - never/rarely made decisions

5.	INDICATORS OF DELIRIUM-PERIODIC DISORDERED THINKING/ AWARE-NESS	*(Code for behavior in the last 7 days.)* [Note: Accurate assessment requires conversations with staff and family who have direct knowledge of resident's behavior over this time]. 0. Behavior not present 1. Behavior present, not of recent onset 2. Behavior present, over last 7 days appears different from resident's usual functioning (e.g., new onset or worsening) a. EASILY DISTRACTED-(e.g., difficulty paying attention; gets sidetracked) b. PERIODS OF ALTERED PERCEPTION OR AWARENESS OF SURROUNDINGS-(e.g., moves lips or talks to someone not present; believes he/she is somewhere else; confuses night and day) c. EPISODES OF DISORGANIZED SPEECH-(e.g., speech is incoherent, nonsensical, irrelevant, or rambling from subject to subject; loses train of thought) d. PERIODS OF RESTLESSNESS-(e.g., fidgeting or picking at skin, clothing, napkins, etc.; frequent position changes; repetitive physical movements or calling out) e. PERIODS OF LETHARGY-(e.g., sluggishness; staring into space; difficult to arouse; little body movement) f. MENTAL FUNCTION VARIES OVER THE COURSE OF THE DAY-(e.g., sometimes better, sometimes worse; behaviors sometimes present, sometimes not)

6.	CHANGE IN COGNITIVE STATUS	Resident's cognitive status, skills, or abilities have changed as compared to status of **90 days ago** (or since last assessment if less than 90 days) 0. No change　　1. Improved　　2. Deteriorated

SECTION C. COMMUNICATION/HEARING PATTERNS

1.	HEARING	*(With hearing appliance, if used)* 0. HEARS ADEQUATELY-normal talk, TV, phone 1. *MINIMAL DIFFICULTY* when not in quiet setting 2. *HEARS IN SPECIAL SITUATIONS ONLY*-speaker has to adjust tonal quality and speak distinctly 3. *HIGHLY IMPAIRED*/absence of useful hearing

2.	COMMUNI-CATION DEVICES/ TECH-NIQUES	*(Check all that apply during last 7 days)* a. Hearing aid, present and used ☐ b. Hearing aid, present and not used regularly ☐ c. Other receptive comm. techniques used (e.g. lip reading) ☐ d. *NONE OF ABOVE* ☐

3.	MODES OF EXPRESSION	*(Check all used by resident to make needs known)* a. Speech ☐　　d. Signs/gestures/sounds ☐ b. Writing messages to express or clarify needs ☐　　e. Communication board ☐ c. American sign language or Braille ☐　　f. Other ☐ g. *NONE OF ABOVE* ☐

4.	MAKING SELF UNDER-STOOD	*(Expressing information content-however able)* 0. UNDERSTOOD 1. *USUALLY UNDERSTOOD*-difficulty finding words or finishing thoughts 2. *SOMETIMES UNDERSTOOD*-ability is limited to making concrete requests 3. *RARELY/NEVER UNDERSTOOD*

5.	SPEECH CLARITY	*(Code for speech in the last 7 days)* 0. *CLEAR SPEECH* - distinct, intelligible words 1. *UNCLEAR SPEECH* - slurred, mumbled words 2. *NO SPEECH* - absence of spoken words

6.	ABILITY TO UNDER-STAND OTHERS	*(Understanding verbal information content-however able)* 0. *UNDERSTANDS* 1. *USUALLY UNDERSTANDS*-may miss some part/intent of message 2. *SOMETIMES UNDERSTANDS*-responds adequately to simple, direct communication 3. *RARELY/NEVER UNDERSTANDS*

7.	CHANGE IN COMMUNI-CATION/ HEARING	Resident's ability to express, understand, or hear information has changed as compared to status of **90 days ago** (or since last assessment if less than 90 days) 0. No change　　1. Improved　　2. Deteriorated

☐ = When box blank, must enter number or letter　　☐ a. = When letter in box, check if condition applies

MDS 2.0 01/30/98

- 3 -

Resident _____   Numeric Identifier _____

SECTION D. VISION PATTERNS

1.	VISION	*(Ability to see in adequate light and with glasses if used)* 0. *ADEQUATE*-sees fine detail, including regular print in newspapers/books 1. *IMPAIRED*-sees large print, but not regular print in newspapers/books 2. *MODERATELY IMPAIRED*-limited vision; not able to see newspaper headlines, but can identify objects 3. *HIGHLY IMPAIRED*-object identification in question, but eyes appear to follow objects 4. *SEVERELY IMPAIRED*-no vision or sees only light, colors, or shapes; eyes do not appear to follow objects	
2.	VISUAL LIMITATIONS /DIFFI-CULTIES	a. Side vision problems-decreased peripheral vision (e.g., leaves food on one side of tray, difficulty traveling, bumps into people and objects, misjudges placement of chair when seating self)	a.
		b. Experiences any of following: sees halos or rings around lights; sees flashes of light; sees "curtains" over eyes	b.
		c. *NONE OF ABOVE*	c.
3.	VISUAL APPLIANCES	Glasses; contact lenses; magnifying glass 0. No 1. Yes	

SECTION E. MOOD AND BEHAVIOR PATTERNS

1.	INDICATORS OF DEPRESSION, ANXIETY, SAD MOOD	*(Code for indicators observed in last 30 days, irrespective of the assumed cause)* 0. Indicator not exhibited in last 30 days 1. Indicator of this type exhibited up to five days a week 2. Indicator of this type exhibited daily or almost daily (6,7 days a week)	

	VERBAL EXPRESSIONS OF DISTRESS		h. Repetitive health complaints-e.g., persistently seeks medical attention, obsessive concern with body functions	
	a. Resident made negative statements-e.g., *"Nothing matters; Would rather be dead; What's the use; Regrets having lived so long; Let me die"*		i. Repetitive anxious complaints/concerns (non-health related) e.g., persistently seeks attention/ reassurance regarding schedules, meals, laundry, clothing, relationship issues	
	b. Repetitive questions-e.g., *"Where do I go; What do I do?"*			
	c. Repetitive verbalizations-e.g., calling out for help, *("God help me")*		SLEEP-CYCLE ISSUES	
			j. Unpleasant mood in morning	
			k. Insomnia/change in usual sleep pattern	
	d. Persistent anger with self or others-e.g., easily annoyed, anger at placement in nursing home; anger at care received		SAD, APATHETIC, ANXIOUS APPEARANCE	
			l. Sad, pained, worried facial expressions-e.g., furrowed brows	
	e. Self deprecation-e.g., *"I am nothing; I am of no use to anyone"*		m. Crying, tearfulness	
	f. Expressions of what appear to be unrealistic fears-e.g., fear of being abandoned, left alone, being with others		n. Repetitive physical movements - e.g., pacing, handwringing, restlessness, fidgeting, picking	
			LOSS OF INTEREST	
	g. Recurrent statements that something terrible is about to happen-e.g., believes he or she is about to die, have a heart attack		o. Withdrawal from activities of interest-e.g., no interest in long standing activities or being with family/ friends	
			p. Reduced social interaction	

2.	MOOD PERSIS-TENCE	One or more indicators of depressed, sad or anxious mood were not easily altered by attempts to "cheer up", console, or reassure the resident over **last 7 days** 0. No mood 1. Indicators present, 2. Indicators present, indicators easily altered not easily altered	
3.	CHANGE IN MOOD	Resident's mood status has changed as compared to status of **90 days ago** (or since last assessment if less than 90 days) 0. No change 1. Improved 2. Deteriorated	

4.	BEHAVIORAL SYMPTOMS	(A) *Behavioral symptom frequency in last 7 days*
		   0. Behavior not exhibited in last 7 days
		   1. Behavior of this type occurred 1 to 3 days in last 7 days
		   2. Behavior of this type occurred 4 to 6 days, but less than daily
		   3. Behavior of this type occurred daily
		(B) *Behavioral symptom alterability in last 7 days*
		   0. Behavior not present OR behavior was easily altered
		   1. Behavior was not easily altered
			(A)	(B)

		a. WANDERING (moved with no rational purpose, seemingly oblivious to needs or safety)		
		b. VERBALLY ABUSIVE BEHAVIORAL SYMPTOMS (others were threatened, screamed at, cursed at)		
		c. PHYSICALLY ABUSIVE BEHAVIORAL SYMPTOMS (others were hit, shoved, scratched, sexually abused)		
		d. SOCIALLY INAPPROPRIATE/DISRUPTIVE BEHAVIORAL SYMPTOMS (made disruptive sounds, noisiness, screaming, self-abusive acts, sexual behavior or disrobing in public, smeared/threw food/feces, hoarding, rummaged through others' belongings)		
		e. RESISTS CARE (resisted taking medications/ injections, ADL assistance, or eating)		

5.	CHANGE IN BEHAVIORAL SYMPTOMS	Resident's behavior status has changed as compared to status of **90 days ago** (or since last assessment if less than 90 days) 0. No change 1. Improved 2. Deteriorated	

SECTION F. PSYCHOSOCIAL WELL-BEING

1.	SENSE OF INITIATIVE/ INVOLVE-MENT	a. At ease interacting with others	a.
		b. At ease doing planned or structured activities	b.
		c. At ease doing self-initiated activities	c.
		d. Establishes own goals	d.
		e. Pursues involvement in life of facility (e.g., makes/ keeps friends; involved in group activities; responds positively to new activities; assists at religious services)	e.
		f. Accepts invitations into most group activities	f.
		g. *NONE OF ABOVE*	g.
2.	UNSETTLED RELATION-SHIPS	a. Covert/open conflict with or repeated criticism of staff	a.
		b. Unhappy with roommate	b.
		c. Unhappy with residents other than roommate	c.
		d. Openly expresses conflict/anger with family/friends	d.
		e. Absence of personal contact with family/friends	e.
		f. Recent loss of close family member/friend	f.
		g. Does not adjust easily to change in routines	g.
		h. *NONE OF ABOVE*	h.
3.	PAST ROLES	a. Strong identification with past roles and life status	a.
		b. Expresses sadness/anger/empty feeling over lost roles/status	b.
		c. Resident perceives that daily routine (customary routine, activities) is very different from prior pattern in the	c.
		d. *NONE OF ABOVE*	d.

SECTION G. PHYSICAL FUNCTIONING AND STRUCTURAL PROBLEMS

1.	(A) ADL SELF-PERFORMANCE - *(Code for resident's PERFORMANCE OVER ALL SHIFTS during last 7 days - Not including setup)*
	0. *INDEPENDENT* - No help or oversight - OR - Help/oversight provided only 1 or 2 times during last 7 days
	1. *SUPERVISION* - Oversight, encouragement or cueing provided 3 or more times during last 7 days - OR - Supervision (3 or more times) plus physical assistance provided only 1 or 2 times during last 7 days
	2. *LIMITED ASSISTANCE* - Resident highly involved in activity; received physical help in guided maneuvering of limbs or other nonweight bearing assistance 3 or more times - OR - More help provided only 1 or 2 times during last 7 days
	3. *EXTENSIVE ASSISTANCE* - While resident performed part of activity, over last 7-day period, help of following type(s) provided 3 or more times:
	   - Weight-bearing support
	   - Full staff performance during part (but not all) of last 7 days
	4. *TOTAL DEPENDENCE* - Full staff performance of activity during entire 7 days
	8. *ACTIVITY DID NOT OCCUR* during entire 7 days			

			(A) SELF-PERF	(B) SUPPORT
	(B) ADL SUPPORT PROVIDED - *(Code for MOST SUPPORT PROVIDED OVER ALL SHIFTS during last 7 days; code regardless of resident's self-performance classification)* 0. No setup or physical help from staff 1. Setup help only 2. One person physical assist 8. ADL activity itself did not 3. Two + persons physical assist occur during entire 7 days			
a.	BED MOBILITY	How resident moves to and from lying position, turns side to side, and positions body while in bed		
b.	TRANSFER	How resident moves between surfaces - to/from: bed, chair, wheelchair, standing position (EXCLUDE to/from bath/toilet)		
c.	WALK IN ROOM	How resident walks between locations in his/her room		
d.	WALK IN CORRIDOR	How resident walks in corridor on unit		
e.	LOCOMO-TION ON UNIT	How resident moves between locations in his/her room and adjacent corridor on same floor. If in wheelchair, self-sufficiency once in chair		
f.	LOCOMO-TION OFF UNIT	How resident moves to and returns from off unit locations (e.g., areas set aside for dining, activities, or treatments). **If facility has only one floor**, how resident moves to and from distant areas on the floor. If in wheelchair, self-sufficiency once in chair		
g.	DRESSING	How resident puts on, fastens, and takes off all items of street clothing, including donning/removing prosthesis		
h.	EATING	How resident eats and drinks (regardless of skill). Includes intake of nourishment by other means (e.g., tube feeding, total parenteral nutrition)		
i.	TOILET USE	How resident uses the toilet room (or commode, bedpan, urinal): transfer on/off toilet, cleanses, changes pad, manages ostomy or catheter, adjusts clothes		
j.	PERSONAL HYGIENE	How resident maintains personal hygiene, including combing hair, brushing teeth, shaving, applying makeup, washing/drying face, hands, and perineum (EXCLUDE baths and showers)		

Resident _____   Numeric Identifier _____

2.	BATHING	How resident takes full-body bath/shower, sponge bath, and transfers in/out of tub/shower (EXCLUDE washing of back and hair.) *Code for most dependent in self-performance and support.*		
		(A) BATHING SELF-PERFORMANCE codes appear below	(A)	(B)
		0. Independent-No help provided		
		1. Supervision-Oversight help only		
		2. Physical help limited to transfer only		
		3. Physical help in part of bathing activity		
		4. Total dependence		
		8. Activity itself did not occur during entire 7 days		
		(Bathing support codes are as defined in Item 1, code B above)		

3.	TEST FOR BALANCE (see training manual)	*(Code for ability during test in the last 7 days)*	
		0. Maintained position as required in test	
		1. Unsteady, but able to rebalance self without physical support	
		2. Partial physical support during test; or stands (sits) but does not follow directions for test	
		3. Not able to attempt test without physical help	
		a. Balance while standing	
		b. Balance while sitting - position, trunk control	

4.	FUNCTIONAL LIMITATION IN RANGE OF MOTION (see training manual)	*(Code for limitations during last 7 days that interfered with daily functions or placed resident at risk of injury)*		
		(A) RANGE OF MOTION	**(B)** VOLUNTARY MOVEMENT	
		0. No limitation	0. No loss	
		1. Limitation on one side	1. Partial loss	
		2. Limitation on both sides	2. Full loss	(A) (B)
		a. Neck		
		b. Arm - Including shoulder or elbow		
		c. Hand - Including wrist or fingers		
		d. Leg - Including hip or knee		
		e. Foot - Including ankle or toes		
		f. Other limitation or loss		

5.	MODES OF LOCOMOTION	*(Check all that apply during last 7 days)*			
		a. Cane/walker/crutch	a.	d. Wheelchair primary mode of locomotion	d.
		b. Wheeled self	b.		
		c. Other person wheeled	c.	e. NONE OF ABOVE	e.

6.	MODES OF TRANSFER	*(Check all that apply during last 7 days)*			
		a. Bedfast all or most of time	a.	d. Lifted mechanically	d.
		b. Bed rails used for bed mobility or transfer	b.	e. Transfer aid (e.g., slide board, trapeze, cane, walker, brace)	e.
		c. Lifted manually	c.	f. NONE OF ABOVE	f.

7.	TASK SEGMENTA-TION	Some or all of ADL activities were broken into subtasks during **last 7 days** so that resident could perform them	
		0. No 1. Yes	

8.	ADL FUNCTIONAL REHABILITA-TION POTENTIAL	a. Resident believes he/she is capable of increased independence in at least some ADLs	a.
		b. Direct care staff believe resident is capable of increased independence in at least some ADLs	b.
		c. Resident able to perform tasks/activity but is very slow	c.
		d. Difference in ADL Self-Performance or ADL Support, comparing mornings to evenings	d.
		e. NONE OF ABOVE	e.

9.	CHANGE IN ADL FUNCTION	Resident's ADL self-performance status has changed as compared to status of **90 days ago** (or since last assessment if less than 90 days)	
		0. No change 1. Improved 2. Deteriorated	

SECTION H. CONTINENCE IN LAST 14 DAYS

1.	CONTINENCE SELF-CONTROL CATEGORIES
	(Code for resident's PERFORMANCE OVER ALL SHIFTS)
	0. *CONTINENT* - Complete control [*includes use of indwelling urinary catheter or ostomy device that does not leak urine or stool*]
	1. *USUALLY CONTINENT* - BLADDER, incontinent episodes once a week or less; BOWEL, less than weekly
	2. *OCCASIONALLY INCONTINENT* - BLADDER, 2 or more times a week but not daily; BOWEL, once a week
	3. *FREQUENTLY INCONTINENT* - BLADDER, tended to be incontinent daily, but some control present (e.g., on day shift); BOWEL, 2-3 times a week
	4. *INCONTINENT* - Had inadequate control BLADDER, multiple daily episodes; BOWEL, all (or almost all) of the time

a.	BOWEL CONTINENCE	Control of bowel movement, with appliance or bowel continence programs, if employed	
b.	BLADDER CONTINENCE	Control of urinary bladder function (if dribbles, volume insufficient to soak through underpants), with appliances (e.g., foley) or continence programs, if employed	

2.	BOWEL ELIMINATION PATTERN	a. Bowel elimination pattern regular - at least one movement every three days	a.	c. Diarrhea	c.
				d. Fecal impaction	d.
		b. Constipation	b.	e. NONE OF ABOVE	e.

3.	APPLIANCES AND PROGRAMS	a. Any scheduled toileting plan	a.	f. Did not use toilet room/commode/urinal	f.
		b. Bladder retraining program	b.	g. Pads/briefs used	g.
		c. External (condom) catheter	c.	h. Enemas/irrigation	h.
		d. Indwelling catheter	d.	i. Ostomy present	i.
		e. Intermittent catheter	e.	j. NONE OF ABOVE	j.

4.	CHANGE IN URINARY CONTINENCE	Resident's urinary continence has changed as compared to status of **90 days ago** (or since last assessment if less than 90 days)	
		0. No change 1. Improved 2. Deteriorated	

SECTION I. DISEASE DIAGNOSES

Check only those diseases that have a relationship to current ADL status, cognitive status, mood and behavior status, medical treatments, nursing monitoring, or risk of death. (Do not list inactive diagnoses)

1.	DISEASES	*(If none apply, CHECK the NONE OF ABOVE box)*			
		ENDOCRINE/METABOLIC/NUTRITIONAL		v. Hemiplegia/Hemiparesis	v.
		a. Diabetes mellitus	a.	w. Multiple sclerosis	w.
		b. Hyperthyroidism	b.	x. Paraplegia	x.
		c. Hypothyroidism	c.	y. Parkinson's disease	y.
		HEART/CIRCULATION		z. Quadriplegia	z.
		d. Arteriosclerotic heart disease (ASHD)	d.	aa. Seizure disorder	aa.
		e. Cardiac dysrhythmias	e.	bb. Transient ischemic attack (TIA)	bb.
		f. Congestive heart failure	f.	cc. Traumatic brain injury	cc.
		g. Deep vein thrombosis	g.	**PSYCHIATRIC/MOOD**	
		h. Hypertension	h.	dd. Anxiety disorder	dd.
		i. Hypotension	i.	ee. Depression	ee.
		j. Peripheral vascular disease	j.	ff. Manic depression (bipolar disease)	ff.
		k. Other cardiovascular disease	k.	gg. Schizophrenia	gg.
		MUSCULOSKELETAL		**PULMONARY**	
		l. Arthritis	l.	hh. Asthma	hh.
		m. Hip fracture	m.	ii. Emphysema/COPD	ii.
		n. Missing limb (e.g., amputation)	n.	**SENSORY**	
		o. Osteoporosis	o.	jj. Cataracts	jj.
		p. Pathological bone fracture	p.	kk. Diabetic retinopathy	kk.
		NEUROLOGICAL		ll. Glaucoma	ll.
		q. Alzheimer's disease	q.	mm. Macular degeneration	mm.
		r. Aphasia	r.	**OTHER**	
		s. Cerebral palsy	s.	nn. Allergies	nn.
		t. Cerebrovascular accident (stroke)	t.	oo. Anemia	oo.
				pp. Cancer	pp.
		u. Dementia other than Alzheimer's disease	u.	qq. Renal failure	qq.
				rr. NONE OF ABOVE	rr.

2.	INFECTIONS	*(If none apply, CHECK the NONE OF ABOVE box)*			
		a. Antibiotic resistant infection (e.g., Methicillin resistant staph)	a.	g. Septicemia	g.
				h. Sexually transmitted diseases	h.
		b. Clostridium difficile (c.diff.)	b.	i. Tuberculosis	i.
		c. Conjunctivitis	c.	j. Urinary tract infection in **last 30 days**	j.
		d. HIV infection	d.	k. Viral hepatitis	k.
		e. Pneumonia	e.	l. Wound infection	l.
		f. Respiratory infection	f.	m. NONE OF ABOVE	m.

3.	OTHER CURRENT OR MORE DETAILED DIAGNOSES AND ICD-9 CODES	a.	
		b.	
		c.	
		d.	
		e.	

SECTION J. HEALTH CONDITIONS

1.	PROBLEM CONDITIONS	*(Check all problems present in last 7 days unless other time frame is indicated)*			
		INDICATORS OF FLUID STATUS		f. Dizziness/Vertigo	f.
				g. Edema	g.
		a. Weight gain or loss of 3 or more pounds within a 7 day period	a.	h. Fever	h.
				i. Hallucinations	i.
		b. Inability to lie flat due to shortness of breath	b.	j. Internal bleeding	j.
		c. Dehydrated; output exceeds input	c.	k. Recurrent lung aspirations in **last 90 days**	k.
		d. Insufficient fluid; did **NOT** consume all/almost all liquids provided during **last 3 days**	d.	l. Shortness of breath	l.
				m. Syncope (fainting)	m.
				n. Unsteady gait	n.
		OTHER		o. Vomiting	o.
		e. Delusions	e.	p. NONE OF ABOVE	p.

Resident _____   Numeric Identifier _____

2.	PAIN SYMPTOMS	*(Code the **highest** level of pain present in the **last 7 days**)*

| a.**FREQUENCY** with which resident complains or shows evidence of pain
0. No pain *(skip to J4)*
1. Pain less than daily
2. Pain daily | | b. **INTENSITY** of pain
1. Mild pain
2. Moderate pain
3. Times when pain is horrible or excruciating | |

3.	PAIN SITE	*(If pain present, check all sites that apply in last 7 days)*			
		a. Back pain	a.	f. Incisional pain	f.
		b. Bone pain	b.	g.Joint pain (other than hip)	g.
		c. Chest pain while doing usual activities	c.	h.Soft tissue pain (e.g. lesion, muscle)	h.
		d. Headache	d.	i. Stomach pain	i.
		e. Hip pain	e.	j. Other	j.

4.	ACCIDENTS	*(Check all that apply)*		c.Hip fracture in **last 180 days**	c.
		a. Fell in **past 30 days**	a.	d.Other fracture in **last 180 days**	d.
		b. Fell in **past 31-180 days**	b.	e.*NONE OF ABOVE*	e.

5.	STABILITY OF CONDITIONS	a. Conditions/diseases make resident's cognitive, ADL, mood or behavior patterns unstable - (fluctuating, precarious, or deteriorating)	a.
		b. Resident experiencing an acute episode or a flare-up of a recurrent or chronic problem	b.
		c. End-stage disease, 6 or fewer months to live	c.
		d. *NONE OF ABOVE*	d.

SECTION K. ORAL/NUTRITIONAL STATUS

1.	ORAL PROBLEMS	a. Chewing problem	a.
		b. Swallowing problem	b.
		c. Mouth pain	c.
		d. *NONE OF ABOVE*	d.

2.	HEIGHT AND WEIGHT	*Record (a.) height in inches and (b.) weight in pounds. Base weight on most recent measure in last 30 days; measure weight consistently in accord with standard facility practice - e.g., in a.m. after voiding, before meal, with shoes off, and in nightclothes*

a.HT (in.)			b.WT (lb.)		

3.	WEIGHT CHANGE	a. **Weight loss** - 5% or more in **last 30 days**; or 10% or more in **last 180 days** 0. No 1. Yes	
		b. **Weight gain** - 5% or more in **last 30 days**; or 10% or more in **last 180 days** 0. No 1. Yes	

4.	NUTRI-TIONAL PROBLEMS	a. Complains about the taste of many foods	a.	c.Leaves 25% or more of food uneaten at most meals	c.
		b. Regular or repetitive complaints of hunger	b.	d.*NONE OF ABOVE*	d.

5.	NUTRI-TIONAL APPROACH-ES	*(Check all that apply in last 7 days)*			
		a.Parenteral IV	a.	f. Dietary supplement between meals	f.
		b.Feeding tube	b.	g.Plate guard, stabilized built-up utensil, etc.	g.
		c.Mechanically altered diet	c.	h.On a planned weight change program	h.
		d.Syringe (oral feeding)	d.	i. *NONE OF ABOVE*	i.
		e.Therapeutic diet	e.		

6.	PARENTERAL OR ENTERAL INTAKE	*(Skip to Section L if neither 5a nor 5b is checked)*
		a. Code the proportion of total calories the resident received through parenteral or tube feedings in the **last 7 days** 0. None 3. 51% to 75% 1. 1% to 25% 4. 76% to 100% 2. 26% to 50%	
		b. Code the average fluid intake per day by IV or tube in **last 7 days** 0. None 3. 1001 to 1500 cc/day 1. 1 to 500 cc/day 4. 1501 to 2000 cc/day 2. 501 to 1000 cc/day 5. 2001 or more cc/day	

SECTION L. ORAL/DENTAL STATUS

1.	ORAL STATUS AND DISEASE PREVENTION	a. Debris (soft, easily movable substances) present in mouth prior to going to bed at night	a.
		b. Has dentures or removable bridge	b.
		c. Some/all natural teeth lost - does not have or does not use dentures (or partial plates)	c.
		d. Broken, loose, or carious teeth	d.
		e. Inflamed gums (gingiva); swollen or bleeding gums; oral abscesses; ulcers or rashes	e.
		f. Daily cleaning of teeth/dentures or daily mouth care - by resident or staff	f.
		g. *NONE OF ABOVE*	g.

SECTION M. SKIN CONDITION

1.	ULCERS (Due to any cause)	*(Record the number of ulcers at each ulcer stage-regardless of cause. If none present at a stage, record "0" (zero). Code all that apply during last 7 days. Code 9 = 9 or more.) [Requires full body exam.]*	Number at Stage
		a. Stage 1. A persistent area of skin redness (without a break in the skin) that does not disappear when pressure is relieved.	
		b. Stage 2. A partial thickness loss of skin layers that presents clinically as an abrasion, blister, or shallow crater.	
		c. Stage 3. A full thickness of skin is lost, exposing the subcutaneous tissues - presents as a deep crater with or without undermining adjacent tissue.	
		d. Stage 4. A full thickness of skin and subcutaneous tissue is lost, exposing muscle or bone.	

2.	TYPE OF ULCER	*(For each type of ulcer, code for the highest stage in the last 7 days using scale in item M1-i.e., 0 = none; stages 1,2,3,4)*	
		a. Pressure ulcer-any lesion caused by pressure resulting in damage of underlying tissue	
		b. Stasis ulcer-open lesion caused by poor circulation in the lower extremities	

3.	HISTORY OF RESOLVED ULCERS	Resident had an ulcer that was resolved or cured in **LAST 90 DAYS** 0. No 1. Yes	

4.	OTHER SKIN PROBLEMS OR LESIONS PRESENT	*(Check all that apply during last 7 days)*	
		a. Abrasions, bruises	a.
		b. Burns (second or third degree)	b.
		c. Open lesions other than ulcers, rashes, cuts (e.g., cancer lesions)	c.
		d. Rashes - e.g., intertrigo, eczema, drug rash, heat rash, herpes zoster	d.
		e. Skin desensitized to pain or pressure	e.
		f. Skin tears or cuts (other than surgery)	f.
		g. Surgical wounds	g.
		h. *NONE OF ABOVE*	h.

5.	SKIN TREAT-MENTS	*(Check all that apply during last 7 days)*	
		a. Pressure relieving device(s) for chair	a.
		b. Pressure relieving device(s) for bed	b.
		c. Turning/repositioning program	c.
		d. Nutrition or hydration intervention to manage skin problems	d.
		e. Ulcer care	e.
		f. Surgical wound care	f.
		g. Application of dressings (with or without topical medications) other than to feet	g.
		h. Application of ointments/medications (other than to feet)	h.
		i. Other preventative or protective skin care (other than to feet)	i.
		j. *NONE OF ABOVE*	j.

6.	FOOT PROBLEMS AND CARE	*(Check all that apply during last 7 days)*	
		a.Resident has one or more foot problems-e.g., corns, calluses, bunions,hammer toes,overlapping toes,pain,structural problems	a.
		b.Infection of the foot-e.g.,cellulitis, purulent drainage	b.
		c.Open lesions on the foot	c.
		d.Nails/calluses trimmed during **last 90 days**	d.
		e.Received preventative or protective foot care (e.g., used special shoes, inserts, pads, toe separators)	e.
		f.Application of dressings (with or without topical medications)	f.
		g. *NONE OF ABOVE*	g.

SECTION N. ACTIVITY PURSUIT PATTERNS

1.	TIME AWAKE	*(Check appropriate time periods over **last 7 days**)* Resident awake all or most of time (i.e., naps no more than one hour per time period) in the:			
		a. Morning	a.	c. Evening	c.
		b. Afternoon	b.	d. *NONE OF ABOVE*	d.

(If resident is comatose, skip to Section O)

2.	AVERAGE TIME INVOLVED IN ACTIVITIES	**(When awake and not receiving treatments or ADL care)** 0. Most-more than 2/3 of time 2.Little-less than 1/3 of time 1. Some-from 1/3 to 2/3 of time 3.None	

3.	PREFERRED ACTIVITY SETTINGS	*(Check all settings in which activities are preferred)*			
		a. Own room	a.	d. Outside facility	d.
		b. Day/activity room	b.	e. *NONE OF ABOVE*	e.
		c. Inside NH/off unit	c.		

4.	GENERAL ACTIVITY PREFER-ENCES (adapted to resident's current abilities)	*(Check all PREFERENCES whether or not activity is currently available to resident)*			
		a.Cards/other games	a.	g.Trips/shopping	g.
		b.Crafts/arts	b.	h.Walking/wheeling outdoors	h.
		c.Exercise/sports	c.	i. Watching TV	i.
		d.Music	d.	j. Gardening or plants	j.
		e.Reading/writing	e.	k.Talking or conversing	k.
		f.Spiritual/religious activities	f.	l. Helping others	l.
				m.*NONE OF ABOVE*	m.

MDS 2.0 01/30/98

Resident _____   Numeric Identifier _____

5.	PREFERS CHANGE IN DAILY ROUTINE	Code for resident preferences in daily routines	
		0. No change 1. Slight change 2. Major change	
		a.Type of activities in which resident is currently involved	
		b.Extent of resident involvement in activities	

SECTION O. MEDICATIONS

1.	NUMBER OF MEDICA-TIONS	*(Record the number of different medications used in the last 7 days; enter "0" if none used)*	
2.	NEW MEDICA-TIONS	*(Resident currently receiving medications that were initiated during the last 90 days)* 0. No 1. Yes	
3.	INJECTIONS	*(Record the number of DAYS injections of any type received during the last 7 days; enter "0" if none used)*	
4.	DAYS RECEIVED THE FOLLOWING MEDICATION	*(Record the number of DAYS during last 7 days; enter "0" if not used. Note - enter "1" for long-acting meds used less than weeklly)*	

a. Antipsychotic		d. Hypnotic	
b. Antianxiety		e. Diuretic	
c. Antidepressant			

SECTION P. SPECIAL TREATMENTS AND PROCEDURES

1.	SPECIAL TREAT-MENTS, PROCE-DURES, AND PROGRAMS	a. SPECIAL CARE - *Check treatments or programs received during the last 14 days*	

TREATMENTS			l. Ventilator or respirator	l.
a. Chemotherapy	a.	**PROGRAMS**		
b. Dialysis	b.	m. Alcohol/drug treatment program	m.
c. IV medication	c.		
d. Intake/output	d.	n. Alzheimer's/dementia special care unit	n.
e. Monitoring acute medical condition	e.	o. Hospice care	o.
f. Ostomy care	f.	p. Pediatric unit	p.
g. Oxygen therapy	g.	q. Respite care	q.
h. Radiation	h.	r. Training in skills required to return to the commu-nity (e.g., taking medica-tions, house work, shop-ping, transportation,ADLs)	r.
i. Suctioning	i.		
j. Tracheotomy care	j.		
k. Transfusions	k.	s. *NONE OF ABOVE*	s.

b. THERAPIES - *Record the number of days and total minutes each of the following therapies was administered (for at least 15 minutes a day) in the last 7 calendar days (Enter 0 if none or less than 15 min. daily)*
[Note - count only post admission therapies]

(A) = # of days administered for **15 minutes or more**
(B) = total # of minutes provided in last 7 days

	DAYS (A)	MIN (B)
a. Speech-language pathology and audiology services		
b. Occupational therapy		
c. Physical therapy		
d. Respiratory therapy		
e. Psychological therapy (by any licensed mental health professional)		

2.	INTERVEN-TION PROGRAMS FOR MOOD, BEHAVIOR, COGNITIVE LOSS	*(Check all interventions or strategies used in* **last 7 days** *- no matter where received)*	
		a. Special behavior symptom evaluation program	a.
		b. Evaluation by a licensed mental health specialist in **last 90 days**	b.
		c. Group therapy	c.
		d. Resident-specific deliberate changes in the environ-ment to address mood/behavior patterns - e.g., providing bureau in which to rummage	d.
		e. Reorientation - e.g., cueing	e.
		f. *NONE OF ABOVE*	f.

3.	NURSING REHABILITA-TION/ RESTOR-ATIVE CARE	*Record the NUMBER OF DAYS each of the following rehabilita-tion or restorative techniques or practices was provided to the resident for more than or equal to 15 minutes per day in the last 7 days* *(Enter 0 if none or less than 15 min. daily.)*	

a.Range of motion (passive)		f. Walking	
b.Range of motion (active)		g. Dressing or grooming	
c.Splint or brace assistance		h. Eating or swallowing	
TRAINING AND SKILL PRACTICE IN:		i. Amputation/ prosthesis care	
d. Bed mobility		j. Communication	
e. Transfer		k. Other	

4.	DEVICES AND RESTRAINTS	*(Use the following codes for last 7 days.)* 0. Not used 1. Used less than daily 2. Used daily	
		Bed rails	
		a. - Full bed rails on all open sides of bed	
		b. - Other types of side rails used (e.g.,half rail, one side)	
		c. Trunk restraint	
		d. Limb restraint	
		e. Chair prevents rising	
5.	HOSPITAL STAY(S)	Record number of times resident was admitted to hospital with an overnight stay **in last 90 days** (or since last assessment if less than 90 days). *(Enter 0 if no hospital admissions)*	
6.	EMERGENCY ROOM (ER) VISIT(S)	Record number of times resident visited ER without an overnight stay **in last 90 days** (or since last assess-ment if less than 90 days). *(Enter 0 if no ER visits)*	
7.	PHYSICIAN VISITS	In the **LAST 14 DAYS** (or since admission if less than 14 days in facility) how many days has the physician (or authorized assistant or practitioner) examined the resident? *(Enter 0 if none)*	
8.	PHYSICIAN ORDERS	In the **LAST 14 DAYS** (or since admission if less than 14 days in facility) how many days has the physician (or authorized assistant or practitioner) changed the resident's orders? *Do not include order renewals without change. (Enter 0 if none)*	
9.	ABNORMAL LAB VALUES	Has the resident had any abnormal lab values during the **last 90 days** (or since admission)? 0. No 1. Yes	

SECTION Q. DISCHARGE POTENTIAL AND OVERALL STATUS

1.	DISCHARGE POTENTIAL	a. Resident expresses/indicates preference to return to the community 0. No 1. Yes	
		b. Resident has a support person who is positive towards discharge 0. No 1. Yes	
		c. Stay projected to be of a short duration - discharge projected **within 90 days** (do no include expected discharge due to death) 0. No 2. Within 31-90 days 1. Within 30 days 3. Discharge status uncertain	
2.	OVERALL CHANGE IN CARE NEEDS	Resident's overall self sufficiency has changed signifi-cantly as compared to status of **90 days ago** (or since last assessment if less than 90 days) 0. No change 1. Improved - receives fewer supports, needs less restrictive level of care 2. Deteriorated - receives more support	

SECTION R. ASSESSMENT INFORMATION

1.	PARTICIPA-TION IN ASSESS-MENT	a. Resident: 0. No 1. Yes	
		b. Family: 0. No 1. Yes 2. No family	
		c. Significant other: 0. No 1. Yes 2. None	

2. SIGNATURES OF PERSONS COMPLETING THE ASSESSMENT:

a. Signature of RN Assessment Coordinator (sign on above line)

b. Date RN Assessment Coordinator signed as complete

	Month	Day	Year

c. Other Signatures	Title	Sections	Date
d.			Date
e.			Date
f.			Date
g.			Date
h.			Date

- 7 -

Resident _____   Numeric Identifier _____

SECTION T. THERAPY SUPPLEMENT FOR MEDICARE PPS

1.	**SPECIAL TREAT-MENTS AND PROCE-DURES**	**a. RECREATION THERAPY** - *Enter number of days and total minutes of recreation therapy administered (for at least 15 minutes a day) in the last 7 days (Enter 0 if none)*

(A) = # of days administered for 15 minutes or more

(B) = total # of minutes provided in last 7 days

	DAYS (A)	MIN (B)

Skip unless this is a Medicare 5 day or Medicare readmission/return assessment.

b. ORDERED THERAPIES - *Has physician ordered any of following therapies to begin in FIRST 14 days of stay-physical therapy, occupational therapy, or speech pathology service?*
   0. No   1. Yes

If not ordered, skip to Item 2

c. Through day 15, provide an estimate of the number of days when at least 1 therapy service can be expected to have been delivered.

d. Through day 15, provide an estimate of the number of therapy minutes (across the therapies) that can be expected to be delivered?

2.	**WALKING WHEN MOST SELF SUFFICIENT**	*Complete item 2 if ADL self-performance score for TRANSFER (G.1.b.A) is 0, 1, 2, or 3 AND at least one of the following are present:*

-Resident received physical therapy involving gait training (P.1.b.c)
-Physical therapy was ordered for the resident involving gait training (T.1.b)
-Resident received nursing rehabilitation for walking (P.3.f)
-Physical therapy involving walking has been discontinued within the past 180 days

Skip to Item 3 if resident did not walk in last 7 days

(FOR FOLLOWING FIVE ITEMS, BASE CODING ON THE EPISODE WHEN THE RESIDENT WALKED THE FARTHEST WITHOUT SITTING DOWN. INCLUDE WALKING DURING REHABILITATION SESSIONS.)

a. Furthest distance walked without sitting down during this episode.
   0. 150+ feet   3. 10-25 feet
   1. 51-149 feet   4. Less than 10 feet
   2. 26-50 feet

b. Time walked without sitting down during this episode.
   0. 1-2 minutes   3. 11-15 minutes
   1. 3-4 minutes   4. 16-30 minutes
   2. 5-10 minutes   5. 31+ minutes

c. Self-Performance in walking during this episode.
   0. *INDEPENDENT* - No help or oversight
   1. *SUPERVISION* - Oversight, encouragement or cueing provided
   2. *LIMITED ASSISTANCE* - Resident highly involved in walking; received physical help in guided maneuvering of limbs or other nonweight bearing assistance
   3. *EXTENSIVE ASSISTANCE* - Resident received weight bearing assistance while walking

d. Walking support provided associated with this episode (code regardless of resident's self-performance classification).
   0. No setup or physical help from staff
   1. Setup help only
   2. One person physical assist
   3. Two+ persons physical assist

e. Parallel bars used by resident in association with this episode.
   0. No   1. Yes

3.	**CASE MIX GROUP**	Medicare [ ][ ][ ][ ][ ] State [ ][ ][ ][ ][ ]

MDS 2.0 01/30/98

*Page 8 of this form is not included because it is relevant only to Texas.

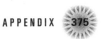

Resident _____   Numeric Identifier _____

SECTION U. MEDICATIONS

List all medications that the resident **received** during the last 7 days. Include scheduled medications that are used regularly, but less than weekly.

1. **Medication Name and Dose Ordered.** Record the name of the medication and dose ordered.

2. **Route of Administration (RA).** Code the Route of Administration using the following list:

1 = by mouth (PO)	5 = subcutaneous (SQ)	8 = inhalation
2 = sub lingual (SL)	6 = rectal (R)	9 = enteral tube
3 = intramuscular (IM)	7 = topical	10 = other
4 = intravenous (IV)		

3. **Frequency.** Code the number of times per day, week, or month the medication is administered using the following list:

PR = (PRN) as necessary	2D = (BID) two times daily	QO = every other day
1H = (QH) every hour	(includes every 12 hrs)	4W = 4 times each week
2H = (Q2H) every two hours	3D = (TID) three times daily	5W = five times each week
3H = (Q3H) every three hours	4D = (QID) four times daily	6W = six times each week
4H = (Q4H) every four hours	5D = five times daily	1M = (Q month) once every month
6H = (Q6H) every six hours	1W = (Q week) once each wk	2M = twice every month
8H = (Q8H) every eight hours	2W = two times every week	C = continuous
1D = (QD or HS) once daily	3W = three times every week	O = other

4. **Amount Administered (AA).** Record the number of tablets, capsules, suppositories, or liquid (any route) **per dose** administered to the resident. Code 999 for topicals, eye drops, inhalants and oral medications that need to be dissolved in water.

5. **PRN-number of days (PRN-n).** If the frequency code for the medication is "PR", record the number of times during the last 7 days each PRN medication was given. Code STAT medications as PRNs given once.

6. **NDC Codes.** Enter the National Drug Code for each medication given. Be sure to enter the correct NDC code for the drug name, strength, and form. The NDC code must match the drug dispensed by the pharmacy.

1. Medication Name and Dose Ordered	2. RA	3. Freq	4. AA	5. PRN-n	6. NDC Codes

MDS 2.0 01/30/98

APPENDIX F Agency List

American Academy of Audiology
8300 Greensboro Drive, Suite 750
McLean, VA 22102
1-800-AAA-2336
http://www.audiology.org

American Academy of Ophthalmology
PO Box 7472
San Francisco, CA 94120-7424
1-800-222-3937
http://www.eyenet.org

American Association for Retired People (AARP)
601 E Street NW
Washington, DC 20049
1-800-424-3410
http://www.aarp.org

American Association of Diabetes Educators
100 West Monroe Street, 4th floor
Chicago, IL 60603-1901
1-312-424-2426
http://www.aadenet.org

American Cancer Society
1-800-ACS-2345
http://www.cancer.org

American Diabetes Association
1701 North Beauregard Street
Alexandria, VA 22311
1-800-DIABETES
http://www.diabetes.org

American Dietetic Association
216 West Jackson Boulevard
Chicago, IL 60666-6995
1-800-887-1600
http://www.eatright.org

American Foundation for the Blind
11 Penn Plaza, Suite 300
New York, NY 10001
1-800-232-5463
http://www.afb.org

American Heart Association
National Center
7272 Greenville Avenue
Dallas, TX 75231
1-800-AHA-USA1
http://www.americanheart.org

American Lung Association
1740 Broadway
New York, NY 10019
1-800-LUNG-USA
http://www.lungusa.org

American Speech-Language-Hearing Association
10801 Rockville Pike
Rockville, MD 20852
888-321-ASHA
http://www.asha.org

American Tinnitus Association
PO Box 5
Portland, OR 97207-0005
1-503-248-9985
http://www.ata.org

Arthritis Foundation
P.O Box 7669
Atlanta, GA 90957-0669
1-800-283-7800
http://www.arthritis.org

Association for Macular Diseases, Inc.
210 East 64th Street
New York, NY 10021
212-605-3719
http://www.macula.org

Asthma and Allergy Foundation of America
1233 20th Street, NW, Suite 402
Washington, DC 20036
1-800-7-ASTHMA
http://www.aafa.org

The Center for the Partially Sighted
12301 Wilshire Blvd, Suite 600
Los Angeles, CA 90025
1-800-481-EXES
http://www.low-vision.org

Choice in Dying
1035 30th Street, NW
Washington, DC 20007
1-800-989-WILL
http://www.choices.org

The Deafness Research Foundation
575 Fifth Avenue, 11th Floor
New York, NY 10017
1-800-535-3323
http://www.drf.org

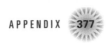

The Glaucoma Foundation
116 John Street, Suite 1605
New York, NY 10038
1-800-GLAUCOMA
http://www.glaucoma-foundation.org

Heath Care Financing Administration
7500 Security Blvd.
Baltimore, MD 21244
460-786-3000
http://www.hfca.gov

Juvenile Diabetes Foundation
120 Wall Street
New York, NY 10005
1-800-JDF-CURE
http://www.jdf.org

National Arthritis and Musculoskeletal and Skin Diseases Information Clearing House
1 AMS Circle
Bethesda, MA 20892-3675
301-495-4484

National Association for Continence
PO Box 8310
Spartanburg, SC 29305-8310
1-800-BLADDER
http://www.nafc.org

National Association for Visually Handicapped
22 West 21st Street
New York, NY 10010
212-889-3141
http://www.navh.org

National Association of Area Agencies on Aging
927 15th Street, 6th floor
Washington, DC 20005
202-296-8130
http://www.n4a.org

National Braille Association
3 Townline Circle
Rochester, NY 14623-2513
716-427-8260
http://members.aol.com/nbaoffice/index.htm

The National Council on the Aging
409 Third Street SW
Washington, DC 20024
202-479-1200
http://www.ncoa.org

National Diabetes Information Clearing House
1 Information Way
Bethesda, MD 20892-3560
301-654-3327
http://www.niddk.nih.gov/health/diabetes/ndic.htm

National Eye Institute/National Institutes of Health
2020 Vision Place
Bethesda, MD 20892-3655
301-496-5248
http://www.nei.nih.gov

National Hearing Society
16880 Middlebelt Road, Suite 4
Livonia, MI 48154
734-522-7200
http://www.hearingihs.org

National Institute on Deafness and Other Communication Disorders
National Institutes of Health
31 Center Drive, MSC 2320
Bethesda, MD 20892-2320
301-496-7243
http://www.nih.gov/nidcd

National Kidney and Urologic Diseases Information Clearinghouse
3 Information Way
Bethesda, MA 20892-3580
301-654-4415
http://www.niddk.nih.gov/health/kidney/nkudic.htm

National League for Nursing
61 Broadway, 33rd floor
New York, NY 10006
1-800-669-1656
http://www.nln.org

National Osteoporosis Foundation
1232 22nd Street, NW
Washington, DC 20037-1292
1-800-223-9994
http://www.nof.org

National Institute of Arthritis and Musculoskeletal and Skin Diseases
Information Office, Building 31, Room 4C-05
31 Center Drive, MSC 2350
Bethesda, MA 20892-2350
http://www.nih.gov/niams

The North American Nursing Diagnosis Association (NANDA)
1211 Locust Street
Philadelphia, PA 19107
215-545-8105
http://www.nanda.org

Self Help for Hard of Hearing People, Inc.
7910 Woodmont Avenue, Suite 1200
Bethesda, MD 20814
301-657-2248
http://www.shhh.org

Website Resources

http://www.census.gov	
http://www.nih.gov/nia	(National Institutes of Health/National Institute on Aging)
http://seniors-site.com/nursing/index.html	(Nursing Home Information)
http://www.hcfa.gov	(OBRA regulations)
http://www.rights.org/deathnet/lwc.html	(The Living Will Center)
http://www.choices.com	(Information on Living Wills and Advanced Directives)
http://www.menopause.org	(North American Menopause Society)
http://www.arthritis.org	(Arthritis Foundation)
http://www.glaucoma-foundation.org/info	(The Glaucoma Foundation)
http://www.eyenet.org	(American Academy of Ophthalmology)
http://www.hfca.com	(Health Care Financing Administration)
http://www.nanda.org	(North American Nursing Diagnosis Association)
http://www.nln.org	(National League for Nursing)
http://www.aarp.org	(American Association for Retired Persons)
http://www.n4a.org	(National Association of Area Agencies on Aging)
http://www.ncoa.org	(National Council on Aging)
http://www.americanheart.org	(American Heart Association)
http://www.cancer.org	(American Cancer Society)
http://www.alcoholicsanonymous.org	(Alcoholics Anonymous)
http://www.nafc.com	(National Association of Continence)

Glossary

adventitious sounds: abnormal lung sounds heard *on auscultation*

agnosia: loss of the ability to recognize familiar objects or people as the result of organic brain damage

agraphia: loss of the ability to write as the result of injury to the language center of the brain

akathisia: extreme restlessness

Alzheimer's disease: a neurologic disease causing progressive decline in cognitive ability

anemia: a decrease in hemoglobin in the blood to levels below the normal range

angina pectoris: pain in the chest area caused by a lack of oxygen to the heart muscle as the result of atherosclerosis

anticoagulant: a substance that prevents or delays the clotting of blood

aphasia: inability to speak as the result of injury to *certain areas* of the brain

apraxia: difficulty or inability performing purposeful acts

aspiration pneumonia: an inflammation in the lungs caused by inhaling foreign particles into the bronchial tree and the lungs

ataxia: impaired ability to coordinate movement; unsteady gait

atherosclerosis: the buildup of yellowish plaques on the inner walls of the arteries causing the lumen of the arteries to become more and more narrow until blood flow is severely limited

atrial fibrillation: an irregularity resulting in a quivering action of the atria of the heart, rather than a pumping action

aura: a recurring sensation that precedes an epileptic seizure

benign: nonmalignant; not cancerous

bradycardia: heart rate lower than 60 beats per minute

bradykinesia: abnormally slow movements

cardiac output: the amount of blood pumped per minute from the left ventricle

carcinogen: a substance that contributes to the development of cancer

central sleep apnea: sleep disorder in which *the person* momentarily ceases to breathe

Crohn's disease: a chronic inflammation of the alimentary tract, usually affecting the walls of the large and small intestine; also called *regional enteritis* and *granulomatous colitis*

circulatory overload: excessive amounts of fluid in the extracellular compartments of the body

cognitive: pertaining to intellectual functioning

contracture: a permanent shortening of a muscle that leaves the limb abnormally shaped and in a fixed position

computed tomography: a painless, noninvasive x-ray technique that produces a detailed cross-section of tissue; formerly called *computerized axial tomography*

conjunctivitis: inflammation of the inner conjunctival sac

cheilosis: scales and fissures on the lips and mouth

convulsion: involuntary muscle relaxation and contraction

cyanosis: a bluish discoloration of the skin, nail beds, or mucous membranes caused by lack of oxygen

clonic: increased, repetitive muscular contractions and relaxations

crepitation: a crackling or grating sound

débridement: removal of dead tissue from a wound

delirium: a temporary, acute confusional state that is a symptom of a treatable medical condition

dementia: a permanent and often progressive loss of cognitive function

detached retina: separation of the sensory layer from the pigmented layer of the retina of the eye

diaphoresis: profuse sweating

drug toxicity: poisonous or dangerous effects of a drug as the result of excessive administration or the inability of the body to excrete the drug

dysarthria: difficulty speaking

epidermis: outer layer of the skin

epistaxis: nosebleed

Escherichia coli: an organism normally found in the intestinal tract that can cause disease in other areas of the body

esophagogastroduodenoscopy: visualization of the esophagus, the stomach, and the duodenum

exacerbation: an increase in intensity of symptoms or severity of a disease

excoriation: an abrasion of the skin

expressive aphasia: the inability to speak words; the person knows what he/she wants to say but cannot state the word

extrapyramidal effects: side effects of medications that affect the extrapyramidal tract of the body resulting in involuntary muscular movement, abnormal posture, and symptoms of parkinsonism

exudate: fluid from a wound that may contain pus, bacteria, or cellular waste

fight or flight response: response to a stressor that prepares the person to deal with or avoid the stress

fistula: passageway from one area to another

functional assessment: assessing the individual's ability to function within the environment and to perform activities of daily living

gerontology: the study of all aspects of aging

global aphasia: loss of the ability to use any form of the written or spoken word

hallucination: a false perception occurring without external sensory stimuli

hemodialysis: method of providing for kidney functioning by circulating blood through tubes made of semipermeable membranes that remove waste substances from the blood; may be used in patients with acute or chronic renal failure

Homans' sign: pain in the calf when the foot is dorsiflexed

hospice: an organization that cares for the dying

hyperkalemia: elevated levels of potassium in the blood

hyperthermia: elevated body temperature

hypokalemia: low levels of potassium in the blood

hypothermia: body temperature below normal

illusion: an incorrect interpretation of stimuli in the environment

infiltration: fluid that collects in the tissues when the catheter is out of the vein

irritable bowel syndrome: increased motility of the large and small intestines causing diarrhea and pain in the lower abdomen

ischemia: decreased blood supply to an area

lactose intolerance: inability to digest protein lactose (found in milk) due to a deficiency of the enzyme *lactase*

lumbar puncture: insertion of a needle into the subarachnoid space of the spinal cord in the lumbar region

magnetic resonance imaging: a method of providing an image using radiofrequency radiation

malignant: serious with the potential to cause death

managed health care: a method of coordinating and delivering health care through entities such as health maintenance organizations (HMOs), preferred provider organizations (PPOs), and provider sponsored organizations (PSOs)

Medicaid: health care benefits administered jointly by federal and state governments for those who cannot afford private health insurance and for older adults whose Medicare benefits have been exhausted

Medicare: health care insurance sponsored by the federal government for individuals on social security

melena: blood in the stool

negligence: act of omission or commission that results in injury to an individual

neurofibrillary tangles: specific type of abnormal neurologic finding in the brains of patients with Alzheimer's disease

nursing facility: care setting for those requiring 24 hour-a-day nursing care; also called a *nursing home*

oliguria: scanty urine output; less than 30 mL per hour

osteoporosis: disease in which the bones become porous and weak

paresthesia: a feeling of numbness or tingling

peritoneal dialysis: removal of toxic substances from the body by perfusing sterile chemical solutions through the peritoneal cavity; used for acute or chronic renal failure and to treat certain poisonings

pernicious anemia: a type of anemia caused by a lack of the intrinsic factor in the gastric secretions and resulting in an inability to absorb vitamin B_{12}

pharyngitis: inflammation of the pharynx

polypharmacy: the taking of many medications, including those prescribed by a physician and over-the-counter drugs

rehabilitation: the process of assisting disabled individuals to regain optimum health and a satisfactory level of independence

reminiscence: remembering past experiences for the purpose of identifying in them new meanings

respite care: a place where caregivers can leave the ill or debilitated for several hours to several weeks of care; allows full-time caregivers to obtain some relief from the stress of a 24-hour day

restorative care: a specialized type of care that helps older adults reach maximum functional capacity—physically, mentally, emotionally, and socially

senile plaques: abnormal findings in the brain tissue of patients with Alzheimer's disease

syncope: fainting

tachycardia: heart rate over 100 beats per minute

ulcer: a open sore or lesion of the skin

urticaria: large red welts or wheals on the skin accompanied by severe itching; also called *hives*

vagotomy: the cutting of a certain portion of the vagus nerve in gastric surgery to decrease the amount of gastric acid secreted and prevent the recurrence of gastric ulcers

vagus nerve: the longest pair of cranial nerves, *functioning* in speech, swallowing, and in the operation of many parts of the body

vertigo: dizziness

wheal: a raised area on the surface of the skin

wheeze: abnormal lung sounds caused by air passing through a narrowed bronchus

Index

Note: Page numbers in *italics* indicate illustrations; those followed by t indicate tables; and those followed by d indicate display material.

A

Abdomen, examination of, 56t
Absorption, drug, 132
Abuse
    by Alzheimer's patients, 205–206, 206d
    elder, 183–185
Acarbose (Precose), 322
Accident prevention. *See* Safety measures
Accommodation, 331
    age-related changes in, 332
ACE inhibitors, for heart failure, 221
Acetaminophen (Tylenol)
    for arthritis, 249, 250t
    for pain, 159t
Acetazolamide (Diamox), for glaucoma, 334
Acetylcholine, in Alzheimer's disease, 203, 204, 205
Acetylsalicylic acid, for arthritis, 249, 250t
Acrochordons, 197t
ACTH, 315t, 316
Actinic keratosis, 197–198
Active assistive range of motion, 95
Active listening, 43, 44d
Active neglect, 184
Activities director, 19
Activities of daily living. *See also* Self-care
    Katz Index of, 67, 69d
Activity. *See* Exercise
Actos (pioglitazone), 322
Acute pain, 156
Acute renal failure, 307–308, 309–311
Adrenal glands, 314, 315, 315t
    age-related changes in, 315
Adrenocorticotropic hormone (ACTH), 315t, 316
Adult day care, 17
    for Alzheimer's patients, 208
Advanced directives, 31–33, 360–362
Adverse drug reactions, 134
Advice, 44
Advil (ibuprofen), 144t
    for arthritis, 249, 250t
    for pain, 159t
Aerobic exercise, 107–108
AeroBid (dexamethasone flunisolide), 265t
Affective functioning, 72–74, 74d, 78, 86–87, 93
Age
    chronological, 13
    functional, 13
Ageism, 8, 9b, 10
Age-related macular degeneration, 332, 332–333
Aggressive behavior, 352t, 352–353
Aging. *See also* Older adults
    activity theory of, 25
    attitudes toward, 8–10, 9d
    biology of, 23d, 23–26
    continuity theory of, 25

    cross-linking theory of, 23d, 24
    disengagement theory of, 25
    free radical theory of, 23d, 24
    genetic theory of, 23d, 23–24
    immunologic theory of, 23d, 24
    in men vs. women, 2
    myths about, 8, 9d
    psychosocial theories of, 25
    realities of, 10, 11d
    senescence and, 23
    theories of, 22–26
    wear and tear theory of, 23d, 24–25
Agitation
    in depression, 174
    management of, 35d–36d
Agnosia, 202
Agraphia, 209
Airway management, in coma, 233
Albumin, in protein-energy malnutrition, 167, 192
Albuterol (Ventolin, Proventil), 264t
Alcohol use/abuse, 103–104, 181–183, 183d
    osteoporosis and, 244d
Aldactone (spironolactone), 144t
Alendronate (Fosamax), for osteoporosis, 244–245
Alginate dressings, for pressure ulcers, 194
Allopurinol (Zyloprim), for gout, 251t, 254
Alpha1-adrenergic blocking agents, for benign prostatic
    hyperplasia, 302–303
Alphagan (brimonidine), for glaucoma, 334
Alprazolam (Xanax), 142t
Alupent (metaproterenol), 264t
Alveoli, 260, 261
    age-related changes in, 260, 262
    in emphysema, 263–266
Alzheimer's disease, 202–208
    assessment in, 209
    behavioral symptoms in, 205–207, 205d
    diagnosis of, 203, 203d
    etiology of, 203–204
    memory loss in, 89, 160t, 202, 203, 204, 204d
    vs. multi-infarct dementia, 208
    nursing care in, 209–211
    prevalence of, 203
    stages of, 204, 204d
    treatment of, 204–208
Amantadine (Symmetrel), 143t
    for parkinsonism, 212
Ambulation. *See* Mobility; Walking
American Association of Retired Persons (AARP), 85
American Nurses Association Code for Nurses, 28, 28d
Amiloride (Midamor), 144t
Aminophylline (Theo-Dur), 264t
Amitriptyline (Elavil), drug interactions with, 136t
Amoxicillin (Amoxil), for urinary tract infections, 297, 298t
Ampicillin (Omnipen, Principen), 143t
    for urinary tract infections, 297, 298t
Analgesics, 158, 158d, 159t
    for arthritis, 249, 250t–251t, 254–255
Anger, communication and, 47–48, 48d

Angina pectoris, 224–225, 226
Angiomas, cherry, 197t
Angiotensin-converting enzyme (ACE) inhibitors, for heart
  failure, 221
Ansaid (flurbiprofen), for arthritis, 250t
Anterior pituitary, 314, 315t, 316
Antianxiety drugs, 142t
Antibiotics, 143t
  superinfections and, 272
  for urinary tract infections, 297, 298t
Anticholinergics
  for gallbladder disease, 288–289
  for respiratory disorders, 264t
Anticipatory grief, 180, 181, 181d
Anticonvulsants, 216
Antidepressants, 143t, 176
Antiembolic stockings, for venous insufficiency, 236, 237, 238
Antihypertensives, 229–230
Anti-infectives, 143t
Antiparkinson drugs, 143t
Antipsychotics, 142t
Antivirals, for influenza, 273
Anxiety, in osteoporosis, 246
Anxiolytics, 142t
Aphakia, 335
Aphasia, 202
  in stroke patients, 231, 234
Apnea, sleep, 274
Apraxia, 202
Aqueous humor, 331, 331
  age-related changes in, 331
Arcus senilis, 331, 332
Area Agencies on Aging, 7d, 7–8
Aricept (donepezil), for Alzheimer's disease, 205
Arrhythmias, pacemaker for, 227–229
Artane (trihexyphenidyl), 143t
Arterial insufficiency, 237–239
Arterial ulcers, 238, 239
Arteriosclerosis. See Atherosclerosis
Arthritis, 247–252
  assessment in, 254
  degenerative, 247–249, 248
  nursing management in, 254–257
  resources for, 255, 257d
  rheumatoid, 248, 249–252
  sexual function and, 126
Artificial nutrition and hydration, in terminal illness, 33,
  365–366
Ascorbic acid, deficiency of, 166, 166t
Aspirin, 144t
  for arthritis, 249, 250t
  for pain, 159t
Assertive behavior, 352t, 353–354
Assessment, 53–58, 54t–57t
  affective, 72–74, 74d, 93
  in care planning, 60–62
  in client/family teaching, 63
  cognitive, 70–72, 73d, 93
  cultural, 81t
  functional, 65–76, 93. See also Functional assessment
  Minimum Data Set for, 58, 61, 62, 66, 367–375
  nutritional, 167, 168d, 169d
    for pressure ulcers, 191–192, 192
  physical health, 66–67
  psychological, 70–75
  psychosocial, 79, 80d
  Resident Assessment Instrument for, 60–62
  of restorative care potential, 93–94
  self-care, 67–70
  social, 74–75, 75d
Assisted living communities, 16
Assistive devices
  for feeding, 98–99, 99
  for mobility, 95–98, 96–99
  for self-care, 98–100, 99
Asthma, 269–270
Atenolol, 144t
Atherosclerosis, 111, 111–112, 223–229. See also Coronary
  artery disease
  arterial insufficiency in, 237–239
  definition of, 223
  stroke and, 230
Ativan (lorazepam), drug interactions with, 136t
Atrophic gastritis, 281–282
Atrovent (ipratropium bromide), 264t
Auranofin (Ridaura), for rheumatoid arthritis, 251t
Aurothioglucose (Solganal), for rheumatoid arthritis, 251t
Autocratic leadership, 348
Autolytic débridement, of pressure ulcers, 193
Avandia (rosiglitazone), 322
Azmacort (triamcinolone), 265t

B
Baby boomers, 4
Bactrim (trimethoprim-sulfamethoxazole), for urinary tract
  infections, 297, 298t
Balance, 339–340
  impairment of, 344
Bandage, elastic, for venous insufficiency, 238
Barrel chest, 261, 263
Barthel Index, 70, 72t
Basal cell carcinoma, 195
Bath, sitz, 286
Bathing
  assistive devices for, 99, 100
  in Katz Index, 67–68
  safety guidelines for, 101d
Beck Depression Inventory, 74, 74d
Beclomethasone (Beclovent, Beconase), 265t
Behavior
  aggressive, 352t, 352–353
  assertive, 352t, 353–354
  passive, 351–354, 352, 352t
Behavioral symptoms, 34–35, 37d
  in Alzheimer's disease, 205–207, 206d, 207d
Belittling, 45
Benemid (probenecid), for gout, 251t, 254
Benign essential tremor, 201
  vs. parkinsonism, 213
Benign prostatic hyperplasia, 301–304
  sexual function and, 126
Benzodiazepines, 142t
Benztropine (Cogentin), 143t
Beta-adrenergic blocking agents, 144t
  for respiratory disorders, 264t, 269–270
Betaxolol (Betoptic), for glaucoma, 334
Bile, 278
Biliary colic, 287
Biopsy, skin, 195
Bipolar disorder, 174
  depression in, 174, 175. See also Depression
  lithium for, 176, 177t
  mania in, 174, 175, 176d
Bisacodyl (Dulcolax), 143t
Bladder, age-related changes in, 296, 296
Bladder training, 154, 154d

Blood glucose monitoring, 322–323
Blood pressure
    assessment of, 56t
    decreased, 201
    elevated, 229–230
Blood vessels, age-related changes in, 219
Body language, 42
Body temperature, regulation of, 201–202
Body weight, desirable, 103, 105t
Bone
    age-related changes in, 241–242
    composition of, 241
Bouchard nodes, 248, 249
Bowel. *See also* under Intestinal
Bowel elimination, in stroke patients, 233
Bowel movements, frequency of, 286
Bradykinesia, in Parkinsonism, 211
Breast, examination of, 56t
Breast cancer
    detection of, 56t, 113, 114
    risk factors for, 113
Breast self-examination, 113, 114
Breathing, 260
    age-related changes in, 260–263, 262
    diaphragmatic, 267
    difficult. *See* Dyspnea
    pursed-lip, 267
Breath sounds, 271t
    assessment of, 56t
Brethaire (terbutaline), 264t
Bricanyl (terbutaline), 264t
Brimonidine (Alphagan), for glaucoma, 334
Bromocriptine (Parlodel), 143t
Bronchi, 260, 261
Bronchitis, chronic, 266–269. *See also* Chronic obstructive
        pulmonary disease (COPD)
Bronchodilators, 263, 264t–265t
    for asthma, 264t–265t, 270
    for chronic obstructive pulmonary disease, 263, 264t–265t
    metered-dose inhalers for, 263, 268, 268d, 270
Bronchopneumonia, 270
Bronchospasm, in chronic obstructive pulmonary
        disease, 263
Bupropion (Wellbutrin), 143t
Bursae, age-related changes in, 242
Buspirone (BuSpar), 142t

C
Calcitonin-salmon (Miacalcin), for osteoporosis, 244–245
Calcium, osteoporosis and, 113–114, 243, 244d
Calcium channel blockers, for angina, 225
Calculi, gallbladder, 287, 288
Cancer
    breast, 113
    detection of, 112d, 112–113
    prevention of, 112–113
    prostate, 305–307, 306
        surgery for, 303d
    skin, 194–197, 196, 196d, 197, 197d
    warning signs of, 112, 112d
Candidiasis superinfection, 272
Cane, 95–96, 96
Capillary refill time, 237
Capsules, administration of, 141
Carbidopa (Lodosyn), 143t
    for parkinsonism, 212, 213
Carbohydrates, recommended intake of, 106
Cardiac arrhythmias, pacemaker for, 227–229

Cardiac glycosides, 143t–144t
Cardiac output, decreased, 222, 222d, 226
Cardiac pacemakers, 227–229
Cardiac rehabilitation, 227, 228
Cardiac valves, 219
    age-related changes in, 220
Cardiovascular disease
    development of, 111
    prevention of, 111–112
    risk factors for, 111–112
Cardiovascular system, 218–239. *See also* Heart
    age-related changes in, 219
    examination of, 55t
Caregiver role strain, 185d, 210
Caregivers, 3, 84–85
    of Alzheimer's patients, 207d, 207–208, 210
    characteristics of, 3
    problems and needs of, 185d, 210
    respite care for, 85, 207
    of stroke patients, 234, 235d
Care plan
    assessment of, 62
    development of, 59, 60d
    evaluation of, 62
    implementation of, 62
Care planning conference, 62
Caring relationship, 14–15, 15d, 49
Carotid pulse, measurement of, 54t
Cartilage
    age-related changes in, 242
    costal, 260–261
Cataracts, 335, 335d
Catechol-O-methyltransferase (COMT) inhibitors, for
        parkinsonism, 212–213
Catheterization, urinary
    for incontinence, 154–155
    infection in, 301
Cefaclor (Ceclor), 143t
Celebrex (celocoxib), 249
Cell-mediated immunity, 24
Celocoxib (Celebrex), 249, 250t
Centenarian, 23
Central nervous system, 201
    age-related changes in, 201–202
Central sleep apnea, 274
Cephalexin (Keflex), 143t
Cephalosporins, 143t
Cerebral ischemia, dementia and, 208
Cerebrovascular accident (CVA), 230–234
Cerumen, 339
    removal of, 341
Challenging, 44–45
Change
    adjusting to, 356
    planned vs. unplanned, 356
Change agent, 356
Change theory, 356
Changing the subject, 45
Charts, for drug monitoring, 146, 147d
Check-off chart, for medications, 146, 147d
Chemical débridement, of pressure ulcers, 193, 193d
Chemical restraints, 33, 34. *See also* Restraints
Cherry angiomas, 197t
Chest, 260–261
    barrel, 261, 263
Chest pain
    in coronary artery disease, 223–224, 225, 226
    in myocardial infarction, 225

Chloral hydrate, 142t
Chlorothiazide (Diuril), 144t
Chlorpromazine (Thorazine), 142t
Choice in Dying, 31, 32
Cholecystectomy, 288
Cholecystitis, 287–288
Cholelithiasis, 287–289, 288
Cholesterol, elevated, 111–112, 112d
Chondroitin, 249
Choroid, 331, 331
Chronic bronchitis, 266–269. *See also* Chronic obstructive
    pulmonary disease (COPD)
Chronic illness, 5
    sexual function and, 126
Chronic insomnia, 155
Chronic obstructive pulmonary disease (COPD), 263–269
    assessment in, 266–267
    chronic bronchitis as, 266–269
    drug therapy for, 263, 264t–265t
    emphysema as, 263–266
    nursing management in, 267–269
    signs and symptoms of, 263
    smoking and, 263
Chronic pain, 156
Chronic renal failure, 308–311
Chronological age, 13
Cigarette smoking
    cardiovascular disease due to, 111
    chronic obstructive pulmonary disease due to, 263
    osteoporosis due to, 244d
Cilia, 260
Ciliary body, 331, 331
Circulation
    age-related changes in, 219–220
    collateral, 220
Circulatory problems, in diabetes, 325
Cirrhosis, 289–291
Clarifying, 47
Client/family teaching
    cognitive function and, 89, 89d
    for medications, 148
    nursing diagnoses for, 63d
    nursing process in, 62–64, 63d
    strategies for, 89d
Clinical nurse specialist (CNS), 15
Clinoril (sulindac), 144t
    for arthritis, 250t
Clorazepate (Tranxene), 142t
Closed-angle glaucoma, 333, 333–335
Clothing, assistive devices for, 99, 99
Cloxacillin (Tegopen), 143t
Cobalamin, deficiency of, 166, 166t
Code for Nurses (ANA), 28, 28d
Code for Nurses (ICN), 28, 29d
Codeine, 159t
Cogentin (benztropine), 143t
Cognex (tacrine), for Alzheimer's disease, 204
Cognitive function, 78, 88–89, 89d
    assessment of, 70–72, 73d, 93
    drugs and, 134
    intelligence and, 88
    memory and, 89
    in stroke patients, 234
Cognitive loss, stress management in, 123
Colace (docusate), 143t
Colchicine, for gout, 251t, 254
Colic, biliary, 287

Colitis, pseudomembranous, 272
Collaborative problems, 58
Collagen, 24
Collateral circulation, 220
Colles fracture, 246
Color coding, for medications, 146–147
Coma
    hepatic, 290–291
    nursing care in, 233–234
Communication, 14, 39–48
    anger and, 47–48, 48d
    definition of, 40
    with grieving person, 180d
    with hearing impaired, 343
    language barriers and, 82, 82d
    limitations to, 44–45
    listening skills in, 43, 44d
    nonverbal, 42–43, 43d
    one-way, 40
    process of, 40–41, 41
    with stroke patients, 234
    therapeutic, 45–47
    tips for, 44, 45, 46, 47
    two-way, 40
    types of, 41–43
    verbal, 41–42
Community senior citizen centers, 17
Compazine (prochlorperazine), 142t
Competence, determination of, 31
Compression stockings, for venous insufficiency, 236,
    237, 238
Compromise, 354
Condom catheter, for incontinence, 154–155
Conductive hearing loss, 340
Conflict resolution, 354, 354
Confusion, 158–161. *See also* Delirium; Dementia
    in diabetes, 323
    drug-related, 134, 161, 162t
    physiologic aspects of, 160–161
    restraints for, 165
Congestive heart failure (CHF), 220d, 220–223, 222d, 223d
Consent, 30
Constipation, 285–286
Contact lenses, 336–337
Continence, in Katz Index, 70
Continuing care retirement communities, 16
Coping strategies, 121–123
    emotionally focused, 118
    problem-focused, 118, 121
Cornea, 331, 331
    age-related changes in, 331
Coronary artery disease, 220, 223–227
    angina in, 224–225, 226
    assessment in, 225–226
    cardiac rehabilitation in, 227, 228
    collateral circulation in, 220
    management of, 226–227
    myocardial infarction and, 225–227
    risk factors for, 224d
Corticosteroids, for respiratory disease, 265t, 270
Cortisol, age-related changes in, 316
Costal cartilage, 260–261
Cough
    in chronic bronchitis, 266, 268
    impaired, 262
    in pneumonia, 271–272
    promotion of, 272

Crackles, 271t
Creatinine clearance, 295
Cromolyn sodium (Intal, Gastrocrom), for asthma, 265t, 270
Cross-linking theory of aging, 23d, 24
Crutches, 96, 96–97, 97
Crystallized intelligence, 89
Cultural aspects, of gerontologic nursing, 15, 80–82
Cultural assessment, 81t
Cuprimine (penicillamine), for arthritis, 251t, 252
Custodial care, vs. restorative care, 94–95
Cystitis, 296–300, 297d, 298t
Cystocele, 311-312

D

Dalmane (flurazepam), 142t
    drug interactions with, 136t
Darvon (propoxyphene), 159t
Data
    objective, 53
    subjective, 53
Day care, adult, 17
Deafness. *See* Hearing loss
Death and dying
    advanced directives and, 31–33, 360–362
    artificial nutrition and hydration in, 33, 365–366
    living wills and, 31–32
    Medical Power of Attorney for Health Care and, 31, 32–33, 363–364
Débridement, of pressure ulcers, 193, 193d
Decadron, for respiratory disorders, 265t
Decerebrate rigidity, 232
Decorticate rigidity, 232
Decubitus ulcers. *See* Pressure ulcers
Deep vein thrombosis (DVT), 237, 238, 239
Defending, 45
Degenerative joint disease, 247–249, 248. *See also* Arthritis
Dehydration, 168–169, 170d
    confusion and, 162t
    in diarrhea, 284, 285
    in terminal illness, 33, 365–366
Delirium, 158–161, 160t, 162t–163t, 163d, 202
    vs. dementia, 160t, 202
Dementia, 202–211
    Alzheimer's, 202–208. *See also* Alzheimer's disease
    assessment in, 209
    behavioral symptoms in, 34–35, 37d
    characteristics of, 160t, 202
    confusion in, 158–161
    definition of, 158, 202
    vs. delirium, 160t, 202
    vs. depression, 160t
    management of, 209–211
    multi-infarct, 208
    normal-pressure hydrocephalus and, 208–209
    restraints in, 33–37
Demerol (meperidine), 159t
Democratic leadership, 348–349
Denial, as coping mechanism, 123
Dental system, age-related changes in, 278, 278
Depression, 173–177
    antidepressants for, 176
    assessment for, 72–74, 74d, 174–175
    in bipolar disorder, 174
    confusion and, 158–161, 160t
    vs. dementia, 160t
    drug-related, 173d, 174
    hopelessness and, 176–177

major, 174
management of, 175–177, 176d
restorative care and, 93–94
risk factors for, 173
signs and symptoms of, 173–174
suicide and, 177–179
types of, 173–174
Dermatitis, 199
    seborrheic, 198
    stasis, 198
DETERMINE Guidelines, for nutritional deficiencies, 169d
Detrol (tolterodine tartrate), for urinary incontinence, 301
Developmental tasks, 78t, 78–79
DEXA (dual-energy x-ray absorptiometry), for osteoporosis, 243
Dexamethasone flunisolide (AeroBid), 265t
Diabetes mellitus, 319–328
    assessment in, 325–326
    blood glucose monitoring in, 322–323
    complications of, 323t, 323–325, 324d, 325d
    diagnosis of, 319, 320
    diet in, 321, 326–327
    exercise in, 320–321
    medications in, 325, 326t
    nursing management in, 326–328
    patient teaching in, 327, 328d
    sexual function and, 126
    treatment of, 319–320
    type I, 319–320
    type II, 320
Diabetic ketoacidosis, 319, 323t, 324, 324d
Diabetic neuropathy, 325
Diabetic retinopathy, 324–325
Diabetic ulcers, 325, 327
Dialysis, 308–309
Diamox (acetazolamide), for glaucoma, 334
Diaphragm, 260, 261
Diaphragmatic breathing, 267
Diaphragmatic hernia, 287, 287
Diarrhea, 284–285
Diastole, 220, 221
Diet. *See also* Eating; Feeding; Nutrition
    altered taste and, 345
    cancer and, 113
    cardiovascular disease and, 110–112
    in constipation, 286
    in diabetes, 321, 326–327
    in diverticulitis, 284
    in dysphagia, 281
    in gallbladder disease, 289
    guidelines for, 103–106, 104
    in hiatal hernia, 287
    low-fat, 103
    osteoporosis and, 243, 244d, 245, 246
    in peptic ulcer disease, 283
Dietician, registered, 19
Diflusinal (Dolobid), 159t
Digestion, 278
    age-related changes in, 278–279, 279
Digital rectal examination, of prostate, 302, 302, 305
Digoxin (Lanoxin), 135t, 143t–144t
    for heart failure, 221
    toxicity of, 221, 285
Disease, chronic, 5
Distribution, drug, 132–133
Diuretics, 144t
    for heart failure, 221, 222
    for hypertension, 230

Diuril (chlorothiazide), 144t
Diverticulitis, 283, 283–284
Diverticulosis, 283, 283–284
Documentation, of drug administration, 139, 141
Docusate (Colace), 143t
Dolobid (diflusinal), 159t
Donepezil (Aricept), for Alzheimer's disease, 205
Dopamine, in parkinsonism, 212
Dorzolamide (Trusopt), for glaucoma, 334
Dosage, drug, 140
Dowager's hump, 242, 243
Dressings
    assistive devices for, 99, 99
    in Katz Index, 68
    for pressure ulcers, 192–194
    wet-to-dry, for débridement, 193
Drug(s)
    absorption of, 132
    adverse reactions to, 134
    alcohol and, 182
    cognitive effects of, 134
    confusion due to, 134, 161, 162t
    containers for, 147–148, 148
    cumulative effects of, 134–135
    depression due to, 173d, 174
    in diabetes mellitus, 325, 326t
    distribution of, 132–133
    dosage of, 140
    excretion of, 133–134
    generic, 140
    lipid solubility of, 132–133
    metabolism of, 133
    ototoxic, 343, 343t
    for pain relief, 158, 158d, 159t
    polypharmacy and, 135–136, 136t, 144
    protein binding of, 132, 133d
    sexual dysfunction due to, 126d
    sleep disturbances due to, 155
    therapeutic levels of, 135, 135t
    toxic effects of, 135, 135d
    undesirable for older patients, 140, 140d
    unusual reactions to, 135
    urinary incontinence due to, 153, 153d, 300, 300d
    xerostomia due to, 280
Drug administration, 138–149
    charts for, 146–147, 147d
    containers for, 148, 148
    documentation of, 139, 141
    implementation of, 141
    intramuscular, 141
    nursing process in, 139–144
    oral, 141
    by patient, 145–148
    monitoring systems for, 146–148, 147d, 148
    with vision problems, 145–146, 146d
    patient/family teaching for, 146–147, 147d
    punch card for, 141
    routes of, 140, 141
    Six Rights of, 139–141
    subcutaneous, 141
    time of, 140–141
Drug-drug interactions, 136, 136t, 144
Drug history, 145, 145d
Drug idiosyncrasy, 135
Drug therapy, noncompliance with, 148–149
Dry mouth, 188, 189, 198, 280
    altered taste and, 344–345
Dry skin, 188, 189, 198

Dual-energy x-ray absorptiometry (DEXA), for osteoporosis, 243
Dulcolax (bisacodyl), 143t
Duodenal ulcers, 282–283
Duodenum, 278
Durable power of attorney for health care, 31, 32, 363–364
Dysfunctional grief, 180, 181, 181d
Dysphagia, 280, 280–281, 281d
    in parkinsonism, 214
    stroke and, 231
Dyspnea
    in asthma, 269
    breathing techniques for, 267
    in emphysema, 266, 267
    in heart failure, 220, 222
Dysrhythmias, pacemaker for, 227–229
Dysthymia, 174, 176

E
Ear
    age-related changes in, 340
    examination of, 54t, 342
    hearing loss and, 340–344
    structure of, 339–340, 340
Ear wax, 339
    removal of, 341
Eating. *See also* Diet; Feeding; Nutrition
    assistive devices for, 98–99, 99
    promotion of, 170d
Economic factors
    in health care access, 5–6, 7
    in noncompliance, 148–149
    in nutrition, 107
    in undernutrition, 169d
Ectropion, 336, 336
Eczema, 199
Edema, pulmonary, 223
Education. *See* Client/family teaching
Elastic stockings, for venous insufficiency, 236, 237, 238
Elavil (amitriptyline), drug interactions with, 136t
Eldepryl (selegiline), for parkinsonism, 212
Elder abuse and neglect, 183–185
Elderly. *See* Older adults
Electroencephalography, in seizure disorders, 216
Electrolyte imbalances, 295
Emotionally focused coping, 118
Empathy, 49
Emphysema, 263–266. *See also* Chronic obstructive pulmonary disease (COPD)
Endocrine disorders, 317–328
Endocrine system, 313–328
    age-related changes in, 316
    glands of, 313–316, 314
    hormones of, 313–316, 315t
    negative feedback in, 314
End-of-life decisions, 31–32
    advanced directives, 31–33, 360–362
End-of-life issues
    artificial nutrition and hydration, 33, 365–366
    living wills, 31–32
    Medical Power of Attorney for Health Care, 31, 32–33, 363–364
Endorphins, 157
Enkephalins, 157
Enteral feeding, 167–168
    in terminal illness, 33, 365–366
Entropion, 336, 336
Environmental modifications, 100, 100, 101d
    for confusion, 163t

for hearing impairment, 343–344
for urinary incontinence, 154
for vision impaired, 337
Enzymatic débridement, of pressure ulcers, 193, 193d
Epilepsy, 215–217
Epithelization, in wound healing, 194
Equilibrium, 339-340
impairment of, 344
Erectile dysfunction, 125, 126. *See also* Sexuality/sexual function
Erickson's developmental tasks, 78t, 78–79
Esidrix (hydrochlorothiazide), 144t
Esmolol, 144t
Esophageal varices, 289
Esophagus, 278, 279
Essential tremor, 201
vs. parkinsonism, 213
Esteem needs, 20
Estrogen, 315t, 316
age-related changes in, 315
osteoporosis and, 242, 243
Estrogen replacement therapy, for osteoporosis, 243–244
Ethical codes, 28d, 28–29
Ethical nursing care, 28d, 28–30
Ethics, definition of, 28
Ethnocentrism, 80–82
Etodolac (Lodine), for arthritis, 250t
Euthyroid state, 318–319
Evaluation
in care planning, 62
in client/family teaching, 64
in nursing process, 59, 60d
Evista (raloxifene), for osteoporosis, 244–245
Excretion, drug, 133–134
Exercise
aerobic, 107–108
benefits of, 107d, 107–108
cardiovascular disease and, 110–112
in diabetes, 320–321
guidelines for, 108–109
health risks of, 109–112
nurse's role in, 108
osteoporosis and, 244d
recommendations for, 108–109
respiratory function and, 263
for strength and flexibility, 109, 110d
in stress management, 121
target zone for, 108d
walking as, 108–109, 109d
Exercises
Kegel, 153–154
range-of-motion, 95, 95d
in arthritis, 255
for strength and flexibility, 109, 110d
Extracapsular cataract extraction, 335
Eye. *See also* Vision
age-related changes in, 331–332
disorders of, 332–339
examination of, 54t
structure and function of, 331, 331
Eye contact, in communication, 42
Eyeglasses, 336–337
Eyelids, disorders of, 336, 336

F

Face, examination of, 54t–55t
Facial expression, in communication, 42
Faith, 127–129

in stress management, 123
Falls, 163–165
fractures and, 163–164
prevention of, 100, 100, 101d, 164d, 164–165
risk factors for, 164
Family
abuse and neglect by, 183–185, 185d
as caregivers, 3, 84–85. *See also* Caregivers
resources for, 376–377
as support system, 3–4, 84–85
teaching for. *See* Client/family teaching
Family conflict, 85, 86d
Family coping, compromised, 85, 86d
Family roles, 84
Fat, dietary, 103, 106
Fecal impaction, 285
Fecal incontinence, in stroke patients, 233
Feedback, 40
Feeding. *See also* Diet; Eating; Nutrition
assistive devices for, 98–99, 99
in dysphagia, 281
enteral, 167–168
in terminal illness, 33, 365–366
in hemiplegia, 233
in Katz Index, 70
in parkinsonism, 214
Feldene (piroxicam), for arthritis, 250t
Fenoprofen (Naflon), 144t, 159t
Fetal tissue transplant, for parkinsonism, 213
Fiber, dietary, 104–105
for constipation, 286
Fibromyalgia, 252–253
Financial abuse, 184
Financial factors
in health care access, 5–6, 7
in noncompliance, 148–149
in nutrition, 107
in undernutrition, 169d
Finasteride (Proscar), for benign prostatic hyperplasia, 303, 304d
Fires, prevention of, 101d
Flexibility, exercise for, 109
Flomax (tamsulosin), for benign prostatic hyperplasia, 302–303, 304d
Fluid intelligence, 89
Fluid management
in dehydration, 168–169, 170d
in diarrhea, 285
in heart failure, 221, 222
in terminal illness, 33, 365–366
Flurazepam (Dalmane), 142t
drug interactions with, 136t
Flurbiprofen (Ansaid), for arthritis, 250t
Folex (methotrexate), for arthritis, 251t, 252
Follicle-stimulating hormone (FSH), 315t, 316
Folstein Mini-Mental State Examination, 72, 73d, 79
Food Guide Pyramid, 103, 104
Foods. *See also* Diet; Nutrition
selection of, 103–106
Footboard, 233
Foot care, in diabetes, 327
Foot ulcers
arterial, 238, 239
diabetic, 325, 327
Foreign language speakers, 82, 82d
Fosamax (alendronate), for osteoporosis, 244–245
Fowler position, 256t
Fractures
Colles, 246

Fractures (*continued*)
  from falls, 163–164
  hip, 246–247, 247
  osteoporosis and, 242, 246–247, 247
Frail elderly, 5, 13
Free radical theory of aging, 23d, 24
Friction, pressure ulcers and, 189–190, 190
Friends, as support system, 85
Functional age, 13
Functional assessment, 65–76, 93
  affective assessment in, 72–74, 74d
  Barthel Index in, 70, 72t
  components of, 66–70
  definition of, 66
  health history in, 67, 68d
  Katz Index in, 67, 69d
  Minimum Data Set in, 66, 367–375
  physical health assessment in, 66–67
  psychological assessment in, 70–75
  PULSES Profile in, 70, 71d, 72d
  self-care assessment in, 67–70
  social assessment in, 74–75, 75d
  termination of, 75–76
  uses of, 66, 66d
Functional incontinence, 151, 300d, 300–301. *See also* Urinary
    incontinence
Furadantin (nitrofurantoin), for urinary tract infections, 297, 298t
Furosemide (Lasix), 144t
  drug interactions with, 136t

G
Gait, crutch walking, 96–97, 97
Gait problems, in parkinsonism, 211, 214
Gallbladder
  age-related changes in, 279
  disorders of, 287–289, 288
  functions of, 278
  surgery of, 288
Gallstones, 279, 287–289, 288
Gantanol (sulfamethoxazole), for urinary tract infections, 297, 298t
Gastric ulcers, 282–283
Gastritis, 281–282
Gastrocrom (cromolyn sodium), 265t
Gastrointestinal system, 276–291
  age-related changes in, 278, 278–279
  examination of, 55t
  function of, 278
  structures of, 277, 277–278
Gastrostomy feeding, 168
  in terminal illness, 365–366
General adaptation syndrome, 118–120, 119, 119d
Generalized seizures, 215–216
Generic drugs, 140
Genetic theory of aging, 23d, 23–24
Genitourinary disorders, 296–312
  resources for, 307d
Genitourinary system, 293–312
  age-related changes in, 294–296, 296
  examination of, 56t–57t
  function of, 294
  structures of, 294, 295
Genuineness, 48–49
Geriatric Depression Scale, 174, 175d
Geriatric nurse practitioner (GNP), 15
Geriatrics, definition of, 13
Gerontocracy, 4
Gerontologic nurse, qualities of, 13d, 13–15

Gerontologic nursing. *See also* Nursing
  care settings for, 16–18
  caring in, 14–15, 15d
  cultural aspects of, 15
  definition of, 2, 13
  holistic care in, 14–15, 15, 15d
  practitioners in, 15
Gestures, in communication, 42
Glasgow Coma Scale, 231, 232
Glaucoma, 333, 333–335
Glomerular filtration rate, 294
  age-related changes in, 295
Glomerulus, 294, 295
Glucagon, 315, 315t
Glucophage (metformin), 321–322
Glucosamine, 249
Glucose monitoring, 322–323
Glucose regulation, in diabetes mellitus, 319
Glycosylated hemoglobin, in diabetes mellitus, 322
Goals, 58–59, 59d
Gold compounds, for rheumatoid arthritis, 251t
Gonads, 314, 315t, 316
  age-related changes in, 315
Gout, 251t, 253–254. *See also* Arthritis
Grab bars, 99, 100
Grandparent role, 84
Graves disease, 318
Grief, 179–181
  anticipatory, 180, 181, 181d
  dysfunctional, 180, 181, 181d
Grooming, assistive devices for, 99, 99
Growth hormone (GH), 315t, 316
Guided imagery, 122
Gum disease, 278, 278
Gurgles, 271t

H
Habit training, 154
Hair
  age-related changes in, 188
  examination of, 54t
Halcion (triazolam), 142t
Halo effect, 356
Haloperidol (Haldol), 142t
  for Alzheimer's disease, 207
  drug interactions with, 136t
Hashimoto thyroiditis, 317
Head and neck, examination of, 54t–55t
Health care, 5–8
  access to, insurance and, 5–6, 7
  transcultural, 80
Health care financing, 5–7
Health history, 67, 68d
Health insurance, Medicare/Medicaid, 5–6, 6d, 7
Health maintenance organizations (HMOs), 6
Healthy elderly, 13
Hearing aids, 341–342, 342d
Hearing loss, 340–344
  assessment of, 342d, 342–343
  conductive, 340
  confusion and, 160–161
  learning and, 89
  management of, 341–344
  noncompliance and, 149
  resources for, 344d
  sensorineural, 340–341
Heart. *See also* under Cardiac; Cardiovascular

age-related changes in, 219–220
function of, 219
structure of, 219, 219
Heart attack, 225–227
Heart disease
    atherosclerotic, 220, 223–227. *See also* Coronary artery disease
    prevention of, 111–112
    risk factors for, 111–112, 112d
Heart failure, 220d, 220–223, 222d, 223d
Heart rate, target zone for, 108d
Heat exhaustion, 110
Heat stroke, 110
Heberden nodes, 248, 248
Height, loss of, 242, 243
Helicobacter pylori, peptic ulcers and, 282
Hemiplegia, 231
Hemodialysis, 308–309
Hemorrhoids, 286–287
Hepatic cirrhosis, 289–291
Hepatic encephalopathy, 290–291
Hepatitis, 291
Hernia, hiatal, 287, 287
Herpes zoster, 198–199
Hiatal hernia, 287, 287
Hierarchy of needs, 19–21, 20
High-density lipoprotein, 112, 112d
Hip fractures, 163–165
    from falls, 163–164
    osteoporosis and, 242, 246–247, 247
    sites of, 247
    treatment of, 247
History
    drug, 145, 145d
    health, 67, 68d
HMOs, 6
Holistic care, 14–15, 15, 15d
Homan sign, 236
Home health care, 16–17
Home modifications. *See* Environmental modifications
Hopelessness, 176–177
Hormone replacement therapy, for osteoporosis, 243–244
Hormones, 313–316, 315t
    age-related changes in, 316
Hose, compression, for venous insufficiency, 236, 237, 238
Hospital care, 17
Humoral immunity, 24
Hydration
    artificial, in terminal illness, 33, 365–366
    management of, 168–169, 170d. *See also* Fluid management
Hydrocephalus, normal-pressure, 208–209
Hydrochlorothiazide (HydroDIURIL, Esidrix), 144t
Hydrocolloid dressings, for pressure ulcers, 194
Hydrogel dressings, for pressure ulcers, 194
Hydroxychloroquine, for rheumatoid arthritis, 250t
Hyperammonemia, hepatic encephalopathy and, 290–291
Hypercholesterolemia, 111–112, 112d
Hyperglycemia
    in diabetes, 319
    drug-related, 325, 326t
Hyperglycemic hyperosmolar nonketotic syndrome, 324, 325d
Hyperkalemia
    delirium and, 161
    in diarrhea, 284, 285
    in renal disease, 295, 308
Hypertension, 111, 229–230
    portal, 289–290
    stroke and, 230

Hyperthyroidism, 318d, 318–319
Hypnotics, 142t
Hypoglycemia
    in diabetes, 323, 323t
    drug-related, 325, 326t
    insulin therapy and, 319–320
Hypoglycemic agents, for type II diabetes, 320, 321–322
Hypokalemia
    delirium and, 161
    in diarrhea, 284, 285
Hyponatremia
    confusion and, 162t
    in renal disease, 295
Hypotension, orthostatic, 201
Hypothermia, 201–202, 202d
Hypothyroidism, 317d, 317–318
    sexual function and, 126
Hypoxia, confusion and, 162t
Hytrin (terazosin), for benign prostatic hyperplasia, 302–304, 304d

I

Ibuprofen (Advil, Motrin), 144t
    for arthritis, 249, 250t
    for pain, 159t
Ichthyosis, 197t
Ileum, 278
Illness, chronic, 5
Imagery, guided, 122
Imipramine (Tofranil), 143t
Immobility. *See* Mobility, impaired
Immunity
    cell–mediated, 24
    humoral, 24
Immunization
    for hepatitis, 291
    for influenza, 272
    for pneumococcal pneumonia, 270
Immunologic theory of aging, 23d, 24
Implementation
    of care plan, 62
    in client/family teaching, 63–64
    in nursing process, 59
Impotence, 125, 126. *See also* Sexuality/sexual function
Incontinence
    in stroke patients, 233
    urinary, 151–155, 300–301. *See also* Urinary incontinence
Increased intraocular pressure, in glaucoma, 333
Independence. *See also* Self-care
    assessment of. *See* Functional assessment
    self-esteem and, 86
Independent living retirement communities, 16
Inderal (propranolol), 144t
    drug interactions with, 136t
Indomethacin (Indocin), 144t
    for arthritis, 250t
Infection
    confusion and, 161, 162t
    of pressure ulcers, prevention of, 194
Influenza, 272–273
Information, in stress management, 122
Information resources, 376–378
Informed consent, 30
Insomnia, 155–156, 156d
    chronic, 155
    in depression, 173
    rebound, 156
    transient, 155

Insulin, 315, 315t
    age-related changes in, 315
    deficiency of, in diabetes mellitus, 319, 320
    for diabetes mellitus, 319–320
    regulation of, 314–315
Insulin-dependent diabetes mellitus, 319–320. *See also*
        Diabetes mellitus
Insurance, Medicare/Medicaid, 5–6, 6d, 7
Intal (cromolyn sodium), 265t
Integumentary system, 187–199. *See also* Hair; Nails; Skin
    age-related changes in, 188–189
    components of, 188
Intelligence
    crystallized, 89
    fluid, 89
Intensive insulin therapy, 319
Intermittent claudication, 237, 238–239
International Council of Nurses Code for Nurses, 28, 29d
Interpreters, 82
Intertrigo, 198
Intestinal absorption, 278
Intestinal function, age-related changes in, 279
Intramuscular drug administration, 141
Intraocular lens implant, 335
Intraocular pressure
    in glaucoma, 333
    measurement of, 334
Intrinsic asthma, 269
Intrinsic factor, deficiency of, 166
Ipratropium bromide (Atrovent), 264t
Iris, 331, *331*
    age-related changes in, 331, *332*
Iron, deficiency of, 166
Ischemia, cerebral, dementia and, 208
Isolation
    of hearing impaired, 343
    of vision impaired, 338
Isoniazid, for tuberculosis, 273, 274

J

Jaundice
    in cirrhosis, 290
    in hepatitis, 291
Jejunostomy tube, 168
Jejunum, 278
Joint replacement surgery, 252
Joints
    age-related changes in, 242
    arthritis of, 247–252. *See also* Arthritis
    synovial, 241
Judgments, 44
Jugular veins, examination of, 54t

K

Katz Index of Activities of Daily Living, 67, 69d
Keflex (cephalexin), 143t
Kegel exercises, 153–154
Keratosis
    actinic, 197–198
    seborrheic, 197t
    senile, 197t
Ketoacidosis, diabetic, 323t, 324, 324d
Ketones, urinary, in diabetes mellitus, 322–323
Ketorolac (Toradol), 159t
Kidney
    age-related changes in, 294
    structure and function of, 294, *295*

Kidney disease, in diabetes, 325
Kidney failure, 307–311
Korsakoff syndrome, 182

L

Labeling, 44
Labetalol, 144t
Lacrimal apparatus, 331
Lactose intolerance, 10
Laennec cirrhosis, 289–291
Laissez-faire leadership, 348
Language barriers, 82, 82d
Lanoxin. *See* Digoxin (Lanoxin)
Laparoscopic cholecystectomy, 288
Large intestine
    age-related changes in, 279
    function of, 278
Larodopa (levodopa), 143t
Lasix (furosemide), 144t
    drug interactions with, 136t
Latanoprost (Xalatan), for glaucoma, 334
Lateral position, 256t
Laxatives, 143t
Leaders
    characteristics of, 347–348
    guidelines for, 351d
Leadership, 347–357
    autocratic, 348
    characteristics of, 347–348
    democratic, 348–349
    goal-oriented, 347
    laissez-faire, 348
    vs. management, 347
    participative, 349
    self-aware, 347
    situational, 349–350, 350t
    styles of, 348–350
Learned helplessness, 94–95
Learning, 89, 89d. *See also* Client/family teaching
Legal issues, 30–37
    advanced directives, 31–33, 360–362
    artificial nutrition and hydration, 33, 365–366
    competence determination, 31
    informed consent, 30
    malpractice, 30
    Medical Power of Attorney for Health Care, 31, 32, 363–364
    negligence, 30
    patient self-determination, 31
    restraints, 33–37, 165, 165d
Leg ulcers
    diabetic, 325, 327
    vascular, 237, 238, 239
Lens, 331, *331*
    age-related changes in, 335
    clouding of, 335
Lens implant, 335
Lentigo senilis, 188, 197d
Levodopa (Larodopa), 143t
    for parkinsonism, 212
Levothyroxine (Synthroid), 317
Libido. *See also* Sexuality/sexual function
    changes in, 126
Licensed practical nurse (LPN), 15
    in nursing homes, 19
Life expectancy, 2, 23
Life review, 87
Lifespan, 23

Lipids, 106
Lipid solubility, of drugs, 132–133
Lipofuscin, 24, 220
Lipoprotein, 111–112, 112d
Lispro insulin, 320
Listening skills, 43, 44d
Lithium, 135t, 176, 177t
Liver
    age-related changes in, 279
    cirrhosis of, 289–291
    disorders of, 289–291
    functions of, 278
Living will, 31–32, 360–362
Lobar pneumonia, 270
Lodine (etodolac), for arthritis, 250t
Lodosyn (carbidopa), 143t
    for parkinsonism, 212, 213
Loneliness, 180–181
Long-term care, Medicaid for, 6
Long-term care facilities, 17–18
    abuse in, 184
    evaluation of, 208
    staff in, 18–19
Long-term goals, 58–59, 59d
Long-term memory, 89
Lorazepam (Ativan), drug interactions with, 136t
Losses
    grief and, 179–181
    loneliness and, 180–181
    role-related, 82–84
Love and belonging needs, 20
Low-density lipoprotein, 112, 112d
Low-fat diet, 103
Lungs, 260, 261. See also under Respiratory
    age-related changes in, 260–263, 262
Lung sounds, 271t
Luteinizing hormone (LH), 315t, 316

M
Macrobid (nitrofurantoin), for urinary tract infections, 297, 298t
Macular degeneration, 332, 332–333
Major depression, 174
Malignant melanoma, 195–197, 196, 196d, 197, 197d
Malnutrition, 165–169. See also Nutritional deficiencies
Malpractice, 30
Managed health care, 6–7
Management, 354–357
    adjusting to change in, 356
    vs. leadership, 347
    performance evaluation in, 355–356
    staff motivation and, 354–355
    of unlicensed assistive personnel, 355
Mania, in bipolar disorder, 174, 175, 176d
    lithium for, 176, 177t
Mantra, 122
Maslow's hierarchy of needs, 19–21, 20
Mast cell inhibitors, for respiratory disorders, 265t
Medicaid, 6
Medical Directive to Physician, 31–32, 33
Medical Power of Attorney for Health Care, 31, 32, 363–364
Medicare, 5–6
    managed care and, 7
Medication Administration Record (MAR), 139
Medications. See Drug(s)
Meditation, 122
Melanin, 188
Melanoma, 195–197, 196, 196d, 197, 197d

Mellaril (thioridazine), 142t
    for Alzheimer's disease, 206–207
Memory, 89, 89d
Memory loss
    in alcoholism, 182
    in Alzheimer's disease, 89, 160t, 202, 203, 204, 204d
    in dementia, 160t, 202
Menopause, 316
    osteoporosis and, 242, 243, 244
    sexuality and, 126
Mental illness
    behavioral symptoms in, 34–35, 37d
    restraints in, 33–37
Meperidine (Demerol), 159t
Message, 40
    unclear, 41
Metabolism, drug, 133
Metamucil, 143t
Metaproterenol (Alupent, Metaprel), 264t
Metered-dose inhalers, 263, 268, 268d, 270
Metformin (Glucophage), 321–322
Methotrexate (Rheumatrex, Folex), for arthritis, 251t, 252
Metoprolol, 144t
Miacalcin (calcitonin-salmon), for osteoporosis, 244–245
Midamor (amiloride), 144t
Milk, lactose intolerance and, 107
Mineralocorticoids, 315, 315t
Minerals, 106
    deficiencies of, 165–166, 166t
Mini-Mental State Examination, 72, 73d, 79
Minimum Data Set (MDS), 58, 61, 62, 367–375
    in functional assessment, 66
    in psychosocial assessment, 79
Mirapex (pramipexole), for parkinsonism, 212, 213
Mixed incontinence, 300d, 300–301
Mobility. See also Exercise; Walking
    assistive devices for, 95–96, 96–99
    impaired
        in arthritis, 233
        in osteoporosis, 246
        in parkinsonism, 211, 214
        in stroke patients, 233
        promotion of, 95–98
        range-of-motion exercises for, 95, 95d, 255
        in vision impairment, 338
Moles, 197t
    melanoma and, 195
Monitoring systems, for drug administration, 146–148, 147d, 148
Monoamine oxidase (MAO) inhibitors, 143t
Motivation, staff, 354–355
Motrin (ibuprofen), 144t
    for arthritis, 249, 250t
    for pain, 159t
Mouth
    dry, 188, 189, 198, 280
    altered taste and, 344–345
    examination of, 56t
Mucus, in chronic bronchitis, 266, 267–268
Multi-infarct dementia, 208
Muscle
    age-related changes in, 242
    structure of, 241
Muscle relaxation techniques, 121–122, 122d
Muscle rigidity, in parkinsonism, 211, 214
Musculoskeletal disorders, 242–257
    resources for, 257d
Musculoskeletal system, 240–257

Musculoskeletal system (*continued*)
age-related changes in, 241–242
examination of, 57t
function of, 241
Myocardial infarction, 110–111, 225–227
Myoclonic seizures, 215

N

Nabumetone (Relafen), for arthritis, 249, 250t
Naflon (fenoprofen), 144t, 159t
Nails, age-related changes in, 188
Naproxen (Naprosyn), 144t, 159t
for arthritis, 249, 250t
Narcotics, for pain, 158, 159t
Nardil (phenelzine), 143t
Nasogastric feeding, 167–168
in gallbladder disease, 288
in terminal illness, 33, 365–366
Nasointestinal feeding, 167–168
in terminal illness, 33, 365–366
National Council on the Aging (NCOA), 8
Neck, examination of, 54t–55t
Negative feedback mechanism, 314
Neglect, elder, 183–185
Negligence, 30
Neopen (penicillamine), for arthritis, 251t, 252
Nephron, 294, *295*
Neurologic disorders, 202–217
Neurologic system, 200–217
age-related changes in, 201–202
Neurons, 201
Neuropathy, diabetic, 325
Nevi, 197t
melanoma and, 195
Niacin, deficiency of, 166t
Nitrates, for angina, 224–225, 226
Nitrofurantoin (Furadantin, Macrobid), for urinary tract
infections, 297, 298t
Nitroglycerin, for angina, 224–225, 226
Noncompliance, with drug therapy, 148–149
Non-English speakers, 82, 82d
Non–insulin-dependent diabetes mellitus, 320. *See also* Diabetes
mellitus
Nonproliferative retinopathy, 324
Nonsteroidal anti-inflammatory drugs (NSAIDs), 144t
for arthritis, 249, 250t
for gout, 254–255
for pain, 158, 159t
Nonverbal communication, 42–43, 43d
Normal-pressure hydrocephalus, 208–209
Nose, examination of, 54t
Nosocomial urinary tract infections, 301, 301d
Nurse(s)
attitudes of toward aging, 10
gerontologic, qualities of, 13d, 13–15
licensed practical, 15
in nursing homes, 18–19
as patient advocate, 29
registered, 15
Nurse-patient relationship
communication in, 39–48. *See also* Communication
developing phase of, 50
terminating phase of, 50–51
therapeutic, 48–49
working phase of, 50
Nursing
gerontologic. *See* Gerontologic nursing

transcultural, 15, 80–82
Nursing assistants, in nursing homes, 19
Nursing diagnoses, 58
for client/family teaching, 63d
Nursing facility, 18. *See also* Nursing homes
Nursing Home Reform Act, 18
Nursing home residents, 18
legal rights of, 29, 30d
Nursing homes, 17–18
abuse in, 184
evaluation of, 207
staff in, 18–19
Nursing process, 52–64
assessment in, 53–58, 54t–57t
in care planning, 60–62
in client/family teaching, 62–64, 63d
definition of, 53
evaluation in, 59, 60d
implementation in, 59
nursing diagnosis in, 58, 58d
planning in, 59, 60d
Nutrients
absorption of, 278
recommended intake of, 105–106
Nutrition, 103–107. *See also* Diet; Eating; Feeding
artificial
legal aspects of, 33
in terminal illness, 33, 365–366
boosting intake in, 170d
in chronic obstructive pulmonary disease, 268
effects of aging on, 106–107
pressure ulcers and, 191–192, *192*, 194
resources for, 107
socioeconomic aspects of, 107
in terminal illness, 33, 365–366
Nutritional assessment, 167, 168d, 169d
for pressure ulcers, 191–192, *192*
Nutritional deficiencies, 165–168
assessment for, 167, 168d, 169d
causes of, 165
management of, 167–168
pressure ulcers and, 191–192, *192*
prevention of, 167, 170d
risk assessment for, 168d, 169d
signs and symptoms of, 166t
types of, 165–167
Nutritional Health Checklist, 168d

O

Obesity, sleep apnea and, 2754
Objective data, 53
Occupational therapist, 19
Occupational therapy, 100
Older adults. *See also* Aging
age-based classification of, 13d
caregivers for, 3. *See also* Caregivers
characteristics of, 2–5
contributions of, 9d, 10d
frail, 13
growing population of, 4, *4*
healthy, 13
illness in, 5
life expectancy of, 2
myths about, 8, 9d
nurse's attitude toward, 14
poverty among, 7
resources for, 7–8

stereotyping of, 8–10, 14
Omnibus Budget Reconciliation Act, 18
Omnipen (ampicillin), 143t
    for urinary tract infections, 297, 298t
One-way communication, 40
Open-angle glaucoma, *333,* 333–335
Oral cavity. *See* Mouth
Oral drug administration, 141
Orientation
    in confusion, 161
    in dementia, 210d
Orthostatic hypotension, 201
Osteoarthritis, 247–249, *248. See also* Arthritis
Osteoblasts, 241
Osteoclasts, 241
Osteocytes, 241
Osteoporosis, 113–114, 242–247
    assessment in, 245
    definition of, 242
    diagnosis of, 243
    diet and, 243, 244d, 245, 246
    dowager's hump and, 242
    fractures and, 242, 246–247, *247*
    nursing management in, 245–246
    pathophysiology of, 242–243
    prevalence of, 242
    prevention of, 244d
    risk factors for, 242, 242d
    signs and symptoms of, 243
    treatment of, 243–245
Ototoxic drugs, 343, 343t
Ovaries, 315t, 316
    age-related changes in, 315
Overflow incontinence, 300d, 300–301
Oxazepam, 142t
Oxybutynin, for urinary incontinence, 301
Oxycodone (Oxycontin), 159t
Oxygen therapy, for chronic obstructive pulmonary disease, 267
Oxytocin, 315t, 316

P
Pacemakers, 227–229
Pain, 156–158
    acute, 156
    in arterial insufficiency, 237
    in arthritis, 248, 249, 252
    assessment of, 157
    chest
        in coronary artery disease, 223–224, 225, 226
        in myocardial infarction, 225
    chronic, 156
    definition of, 156
    in fibromyalgia, 252–253
    in gallbladder disease, 287, 288
    in gout, 253–255
    management of, 157d, 157–158, 158d, 159t
    manifestations of, 157
    physiologic aspects of, 156–157
    in urinary tract infection, 299
Pancreas
    digestive functions of, 278
    endocrine functions of, *314,* 315, 315t
Papillomas, senile, 197t
Paralysis, in stroke, 233–235
Parathormone, 315, 315t
Parathyroid gland, *314,* 315, 315t
Parkinsonism, 211–215

Parlodel (bromocriptine), 143t
Parnate (tranylcypromide), 143t
Partial seizures, 215
Participative leadership, 349
Passive behavior, 352, 352t
Passive neglect, 184
Passive suicide, 178
Patient advocate, 29
Patient Bill of Rights, 358–359
Patient Self-Determination Act, 31
Peak flow meter, 269
Pelvic floor exercises, 153–154
Penicillamine (Cuprimine, Neopen), for arthritis, 251t, 252
Penicillins, 143t
Penssaid Topical, for arthritis, 255
Pentazocine (Talwin), 159t
Peptic ulcer disease, 282–283
Performance evaluation, 355–356
Periodontal disease, 278, *278*
Peripheral nervous system, 201
    age-related changes in, 201–202
Peripheral neuropathy, in diabetes, 325
Peripheral vascular disease, 235–239
    arterial insufficiency in, 237–239
    venous insufficiency in, 235–237, 238, 239
Peritoneal dialysis, 308–309
Perphenazine (Trilafon), 142t
Personality traits, 87, 88d
Pessary, 311
Phacoemulsification, 335
Pharmacist, 19
Pharmacokinetics, 132–134
Phenazopyridine (Pyridium), in urinary tract infection, 299
Phenelzine (Nardil), 143t
Phenylbutazone, 144t
Phenytoin, 135t
Physical abuse, 184
Physical examination, 53–58, 54t–57t
    of cardiovascular system, 55t
    of gastrointestinal system, 56t
    of genitourinary system, 56t–57t
    of head and neck, 54t–55t
    of musculoskeletal system, 57t
    of respiratory system, 55t
Physical therapist, 19
Physical therapy, 100
Physiologic needs, 20
Pickup walkers, 97–98, *98*
Pilocarpine, for glaucoma, 334
Pioglitazone (Actos), 322
Piroxicam (Feldene), for arthritis, 250t
Pituitary gland, *314,* 315t, 316
    age-related changes in, 315
Planning. *See also* Care plan
    in client/family teaching, 63
    in nursing process, 59, 60d
Planning conference, 62
Plaques
    in Alzheimer's disease, 203
    in atherosclerosis, 223–224
Pleura, 260, *261*
Pneumonia, 270–272
    in chronic obstructive pulmonary disease, 268
Polypharmacy, 135, 144
    drug interactions and, 136, 136t
Portal hypertension, 289
Positioning

Positioning (*continued*)
  of comatose patients, 233
  guidelines for, 256t
  in wheelchairs, 98, *98*
Positions, 256t
Positive "I" statements, 87
Posterior pituitary, *314*, 315t, 316
Postfall syndrome, 164
Potassium
  deficiency of
    delirium and, 161
    in diarrhea, 284, 285
  excess of
    in acute renal failure, 308
    delirium and, 161
    in diarrhea, 284, 285
    in renal disease, 295, 308
Poverty, 7
Power of attorney for health care, 31, 32, 363–364
PPOs, 6–7
Pramipexole (Mirapex), for parkinsonism, 212, 213
Precose (acarbose), 322
Prednisone, for respiratory disorders, 265t
Preferred provider organizations (PPOs), 6–7
Presbycusis, 340-341. *See also* Hearing loss
Presbyopia, 332
Pressure ulcers, 189–194
  assessment of, 190–192, *191, 192*
  causes of, 189–190, *190*
  débridement of, 193, 193d
  dressings for, 192–194
  infection of, prevention of, 194
  location of, 189, *190*
  management of, 192–194
  prevention of, 190d, 233
  risk factors for, 189, *190*
Primary memory, 89
Principen (ampicillin), 143t
  for urinary tract infections, 297, 298t
Probenecid (Benemid), for gout, 251t, 254
Problem-focused coping, 118, 121
Problem-solving, 350–351
Prochlorperazine (Compazine), 142t
Progressive muscle relaxation, 121–122, 122d
Proliferative retinopathy, 324–325
Proloprim (trimethoprim-sulfamethoxazole), for urinary tract
    infections, 297, 298t
Propoxyphene (Darvon), 159t
Propranolol (Inderal), 144t
  drug interactions with, 136t
Proscar (finasteride), for benign prostatic hyperplasia, 303, 304d
Prostate gland, 294
  cancer of, 305–307, *306*
  surgery for, 303d, 305–306
  disorders of, sexual function and, 126
  palpation of, 302, *302,* 305
  surgery of, 303d, 305–306
    sexual function after, 307
  transurethral resection of, 302, 303d
Prostate-specific antigen (PSA), 305
Prostatitis, 304–305
Protein
  deficiency of, 166–167
    pressure ulcers and, 192, *192*
  recommended intake of, 105
Protein binding, of drugs, 132, 133d
Proventil (albuterol), 264t

Provider sponsored organizations (PSOs), 6–7
Proxy, 32, 33
Pseudomembranous colitis, 272
Psoriasis, 198
PSOs, 6–7
Psychiatric disorders
  behavioral symptoms in, 34–35, 37d
  restraints in, 33–37
Psychological abuse, 184
Psychological adjustments, 86–87
Psychomotor agitation, 174
Psychomotor retardation, in depression, 174
Psychosocial adjustments, 82–84
Psychosocial assessment, 79, 80d
Psychosocial care, cultural aspects of, 80–82
Psychosocial development, 78–79
Psychosocial problems, 78d, 172–185
Psyllium preparations, 143t
Pulmonary edema, 223
Pulse, measurement of, 54t, 55t
PULSES Profile, 70, 71d, 72d
Punch card, for drug administration, 141
Pupil, 331, *331*
  age-related changes in, 331–332
Purpura, senile, 188, 197t
Pursed-lip breathing, 267
Pyelonephritis, 296–300, 297d, 298t
Pyridium (phenazopyridine), in urinary tract infection, 299
Pyridoxine, deficiency of, 166, 166t

Q
Quarterly review, 61
Questions, improper, 45
Quinidine, 135t

R
Rales, 271t
Raloxifene (Evista), for osteoporosis, 244–245
Range-of-motion exercises, 95, 95d
  in arthritis, 255
Reactive drinkers, 182
Reality orientation, 161, 210d
Reassurance, inappropriate, 44
Rebound insomnia, 156
Receiver, 40
Recruitment, 341
Rectocele, 311
Reflecting, 47
Reflex
  cough. *See* Cough
  swallowing, assessment of, 280
Reflux incontinence, 151. *See also* Urinary incontinence
Refraction, in vision, 331
Registered dietician, 19
Registered nurse, 15. *See also* Nurse(s)
  in nursing homes, 18–19
Rehabilitation, 92–95. *See also* Restorative care
  cardiac, 227, 228
  care settings for, 92
  definition of, 92
  after stroke, 234, *236*
Relafen (nabumetone), for arthritis, 249, 250t
Relaxation techniques, 121–122, 122d
Relenza (zanamivir), for influenza, 273
Religious faith, 127–129
  in stress management, 123
Remicade, for rheumatoid arthritis, 252

Reminiscence, 86–87
REM sleep, 155
Renal disease, in diabetes, 325
Renal failure, 307–311
Reporting, of abuse, 185
Resident Assessment Instrument (RIA), 60–61
    Minimum Data Set in, 58, 61, 62, 367–375
    Resident Assessment Protocols in, 61–62
Resident Assessment Protocols (RAPs), 61–62
Residents, nursing home. *See* Nursing home residents
Residual volume, urinary, 151
Resources, patient/family, 376–377
Respiration, 260. *See also* Breathing
    age-related changes in, 260–263, *262*
Respiratory disorders, 263–274
    resources for, 274d
Respiratory infections, 270–272
    superinfection, 272
Respiratory system, 259–274
    age-related changes in, 260–263
    examination of, 55t
    function of, 260
    structures of, 260, *261*
Respite care, 85, 207
Restating, 47
Restlessness, management of, 35d–36d
Restorative care, 19, 91–101
    assistive devices in
        for feeding, 98–99, *99*
        for mobility, 95–98, *96–98*
        for self-care, 99, *99*, 100
    care settings for, 92
    vs. custodial care, 94–95
    definition of, 92
    guidelines for, 94
    home management and, 100
    multidisciplinary team in, 92–93
    nurse's role in, 94
    potential for, assessment of, 93–94
    promoting mobility in, 95, 95d
    promoting self-care in, 98–99
    rehabilitation and, 92–95. *See also* Rehabilitation
Restoril (temazepam), 142t
Restraints, 33–37, 165, 165d
    alternatives to, 35d–36d, 165
    behavioral symptoms and, 34–35, 37d
    chemical, 3334
    in confusion, 165
    disadvantages of, 33–34, 34d
    guidelines for, 33, 34, 37, 37d, 165d
    physical, 33, 34
Retina, 331, *331*
Retinopathy, diabetic, 324–325
Retirement, 83–84
    Social Security and, 2–3
Rheumatoid arthritis, *248*, 249–252. *See also* Arthritis
Rheumatrex (methotrexate), for arthritis, 251t, 252
Rhonchi, 271t
Riboflavin, deficiency of, 165–166, 166t
Ribs, 261
Ridaura (auranofin), for rheumatoid arthritis, 251t
Rigidity, in parkinsonism, 211, 214
Rinne test, 342–343
Rofecoxib (Vioxx), for arthritis, 250t, 254–255
Role-related adjustments, 82–84
Rolling walkers, 97–98
Rosiglitazone (Avandia), 322

S
Safety measures, 20
    in dementia, 210
    environmental modifications as, 100, *100*, 101d. *See also*
        Environmental modifications
    for falls, 164d, 164–165
    in parkinsonism, 214
    restraints as. *See* Restraints
    for seizures, 216–217
    for vision impairment, 338
Salicylates, for arthritis, 249, 250t
Salivary gland dysfunction, 280
Salt, 105
Sandwich generation, 3
Scabies, 199, 199d
Scalp, examination of, 54t
Sclera, 331, *331*
Scolding, 45
Sebaceous glands, age-related changes in, 188
Seborrheic dermatitis, 198
Seborrheic keratosis, 197t
Secondary memory, 89
Security needs, 20
Sedatives, 142t
Seizures, 215–217
    generalized, 215–216
    myoclonic, 215
    partial, 215
    tonic-clonic, 215
Selegiline (Eldepryl), for parkinsonism, 212
Self-actualization, 20–21
Self-assessment, skin, 195, *196*
Self-care
    assistive devices for, 98–100, *99*
    environmental modifications for, 100, *100*, 101d
    promotion of, 177d
    by stroke patients, 234
    in vision impairment, 337
Self-care assessment, 67–70
    Barthel Index in, 70, 72t
    Katz Index in, 67–70, 68d
    PULSES Profile in, 70, 71d, 72d
Self-esteem, 20, 86–87, 87d, 88
    definition of, 124
    promotion of, 124–125, 125d
Self-examination, breast, 113, *114*
Self-neglect, 184
Sender, 40
Senescence, 23
Senile keratosis, 197t
Senile papillomas, 197t
Senilis purpura, 188, 197t
Sensorineural hearing loss, 340–341
Sensory deficits. *See also* Hearing loss; Vision loss
    confusion and, 160–161, 163t
Sensory overload, confusion and, 160–161, 163t
Sensory system, 330–345
Septra (trimethoprim-sulfamethoxazole), for urinary tract
        infections, 297, 298t
Sertraline (Zoloft), 143t
Serum albumin, in protein-energy malnutrition, 167, 192
Sex hormones, 315t, 316
Sexual abuse, 184
Sexual activity, barriers to, 127
Sexuality/sexual function, 9d, 83
    age-related changes in, 126, 316
    benign prostatic hypertrophy and, 304

Sexuality/sexual function (*continued*)
  chronic illness and, 126
  drugs affecting, 126d
  in heart disease, 226
  nurse's attitudes toward, 127, 127d
  nursing process and, 127
  promotion of, 125–127, 128d
  after prostate surgery, 307
Sharp débridement, of pressure ulcers, 193
Shear, pressure ulcers and, 189–190, *190*
Shingles, 199
Short-term goals, 58–59, 59d
Short-term memory, 89
Showering, assistive devices for, 99, *100*
Silence
  in communication, 42–43
  in therapeutic communication, 47
Sims position, 256t
Sinemet, for parkinsonism, 212, 213
Sinoatrial node, 220
Sitting position, 256t
Situational leadership theory, 349–350, 350t
Sitz bath, 286
Six Rights of drug administration, 139–141
Skin
  age-related changes in, 188
  biopsy of, 195
  dry, 188, 189, 198
  structure of, 188, *189*
Skin cancer, 194–197, *196*, 196d, *197*, 197d
Skin care, in diabetes, 325–326, 327
Skin color, 188
Skin lesions
  common, 197d, 197–199
  terminology for, 197d
Skin turgor, in dehydration, 169
Sleep, age-related changes in, 155
Sleep apnea, 274
Sleep disturbances, 155–156, 156d
  in depression, 173
Sliding hiatal hernia, 287, *287*
Small intestine, absorption in, 278
Smell, 344–345
Smoking
  cardiovascular disease due to, 111
  chronic obstructive pulmonary disease due to, 263
  osteoporosis due to, 244d
Snellen E chart, 336
Social assessment, 74–75, 75d
Social Dysfunction Rating Scale, 75, 75d, 79
Social interaction, promotion of, 177d
Social isolation
  of hearing impaired, 343
  of vision impaired, 338
Social Security, 2–3
Social support, 84–85
  from family, 3–4, 84–85, 86d
  from friends, 85
  in stress management, 123
Social workers, 19
Socioeconomic aspects, of nutrition, 107
Sodium, deficiency of
  confusion and, 162t
  in renal disease, 295
Solganal (aurothioglucose), for rheumatoid arthritis, 251t
Spine, 241
  age-related changes in, 241

osteoarthritis of, 249
  thoracic, 261
Spiritual distress, 129, 129d
Spirituality
  promotion of, 127–128
  in stress management, 123
Spironolactone (Aldactone), 144t
Spondylosis, 249
Spousal role. *See also* Widows/widowers
  loss of, 83
Sputum, in chronic bronchitis, 266, 267–268
Squamous cell carcinoma, of skin, 195
Staff motivation, 354–355
Standards of care, negligence and, 30
Stasis dermatitis, 198
Status asthmaticus, 269
Status epilepticus, 216
Stereotypes, of elderly, 14
Sternum, 261
Steroids, for respiratory disease, 265t, 270
Stockings, compression, for venous insufficiency, 236, 237, 238
Stomach
  age-related changes in, 279
  functions of, 278
  inflammation of, 281–282
  ulcers of, 282–283
Stool, impacted, 285
Stool softeners, 143t
Strength, exercises for, 109, 109d
Stress, 118–124
  adaptation to, 118–120, *119,* 119d
  caregiver, 185d
  coping strategies for, 121–123
  physiologic response to, 118–121, *120,* 120d
  sources of, 118, *119*
  transactional model of, 118, *119*
Stress incontinence, 151, 300d, 300–301. *See also* Urinary
    incontinence
Stress management, 121–123
  nursing process in, 123–124
Stroke, 230–234
Subcutaneous drug administration, 141
Subjective data, 53
Substance abuse, 181–183
Sugar, 105
Suicidal ideation, 178
Suicide, 177–179, 178d, 179d
Sulfamethoxazole (Gantanol, Urobak), for urinary tract
    infections, 297, 298t
Sulfatrim (trimethoprim-sulfamethoxazole), for urinary tract
    infections, 297, 298t
Sulfonylureas, for diabetes, 321
Sulindac (Clinoril), 144t
  for arthritis, 250t
Sundown syndrome, in Alzheimer's disease, 205, 206d
Superinfections, 272
Support. *See* Social support
Support groups, 123, 376–377. *See also* Social support
Surgery
  gallbladder, 288
  joint replacement, 252
  prostate, 302, 303d, 305–306
  sexual function after, 307
Surgical incontinence, 300d, 300–301
Swallowing, difficult, *280,* 280–281, 281d
  in parkinsonism, 214
Sweat glands, age-related changes in, 188

Symmetrel (amantadine), 143t
for parkinsonism, 212
Synovial joints, 241
age-related changes in, 242
Synovitis, in rheumatoid arthritis, 249
Synthroid (levothyroxine), 317
Systole, 220, *221*

T

Tablets, administration of, 141
Tacrine (Cognex), for Alzheimer's disease, 204
Talwin (pentazocine), 159t
Tamsulosin (Flomax), for benign prostatic hyperplasia, 302–303, 304d
Tasmar (tolcapone), for parkinsonism, 212–213
Taste, 344–345
T cells, 24
Teaching plan, 62–64, 63d. *See also* Client/family teaching
Teeth, age-related changes in, 278, *278*
Tegopen (cloxacillin), 143t
Temazepam (Restoril), 142t
Temperature, regulation of, 201–202
TENS (transcutaneous electrical nerve stimulation), for pain, 158
Terazosin (Hytrin), for benign prostatic hyperplasia, 302–304, 304d
Terbutaline (Brethaire), 264t
Terminal illness
advanced directives and, 31–33, 360–362
artificial nutrition and hydration in, 33, 365–366
living wills and, 31–32
Medical Power of Attorney for Health Care and, 31, 32–33, 363–364
Testes, 315t, 316
age-related changes in, 315
examination of, 56t
Testosterone, 315t, 316
age-related changes in, 315
Theo-Dur (aminophylline), 264t
Theophylline, 135t
Therapeutic communication, 45–47
Therapeutic drug levels, 135, 135t
Therapeutic relationship, 13, 48–49
Thermoregulation, 201–202
Thiazolidinediones, 322
Thinking. *See* Cognitive function
Thioridazine (Mellaril), 142t
for Alzheimer's disease, 206–207
Thoracic cage, 260–261
deformity of, 261, *263*
Thorazine (chlorpromazine), 142t
Thought processes. *See* Cognitive function
Thrombophlebitis, 236–237, 238, 239
Thrombosis, deep vein, 237, 238, 239
Thyroid crisis, 318
Thyroid disorders, 317–319
sexual function and, 126
Thyroid gland, *314,* 315, 315t
age-related changes in, 315
Thyroiditis, Hashimoto, 317
Thyroid nodules, 318
Thyroid-stimulating hormone (TSH), 315t, 316
Thyroxine (T4), 315, 315t
Timolol (Timoptic), 144t
for glaucoma, 334
Tinnitus, 341, 343
Tofranil (imipramine), 143t

Toileting
assistive devices for, 99, 100
in Katz Index, 68–70
Tolcapone (Tasmar), for parkinsonism, 212–213
Tolterodine tartrate (Detrol), for urinary incontinence, 301
Tonic-clonic seizures, 215
Tonometer, 334
Tooth problems, 278, *278*
Tophi, 253, *253*
Toradol (ketorolac), 159t
Total incontinence, 151. *See also* Urinary incontinence
Total joint replacement, 252
Touch, 345
Trabeculectomy, 334
Trabeculoplasty, 334
Trachea, 260, *261*
Transactional stress model, 118, *119*
Transcultural health care, 15, 80
Transcultural nursing, 15, 80–82
Transcutaneous electrical nerve stimulation (TENS), for pain, 158
Transfer, in Katz Index, 70
Transient insomnia, 155
Transient ischemic attacks (TIAs), 231, 231d
dementia and, 208
Transitional care settings, 17
Transplantation, fetal tissue, for parkinsonism, 213
Transurethral incision of prostate (TUIP), 302, 303d
Transurethral resection of prostate (TURP), 302, 303d
Tranxene (clorazepate), 142t
Tranylcypromide (Parnate), 143t
Tremor
benign essential, 201
vs. parkinsonism, 213
in parkinsonism, 211, 213
Triamcinolone (Azmacort), 265t
Triazolam (Halcion), 142t
Tricyclic antidepressants, 143t
Trihexyphenidyl (Artane), 143t
Triiodothyronine (T3), 315, 315t
age-related changes in, 315t, 316
Triiodothyronine (Triostat), 317-318
Trilafon (perphenazine), 142t
Trimethoprim (Proloprim, Trimpex), for urinary tract infections, 297, 298t
Trimethoprim-sulfamethoxazole (Bactrim), for urinary tract infections, 297, 298t
Triostat, 317–318
Trusopt (dorzolamide), for glaucoma, 334
Tube feeding, 167–168
in terminal illness, 33, 365–366
Tuberculosis, 273–274, 275d, 275t
Tuning fork tests, 342–343
Two-way communication, 40
Tylenol (acetaminophen)
for arthritis, 249, 250t
for pain, 159t
Type A gastritis, 281–282
Type B gastritis, 281–282
Type I diabetes mellitus, 319–320. *See also* Diabetes mellitus
Type II diabetes mellitus, 320. *See also* Diabetes mellitus

U

Ulcers
arterial, 238, 239
diabetic, 325, 327
peptic, 282–283
pressure, 189–194. *See also* Pressure ulcers

Ulcers (*continued*)
venous (stasis), 199, 237, 238, 239
Undernutrition, 165–169. *See also* Nutritional deficiencies
Unlicensed assistive personnel, 355
Unna boot, 237
Ureters, 294, *295*
Urethra, 294, *295*
Urge incontinence, 151, 300d, 300–301. *See also* Urinary incontinence
Uric acid, in gout, 253
Urinalysis, 297
Urinary catheterization
for incontinence, 154–155
infection in, 301
Urinary elimination
age-related changes in, 151, 296
in benign prostatic hyperplasia, 301–302, 303
in stoke patients, 151
Urinary incontinence, 151–155, 300–301
assessment of, 151–153, 152d, 153d
cystocele and, 311
definition of, 151
drug-related, 153, 153d
management of, 153d, 153–155
nursing process in, 151–153
in stroke patients, 233
types of, 151
Urinary retention, 301
Urinary system
age-related changes in, 294–296, *296*
function of, 294
structures of, 294, *295*
Urinary system disorders, 296–312
resources for, 307d
Urinary tract infections, 296–300, 297d, 298t
confusion and, 161, 162t
nosocomial, 301, 301d
prostatitis and, 304–305
Urine
formation of, 294
residual volume of, 151
Urine tests, in diabetes mellitus, 322–323
Urobak (sulfamethoxazole), for urinary tract infections, 297, 298t

V

Vaccination
for hepatitis, 291
for influenza, 272
for pneumococcal pneumonia, 270
Validation therapy, 210d
Valsalva maneuver, 226
Varices, esophageal, 289–290
Varicose veins, 235, 238, 239
Vascular dementia, 208
Vasopressin, 315t, 316
Veins, varicose, 235, 238, 239
Venous insufficiency, 235–237, 238, 239
Venous thrombosis, 237, 238, 239
Venous ulcers, 199, 237, 238, 239
Ventolin (albuterol), 264t
Ventricular failure, 220–223
Verbal abuse, by Alzheimer's patients, 205–206, 206d
Verbal communication, 41–42
Vertebrae, 241
age-related changes in, 241

osteoarthritis of, 249
thoracic, 261
Vertigo, 344
Vioxx (rofecoxib), for arthritis, 250t, 254–255
Viral hepatitis, 291
Vision
age-related changes in, 332–339
normal, 331
Vision loss, 332–339
assessment in, 336–337, 337d
cataracts and, 335
confusion and, 160–161
in diabetes, 324–325
drug administration and, 145–146, 146d
in glaucoma, *333,* 333–335
learning and, 89
in macular degeneration, *332,* 332–333
nursing management in, 337–339
resources for, 337, 339d
Visual acuity, assessment of, 336, 337d
Visualization techniques, 121–122
Vitamins, 106
deficiencies of, 165–166, 166t
Vitreous body, 331, 331
age-related changes in, 331
Voiding. *See* Urinary elimination
Voiding and incontinence record, 152d
Voluntary associations, 376–377

W

Walkers, 97–98, *98*
Walking
with cane, 95–96, *96*
with crutches, *96,* 96–97, *97*
for exercise, 108–109, 109d
vertigo and, 344
with vision impaired patient, 338
with walker, 97–98, *98*
Wandering
in Alzheimer's disease, 205, 206d
management of, 35d–36d
Wear and tear theory of aging, 23d, 24–25
Weber test, 342–343
Websites, 378
Weight, desirable, 103, 105t
Weight loss, 103
pressure ulcers and, 191–192, **192**
Wellbutrin (bupropion), 143t
Wernicke encephalopathy, 182
Wet-to-dry dressing débridement, of pressure ulcers, 193
Wheelchairs, 98, *98*
Wheezing, 271t
in asthma, 269
Whisper test, 342
Widows/widowers, 83
grieving by, 179–181
loneliness of, 180–181
Work role, loss of, 83–84
Wound care, for pressure ulcers, 193
Wound healing, epithelization in, 194
Wrist fracture, 246

X

Xalatan (latanoprost), for glaucoma, 334
Xanax (alprazolam), 142t

Xanthines, for respiratory disorders, 264t
Xerosis, 188, 189, 198
Xerostomia, 280
    altered taste and, 344–345

Y
Yeast infection, as superinfection, 272
Yoga, 122

Z
Zanamivir (Relenza), for influenza, 273
Zinc, deficiency of, 166t
Zoloft (sertraline), 143t
Zyloprim (allopurinol), for gout, 251t, 254

M.Bayly 1/26/02